Principles of Assessment and Outcome Measurement for Occupational Therapists and Physiotherapists

Principles of Assessment and Outcome Measurement for Occupational Therapists and Physiotherapists

Theory, Skills and Application

by

Alison J. Laver Fawcett PhD, DipCOT, OT(C)

Modernisation Manager (Older People's Mental Health Services)
North Yorkshire and York Primary Care Trust
North Yorkshire, England

BICENTENNIAL
1807
⊛WILEY
2007
BICENTENNIAL

John Wiley & Sons, Ltd

Reprinted January 2008, December 2009

Other Wiley Editorial Offices

John Wiley & Sons Inc., 111 River Street, Hoboken, NJ 07030, USA
Jossey-Bass, 989 Market Street, San Francisco, CA 94103-1741, USA
Wiley-VCH Verlag GmbH, Boschstr. 12, D-69469 Weinheim, Germany
John Wiley & Sons Australia Ltd, 42 McDougall Street, Milton, Queensland 4064, Australia
John Wiley & Sons (Asia) Pte Ltd, 2 Clementi Loop #02-01, Jin Xing Distripark, Singapore 129809
John Wiley & Sons Canada Ltd, 6045 Freemont Blvd, Mississauga, ONT, L5R 4J3.

Anniversary Logo Design: Richard J. Pacifico

Library of Congress Cataloging-in-Publication Data
Fawcett, Alison J. Laver.
  Principles of assessment and outcome measurement for occupational therapists and physiotherapists / Theory, skills and application by Alison J. Laver Fawcett.
     p. ; cm.
  Includes bibliographical references and index.
  ISBN: 978-1-86156-480-1 (pbk. : alk. paper)
  1. Physical therapy. 2. Occupational therapy. 3. Disability evaluation. I. Title.
  [DNLM: 1. Occupational Therapy. 2. Needs Assessment. 3. Physical Therapy Modalities. WB 555 F278p 2007]
  RM701.F39 2007
  615.8'2--dc22
                        2006030650
A catalogue record for this book is available from the British Library

ISBN   978-1-86156480-1   (P/B)

Printed and bound in Great Britain by CPI Antony Rowe, Chippenham, Wiltshire

Dedication

This book is dedicated to my husband, Alexander Hamilton Fawcett, and our two wonderful children, Lucas and Beatrix.

It is also dedicated to the talented occupational therapists and physiotherapists who have contributed case examples for the text, in grateful thanks for sharing your practice, expertise and insights.

Contents

Contributors

Gail P. Brooke Dip Phys, Cert in Health Service Management

Gail qualified as a Physiotherapist in 1973 and originally specialised in musculoskeletal work. After working at a number of mental health settings in the north of England, Gail became the Superintendent Physiotherapist at Harrogate District Hospital in 1990. In 1993, she and a colleague piloted several outpatient chronic pain management programmes using a cognitive behavioural approach, which were soon funded by the regional health authority and, in 1995, led to an extended multidisciplinary service, which Gail currently manages. She is also involved in undergraduate recruitment and training at several universities. She manages the Chronic Fatigue Service and the Chronic Pain Service in addition to being Head of Physiotherapy for the Harrogate rural locality of North Yorkshire and York Primary Care Trust.

Rachel Hargreaves BSc (Hons), SROT

Rachel Hargreaves graduated as an Occupational Therapist in 1996 from Coventry University. She initially worked in a large teaching hospital in Leeds, until specialising in Neurology. In 1998/9, she worked in Australia in an Outback Base Hospital, and also worked in inner-city Sydney developing a service in a Nursing Home. On return to the UK, she specialised in Older Adult Mental Health services and currently works as a core member of a Community Mental Health Team, with a special interest in the Memory Clinic Service. At present, she is undertaking a Master's in Professional Health Studies at York St John University College.

Claire Howell BSc OT (Hons)

Claire graduated from Coventry University in 1996 and has worked clinically within the West Midlands since this date. After qualifying, Claire started working in Adult Rehabilitation before moving into the field of Paediatrics in 1998, where she has since specialised. Claire has a varied experience within Paediatrics, both hospital- and community-based, and is currently working for Solihull Primary Care Trust.

Karen Innes BSc OT, Dip in Management Studies, Cert in Counselling

After qualifying as an Occupational Therapist in 1999, Karen completed 18 months' basic grade mixed rotation before gaining Senior II in the physical field as a Hand Therapist working in Rheumatology and Community Services. Karen then worked for six months in Elderly Psychiatry and Acute Assessment before achieving a Senior I post in Ripon Community Mental Health Team. Karen uses the Assessment of Motor and Process Skills to assess clients attending Memory Clinics and has helped set up multidisciplinary community-based groups for people with memory problems and early-diagnosis dementia, for which she presented a poster at the College of Occupational Therapists' annual conference in 2004. She is an Alzheimer's Society committee member and works with Age Concern on a number of projects. She is currently employed by North Yorkshire and York Primary Care Trust.

David Jelley BA (Hons), BSc (Hons)

David is a Superintendent Physiotherapist and Team Leader of the Fast Response Service. He qualified in Leeds in 1993 and since then has spent much of his career working with the elderly client group. David is currently part way through a Master's in Rehabilitation Studies at Bradford University, where he also teaches a session on applying exercise theory to neurological patients. He is employed by North Yorkshire and York Primary Care Trust.

Alison J. Laver Fawcett PhD, OT(C), DipCOT

Alison graduated as an Occupational Therapist in 1986 and, while working in a number of clinical posts in London, developed a joint physiotherapy and occupational therapy initial assessment process with a physiotherapist colleague in a day hospital for older people. In 1990, she became a full-time research occupational therapist in the Department of Geriatric Medicine at St George's Hospital, London. *The Structured Observational Test of Function* (Laver and Powell, 1995) was based on her PhD research and led to her being commissioned to undertake and publish research on the use of the Chessington Occupational Therapy Neurological and Assessment Battery (COTNAB) with older people. She has held senior academic posts at universities in the UK, Canada and the US including McMaster University and Washington University School of Medicine. Following the birth of her first child, Alison became a part-time Mental Health Project Worker, a jointly funded health and social care post with responsibility for evaluating statutory and non-statutory services for older people with mental health problems. Since 2003, Alison has worked as the Modernisation Manager for Older People's Mental Health Services (North Yorkshire and York Primary Care Trust). As part of her service improvement leadership responsibilities, she is currently Project Manager for the Harrogate and Rural District Dementia Services Collaborative team.

Sally Payne MSc, BSc, DipCOT

Sally graduated from Dorset House School of Occupational Therapy, Oxford in 1989. She has worked in the West Midlands ever since in both clinical and research roles. Between 1997 and 1999, Sally took the lead role in developing an outcome tool for use within an interdisciplinary child development team, the results of which were presented at conferences both nationally and internationally. Clinically, Sally has worked with adults and children, before finally specialising in work with children and families. She obtained an MSc in Occupational Therapy from Coventry University in 2004, where she completed her dissertation, *Being the Parent of a Child with Developmental Coordination Disorder*. Sally is currently Head Paediatric Occupational Therapist for Solihull Primary Care Trust.

Heather G. Shaw DipCOT

Heather graduated as an Occupational Therapist from York School of Occupational Therapy in 1979. Having held posts in two acute mental settings, she took up the post in the specialist area of Pain Management in Harrogate in 1996. At that time, it was a fledgling service and Heather has been involved in the development of the service; extra staff have since been recruited and dedicated accommodation for the service achieved. There are now plans to offer a service in Primary Care and expand to surrounding areas. A primary objective of the service has been to educate others. Heather has a particular interest in education, and completed a City & Guilds Certificate in Teaching. She has presented to undergraduates, graduates, peers and GP groups about the theory and practice of pain management.

Foreword

I was delighted when Alison asked me to write the foreword to what is a very comprehensive text concerning assessment and outcome measurement specifically targeted at occupational therapists and physiotherapists. The key feature of this book lies in the exhaustive information contained in all the elements it addresses. The level of detail is impressive, and therefore will serve to inform not only the undergraduate student in the basic tenets of assessment but also the novice practitioner who is seeking more detailed knowledge to inform their practice and the Master's student who searches for more in-depth information relating to their research, and even the expert practitioner or those embarking upon PhD studies will find it to be a stimulus to new and creative thinking in practice, evaluation and research.

The text takes us through the rationale around the need for comprehensive assessment in health and social care settings, describes the methods and sources of assessment data and then challenges the practitioner to consider to what use the collected assessment data within his/her own practice domain is put. The next section of the book details levels (types) of data, making clear reference to assessment examples used in everyday practice, as well as explaining standardisation of assessments and the concepts of validity and reliability. The third section of the book relates to application in practice, including the practicalities of assessment administration, as well as applying models of practice to assessment and, finally, explores clinical reasoning and reflection as parts of the assessment process. Thus the book brings together the totality of the practice process.

A welcome feature of the book is the focus on, and reference to, very detailed case studies that illustrate the elements of practice that the chapter has concentrated upon. Often students and novice practitioners are frustrated by the mini-vignettes that may appear in textbooks, and they cry out for more explicit and detailed examples of practice. In this textbook they have been provided, and make excellent learning tools for the reader. So too are the worksheets that have been supplied, such that individual, group or departmental CPD exercises could be carried out using these tools. In addition, the reader has the opportunity to review the learning achieved by the use of study questions in each chapter, with outline answers available at the end of the book.

This reference text can be used at various levels and therefore should provide useful information for the individual, the team, the group or the library and be a source of inspiration for practice reflection for many years.

Jenny Butler, PhD
Professor of Occupational Therapy
Oxford Brookes University

Preface

Principles of Assessment and Outcome Measurement for Occupational Therapists and Physio-therapists: Theory, Skills and Application aims to provide a comprehensive text on assessment, evaluation and outcome measurement for occupational therapy and physiotherapy students, therapists, managers and educators. The book explores the core principles that underpin effective and efficient therapy assessment processes across a wide range of diagnoses, age groups and practice settings.

Much of the literature, in therapy journals and health and social care policy, now extols the need for evidence-based practice, including the need for well-defined and measured outcomes, the application of evidence-based standardised tests and the development of rigorous assessment processes. Few therapists will disagree with this in principle, yet many struggle to apply this to their own practice. I continue to be alarmed by the number of clinicians who find it difficult to explain the differences between various types of validity or reliability or to understand why these are so important to their selection of tests. There are still far too few clinicians who can undertake a detailed search for evidence-based measures and rigorously critique those identified. Making this important shift in our professional practice has to occur at many levels: amongst educators, clinicians, managers and researchers. It is a shift I became committed to early in my career and became even more passionate about during my doctoral studies and the development of the Structured Observational Test of Function (Laver and Powell, 1995). This mission was further fuelled when exploring the topic further as an author who was invited to contribute chapters on assessment (Laver Fawcett, 2002; Laver and Unsworth, 1999; Laver, 1996). I have written this book in the hope that the information provided can help in our profession's move towards evidence-based measurement through the education of our students. I also hope that clinicians who wish to develop more knowledge and confidence in this area will find the book informative and practical.

In my role as an occupational therapy educator (1991–1999), I searched on a number of occasions for a definitive text that would introduce my students to the importance of assessment and measurement in their practice. I wanted a text that would help them get to grips with psychometrics, test critique and the principles of test administration and reporting. I also looked for a text that provided detailed case examples that unpackaged the therapist's clinical reasoning during assessment and showed the student, step by step, how to apply the principles of rigorous assessment and measurement to practice. Psychometric texts were usually too detailed and dry as a starting point for students. Many therapy texts had chapters on assessment, but the sections on psychometrics were often limited to a few paragraphs and lacked the depth required. Other texts were focused on assessment and evaluation with a particular population, such as children or people who have had a stroke. As I result, I ended up with an extensive reading list, with chapters and articles taken from a wide range of sources, and sometimes suffered complaints from students about the lack of a key set text. As I have worked on this book, I have held in the back of my mind the requirements I had as an educator and tried to pull these elements together into one text.

Over the years, I developed a number of worksheets that I have used with students and clinicians to help them apply the key principles of assessment and gain the confidence to put this knowledge into practice. Feedback received showed that students and colleagues found these helpful and so I have included them in the text.

The purpose of this book is to enable undergraduate and postgraduate students of occupational therapy and physiotherapy, as well as qualified physiotherapists and occupational therapists (clinicians, managers, educators and researchers), to:

- develop a comprehensive and effective assessment process for their clients; this involves integrating the application and interpretation of a range of data-collection methods to achieve a thorough, meaningful, valid and reliable assessment experience for users of therapy services
- select and implement appropriate standardised measures; this involves understanding the meaning and relevance of psychometric properties and being able to analyse data on psychometric properties in order to select the best evidence-based standardised tests and outcome measures for a client group or research population.

It is hoped that *Principles of Assessment and Outcome Measurement for Occupational Therapists and Physiotherapists: Theory, Skills and Application* will encourage and assist students and therapists to reflect upon and improve the quality of their assessment and measurement approaches.

Alison Laver Fawcett

Acknowledgements

I would like to give my heartfelt thanks to those therapists who have contributed to the case studies and clinical examples in this book. While the therapists who have assisted in the development of chapters in some specific way are acknowledged in the Contents as authors at the start of the chapter to which they contributed, I would also like to acknowledge each of the contributors personally here.

Grateful thanks go to Karen Innes, not only for contributing so much to the case studies in Chapter 3 and Chapter 10 of this book but also for her enthusiasm for this project and the interest and support she has shown during the long writing process.

Many thanks to Gail Brooke and Heather Shaw, who gave up their time so I could interview them in depth for the final case study, 'Carol', which appears in Chapter 12. They also engaged in the writing process by reviewing my drafts, adding details and providing additional data. I feel their contribution of such a detailed description of their multidisciplinary practice is a real gift and inspiration to our professions. Gail also leant me a number of useful texts on physiotherapy, measurement and pain.

Many thanks to David Jelley, who has supported the development of this book in a number of ways. David shared his practice in a detailed interview that became the basis for the case study 'Mary', which appears in Chapter 9. He also engaged in the writing process by reviewing my drafts, adding details and providing additional data. David organised for me to observe and interview several of his physiotherapy colleagues in the outpatient and Fast Response services he manages. He also leant me a number of useful physiotherapy texts.

Many thanks to Claire Howell and Sally Payne, who have provided the case study 'Scott' that appears in Chapter 2. Claire and Sally's case provides an excellent example of the different data-collection methods used for a comprehensive therapy assessment process.

Many thanks are also owed to Rachel Hargreaves, who was a natural choice when I wanted an example of a test report for Chapter 8 because of her enthusiasm for implementing a standardised assessment into a memory assessment service for people with suspected dementia. I am grateful to Rachel for providing an excellent example of a comprehensive report related to standardised test results.

I was delighted when Professor Jenny Butler, Professor in Occupational Therapy at Oxford Brookes University, agreed to contribute the Foreword to this book, and I want to express my grateful thanks to Jenny for giving up her time to review the manuscript and for supporting my endeavour in this way.

I am very grateful to Dr Diane Cox for encouraging me to write this book and for providing practical help with the literature search, in particular raiding her husband's physiotherapy journals. I also want to thank her for reviewing chapters early on in the writing process from her perspective as an educator and for her valuable feedback and encouragement.

I would like to thank Colin Whurr, who originally approached me to write a textbook and believed in my book proposal, and Margaret Gallagher, my editor at Whurr Publishers Limited, for her advice and encouragement in the early stages of writing.

Emma Hatfield became my editor when Whurr was acquired by John Wiley & Sons Limited. I have to admit I was nervous about changing editors halfway through the writing process, but I needn't have been. Emma has been an enthusiastic, supportive and very understanding editor and I am extremely grateful for her contribution, and especially for her patience. I also want to thank Dave Thompson, whose artistic talents have resulted in the great illustrations, and Laura Ferrier, who checked and double-checked we had all the necessary permissions.

I want to say a big thank-you to my copy editor, Tim Bettsworth, whose observant and insightful queries have led to a more polished manuscript. I was delighted to learn what *stet* meant (a publishing term for 'let it stand'), but the fact I could rarely use it in response to Tim's queries is testament to how good he is at his job!

Grateful thanks to David Brown (Director of Mental Health) and Tom Welsh (General Manager) at Craven, Harrogate and Rural District (now North Yorkshire and York) Primary Care Trust, who granted me study leave during the summer of 2004 so that I could get focused on the text and make significant progress on the work. I would also like to thank my current employer, North Yorkshire and York Primary Care Trust, for granting me study leave to proofread and index this text. David, I really appreciate not only your authorising my study leave but also your support and for patiently waiting for the book to finally make it to print – and not losing faith that these two periods of study leave would help contribute to my finally producing a worthwhile book.

Thank you to the physiotherapists, particularly David May and Rachel Stuart, at Ripon Community Hospital who allowed me to observe their interviews and assessments and who answered my many questions. Thank you also to the occupational therapists at Harrogate District Hospital, particularly those in the Child Development Unit who described their practice and gave me access to their standardised tests.

Many thanks to Lesley Munro and Lucy Do at Harcourt Assessment for organising for me to be loaned a number of the tests published by Harcourt for review. A number of these texts proved relevant and have been included as examples in the text.

Annie Turner invited me to write a chapter on assessment for the fifth edition of *Occupational Therapy and Physical Dysfunction: Principles, Skills and Practice* (Laver Fawcett, 2002). I'm grateful to Annie for the opportunity to write this chapter because it sowed the seeds for this present book. Having Annie as an editor back then was a fantastic experience and I learnt a lot from her expertise as an occupational therapy educator, writer and editor. Working on the chapter with her convinced me to take the next step and attempt a book on the subject. Annie also helped me to obtain permission from Churchill Livingstone to reproduce a number of figures I developed for the chapter on assessment in this book.

I would also like to acknowledge some special colleagues who have supported, taught, empowered and inspired me throughout my career – each of you in your own way has helped me reach the place where embarking on this textbook was possible: Dr Carolyn Baum, Dr Mary Law, Dr Barbara Cooper, Jennifer Creek, Dr Carolyn Unsworth, Professor Peter Millard, Beryl Steeden and Julia Gosden.

On a more personal note I would like to thank my father, Philip Laver (aka 'Pops'), for helping me to find my missing or incomplete references and particularly for finding missing issue numbers – it was a tedious labour of love and I really appreciated your help. I also want to thank Pops for dealing with my innumerable emails containing the many various drafts of this book attached and for then archiving and backing up all of them on his computer. He has responded to my emails and attachments with numerous encouraging messages, and his belief in my writing endeavour has been very validating. He has also applied his enthusiasm for computing to solve a number of formatting problems for me, particularly when other authors have given me permission to reproduce figures and I have struggled to edit the files they have sent or to create sharp enough reproductions. Above all, I must apologise to my mother, Diane, for providing my father with an ongoing excuse for spending even more time at his computer!

I must acknowledge that this book would not have been finished without the support of my husband, Alex, who has continued to encourage me in this endeavour (even as the years have ticked by) from the envisaged two, to three, then four and now five years working on this text. He has patiently supported me both by taking our children out on numerous occasions so I could have time and peace to write and by putting up with my spending many late nights shut away in my study. I also wish to thank our two children, Lucas and Beatrix, whose thirst for knowledge and frequent 'Why…?' questions keep me on my toes and who helped me to keep life in perspective when the writing process became challenging. To Alex, Lucas and Beatrix I now promise to put some of my occupational therapy knowledge about life balance into practice and become a more active participant in family activities – it is time to put my computer in its place and have more fun!

Alison Laver Fawcett

Introduction

The purpose of this book is to enable students of occupational therapy and physiotherapy, as well as qualified physiotherapists and occupational therapists, to understand the complex art and science of assessment processes, to be familiar with psychometric terms and to be able to identify the properties of tests in order to select and confidently implement the use of appropriate standardised tests and outcome measures in their clinical practice and research.

This introduction briefly describes, chapter by chapter, what is going to be examined in this book. The introduction also discusses and defines the key terminology to be used in the text (including assessment, evaluation, outcome and measurement). Chapter 1 focuses on the importance of accurate assessment (including the advantages and disadvantages of informal versus standardised methods). Methods of assessment such as self-report, proxy and observational approaches are investigated in Chapter 2. In Chapter 3, the different purposes of assessment (such as descriptive, discriminative, predictive and evaluative) are explored and the timing of assessments (including initial, baseline, monitoring and outcome) are considered. Chapter 4 addresses the question of 'What is measurement?' and provides definitions and examples of four levels of measurement (nominal, ordinal, interval and ratio). Test development, standardisation, norm-referenced and criterion-referenced tests are then examined in Chapter 5. Chapter 6 focuses on the topic of validity and concludes with an exploration of face validity and clinical utility. Reliability is then examined in Chapter 7, and this includes an explanation of the different types of reliability statistics used to examine levels of reliability and concepts such as test specificity, sensitivity, error of measurement and floor and ceiling effects. Chapter 8 explains the process of test administration and makes suggestions for reporting and recording test results. The application of models of function to therapy assessment and measurement is explored in Chapter 9 and illustrated with a number of examples, including the World Health Organization's International Classification of Functioning, Disability and Health. Chapter 10 explains the importance of clinical reasoning and reflective practice in effective assessment and discusses different types of clinical reasoning (including diagnostic, interactive, pragmatic, procedural, narrative and ethical reasoning). Advice on implementing the optimum assessment and measurement approach is provided in Chapter 11, along with a detailed example of a test critique and suggestions for examining your current assessment practice and planning improvements to your assessment process. The book ends with a very detailed case study in Chapter 12; this case describes the role of an occupational therapist and a physiotherapist working with a person who is being supported by a Chronic Pain Service and illustrates many of the principles, skills and issues discussed in previous chapters.

Throughout the book, examples of standardised tests along with clinical examples, case vignettes and case histories are used to help the reader see how to apply the principles and skills described to their practice. Worksheets have also been developed to facilitate the reader to start to apply the principles and skills to their own practice. Study questions and brief answers are provided to help the reader check whether they have grasped the key concepts from each chapter.

This introduction will consider the role of occupational therapy and physiotherapy. It provides a review of definitions for key terms used in everyday therapy practice: assessment, evaluation, scale, outcome and measurement. It concludes by presenting the definitions of these key terms that have been developed or selected as a foundation for this text.

OCCUPATIONAL THERAPY AND PHYSIOTHERAPY

This book is written for both occupational therapists and physiotherapists. In exploring assessment and measurement within these professions, it is critical to understand what these two groups of therapists are trying to achieve. In North America, the term *physical therapists* (as opposed to physiotherapists) is used, and these two terms will be used interchangeably in this book depending upon the source of any quoted material. Physiotherapy/physical therapy can be defined as the treatment of physical dysfunction or injury by the use of therapeutic exercises and the application of modalities intended to restore or facilitate normal function or development. The World Confederation for Physical Therapy (WCPT) states:

> The aim of physical therapists is to identify and maximise human movement potential within the spheres of promotion, prevention, treatment and rehabilitation, in partnership with their clients. (World Confederation for Physical Therapy, 2006b)

Occupational therapy is defined by the College of Occupational Therapists (COT) as:

> Occupational therapists work in partnership with people of all ages to find ways of helping them to carry out activities they need or choose to do in order to achieve satisfaction in their daily lives. Occupational therapy assists people to participate in the occupations they need or choose to do through the therapeutic use of activities that are analysed, chosen and adapted to suit the needs and preferences of individuals. (College of Occupational Therapists, 2005a, Appendix 7)

The World Federation of Occupational Therapists (WFOT) provides a definition of occupational therapy that was agreed at a WFOT council meeting in 2004, and can be found on its website supplied with its reference. This definition begins by stating:

> Occupational therapy is a profession concerned with promoting health and wellbeing through occupation. The primary goal of occupational therapy is to enable people to participate in the activities of everyday life. Occupational therapists achieve this outcome by enabling people to do things that will enhance their ability to participate or by modifying the environment to better support participation. (World Federation of Occupational Therapists, 2005)

The major goal of both physiotherapy and occupational therapy is to help people to maximise their potential by reducing the impact of any impairments and limiting the resulting disability and/or handicap. Therapists work with people to help them to obtain their highest levels of activity and participation in order to enhance their quality of life. When a person has a progressive or terminal illness, the goal may be to maintain function for as long as possible and reduce the negative impact of pathology on their quality of life. Therefore, the major objective of both occupational therapy and physiotherapy assessment is to gain a clear picture of the individual in order to develop an intervention plan that will result in improved, or maintained, function and enhanced quality of life. Therapists strive to ensure that these interventions are effective, efficient and economical in order to provide quality services to clients and their carers. Therapists need to use outcome measures to evaluate the effects of their interventions.

Occupational therapists and physiotherapists work in a wide range of settings, including hospitals, health centres, service users' own homes, schools, supported housing and work environments. The vast majority of therapists work within health care services. Health care services are provided in order to prevent, diagnose and treat illness and include services to promote and protect public health (Department of Health, 2004).

LABELS USED FOR PROVIDERS AND RECIPIENTS OF THERAPY SERVICES

Throughout this text, the term *therapist* will be used to include both occupational therapists and physiotherapists. The terms *clinician* and *health care professional* are also used as per the Department of Health's (DoH; 2004) definitions:

- A clinician is defined as a 'professionally qualified staff providing clinical care to patients' (p. 30).
- A health care professional is defined as 'a person who is a member of a profession regulated body' (p. 31).

The terms *patient* (a person receiving health care), *client*, *service user* and *person* will be used interchangeably throughout the text to indicate a recipient of occupational therapy and/or physiotherapy services.

- The word patient stems from the Latin word *pati*, which means 'to suffer' and is still used in medical settings, such as in-patient hospital care (Turner, 2002, p. 355).
- In community settings, the term client is more frequently used, but, like Turner, I feel the derivation of this word from the Latin *cluere*, which means 'to obey' or 'hear', does not reflect concepts of person-centred working, which are becoming more prominent amongst therapy literature.
- Over the past decade, an emphasis on the rights of people receiving health care, and the move away from viewing patients as passive recipients of care, has led to the use of the term service user (Turner, 2002). The DoH defines a service user as 'an individual who uses a health care service, including those who are not in need of treatment, such as blood donors, carers or those using screening services' (Department of Health, 2004, p. 34).

Turner (2002) recommends that as proponents of partnership and person-centred working we should use the terms people and person, as opposed to client or patient. Where the context allows and the meaning is clear, the term person will be used in this book to denote the recipient of therapy services.

The term *carer* is used by the DoH to describe a friend/relative who helps out with the care of another person; for the purposes of this book a carer is defined as 'a person, usually a relative or friend, who provides care on a voluntary basis implicit in relationships between family members' (Department of Health, 2001a, p. 153). It should be noted that in some instances within health and social care settings the term carer can be used to describe a paid staff member delivering care.

To improve the flow of the text, the therapist will be referred to as female and the service user as male in the majority of this book (certain case studies reverse this general rule).

THE IMPORTANCE OF THE SELECTION AND APPLICATION OF TERMINOLOGY IN PRACTICE

It is important to begin a book on assessment and outcome measurement with clear definitions of the key terminology to be used within the text. However, this is far from being a simple exercise. Assessment, evaluation, scales, outcome, measurement and outcome measurement mean different things to different people (Stokes and O'Neill, 1999), and there is some discrepancy in the use of these terms within the physiotherapy and occupational therapy literature. Therapists do not necessarily have a common vocabulary to describe some of their key concepts; for example, Mosey (1991) states that a 'lack of common vocabulary – the result of marked inattention to concept-definition-label consistency – is a serious problem in occupational therapy' (p. 67). More recently, Denshire and Mullavey-O'Byrne (2003) report that 'finding a congruent language to give meaning to practice remains a contentious issue in the literature' (p. 519). To add to the confusion, both everyday and professional vocabulary can have very different meanings on opposite sides of the Atlantic. (As a British therapist working in the USA and Canada for several years, I had personal experience of this – sometimes with embarrassing or amusing consequences!)

The selection and application of terms to describe therapy practices is important because the language we use gives our practice a public face and enables us to share ideas and information. In the area of assessment and measurement, therapists need to obtain a clear understanding of what is meant by frequently used terms in order to communicate effectively about the assessment process and its results with service users and their carers, other health care professionals, referral sources, discharge destinations, managers and policy developers.

The College of Occupational Therapists (2005a) commissioned the *Standard Terminology Project* to represent the understanding of key terms of the majority of members of the occupational therapy profession in the UK. An earlier piece of work was undertaken by the American Occupational Therapy Association (AOTA), who produced the *Uniform Terminology for Reporting Occupational Therapy Services* (American Occupational Therapy Association, 1979). The WCPT and the Chartered Society of Physiotherapy (CSP) provide some definitions and descriptions on their websites. As we find competing and overlapping definitions of terms related to assessment and measurement in the therapy, it is helpful to start with dictionary definitions and see how these terms are used in everyday language. I shall begin with dictionary definitions of key terms. I have used my dependable *Concise Oxford Dictionary* (Sykes, 1983), which I was given when I started my occupational therapy training (now that ages me!) and, as definitions can change over time, I shall also use a much more up-to-date resource: the range of excellent free dictionary and encyclopaedia services that are available on the World Wide Web. I will then explore the use of these words (assessment, evaluation, scale, measurement, outcome and outcome measure) within the therapy and health care literature nationally and internationally in order to gain a deeper understanding of the meanings ascribed to these terms by therapists and in an attempt to give a definitive definition.

DEFINITIONS OF KEY TERMS

ASSESSMENT

Sykes (1983) defines *assess* as 'fix amount of and impose (on person or community); . . . estimate magnitude or quality of'. In the health care literature it has been defined as 'to identify, describe, evaluate and validate information' (Centre for Advanced Palliative Care, 2005). An online dictionary definition for *assessment* calls it 'the act or result of judging the worth or value of something or someone' and gives related words, including *evaluation* and *judgment* (http://www.answers.com/library/Dictionary, accessed 26.10.05).

There are numerous definitions of assessment in the rehabilitation literature. The DoH defines assessment as 'a process whereby the needs of an individual are identified and quality of life is evaluated' (Department of Health, 2001a, p. 151). The AOTA (1979) also calls it a process; in this case it describes assessment as the process of determining the need for, nature of and estimated time of treatment, as well as coordinating with other professionals involved. In the UK, the COT also defines assessment as a process and says it is 'the process of collecting accurate and relevant information about the client in order to set baselines and to monitor and measure the outcomes of therapy or intervention' (College of Occupational Therapists, 2003a, p. 50).

The WCPT describes assessment as the first stage of the physiotherapy process.

> Assessment includes both the examination of individuals or groups with actual or potential impairments, functional limitations, disabilities, or other conditions of health by history taking, screening and the use of specific tests and measures and evaluation of the results of the examination through analysis and synthesis within a process of clinical reasoning. (http://www.fisionline.org/WCPT.html#Iniziale2, accessed 27.10.05)

Two American authors define assessment simply as 'a process by which data are gathered, hypotheses formulated, and decisions made for further action' (Christiansen and Baum, 1991, p. 848). Two other American occupational therapy authors describe assessment as 'the planned collection, interpretation, and documentation of the functional status of an individual related to the individual's capacity to perform valued or required self-care, work or leisure tasks' (Rogers and Holm, 1989, p. 6). The Royal College of Physicians (RCP) also perceives assessment as including 'both the collection of data and the interpretation of those data in order to inform decision' (Royal College of Physicians, 2002, section 4.1). Law and Letts (1989) describe it as an essential component of the therapy process and say assessment is used to describe the person's strengths and problems, formulate a prognosis and evaluate the effects of therapy interventions.

Another description of physiotherapy assessment refers to a range of methods and embeds measurement as part of the process.

> A physiotherapist will initially conduct a subjective examination (interview) of a patient's medical history, and then go on to the objective assessment (physical examination). The subjective examination is guided by the presenting system and complaint, and the objective assessment is in turn guided by the history. This semistructured process is used to rule out serious pathology (so-called red flags), establish functional limitations, refine the diagnosis, guide therapy, and establish a baseline for monitoring progress. As such, the objective exam will then use certain quantifiable measurements to both guide diagnosis and for progress monitoring. These depend upon the system (and area) being managed. (http://en.wikipedia.org/wiki/Physical_therapy#Assessment, accessed 27.10.05)

Some themes about the nature of assessment that emerge from these definitions are:

- assessment is a process
- assessment involves multiple methods of obtaining and interpreting information/data
- information obtained through assessment enables therapists to decide whether therapy is required, to set a baseline for treatment and to evaluate the results of that treatment
- assessment is a process that encompasses the evaluation and measurement of outcomes.

For the purposes of this book, *assessment* will be defined as:

Definition of assessment

Assessment is the overall process of selecting and using multiple data-collection tools and various sources of information to inform decisions required for guiding therapeutic intervention during the whole therapy process. It involves interpreting information collected to make clinical decisions related to the needs of the person and the appropriateness and nature of their therapy. Assessment involves the evaluation of the outcomes of therapeutic interventions.

EVALUATION

Jacobs (1993) notes that 'often, the term assessment is incorrectly thought to be synonymous with evaluation' and goes on to say that 'assessment encompasses evaluation as one of its . . . phases' (p. 228). The word *evaluation* is a noun; related words used by therapists include *to evaluate* (verb) and *evaluative* (adjective). Evaluation is 'the act or result of evaluating' (from CancerWeb at: http://cancerweb.ncl.ac.uk/cgi-bin/omd?query=evaluation, accessed 27.10.05). Sykes (1983) defines evaluate as 'ascertain amount of; find numerical expression for; appraise; assess'. An online dictionary (http://dictionary.reference.com/search?q=evaluate, accessed 27.10.05) provides three definitions for the word evaluate:

- to ascertain or fix the value or worth of
- to examine and judge carefully; appraise
- mathematics: to calculate the numerical value of; express numerically.

The COT defines evaluation as 'the process of using clinical reasoning, problem-analysis, self-appraisal and review to interpret the results of assessment in order to make judgements about the situation or needs of an individual, the success of occupational therapy or the therapist's own performance' (College of Occupational Therapists, 2003a, p. 53). So evaluation is also applied to service review as well as to individual client work. Corr (2003) states that 'a service might be very good, but without evaluation its value diminishes because there is no objective measure of it being "very good"' (p. 235).

The WCPT states that the stage of evaluation in the physical therapy process 'necessitates re-examination for the purpose of evaluating outcomes' (http://www.fisionline.org/WCPT. html#Iniziale2, accessed 27.10.05).

Some ideas about evaluation that appear in these definitions are:

- evaluation involves examining or judging the amount or value of something
- evaluation can be viewed as a subcomponent of a broader assessment process
- evaluation is undertaken to enable a therapist to make a clinical judgement about her client or a judgement about the value of her service
- evaluation of outcomes requires re-examination, and so a therapist has to obtain the same information/data on two occasions to evaluate any change in the outcome of interest
- evaluation can involve expressing something numerically.

For the purposes of this book, *evaluation* will be defined as:

Definition of evaluation

Evaluation is a component of a broader assessment process. It involves the collection of data to enable the therapist to make a judgement about the amount of a specific construct of interest (such as degree of range of movement or level of independence in an activity of daily living) or to make a judgement about the value of an intervention for delivering the desired outcome for a person or the value of a service for delivering outcomes of relevance to the client population. Evaluation often involves data being collected at two time points in order to measure effect and also can involve the translation of observations to numerical scores.

SCALE

Within therapy and rehabilitation literature, we also see the terms *scale, rating scales* and *measurement scales*. The word scale appears in quite a lot of standardised health and therapy tests, for example the Beck Scale for Suicide Ideation (Beck and Steer, 1991). So what do therapists mean by scale? Sykes (1983) defines it as a 'series of degrees, ladder-like arrangement or classification, graded system' and notes that in the context of arithmetic a scale is the 'basis of numerical system as shown by ratio between units in adjacent places of number'. So a scale provides a means of recording something that might be defined in terms of levels, amounts or degrees, and it may also involve numbers.

An online dictionary defines scale in the following way: 'a *scale* is either a weighing scale used for measurement of weight (mass or force), or a series of ratios against which different measurements can be compared. The latter need not always be a linear ratio, and is often logarithmic. *Scaling* is the measurement of a variable in such a way that it can be expressed on a continuum. Rating your preference for a product from 1 to 10 is an example of a scale' (http://www.answers. com/library/Dictionary, accessed 26.10.05).

This dictionary further differentiates between comparative and non-comparative scaling. With *comparative* scaling, the items are directly compared with each other (for example: 'Do you prefer the colour blue or red?'). In *non-comparative* scaling, each item is scaled independently of the others (for example: 'How do you feel about the colour red?') (http://www.answers.com/library/Dictionary, accessed 26.10.05).

The DoH states that 'a scale is a means of identifying the presence and/or severity of a particular problem, such as depression or difficulties with personal care. It is important that scales are used in support of professional judgement, and are valid, reliable and culturally sensitive. A scale is valid if it actually measures what it is supposed to measure. It is reliable if trust can be placed on it when used by different assessors or over time. A scale is culturally sensitive, if questions and the interpretation of responses are not prejudiced against people from specific cultures and backgrounds' (Department of Health, 2006b).

Stevens (1946) describes a well-accepted and well-used model of four levels of measurement scales that differ in the extent to which their scale values retain the properties of the real number line. The four levels are called nominal, ordinal, interval and ratio scales (see Chapter 4 for details).

Ideas about scales that appear in these definitions are:

- a scale provides a means of recording something that might be defined in terms of levels, amounts or degrees
- in health care settings, scales are often used to rate the presence or severity of a problem, for example a symptom or the level of independence in a daily activity, such as personal care
- scales may also involve the use of numbers assigned as scores
- there is an accepted categorisation of scales into four levels of measurement.

For the purposes of this book, *scale* will be defined as:

Definition of scale

A scale provides a means of recording something that can be rated in terms of levels, amounts or degrees. Therapists use scales to rate the presence or severity of a problem, such as a symptom, or to rate the person's level of independence in a needed or chosen occupation, activity or task. Scales can be categorised into one of four levels of measurement: nominal, ordinal, interval or ratio. Numbers are frequently assigned as scores in scales. How these numerical scores can be used and interpreted depends upon the level of measurement used in the scale.

For the purposes of this book, *comparative* and *non-comparative* scaling will be defined as:

Definition of comparative scaling

With comparative scaling, items being rated are directly compared with each other in some way. They may be rated in terms of which are the best, or the most difficult, or the most frequently occurring, or the preferred option (for example: 'Do you prefer coffee or tea?').

Definition of non-comparative scaling

With non-comparative scaling, each item in the scale is rated/scored independently of all the other items. This might be in terms of how well the item can be performed, how frequently the item occurs or how the person feels about that item (for example: 'How well can you get dressed?' 'How often to you go out with friends?' 'How do you feel about caring for your loved one?').

ALTERNATIVE TERMS FOR SCALE

Other terms that are sometimes used in a similar context are *instrument, index, indexes, indices, typology* and *profile*. These terms appear in the literature and are also used in the titles of some standardised health and therapy tests, for example the Barthel Index (Mahoney and Barthel, 1965), the Caregiver Strain Index (Robinson, 1983), the Capabilities of Upper Extremity Instrument (Marino, Shea and Stineman, 1998), the Functional Assessment of Multiple Sclerosis Quality of Life Instrument (FAMS; Cella *et al.*, 1996), the Physiotherapy Functional Mobility Profile (Platt, Bell and Kozak, 1998) and the Abbreviated Functional Limitations Profile (UK) SIP-68 (de Bruin *et al.*, 1994).

An *instrument* is 'a device for recording or measuring' (Hopkins and Smith, 1993a, p. 914). The term *index* is used when multiple indicators of a variable are combined into a single measure. For example, the Barthel Index (Mahoney and Barthel, 1965) uses a series of measures of aspects of a person's level of independence in activities of daily living (ADL) to form a combined measure of ADL function. The plural of index is sometimes given as *indexes* and sometimes as *indices*. A *typology* is similar to an index except the variable is measured at the nominal level (any numbers used in a nominal scale are merely labels and express no mathematical properties – see Chapter 4). The word *profile* has many definitions, but in relation to measurement it is defined as 'a graphical representation of an individual's standing, or level, in a series of tests. If it is a psychological or mental profile these tests would be "measuring various aspects of his mentality"' (Drever, 1973, p. 225). Therapists are often interested in interpreting the *score profile* of a person on a standardised test, for example to compare, contrast and understand the range of scores obtained on a measure that has subtests across a range of constructs (a *construct* is an unobservable, internal process such as short-term memory, figure ground discrimination, colour recognition). To aid interpretation, subtest scores may be plotted on a graph; an example is the Rivermead Perceptual Assessment Battery (RPAB; Whiting *et al.*, 1985). With normative tests, the results may be graphed using percentiles or standard deviations from the mean to provide a score profile that can be used to help the therapist decide whether the person's scores represent abnormal performance or signs of pathology (see Chapter 5 for more information about normative tests, percentiles and standard deviation).

TESTS

Measurement tools developed for use by therapists are given a wide range of names and may include terms like instrument, scale, profile, index and indices in their titles. As so many different terms abound, throughout this book the term *test* will be used to refer to standard-ised measurement tools, expect in cases where a particular published test is being discussed, in which case the term used by the test developers in the test's name will be used. Test is a useful umbrella term that includes in its meaning 'critical examination . . . of a person's or thing's qualities', a 'means of examining, standard for comparison' and 'ground of admission or rejection' (Sykes, 1983). In measurement a test is defined as:

> A standardized type of examination; given to a group or individual; it may be qualitative or quantitative, i.e. determine presence or absence of a particular capacity, knowledge or skill, or determine the degree in which such is present; in the latter case, the degree may be determined by the relative position of an individual in the group or whole population, or by assigning a definite numerical value in terms of some selected unit. (Drever, 1973, p. 296)

OUTCOME

The term *outcome* is being used more and more frequently in health, social care, therapy and rehabilitation literature; so it is a very important term to understand. Sykes (1983) defines it as a 'result, visible effect', and this definition is supported by an online dictionary's, which is 'an end result; a consequence' and also provides a synonym, *effect* (http://www.answers.com/outcome, accessed 26.10.05). In the health care literature, outcome has been defined as 'a measurable end result or consequence of a specific action or essential step' (Centre for Advanced Palliative Care, 2005).

Physiotherapy and occupational therapy services can only be considered valuable if they provide demonstrable benefits. In rehabilitation, an outcome is perceived as the end result of the therapeutic process; for example, Stokes and O'Neill state, 'with respect to physiotherapy, outcome is the end result of intervention' (1999, p. 562). In both occupational therapy and physiotherapy, the therapist works with the client to achieve agreed goals, and these are the desired outcomes of the intervention. The COT states, 'outcomes should relate closely to the client's social, psychological, emotional and cultural needs in relation to occupational per-formance' (College of Occupational Therapists, 2003a, p. 25). The desired outcome of therapy could be improved occupational performance, function or successful adaptation (Henderson, 1991, p. 13). The WCPT highlights the importance of 'including measurable outcome goals negotiated in collaboration with the patient/client, family or care giver' as part of the 'devel-opment of a plan of intervention' (http://www.fisionline.org/WCPT.html#Iniziale2, accessed 27.10.05).

Outcome and process assessment have been defined as 'evaluation procedures that focus on both the outcome or status (outcome assessment) of the patient at the end of an episode of care – presence of symptoms, level of activity, and mortality; and the process (process assessment) – what is done for the patient diagnostically and therapeutically' (taken from CancerWeb at: http://cancerweb.ncl.ac.uk/cgi-bin/omd?query=outcome, accessed 27.10.05).

Some ideas about what an outcome is, which are found in these definitions, are:

- an outcome is the consequence of some sort of action or occurrence
- in therapy, an outcome is the end result of intervention
- the therapist should agree with the service user at the start of therapy what the desired outcome(s) of therapy should be
- outcomes are visible effects, and so are things that can be observed and/or measured.

For the purposes of this book, *outcome* will be defined as:

Definition of outcome

An outcome is the observed or measured consequence of an action or occurrence. In a therapeutic process, the outcome is the end result of the therapeutic intervention.

MEASUREMENT

In the *Concise Oxford Dictionary* (Sykes, 1983) the verb *to measure* is listed as having a number of different meanings, including:

- 'ascertain extent or quantity of (thing) by comparison with fixed unit or with object of known size
- ascertain size and proportions of (person) for clothes
- estimate (quality, person's character, etc.) by some standard or rule
- take measurements
- be of specified size
- have necessary qualification for'.

The dictionary goes on to define *measurement* as the 'act or result of measuring; detailed dimensions'. An online dictionary also provides several definitions, including:

- the act of measuring or the process of being measured
- a system of measuring: *measurement in miles*
- the dimension, quantity or capacity determined by measuring: the measurements of a room (http://www.answers.com/measurement, accessed 26.10.05).

Another online search yielded the following explanation: '*Measurement* of some attribute of a set of things is the process of assigning numbers or other symbols to the things in such a way that relationships of the numbers or symbols reflect relationships of the attributes of the things being measured. A particular way of assigning numbers or symbols to measure something is called a scale of measurement' (Sarle, 1997).

In the *National Clinical Guidelines for Stroke* (Royal College of Physicians, 2002) measurement is defined as 'the comparison of some of the obtained data against some standard or "metric", in order to give the data an absolute relative meaning'.

McDowell and Newell (1996, cited in Stokes and O'Neill, 1999) describe measurement as 'the application of standard scales to variables, giving a numerical score which may be combined for each variable to give an overall score. In the measurement of functional ability, the overall score gives an indication of the level of ability of the individual' (p. 560). (*Note:* the ability to combine individual item scores to form a total score depends on the level of measurement used in the scale – see Chapter 4.) Nunnally and Bernstein (1995, cited in Polgar, 1998, p. 169) also talk about measurement relating to the production of a numerical score and define it as the process of assigning numbers to represent quantities of a trait, attribute or characteristic or to classify objects.

According to the RCP, 'measurement and assessment are linked but not synonymous' (Royal College of Physicians, 2002, section 4.1). Stokes and O'Neill (1999) clarify that 'assessment is the process of understanding the measurement within a specific context' (p. 560).

Concepts about measurement that are found in these definitions are:

- measurement is a component of a wider assessment process
- the assessment provides a context for understanding the relevance of measures obtained
- measuring is used to ascertain the dimensions (size), quantity (amount) or capacity of an aspect of the person of interest to the therapist
- a measurement is the data obtained by measuring
- measurement involves assigning numbers to represent quantities of a trait, attribute or characteristic, or to classify objects
- a measurement is obtained by applying a standard scale to variables to provide a numerical score.

For the purposes of this book, *measurement* will be defined as:

Definition of measurement

A measurement is the data obtained by measuring. Measuring is undertaken by therapists to ascertain the dimensions (size), quantity (amount) or capacity of a trait, attribute or characteristic of a person that is required by the therapist to develop an accurate picture of the person's needs and problems to form a baseline for therapeutic intervention and/or to provide a measure of outcome. A measurement is obtained by applying a standard scale to variables, thus translating direct observations or client/proxy reports to a numerical scoring system.

OUTCOME MEASURE/MEASURES OF OUTCOME

The CSP (2005), on its website section on 'Outcome measures', cites the definition of *outcome measure* used by Mayo *et al.*, (1994): 'a physical therapy outcome measure is a test or scale administered and interpreted by physical therapists that has been shown to measure accurately a particular attribute of interest to patients and therapists and is expected to be influenced by intervention'. Cole *et al.* (1995) state that an outcome measure is 'a measurement tool (instrument, questionnaire, rating form etc.) used to document change in one or more patient characteristic over time' (p. 22) and say that outcome measures are used to evaluate therapy services. It is also defined as 'an instrument designed to gather information on the efficacy of service programs; a means for determining if goals or objectives have been met' (Christiansen and Baum, 1991, p. 855). While the term is defined by the CAPC as: 'the tabulation, calculation, or recording of activity or effort that can be expressed in a quantitative or qualitative manner (when attempting to measure shifts or progress toward desired levels of quality)' (Centre for Advanced Palliative Care, 2005).

Change is not always the object of intervention and 'outcome measures need to be sensitive to protective and preventive effects as well as to improvements' (Heaton and Bamford, 2001, p. 347). It is important to note that 'clinical outcome measures in general document change over time but do not explain why the change has occurred' (Cole *et al.*, 1995, p. vi). So outcome measures are not the be-all-and-end-all solution; we also need to include in our overall assessment process methods for exploring the mechanisms underlying a desired or observed change.

We saw in the discussion on the term outcome that the therapist should agree with the service user at the start of therapy what the desired outcome(s) of therapy should be and should take measurements at the beginning and end of therapy in order to establish whether this desired outcome was indeed achieved. A robust outcome measure is required to take these pre- and post-intervention measurements in a standardised, valid and reliable way.

Some themes that emerge from these definitions of outcome measures are:

- outcome measures are used to document change in one or more client trait, attribute or characteristic over time
- outcome measures are applied to establish whether the desired outcome (the therapy goals or objectives agreed prior to therapeutic intervention) have been achieved
- the desired outcome might be an improvement or the maintenance of some area of function, and the outcome measure needs to be sensitive to the type and degree of anticipated change.

For the purposes of this book, *outcome measure* and *outcome measurement* will be defined as:

Definition of outcome measure

An outcome measure is a standardised instrument used by therapists to establish whether their desired therapeutic outcomes have been achieved.

Definition of outcome measurement

Outcome measurement is a process undertaken to establish the effects of an intervention on an individual or the effectiveness of a service on a defined aspect of the health or well-being of a specified population. Outcome measurement is achieved by administering an outcome measure on at least two occasions to document change over time in one or more trait, attribute or characteristic to establish whether that trait/attribute/characteristic has been influenced by the intervention to the anticipated degree to achieve the desired outcome.

SUMMARY OF DEFINITIONS

This concluding section draws together some of the key definitions in order to show the inter-relationship between assessment, evaluation, measurement and outcome measurement.

In occupational therapy and physiotherapy *assessment* is the overall process of selecting and using multiple data-collection tools and various sources of information. The therapist interprets the collected data/information to guide clinical decisions related to the needs of the person and the appropriateness and nature of therapy. The assessment process is often broad in nature, particularly at the onset of the therapeutic process. Information collected as part of a broad assessment process provides a *context* for understanding the relevance of any specific measures obtained. As the person's needs are defined, the therapist may focus the assessment on specific areas of function. At this stage, the therapist makes a judgement about a specific construct of interest or one concerning the value of an intervention for delivering the desired outcome. This is termed *evaluation*.

Measurement helps the therapist to record the presence or degree of something. In particular, robust measurement techniques help the therapist to ascertain the dimensions (size), quantity (amount) or capacity of a trait, attribute or characteristic. Therapists undertake *outcome measurement* as part of a wider assessment process when they need to establish the effects of an intervention on an individual. They may also undertake outcome measurement to examine the effectiveness of their therapy service. The therapist should agree with the person at the start of therapy what the *desired outcome(s)* of therapy should be. To establish whether this desired outcome was indeed achieved, the outcome measure has to be administered on at least two occasions; usually this is at the beginning and end of the therapeutic intervention. Therapists must carefully define the outcome they have been working towards and ensure the outcome measure selected really does measure the desired outcome (this is a question of validity – see Chapter 6). They also need to check the measure will be sensitive to the degree of change expected (this is a question of sensitivity – see Chapter 7).

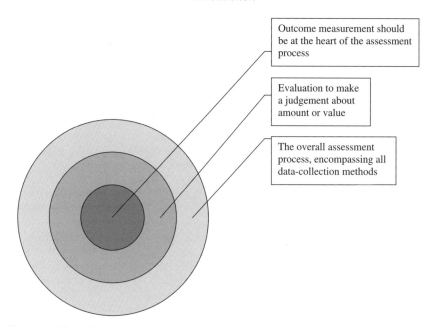

Outcome measurement should be at the heart of the assessment process

Evaluation to make a judgement about amount or value

The overall assessment process, encompassing all data-collection methods

Figure A The relationship between assessment, evaluation and outcome measurement.

Figure A illustrates how assessment is the whole data-gathering and data-interpreting process, within which evaluation and outcome measurement nest. Assessment should be understood as a broad, holistic analysis using multiple types of data (some of which are qualitative and arise from informal observations), whereas evaluation prompts a need for greater specificity and so the focus narrows – and for outcome measurement it becomes clearly defined and requires a robust standardised measure.

1

The Importance of Accurate Assessment and Outcome Measurement

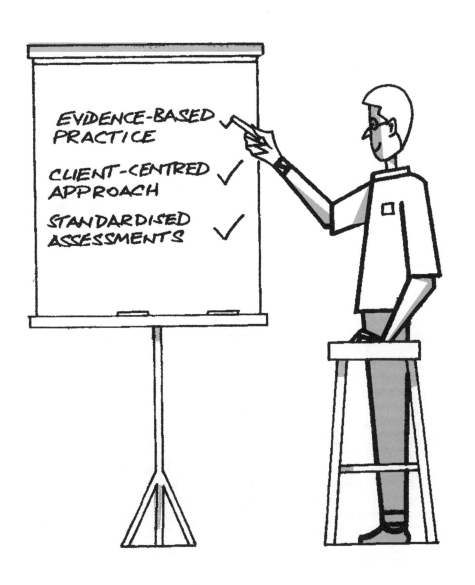

CHAPTER SUMMARY

This chapter focuses on the requirement of therapists to undertake thorough and accurate assessment and measurement. The chapter will describe some developments and policy directions in health and social care practice that have affected occupational therapy and physiotherapy assessment, including:

- a demand for evidence-based practice
- a shift towards the use of standardised assessments
- a requirement to measure outcomes and demonstrate effectiveness
- a focus on client-centred practice
- a demand for robust clinical governance and clinical audit activities
- the use of standards, care pathways, protocols and guidelines.

It also examines the impact of such developments on physiotherapy and occupational therapy assessment, for example the emphasis on demonstrating that intervention is effective leads to a need for reliable, valid and sensitive outcome measures that enable therapists to measure clinically relevant change. In light of a call for standardised measurement, the chapter will discuss some of the advantages and limitations of standardised versus non-standardised tests. This introductory chapter will also explore the complexity of assessment, including the challenges of measuring human behaviour and the impact of the environment, and reflect upon how such complexities influence what can be measured by therapists and the adequacy of these measurements. The chapter concludes by presenting a series of questions about assessment and measurement, which will then be addressed in detail in the following chapters.

ASSESSMENT AS A CORE PART OF THE THERAPY PROCESS

Assessment was defined in the Introduction as the overall process of selecting and using multiple data-collection tools and various sources of information to inform decisions required for guiding therapeutic intervention during the whole therapy process. Assessment involves interpreting information collected to make clinical decisions related to the needs of the person and the appropriateness and nature of their therapy. Assessment involves the evaluation of the outcomes of therapeutic interventions.

Assessment is a core component of health care and therapy processes. It is recognised by health care professionals that assessment is an essential part of a quality service, for example the Royal College of Physicians (RCP; 2002) states that 'assessment is central to the management of any disability'. Assessment is embedded as an essential component of the health care process. The health care process can be simply described as the (Austin and Clark, 1993):

- needs analysis of the client
- identification of what service needs to be provided
- identification of the provider of the service
- provision of the service
- evaluation of the service provided.

Assessment is the first step in the health care process and provides the foundation for effective treatment. Assessment occurs again at the end of the health care process in the form of evaluation. It is also necessary to undertake a re-assessment at several stages during stage four of the process, service provision, because without thorough and accurate assessment the intervention selected may prove inappropriate and/or ineffective.

THE IMPACT OF HEALTH AND SOCIAL CARE POLICY ON ASSESSMENT PRACTICE

The organisational and policy context for health and social care has been under frequent change and reform, particularly over the last decade. In recent years, the provision of health and social care has been exposed to a more market-orientated approach in which government fund-holders and organisations who purchase therapy services have become more concerned about value for money and require assurances that the service provided is both clinically effective and cost-effective. The demand for cost-effective health care is forcing rehabilitation professionals to be able to prove the efficacy and efficiency of their interventions. In the current policy context that focuses on quality, national standards, best value and evidence-based practice (EBP), the ability to demonstrate service outcomes has become increasingly important; for example, the Department of Health (DoH; 1998a) states that the modernisation of care 'moves the focus away from who provides the care, and places it firmly on the quality of services experienced by, and the outcomes achieved for, individuals and their carers and families' (paragraph 1.7).

An emphasis on clinical governance means that therapists are more overtly responsible for the quality of their practice, and this is reflected in an increased interest in EBP. Sheelagh Richards, Secretary of the College of Occupational Therapists (COT), states:

> Now critical appraisal, reflective practice, systematic audit, peer review, best value review, service evaluation, clinical governance and a host of other methodologies are accepted parts of the professional's landscape. The need to deliver evidence-based practice is well understood and all professionals have to play their part in the 'total quality management' of service delivery. (Richards, 2002, p. xvii)

The Chartered Society of Physiotherapy (CSP; 2001a) also highlights these changes to its members and recognises that therapists, and all health care practitioners, are being put under increasing 'pressure to demonstrate the added value of the service they provide' (p. 2). The CSP appreciates that the clinical governance agenda has led to an increased demand for results and proven outcomes and that this helps to inform required service improvements. In order to meet these demands, physiotherapists are being encouraged to learn about measurement and to adopt appropriate outcome measures in their daily practice. This has been made explicit through the introduction of the use of outcome measures into the CSP's revised standards of practice (Chartered Society of Physiotherapy, 2000), and this is helping to raise the profile of outcome measurement within the physiotherapy profession. For occupational therapists, the COT on its website states:

> Every individual providing an occupational therapy service has a responsibility to maintain and improve effectiveness and efficiency through the use of outcomes measures and audit. Occupational therapists should employ a range of quality activities including: evidence-based practice, adherence to national and professional standards and guidelines, risk-management, continuing professional development and listening to the views of those who use the service. (http://www.cot.org.uk/members/ profpractice/quality/intro.php, accessed 4.12.05)

In a paper on the use of standardised assessments by physiotherapists, Stokes and O'Neill (1999) state that 'clinical effectiveness, evidence-based practice, outcome measures and clinical audit are the "buzz words" of today's researcher and practitioner. They are the markers of an aspiration for accountability, productivity and objectivity within the provision of health care' (p. 560). This continues to be true today.

Therapists need to be aware of the reasons that drive their practice. It is only reasonable to be influenced by financial and political drivers when the resultant change in practice yields true benefits for clients. Unsworth (2000) notes: 'current pressures to document outcomes and demonstrate the efficacy of occupational therapy intervention arise from fiscal restraints as much as from the humanitarian desire to provide the best quality health care to consumers. However, measuring outcomes is important in facilitating mutual goal setting, increasing the focus of therapy on the client, monitoring client progress, as well as demonstrating that therapy is valuable' (p. 147).

THE DEMAND FOR EVIDENCE-BASED PRACTICE

The World Confederation of Physical Therapy (WCPT), which was founded in 1951 to represent physical therapists internationally, 'champions the principle that every individual is entitled to the highest possible standard of culturally-appropriate health care provided in an atmosphere of trust and respect for human dignity and underpinned by sound clinical reasoning and scientific evidence' (World Confederation for Physical Therapy, 2006a). In its description of physical therapy the WCPT lists 'principles' supporting the description of physical therapy, and these include emphasising 'the need for practice to be evidence based whenever possible' (http://www.fisionline.org/WCPT.html#Iniziale2, accessed 27.10.05). The CSP, in the effective practice section of its website, begins by telling therapists that 'whatever your occupational role – clinical physiotherapist, assistant, manager, researcher, educator or student – you need to use the best available evidence to inform your practice' (http://www.csp.org.uk/director/effectivepractice.cfm, accessed 27.11.05). While the COT states that 'occupational therapists should be delivering effective practice that is evidence-based where possible' (College of Occupational Therapists, 2005c, p. 1).

SO WHAT IS EVIDENCE-BASED MEDICINE?

Therapists should explicitly be working towards achieving EBP in all areas of their practice. EBP has developed from work on evidence-based medicine (EBM), and expands the concept of EBM to apply across all health care professionals. *EBM* has been defined as:

> the conscientious, explicit, and judicious use of current best evidence in making decisions about the care of individual patients. The practice of evidence based medicine means integrating individual clinical expertise with the best available external clinical evidence from systematic research. (Sackett *et al.*, 1996, p. 71)

Sackett and his colleagues further describe individual clinical expertise as the 'proficiency and judgment that individual clinicians acquire through clinical experience and clinical practice' (p. 71). They state that a clinician's increasing expertise can be demonstrated in a number of ways 'especially in more effective and efficient diagnosis and in the more thoughtful identification and compassionate use of individual patients' predicaments, rights, and preferences in making clinical decisions about their care' (p. 71). Belsey and Snell (2003) have written a useful fact sheet, *What is evidence-based medicine?*, which can be downloaded as a free pdf file from the EBM website at: www.evidence-based-medicine.co.uk/ebmfiles/whatisebm.pdf (accessed, 15.12.05). Belsey and Snell describe EBM as a 'multifaceted process of assuring clinical effectiveness' (p. 1) and describe four main elements:

- 'Production of evidence through research and scientific review.
- Production and dissemination of evidence-based clinical guidelines.
- Implementation of evidence-based, cost-effective practice through education and management of change.
- Evaluation of compliance with agreed practice guidance and patient outcomes – this process includes clinical audit.'

SO WHAT IS EVIDENCE-BASED PRACTICE?

The College of Occupational Therapists Research and Development Group has defined EBP as the explicit use of the best evidence of clinical and cost-effectiveness when working with a particular client. It combines clinical reasoning, existing research and client choice (Research and Development Group, 1997). 'Evidence-based practice encourages the integration of high quality quantitative and qualitative research, with the clinician's clinical expertise and the client's background, preferences and values. It involves the client in making informed decisions and should build on, not replace, clinical judgement and experience' (OTseeker, 2005).

To identify the best available external clinical evidence, clinicians need to seek clinically relevant research, and therapists should particularly seek client-centred clinical research into the accuracy and precision of standardised tests and the efficacy of therapeutic interventions. When new evidence is acknowledged, it sometimes can invalidate previously accepted tests and treatments, and therapists are beholden to replace old unsubstantiated practices with evidence-based practices that are more effective, more accurate, more efficacious and safer (Sackett *et al.*, 1996).

The WCPT provides a two-page overview on EBP for physiotherapists (World Confederation for Physical Therapy, 2003). This document equally applies to occupational therapists and is a good starting point. Like EBM, EBP is achieved through the integration of three factors, which are:

- the best available research
- clinical experience
- client's beliefs and values.

This means that EBP 'requires a combination of art and science' (p. 2). The WCPT describes the rationale for EBP and asserts that undertaking EBP helps therapists to:

- 'improve the care of patients, carers and communities
- reduce variations in practice
- use evidence from high quality research to inform practice, balancing known benefits and risks
- challenge views based on beliefs rather than evidence
- make decision making more transparent
- integrate patient preferences into decision-making
- ensure that knowledge continues to inform practice through life-long learning' (World Confederation for Physical Therapy, 2003, p. 1).

IMPLEMENTATION OF EVIDENCE-BASED PRACTICE

In busy clinical settings, implementing EBP may be difficult. There are many potential barriers to the full implementation of EBP, including lack of time, lack of access to literature and lack of skills in finding and interpreting research. Some of the strategies that have been suggested (OTseeker, 2005) for supporting EBP in clinical environments include:

- fostering a supportive environment in the workplace for EBP
- providing continuing education to develop skills in literature searching, critical appraisal and research methods
- collaborating/participating in research evaluating therapy interventions
- participating in or establishing a journal club
- focusing on reading research articles that have a rigorous study design or reviews that have been critically appraised
- seeking out evidence-based clinical guidelines.

In order to use evidence, it is necessary to undertake a number of tasks.

- Search for and locate the evidence related to a specific clinical question.
- Appraise the evidence collected.
- Store and retrieve the evidence when required.
- Ensure the body of evidence used to inform clinical decisions is kept updated.
- Communicate the findings from the evidence and use these findings in clinical practice.
  (Belsey and Snell, 2003)

SO HOW DO YOU TRACK DOWN THE BEST EVIDENCE?

The COT has published a guide on finding and using evidence bases (Mountain and Lepley, 1998) that provides a useful starting point for therapists.

THE COCHRANE LIBRARY

In terms of databases, a good place to start is the Cochrane Library, which provides a collection of separate databases. Five of these provide coverage of EBM, and the other two provide information on research methodology. The databases are:

- the Cochrane Database of Systematic Reviews
- the Database of Abstracts of Reviews of Effectiveness (DARE)
- the Cochrane Controlled Trials Register
- the Cochrane Database of Methodology Reviews
- the Cochrane Methodology Register
- the Health Technology Assessment Database
- the NHS Economic Evaluation Database.

DARE includes structured abstracts of systematic reviews that have been critically appraised by reviewers at the NHS Centre for Reviews and Dissemination in York and by other people, for example from the American College of Physicians' Journal Club and the journal *Evidence-Based Medicine*.

THE SCOTTISH INTERCOLLEGIATE GUIDELINES NETWORK (SIGN)

The SIGN has published over 80 clinical guidelines, some of which are of relevance to occupational therapists and/or physiotherapists. These can be accessed at: http://www.sign. ac.uk/ (accessed 10.12.05). For example, the guideline for the prevention and management of hip fracture on older people, 'Section 9: rehabilitation and discharge' states:

> 9.1 Early assessment: Early assessment by medical and nursing staff, physiotherapist and occupational therapist to formulate appropriate preliminary rehabilitation plans has been shown to facilitate rehabilitation and discharge. *Evidence level 2+.* (http://www.sign.ac.uk/guidelines/fulltext/56/section9.html, accessed 10.12.05)

The role of the physiotherapist and occupational therapist is also indicated in Section 9.22: 'multidisciplinary rehabilitation', which states:

> Multidisciplinary team working is generally considered to be effective in the delivery of hip fracture rehabilitation. The professions, grades and interrelationships of members of the 'multidisciplinary team' vary between studies and, because these characteristics are rarely described in detail, the effectiveness of different approaches

to team working is not yet well understood. Rehabilitation should be commenced early to promote independent mobility and function. The initial emphasis should be on walking and activities of daily living (ADL) e.g. transferring, washing, dressing, and toileting. Balance and gait are essential components of mobility and are useful predictors in the assessment of functional independence. *Evidence level 2++*. (http://www.sign.ac.uk/guidelines/fulltext/56/section9.html, accessed 10.12.05)

OCCUPATIONAL THERAPY SYSTEMATIC EVALUATION OF EVIDENCE (OTseeker)

OTseeker is a database that contains abstracts of systematic reviews and randomised controlled trials relevant to occupational therapy. It provides therapists with easy access to trials from a wide range of sources. The trials included have been critically appraised and rated to assist therapists to evaluate their validity and interpretability. These ratings will help therapists to judge the quality and usefulness of trials for informing their clinical interventions (http://www.otseeker.com/, accessed 26.10.05).

PHYSIOTHERAPY EVIDENCE DATABASE (PEDro)

PEDro is an initiative of the Centre for Evidence-Based Physiotherapy (CEBP). It has been developed to give rapid access to bibliographic details and abstracts of randomised controlled trials, systematic reviews and evidence-based clinical practice guidelines in physiotherapy. Most trials on the database have been rated for quality to help therapists quickly discriminate between trials that are likely to be valid and interpretable and those that are not. The PEDro site has been supported by a number of organisations, including the Australian Physiotherapy Association, the School of Physiotherapy at the University of Sydney, the Cochrane Collaboration and New South Wales' Department of Health. The site can be found at: http://www.pedro.fhs.usyd.edu.au/index.html (accessed 26.10.05). It also contains two useful tutorials:

- Part I: Are the findings of this trial likely to be valid?
- Part II: Is the therapy clinically useful?

Do not forget that a significant amount of therapy research still remains unpublished but may be accessible, for example the COT's library holds a significant number of occupational therapy PhD and Master's theses and offers a loan service. Carr (1999) examines this collection in her publication *Thesis Collection: The National Collection of Unpublished Occupational Therapy Research*.

LEVELS OF EVIDENCE AND GRADES OF RECOMMENDATIONS

When examining and reporting on evidence, researchers and clinicians apply a grading system, for example the system proposed by Muir Gray (2001):

- Level I: systematic review of multiple well-designed randomised controlled trials (RCTs); the term meta-analysis is used to describe quantitative approaches to synthesising evidence from multiple RCTs
- Level II: one properly designed RCT of appropriate size
- Level III: well-designed trials without randomisation single group pre- and post-cohort, time series or matched control studies
- Level IV: well-designed non-experimental studies from more than one centre or research group
- Level V: opinions of respected authorities, based on clinical evidence, descriptive studies or reports of expert committees

Muir Gray's system has been used in a number of therapy guidelines, such as those produced by the National Association of Rheumatology Occupational Therapists (NAROT; 2005).

The key to using the evidence is the ability to critically appraise the evidence and make decisions as to whether the evidence is robust and whether it applies to your clinical situation and should be used to influence your practice. Critical appraisal has been defined as 'a method of assessing and interpreting the evidence by systematically considering its validity, results and relevance to the area of work considered' (Belsey and Snell, 2003, p. 2). Criteria for examining the quality of research studies in order to assess the evidence are provided by the SIGN (www.sign.ac.uk, accessed 10.12.05) and are:

- clear aim stated
- appropriate sampling strategy applied
- valid and reliable measurement tools used
- adequate literature review provided
- all participants accounted for adequately
- statistical methods described fully and were appropriate
- statistical significance assessed
- outcomes clearly stated
- population similar to the clinical group of interest
- bias addressed.

Assessment is complex, and the therapist needs to take many inter-relating factors into consideration. Therefore, assessment requires careful planning and conscious decision-making in order to select the optimum assessment strategy for a particular client's needs. No one assessment strategy will be suitable for all people with a particular diagnosis; so the therapist needs to combine the best evidence with a client-centred approach. Now we have explored what EBP is, you can reflect upon your own assessment practice, or the assessment approaches you have observed while on clinical placement if you are a student. To assist you with reflecting on how much your practice is based on evidence, please turn to Worksheet 1: Evidence-based practice, which you will find towards the end of this book (page 396).

THE APPLICATION OF STANDARDISED ASSESSMENTS

Standardisation is defined by the American Occupational Therapy Association (AOTA) as:

> made standard or uniform; to be used without variation; suggests an invariable way in which a test is to be used, as well as denoting the extent to which the results of the test may be considered to be both valid and reliable. (Hopkins and Smith, 1993b, p. 914)

Standardised test/measure/assessment/instrument is defined as a:

> published measurement tool, designed for a specific purpose in a given population, with detailed instructions provided as to when and how it is to be administered and scored, interpretation of the scores, and results of investigations or reliability and validity. (Cole *et al.*, 1995, p. 22)

A standardised assessment 'has a set, unchanging procedure' (College of Occupational Therapists, 2005c, p. 1) that the therapist must follow precisely when administering it, and standardised assessments also require 'a consistent system for scoring' (p. 1). The use of standardised assessments helps to 'ensure minimal variation in the way [tests are] carried out at different times and by different testers' (p. 1). Reducing the amount of variation in test administration helps to make a test more reliable when it is applied over time or used by different therapists. Test scores need to be stable over time and across therapist testers if the results are to be used to measure clinical change in order to evaluate therapy outcomes. (For more details about standardisation see Chapter 5.)

The last decade has seen considerable changes in physiotherapy and occupational therapy assessment practice. For example, historically, therapists have favoured the use of non-standardised assessments, particularly informal interview and unstructured observation (for example of movements, posture and the performance of ADL). Therapists have adapted existing standardised tests to suit their clinical environment (for example see Shanahan, 1992). There has been a trend towards the development of assessments on an individual department or service basis. This has the advantage that the assessment process can be tailored to the particular client group and to the practice environment. However, a major limitation is that majority assessments 'home grown' in individual physiotherapy and occupational therapy departments are not rigorously standardised, nor are they backed by research that examines their reliability and validity.

In the current environment of EBP, therapists are being encouraged to utilise more standardised assessments in their practice in order to ensure that their assessments are as valid and reliable as possible and to enable the measurement of treatment outcomes. Previously, many of the standardised tests that therapists adopted were not developed by occupational therapists or physiotherapists and were borrowed from other fields, such as experimental and clinical psychology (for example see McFayden and Pratt, 1997). A disadvantage of this practice of borrowing tests from other disciplines was that the tests did not always fit well with therapists' philosophies and practices, and the use of standardised tests was often rejected because they lacked good clinical utility and face validity (see Chapter 6). As a result, there was a need for therapists to develop valid, reliable, sensitive and clinically useful assessments of people's functional performance (Fisher and Short-DeGraff, 1993). The last decade has seen developments in both physiotherapy and occupational therapy research that has led to an increase in the number of standardised assessments that have been developed by therapists. Clinicians now have a much wider choice of suitable standardised assessments from which to select appropriate measures for their client group.

In the past, therapists have tended to undertake a formal assessment on referral and then informally monitor the person's progress during treatment. With the emphasis on EBP, it is no longer sufficient for therapists to undertake one assessment to provide a baseline from which to plan treatment; ongoing evaluative assessment also is required to monitor the effectiveness of intervention in a reliable and sensitive manner.

THE USE OF STANDARDISED VERSUS NON-STANDARDISED ASSESSMENTS

In the past, each therapist or institution often took responsibility for developing their own assessment tasks and protocols. Assessment was subjective and decentralised and 'the norms against which the patient's performance was judged were based upon the therapist's testing and treatment experiences with previous patients' (Borg and Bruce, 1991, p. 541). As the therapy professions developed and strived to build a more scientific foundation for practice, there was an identified need for assessment processes to become standardised, evidence-based and more centralised. However, even today a significant proportion of therapists continue to adopt predominately non-standardised forms of assessment. Several authors (for example Eakin, 1989a; McAvoy, 1991) have discussed the trend for therapists to continually re-invent the wheel in terms of the assessment tools they use. This is exemplified by the numerous home-grown checklists that litter our practice and the tendency to 'adaptation syndrome', whereby the standardised assessments that are used are altered almost at whim. There are a number of reasons why therapists continue to use non-standardised assessments. For example, therapists have reported the following reasons (Chia, 1996; Laver, 1994):

- a lack of appropriate standardised assessments
- poor resources limit their ability to purchase standardised measures
- standardised assessments can be lengthy to administer and therapists report they do not have the time or that the length makes the test too tiring for clients
- non-standardised assessments are flexible in terms of procedures, settings and the manner in which the assessment is administered and are, therefore, perceived as being more client-centred
- non-standardised assessments are seen as useful for observing functional ability in the person's home environment, for addressing the qualitative aspects of performance and for exploring the dynamics between the client and carer.

Tallis (1998, cited in Stokes and O'Neill, 1999) discusses the reasons why measurement was not being undertaken by rehabilitation therapists; these included: 'misplaced confidence; misinterpretation of negative findings; the length of time taken to use the measurement; ideological hostility, i.e. the perceived disparity between measurement and assessment; the difficulty identifying true change (signal to noise ratio); and the pitfalls of communicating assessment findings' (Stokes and O'Neill, 1999, p. 560).

Neale (2004) writes about why she has difficulty with standardised assessments and outcome measures. First, she reports that, in her work setting comprising a rehabilitation ward and stroke unit, her team 'use the Barthel ADL Index . . . which is completed at the weekly multi-disciplinary meeting . . . but it is not sensitive to the changes we see in patients during rehabilitation . . . the person can have the same score but still be showing marked improvement. We bemoan the Barthel, but the same difficulty arises with the other ADL assessments' (Neale, 2004, pp. 25–26). Second, she comments on the issue of time: 'using a test takes up at least one treatment session to administer and more time to evaluate' (p. 25).

However, she also provides an example of how the use of a standardised assessment helped to identify a previously undiagnosed deficit.

> I have acquired various standardised assessments for the department over the years. I do not use any with every patient. I learnt early that this may mean I miss things – when I first had the Balloons Test [Edgeworth, Robertson and McMillan, 1998], I practised on one 'well recovering' stroke patient. Neither she nor I had noticed any indication of inattention in hospital. The test showed she missed the bottom left quadrant – and she subsequently reported the effects when serving food/covering a pie when at home. (Neale, 2004, p. 25)

Standardised tests can help to confirm hypotheses or suspicions about underlying deficits indicated by the person's performance on unstandardised tasks: 'We have the Rivermead Perceptual Assessment Battery [Whiting *et al.*, 1985] and I tend to use a shortened form [Lincoln and Edmans, 1989]. This is usually to confirm a suspicion I have formed during a functional activity, as it feels useful to have these suspicions confirmed' (Neale, 2004, p. 25).

Another common practice is to take different parts of standardised tests or individual test items and integrate these into a therapist-constructed, tailored assessment battery for a specific client group or service (Chia, 1996). However, once the standard procedure for test administration and scoring has been changed, even in a small way, the reliability and validity of that part of the test or test item can no longer be guaranteed. Therefore, although the test items might have been generated from a standardised test the ensuing therapist-made assessment cannot be viewed as being standardised. A further limitation of this practice, of using test items/parts drawn from standardised tests, is that the original source of, or reference for, the test item is rarely recorded on the tailored assessment and forms. This means that, once the therapists involved in developing the tailored assessment leave the service, the therapists who replace them are unaware of the original sources and the rationale for the development of the tailored therapist-constructed assessment battery. Consequently, therapists using inherited therapist-constructed assessments can find it difficult to justify the reasons for carrying out these non-standardised assessments (Chia, 1996).

If therapists are to use non-standardised assessments, it is critical that they are fully aware of their limitations. The findings from a non-standardised assessment are open to interpretation and are, therefore, much more subjective than the findings gained from a standardised measure. Furthermore, because detailed procedures for administering and scoring the test are rarely available for non-standardised assessments, it is not possible for the therapist to reliably repeat the assessment with the client in order to evaluate the effects of treatment. It is even more unreliable if another therapist tries to repeat the assessment with the same client at a later date.

Therapists should not underestimate the consequences of continuing to use non-standardised assessments where standardised measures of the same construct or area of function exist. This has been demonstrated in a study by Stewart (1999). Stewart compared the results of a non-standardised assessment with a standardised measure of severity of disability in a group of elderly people. The purpose of her study was to examine if there were differences in outcomes and explore the consequences for service entitlement. The results of the study indicated that the non-standardised measure had 'restricted ability to identify and measure accurately the degree of disability of older people' and 'that because of the limited psychometric rigour of the [non-standardised measure] one consequence for service provision may be that a vulnerable group, elderly frail people, are denied services unnecessarily' (p. 422). Stewart concludes that 'when clinical judgement is based on objective assessment arising from the use of standardised instruments rather than intuitive guesswork, occupational therapists' decision making can be seen to be more rational and consequently defensible' (p. 422).

BENEFITS OF APPLYING STANDARDISED MEASURES

The use of improved, appropriate, sensitive and standardised measures within occupational therapy and physiotherapy research and clinical practice would aid these professions at several different levels (Stokes and O'Neill, 1999).

- Health care policy level: in a wide sense, the principles of current health care (clinical governance, EBP, demonstrable effectiveness) demand accountability and quality of service; funding for services is becoming increasingly linked to evidence of effectiveness and efficiency.
- Perception of the professions of occupational therapy and physiotherapy: it is essential that therapists present their assessment data, interventions and outcome data in a format that educates other professionals, clients and lay persons about the unique roles that occupational therapists and physiotherapists have in the interdisciplinary team.
- Research/theory–practice gap within the professions: both physiotherapy and occupational therapy continue to experience a gap between theory and related research and what is actually occurring in clinical practice.
- Standardised assessments and outcome measures: these are used in research and results are disseminated in professional literature; however, the findings of these studies may be incorporated into clinical practice more easily if similar scales are already in use in practice and therapists are comfortable with implementing different standardised tools.
- Clinical research endeavours: a vast majority of therapy research involves small sample sizes and research undertaken at a single site or in non-practice settings (for example simulated environments within university programmes); if outcomes measures were a routine aspect of therapy, then clinically based research and multicentre trials would be much easier to undertake.

- Therapist level: the use of standardised measures can improve communication among practitioners, foster consistency and reaffirm knowledge and skill (Lewis and Bottomley, 1994).
- Client level: the client receives an improved service in which assessment and outcome data are based on reliable, valid and sensitive measures.

In conclusion, many non-standardised, therapist-constructed assessments continue to be used in practice and have both strengths and limitations. Therapists should be clear as to the theoretical foundations of all their assessment procedures, including both standardised and non-standardised tests. Where components of standardised tests are used in a therapist-constructed assessment battery, therapists should be able to quote the original source and the rationale for the test item's use in the ensuing non-standardised assessment. In cases where non-standardised assessments are used without such theoretical underpinning or rationale, professional credibility and client welfare can be at risk. Inadequate, and even inaccurate, decisions may be made from non-standardised assessments that can have negative consequences for both individual client care and, where the effectiveness of physiotherapy and occupational therapy intervention cannot be reliably demonstrated, for the service provision as a whole.

THE REQUIREMENT TO DEMONSTRATE EFFECTIVENESS

SO WHAT DO WE MEAN BY THE TERM *EFFECTIVENESS*?

An effect is the power to produce an outcome or achieve a result. Effectiveness, in a clinical setting, relates to whether or not the anticipated therapeutic outcome is achieved during the therapeutic process. So the effect of therapy is the identifiable outcome that can be recorded at an agreed point (often the end) of the therapeutic process. Clinical effectiveness (also referred to as effective practice) 'is achieved when an action, intervention or system does what it is intended to do' (College of Occupational Therapists, 2005d, p. 1).

Two related, but significantly different, terms are *efficacy* and *efficiency*. These are also important for therapists to consider and are defined briefly, along with some other terms related to effectiveness and outcome measurement, in Table 1.1 (below).

WHY DO WE NEED TO DEMONSTRATE EFFECTIVENESS?

'All professions that hope to advance their practices must take three giant leaps forward to achieve their goals. They must first document the status and process of practice, then develop valid standards of practice and always they must test the outcome of their actions on behalf of their clients' (Cole *et al.*, 1995, p. 2). As Cole *et al.* also point out, 'not everything we do in the name of therapy is successful or the final word' (p. 5). We may use practices that have been handed down from generation to generation of therapists because they appear beneficial and we feel they make a difference, but nowadays 'clients should be ensured some appropriate level of outcome measurement' (p. 4) and 'individual therapists must determine what procedures are truly beneficial and directly related to outcomes' (p. 5).

SO HOW DO WE DEMONSTRATE EFFECTIVENESS?

Standardised outcome measures are used to demonstrate whether or not your interventions are effective. Outcome data collected routinely will allow you to form a clearer idea over time about what aspects of your practice are effective and what aspects need to be changed so you can base future treatment on the results of your findings with similar clients. Outcome measurement is undertaken by administering an outcome measure on at least two occasions. This is done to document change over time in the agreed focus of therapy in order to establish whether it has been influenced by the intervention to the anticipated degree and has achieved the desired outcome.

Table 1.1 Definition of terms related to effectiveness and outcome measurement

Term	Definition
Effectiveness	Whether treatments do more good than harm in those to whom they are offered under the usual conditions of care, which may differ from those in the experimental situation. Effectiveness is the measure of the ability of a programme, project or work task to produce a specific desired effect or result that can be measured. Relates to outcomes, not the efficiency of performance (Centre for Advanced Palliative Care, 2005).
Clinical effectiveness	'The degree to which a therapeutic outcome is achieved in real-world patient populations under actual or average condition of treatment provision' (Maniadakis and Gray, 2004, p. 27).
Cost-effectiveness analysis	Is an analysis that 'compares the costs and health effects of an intervention to assess whether it is worth doing from the economic perspective' (Phillips and Thompson, 2003, p. 1). Costs are categorised as: *direct costs* for the service and patient, *service costs*: staff time, equipment, drugs, *patient costs*: transport, out-of-pocket expenses, *indirect costs*: production losses, other uses of time, *intangibles*: e.g. pain, suffering, adverse effects (p. 2).
Efficiency	Measure of production or productivity relative to input resources. Efficiency refers to operating a programme or project, or performing work tasks economically. Relates to resources expended or saved, not the effectiveness of performance.
Efficacy	This involves assessing whether a treatment actually works for those who receive it under ideal conditions and is the province of research. It has been defined as 'the degree to which a therapeutic outcome is achieved in a patient population under rigorously controlled and monitored circumstances, such as controlled clinical trials' (Maniadakis and Gray, 2004, p. 27).
Outcome measure	A standardised instrument used by therapists to establish whether their desired therapeutic outcomes have been achieved.
Outcome measurement	Is the process undertaken to establish the effects of an intervention on an individual or the effectiveness of a service on a defined aspect of the health or well-being of a specified population.
Performance measure	Generic term used to describe a particular value or characteristic designated to measure input, output, outcome, efficiency or effectiveness. Performance measures are composed of a number and a unit of measure. The number provides the magnitude (how much) and the unit is what gives the number its meaning (what) (Centre for Advanced Palliative Care, 2005).
Performance measurement	A management tool for enhancing decision-making and accountability. Performance measurement as a strategic process is used to assess accomplishment of organisational strategic goals and objectives (Centre for Advanced Palliative Care, 2005).

Cole *et al.* (1995) identify three basic standards for users of outcome measures, these are:

- 'selecting the appropriate measure for a given population based on scientific evidence
- administering the measure according to the developer's procedure
- interpreting the results consistent with evidence of reliability and validity, and comparison to empirically derived norms of comparison group' (p. 171).

(For more information see Chapter 3 and Chapter 8 of this book.)

A FOCUS ON CLIENT-CENTRED PRACTICE

The World Health Organization (WHO; 2002) emphasises that all health professionals should pay attention to insider perspectives of people with disability. In recent years, policy in the UK has had a greater focus on the client being given adequate information to make an informed choice about his health and/or social care. Health and social care professionals are mandated to listen to the needs of the client and respond to these identified needs as an integral part of any care package or therapeutic process (Clouston, 2003). A series of National Service Frameworks (NSFs) have been drawn up by the Department of Health (DoH) that put an emphasis on placing the client and his family at the centre of the health care process, and not just as a service recipient.

The COT (College of Occupational Therapists, 2003a) describes the 'principles of client-centred practice' as including:

- 'respecting diversity
- recognising the client has rights
- clarifying role expectations within the therapeutic encounter
- building collaborative therapist–client relationships
- focusing on the client's needs, problems and priorities
- negotiating problems and goals with the client and/or carer
- incorporating the client's perspective at all stages of intervention
- sharing power and decision making with the client and/or carer
- promoting client autonomy and choice through providing information
- ensuring that interventions are congruent with the client's life world and context' (p. 30).

Applying these principles means that the therapeutic intervention, while it may be influenced by guidelines, protocols or standards, is not the same for each client with the same diagnosis. Therapists now have to consistently use self-report and proxy assessment methods to seek information about the wishes, needs, priorities, problems and goals of the client (and where appropriate the carer). Therapists have to analyse traditional observational assessment data in the light of self-report and proxy data and then negotiate the desired outcomes and therapeutic approach with the person. Therapists have needed to develop client-centred outcome measures to capture self-report data reliably and provide robust evaluative measures of the client's and carer's perceptions and experience of the therapeutic outcome. (For more information see Chapter 2.)

THE DEMAND FOR ROBUST CLINICAL GOVERNANCE

'Clinical governance is a system for improving the standard of clinical practice' (Starey, 2003, p. 1). *Clinical governance* was first described by the DoH in the White Paper *The New NHS: Modern, Dependable* (1998b) in which it was described as a system to ensure that clinical standards were met and that processes were in place to ensure continuous improvement in service delivery. The DoH has since defined clinical governance as a framework 'through which NHS organisations are accountable for continuously improving the quality of their services and safeguarding high standards of care, by creating an environment in which clinical excellence will flourish' (Department of Health, 2004, p. 29). Clinical governance emphasises the responsibility that health organisations and their staff have to monitor the quality of their services and to continually work towards modernisation and improvement. Similar responsibilities are held by social care organisations and their staff, as outlined in Department of Health (1998a); this document outlines three main priorities: promoting independence, improving protection and raising standards. An aspect of this is *best value*, which means that staff have to provide their services based on clear standards related to both the quality and the cost of the service and that services have to be delivered in the most effective, economic and efficient way.

The COT summarises the 'core elements' of clinical governance as including:

- continued professional development and professional performance management
- implementation and monitoring of national standards
- research and development
- evidence-based practice including clinical and cost-effectiveness
- clinical audit
- risk management including critical incident reporting and complaints procedures
- learning from experience
- clear lines of responsibility and accountability
- team working
- participation in national 'confidential inquiries'
- appropriate safeguards to govern access and storage of confidential service user information (College of Occupational Therapists, 2005e, pp. 1–2).

For more information see the DoH's website (http://www.dh.gov.uk), and also the Clinical Governance Assessment Toolkit (CGAT), which has been produced by the NHS Information Authority (2003). The Health and Social Care Information Centre is a special health authority that became a statutory body on 1 April 2005. The authority took on some of the information related to functions of the former NHS Information Authority and some statistics and information management functions of the DoH, including social care. Its website can be accessed at: http://www.icservices.nhs.uk/servicecat/services.asp. Within this website is a useful section on clinical governance information. This part of the website defines who is likely to ask health and social care organisations for clinical governance information and describes the reporting arrangements in place. Links to all relevant information are held in one place, making it easier for therapists and managers of therapy services to find out what is relevant to their organisation. This part of the website can be accessed at: http://www.icservices.nhs.uk/clinicalgovernance.

CLINICAL AUDIT

Clinical audit has been defined as:

> a quality improvement process that seeks to improve patient care and outcomes through a systematic review of care against explicit criteria and the implementation of change. Aspects of the structure, processes, and outcomes of care are selected and systematically evaluated against specific criteria. Where indicated, changes are implemented at an individual, team, or service level and further monitoring is used to confirm improvement in healthcare delivery. (Department of Health, 2004, p. 29)

Audit is the 'systematic and critical analysis of the quality of clinical care including diagnostic and treatment procedures, associated use of resources, outcomes and quality of life for clients' (College of Occupational Therapists, 2003a, p. 50). Audit is a quality process that compares actual performance in a specific setting against agreed standards of practice (Research and Development Group, 1997). For more information, the COT publishes the useful *Clinical Audit Information Pack* (Sealey, 1998).

THE USE OF STANDARDS, PROTOCOLS, GUIDELINES AND CARE PATHWAYS

What is the difference between a standard, a guideline and a protocol? These three terms are defined briefly, along with some other relevant terms, in Table 1.2 (below).

Guidelines, protocols and standards all provide explicit statements of expected practice performance (Bury and Mead, 1998).

Table 1.2 Definitions related to standards, protocols and guidelines

Term	Definition
Care pathway	Is 'a pathway for a specific user group which determines locally agreed, multidisciplinary health practice and is based on the available guidelines and evidence' (Department of Health, 2004, p. 29).
Standards	Are a basis for measurement. They provide a definite level of excellence. The Centre for Advanced Palliative Care (2005) defines a standard as an established measurable condition or state used as a basis for comparison for quality and quantity.
Protocols	Are plans of care for clients presenting with similar conditions, diagnoses or problems. The DoH (2001a) defines a protocol as 'a plan detailing the steps that will be taken in the care or treatment of an individual' (p. 158).
Guidelines	*Clinical* guidelines are systematically developed statements that assist clinicians and clients in making decisions about appropriate treatments for specific conditions (NHS Executive, 1996). *Preferred practice* guidelines provide the recommended approach to guide the provision of care related to a particular issue. They must be flexible to take into account the exceptions/variations needed to meet the wide range of client/family expectations and needs. Guidelines may be consensus- or evidence-based. (Centre for Advanced Palliative Care, 2005).
Care management	The DoH (2001a) defines this as 'a process whereby an individual's needs are assessed and evaluated, eligibility for service is determined, care plans are drafted and implemented, and needs are monitored and reassessed' (p. 152).
Care planning	Is 'a process based on an assessment of an individual's assessed need that involves determining the level and type of support to meet those needs, and the objectives and potential outcomes that can be achieved' (Department of Health, 2001a, p. 152).
Care package	Comprises 'a combination of services designed to meet a person's assessed needs' (Department of Health, 2001a, p. 152).

The term *standard* refers to a high level of quality, skill, ability or achievement by which someone is judged. Sykes (1983) defines it as a 'weight or measure to which others conform or by which the accuracy or quality of others is judged'.

A *guideline* is a systematically developed statement to assist clients' and therapists' decisions about appropriate health care for specific circumstances (Field and Lohr, 1992). Clinical guidelines are based on the best available evidence and provide recommendations for practice about specific clinical interventions for specific client populations.

A *protocol* is a step-by-step outline for undertaking a specific task. They normally have to be followed exactly, whereas with a guideline the recommendations need to be considered in the light of the particular client and setting as well as the strength of the evidence base (http://www.csp.org.uk/director/effectivepractice/standards.cfm, accessed 27.11.05).

CLINICAL PRACTICE GUIDELINES

Clinical practice guidelines form part of the evidence base from which therapists should work. They are written on a clearly defined topic and require a systematic search in order to be based on the best available evidence. The development of clinical practice guidelines involves the collection and review of:

- scientific evidence (literature reviews, meta-analyses, literature synthesis)
- professional opinions (experts)
- practice experience
- cost concerns.

Once this information has been collected, draft guidelines are drawn up and a consensus and refining process is undertaken. This might involve:

- the input of experts
- consensus conferences (usually involving representatives of the full range of stakeholders)
- methods for obtaining official commitment and sign-up from stakeholder organisations to the proposed guidelines
- seeking any additional evidence and adding value judgements.

The output from this process usually would comprise:

- the clinical guidelines being formatted as a written document
- publication and distribution of the guideline to all relevant staff/organisations
- an implementation strategy to ensure that the guidelines lead to changes in practice where required.

CRITERIA FOR ACCEPTABLE GUIDELINES

Reinauer (1998) cites the work of Lohr (1997), who gives the following criteria for judging the quality of guidelines:

- reliability and reproducibility
- scientific validity
- clinical applicability
- clinical flexibility
- clarity
- multidisciplinary approach
- scheduled review
- documentation of procedures, evidence etc.

Many clinical guidelines and statements of good practice highlight the importance of assessment. For example, the *National Clinical Guidelines for Stroke*, which were developed by the Intercollegiate Working Party for Stroke (Royal College of Physicians, 2002, section 4.1) state that:

- clinicians should use assessments or measures appropriate to their needs (i.e. to help make a clinical decision)
- where possible and available, clinicians should use assessments or measures that have been studied in terms of validity (appropriateness for the purpose) and reliability (extent of variability)
- routine assessments should be minimised, and each considered critically
- patients should be reassessed at appropriate intervals.

The CSP refers its members to physiotherapy guidelines found on its website and to the National Institute for Clinical Excellence (NICE) and SIGN (http://www.csp.org.uk/director/effectivepractice.cfm, accessed 27.11.05). Two examples of physiotherapy guidelines are:

- evidence-based clinical guidelines for the diagnosis, assessment and physiotherapy management of shoulder impingement syndrome. These guidelines address the clinical question: 'What is best practice in the physiotherapy diagnosis, assessment and management of shoulder impingement syndrome?'
- clinical guidelines for the physiotherapy management of whiplash-associated disorder (WAD). These clinical guidelines demonstrate how physiotherapy can be effective in

the management of people with whiplash injuries and are a valuable resource for doctors, patients, managers and other professionals.

These guidelines can be accessed from the CSP website (http://www.csp.org.uk/director/ effectivepractice/clinicalguidelines.cfm, accessed 1.12.05).

An example of guidelines for occupational therapy is 'Occupational therapy in the management of inflammatory rheumatic diseases' produced by NAROT and available free to British Association of Occupational Therapists/COT members on the COT website at: http://www. cot.co.uk/members/publications/guidelines/pdf/inflamatory1.pdf (accessed 10.12.05).

The COT (2000) has developed a document for therapists entitled *Producing Clinical Guidelines for Occupational Therapy Practice*. This provides a step-by-step outline description of how to produce, test and apply clinical guidelines to occupational therapy practice. SIGN has developed the 'Guideline developers' handbook', which was last updated in May 2004 and can be accessed online at: http://www.sign.ac.uk/guidelines/fulltext/50/index.html (accessed 1.01.06).

The CSP has published *Standards of Physiotherapy Practice* (SOPP; Chartered Society of Physiotherapy, 2005b). These reflect the achievable standards for the practice of physiotherapy. Thus the SOPP allow therapists to measure their practice and from the results make decisions about how best to improve their practice in their own particular area of work. These standards provide a collection of documents that describe the professional consensus on the practice of physiotherapy for members of the CSP working in any occupational setting. They reflect the collective judgement of the profession at a given point in time. As the practice of physiotherapy is constantly developing, the standards will, by definition, change over time to reflect these developments. The CSP states that SOPP:

- make an important contribution to the excellence and consistency in clinical practice through clinical governance
- reflect all practice areas, settings and specialities
- set the national standards against which individuals and services can compare their performance
- provide audit tools to enable a measurement of compliance with the standards.

The SOPP pack comprises:

- core standards – the responsibility of individual members
- service standards – the responsibility of organisations and practices
- audit tools – tools to measure the implementation of the core standards.

THE COMPLEXITY OF ASSESSMENT

Physiotherapy and occupational therapy assessment involve highly complex skills that combine knowledge, experience, creativity and original thought. From an outsider's viewpoint, physiotherapy and occupational therapy assessment might look easy: an observer may think that it does not require a person to hold a degree in order to watch someone get dressed and to say whether he can do it or not, or to watch someone walk across a room and say whether he has problems with balance. Creek (1996a) discusses the complexity of simple everyday activities, such as making a cup of tea, and explains how the therapeutic use of such activities requires training at degree level. Therapy assessment is actually very multifaceted and intricate. The therapist needs to observe *how* the person performs and specify *where* and *when* he struggles. The therapist then hypothesises the underlying causes for the problems observed and records *how* the person responds to different prompts and cues. It is not enough to know that a person cannot manage a task; the therapist must also understand *why* in order to plan the appropriate treatment. For example, treatment will be very different for a person following a stroke who cannot dress owing to spasticity and reduced sensation in one arm compared to a person unable to dress because of unilateral spatial neglect and body-scheme deficits, although at first glance both the diagnosis and the functional problem may appear similar. The therapist has to use all of the available information and observations to estimate the person's underlying capacity; she then considers her observations and proxy report data about the person's current function and forms hypotheses for any discrepancy between likely capacity and actual functional performance. Then the therapist plans an intervention to support the person to maximise his capacity and reach his full potential. When developing an intervention, the therapist has to predict future outcomes and plan *how* and *when* these outcomes will be measured in order to evaluate the effectiveness of the intervention.

There are several key reasons why physiotherapy and occupational therapy assessment is complex and needs to be multifaceted. These relate to the:

- nature of therapeutic practice
- nature of human occupation and occupational performance
- complexity of measuring human function
- influence of the level of task demand
- impact of familiarity on performance
- influence of environment on performance
- constraints of the practice setting.

These issues will now be explored briefly.

THE NATURE OF THERAPEUTIC PRACTICE

> The evolution of medicine and rehabilitation has been a mixture of science, philosophy, sociology, and intuition. Some of the finest practitioners may be some of the worst scientists. However, they may have an extraordinary intuitive science. Because of this fine mixture, it is difficult to quantify assessments, treatments, and outcomes. Nevertheless, this needs to be done. (Lewis and Bottomley, 1994, p. 139)

Physiotherapists and occupational therapists are focused upon rehabilitation and remediation. The rehabilitation of individuals with disabilities and the remediation of their functional deficits are addressed through therapeutic interventions. Physiotherapy and occupational therapy practice comprise a combination of art and science. Therefore, therapists tend to use both quantitative and qualitative approaches to assessment. Consequently, some aspects of therapy assessment are standardised, specific and meticulous, while other aspects are intuitive, fluid and creative. Therapists have to balance, reconcile and incorporate information from both approaches into the overall assessment process and resulting documentation. The proportion of art and science varies from therapist to therapist and is influenced by the emphasis of their pre-registration education and training, the influence of supervisors, mentors and peers, the nature of their continuing professional development (CPD), the clinical setting in which they work and the type of client group they serve.

Both physiotherapy and occupational therapy are holistic therapies in which the therapist is trying to consider the whole person during the assessment process. Therefore, the domain of concern for a therapy assessment is very broad and covers different levels of function from pathophysiology to societal limitation (see Chapter 9). A therapist considers macro issues, such as the person's environment, family support, roles and values, in addition to undertaking micro-level assessment of very specific areas, such as range of motion and muscle tone.

The therapeutic process is client-centred. This means that each assessment should be individually tailored to the client and should lead to an individualised intervention programme. More frequently, services are developing protocols for people with similar diagnoses or problems, and therapists will use such protocols to guide their choice of assessment tools and interventions for a client group. The therapist needs to gain a clear picture of the individual, which includes his past life, present situation and hopes for the future, and his roles, motivation, locus of control, attitudes towards his condition and towards therapy. The therapist uses this information to understand how the medical diagnosis and prognosis may affect that person's quality of life. As the assessment progresses, and the unique aspects of the person's presentation emerge, the therapist refines the assessment in order to target the specific therapeutic needs and goals of the person.

Therapists work in a wide variety of practice settings; so they need to be able to conduct assessments in a range of environments. This might involve undertaking an assessment in a person's home or workplace, a hospital ward or outpatient clinic, a therapy department, a GP's practice, a school classroom or a nursing home. Therapists do not always have easy access to all the environments of relevance to a client and will use simulated environments for assessment. The accuracy of the simulated environment will have a significant impact on the usefulness of the assessment scores for the prediction of the person's likely functioning in his natural environment (Austin and Clark, 1993). For example, a mobility assessment undertaken on an expanse of level lino flooring in a physiotherapy department may not produce a good predictor of the person's safety when moving on different types of flooring in the cluttered environment of his home.

Physiotherapy and occupational therapy are frequently provided within a multidisciplinary context. Therapists needs to liaise with other professionals and share the assessment process and results obtained for each client and for the client group as a whole. When working in a team, it is important not to have too much overlap, such that the person is asked the same questions by several members of the team; nor should there be any gaps in the assessment, where members of the team assume that another professional has assessed that area. This means that good communication and a clear understanding of the role of each member of the team is critical for an efficient, effective and thorough multidisciplinary assessment. Another factor that complicates assessment in a multidisciplinary setting is that of attempting to evaluate therapy outcomes. How can you be sure that your therapy intervention has led to the observed changes in function, rather than the intervention performed by another team member or combination of interventions working in conjunction? This causes a real problem for therapists: on the one hand we are being encouraged to measure outcomes and demonstrate the effectiveness of our physiotherapy or occupational therapy intervention, but on the other hand, in many instances, we believe that our clients benefit from a multidisciplinary approach and that it would be unethical to withhold another intervention in order to limit potential confounding variables when measuring outcomes. The client's perspective in this has been well described by Sherr Klein (1997) in her book *Slow Dance*, in which she describes her experience after having suffered a stroke:

> After my exalted [physiotherapist] told me I should stop my acupuncture sessions with Bernard, I didn't have much faith in him either. 'If you do so many therapies at once, how can we tell which one is working?' he asked. 'I don't give a damn which one works,' I muttered to myself. 'I just want to get better.' It seemed like typical professional chauvinism. Bernard said no one thing was responsible for my progress; we were a team, all of us, including me. (Sherr Klein, 1997, p. 220)

THE NATURE OF HUMAN OCCUPATION AND OCCUPATIONAL PERFORMANCE

Human behaviour is organised by roles. A *role* is 'a part played or a position held in a social context that fulfils an expected and/or chosen function' (College of Occupational Therapists, 2005a, p. 2), and these roles are fulfilled through the performance of tasks, activities and occupations.

For therapists, *human occupation* means much more than the commonplace understanding of occupation meaning work or productivity (Watson and Fourie, 2004); therapists define occupation more broadly to include 'an activity or group of activities that engages a person in everyday life, has personal meaning and provides structure to time. Occupations are seen by the individual as part of her/his identity, and they can be categorised in terms of self-care, productivity and/or leisure occupations' (College of Occupational Therapists, 2005a, p. 9). An *activity* is 'a task or sequence of tasks performed by an individual or a group that may contribute to an occupation or occupations' (p. 2). While a *task* is defined as 'a self-contained stage in an activity; a definable piece of performance with a completed purpose or product; a constituent part of an activity' (College of Occupational Therapists, 2003a, p. 60).

Box 1.1 Relationship between occupation, activity and task

As an example, a person may have the *occupation* of providing meals for the family.

This occupation will be formed by a number of *activities*, such as planning meals for the week, shopping for ingredients, preparing and cooking meals and packing lunchboxes.

These activities will be formed by a number of *tasks*, such as peeling the vegetables, boiling the vegetables, making gravy, preparing the meat, roasting the meat, dishing up the meal onto plates and laying the table.

Occupational performance occurs during the interaction of the individual with the environment through the selection, planning and carrying out of activities that form occupations and contribute to roles (College of Occupational Therapists, 2005a). Like occupation, for therapists *environment* means much more than the commonplace understanding of environment as our physical surroundings; rather environment is defined as 'the set of circumstances and conditions (e.g. physical, social, cultural) in which a person lives, works and develops, that can shape and be shaped by occupational performance' (College of Occupational Therapists, 2005a, p. 2).

The performance of tasks, activities and occupations can form everyday routines, which are habitual chains of behaviour with a fixed sequence, such as getting up, washed, dressed and eating breakfast. Tasks, activities and occupations also contribute to less frequent life events, such as giving birth to a child, planning a marriage ceremony or achieving a qualification. Human behaviour is also organised in this way to enable some people to achieve exceptional things, such as a mountaineer climbing Everest, an athlete winning a race and becoming an Olympic medallist or a person fighting for their life in a war zone. The ordinary or extraordinary things that people engage in each day are central to the manner in which each person lives their life. There are many factors that influence the occupations, activities and tasks that people choose or feel compelled to do and which support or restrict their occupational performance. These factors include wider environmental factors, such as culture, norms and values and the person's social and physical environment, and personal factors, such as age, gender, personal capacity and the impact of illness and adversity (Watson, 2004). So not only must the therapist decide whether she will assess the person's ability through consideration of occupations and/or activities and/or tasks but also she has to assess the person's environment and evaluate the impact (whether supporting or limiting) of that environment on the person's ability to perform desired and necessary tasks, activities and occupations.

The tasks, activities and occupations we perform shape who we are, what we are, who we become and how we achieve our dreams and aspirations. However, the tasks, activities and occupations we end up doing can also limit our potential and prevent us from achieving our goals and fulfilling our potential. Sometimes this is our choice, but for many people this results from a lack of opportunity. The constraints of their physical and sociocultural environment limit the variety and choice of their occupations (Watson, 2004). As therapists, we obviously need to consider how this affects our clients, but we should also consider how this influences the way in which we achieve our roles as therapists. For example, are we doing tasks and activities that could be delegated to a technician or support worker? Is there an expectation to discharge patients in a set time frame that limits a full and personalised assessment process for each client? Are the financial constraints of our organisation preventing us from purchasing a well-evidenced standardised assessment that we have identified as a valid and reliable outcome measure?

Each person enters therapy with a unique set of past experiences, values, norms and expectations, and these factors contribute to the nature of the therapeutic relationship formed between the client and therapist (Austin and Clark, 1993, p. 22). People come to therapy with a unique set of roles, occupations, activities and tasks. Although there are activities that everyone needs to do in some form or another, such as eating, sleeping, washing, toileting and finding a way to move around (see Maslow, 1943; for use of Maslow's hierarchy by therapists see Lewis and Bottomley, 1994, pp. 70–71), a large percentage of our activities are culturally and personally determined. This means that therapists need to tailor their assessments to individual clients' needs and cannot develop a standard process for assessment that can be applied in its entirety to every single client.

THE COMPLEXITY OF MEASURING HUMAN FUNCTION

For therapists, *function* is defined as the ability to perform tasks, activities and/or occupations to expected levels of competency. *Dysfunction* occurs when a person cannot perform tasks, activities and/or occupations to these normal standards of proficiency. Function is achieved through the interaction of performance components. These are subsystems within the individual, such as the motor system, the sensory system or the cognitive and perceptual systems. As the interaction between the motor, sensory, perceptual and cognitive systems is complex, the definition of each system implicitly refers to the functioning of other systems. For example, Allport (1955) defines *perception* as relating to our awareness of the objects or conditions about us and the impression objects make upon our senses. Perception relates to the way things look or the way they sound, feel, taste or smell. Perception involves, to some degree, an understanding awareness, a *meaning* or a *recognition* of objects and the awareness of complex environmental situations as well as single objects. This definition implicitly refers to both the sensory and cognitive systems, that is before an awareness of objects and conditions is registered sensory stimuli have been received from the environment and transmitted by the visual, auditory, gustatory, olfactory and/or somatic sensory systems to the brain, and the cognitive system is involved with accessing information, stored in the memory, required to recognise stimuli in the context of past experience. It appears that tightly defined experimental conditions are required in order to attempt to evaluate the discrete functioning of any one system. In clinical settings, where the aim is to assess the individual in their everyday context, the imposition of such experimental conditions impinges on the ecological validity of assessment. Therefore, during clinical evaluation, it is preferable to evaluate the motor, sensory, perceptual and cognitive systems together.

Function is dynamic, not static, and this can make it challenging to obtain a 'true' baseline of function at the start of the therapy process. Health professionals are being encouraged to embrace EBP. This means that therapists need to evaluate the effects of their intervention using outcome measures. When undertaking assessment to evaluate the effects of an intervention, the therapist needs to be aware that the person's scores on an outcome measure are open to a degree of error, and she will need to take any confounding variables into consideration when interpreting the person's performance on the outcome measure. A person's functioning can be influenced by several factors, for example:

- changing levels of pain
- concentration

- anxiety
- fatigue
- response to a drug regimen
- level of stiffness.

Therefore, a single assessment might not present a true and complete picture of the person's ability. Variability in a person's function can be more extreme for certain diagnoses. People with Parkinson's disease, for example, may have very different levels of functional independence depending on the timing and effects of their medication. A therapist should try to undertake different parts of the assessment on different occasions, varying the time of day and the assessment environment. Test anxiety can affect performance, and a client's performance often improves as their therapist becomes familiar and good rapport is established.

When evaluating the outcome of intervention, the therapist must be aware that a person's function may change for many reasons. For example, improvements may be observed as a result of a specific intervention or the success of a combination of interventions. This is important because physiotherapy, or occupational therapy, is rarely the sole intervention and often is provided in a multidisciplinary context. Other factors that might result in observed improvements in function include:

- belief/hope that change in function is possible
- placebo effect
- strong sense of locus of control
- good copying strategies
- high motivation
- good rapport with the therapist
- feelings of acceptance and support.

When undertaking assessment to provide an accurate baseline and/or evaluate the effects of an intervention, the therapist needs to define the specific area to be measured and will need to take any confounding variables into consideration when interpreting the person's performance on the outcome measure.

Another factor that can complicate the measurement of outcomes is the person's level of insight. The therapist needs to assess whether the person has insight into the nature and severity of his condition, because the need for insight is fundamental to the success of the therapeutic process. A lack of insight can affect the accuracy of any self-report data collected from the client and can hinder the negotiation of treatment goals and the formulation of an agreed plan for intervention. Insight may improve during the intervention, and this can enable a more realistic treatment plan to be renegotiated. However, when therapy goals are renegotiated mid-intervention, the baseline assessment, which founded the original treatment goals, may no longer be accurate or appropriate to the renegotiated treatment goals, and this can lead to serious complications in the interpretation of any measures of outcome (Austin and Clark, 1993).

Therapy sometimes spans several weeks, months or even years. Therapists should, therefore, be aware that habituation effects may affect self-report and proxy data when measuring outcomes over a long period. Some people progress through the intervention period constantly adapting to the changes in their ability or symptoms; because of these adaptations in response to treatment, the client and carer may lose sight of the client's original level of function and not notice the degree of change that has occurred since the baseline assessment (Austin and Clark, 1993).

Timing the evaluation is an important consideration. For example, if therapists are concerned with the long-term benefits of intervention for their clients, then a final assessment at discharge does not provide the whole picture when measuring outcomes. One must not assume that function will always plateau post discharge. Sometimes some of the progress achieved during treatment can be lost post discharge when the client no longer has the therapist for support and encouragement or fails to keep up with an exercise programme once therapy is terminated. For other people, the skills, abilities and attitudes they acquired during the intervention period can inspire progress, and function continues to improve over time (Austin and Clark, 1993). When measuring outcomes, it is important to consider the intervention period or number of therapy sessions that are anticipated in order to obtain the desired change. The timings of measurements are critical, and the therapist needs to judge the spacing of measurement and not undertake the final measurement too early before the client has had the opportunity to gain the maximum change possible.

THE INFLUENCE OF THE LEVEL OF TASK DEMAND

Performance is affected by how demanding or difficult a task is and by the person's capacity, motivation, experience and knowledge. Therapists need to take these factors into account during assessment. Experience, knowledge and capacity are inter-related. This relationship is complex and subject to individual variation; so these factors are difficult to separate and assess in isolation. How the therapist structures the assessment and her reasoning behind her interpretation of assessment data is critical to her ability to untangle these complex influences upon performance. *Task demand* is defined as 'the amount of cognitive and physical skill required to perform the task' (Hilko Culler, 1993, p. 218). When a person goes to perform a task, he first obtains factual information about the demands of that task. From this information, he develops ideas, insights and beliefs related to the task, and he then creates strategies to complete the task more efficiently.

A person's capacity, defined in terms of the amount of information that the central nervous system can handle and process, is limited. The brain has limits for the quantity of sensory information (experienced through the visual, tactile, auditory, olfactory, gustatory and somatic sensory systems) that it can process at a time. For example, the auditory system can only process a certain amount of auditory stimulation at a time, which is why it is hard to concentrate on two people speaking simultaneously. All tasks place demands on the capacity of at least some of the body's sensory systems and, consequently, on the brain's ability to process sensory stimulation. The level and quality of a person's performance will be determined by the demands of a task if the demands of that task are within a person's capacity. For example, a person may have the capacity to perform two different tasks, such as eating cereal from a bowl with a spoon and eating a meal using a knife and fork. Although the person can do both tasks, he will eat his cereal with greater ease because it is a less demanding, easier, task. If the person reaches the maximum level of his capacity, then performance will be limited by his capacity, not by the task demands.

Capacity alters in relation to both the normal developmental processes and to pathology. In terms of normal development, infants learn to use spoons before they learn to use knives and forks. Although organically based capacities decrease with age, many everyday tasks are considered to make relatively few demands, and on these tasks it is expected that performance will not vary with age (Welford, 1993). However, some more complex tasks may demand more than the person's capacity allows, and then performance can be a function of age. The onset of any limitation depends on the nature of the task demands, the individual's capacity and the rate at which capacities decline; that is the greater the capacity and the slower the rate of decline, the later will performance begin to decrease as a function of age (Welford, 1993; Craik, 1977). Capacity can be reduced as the result of an injury or illness. For example, a person who has experienced a stroke and who has associated motor and sensory deficits and a resultant limited capacity in the motor and sensory systems may be unable to either eat using a spoon or a knife and fork. The difference in task demand is not the issue, in this example, because the problems in task performance are related to the person's reduced motor and sensory capacity.

Performance at all ages is affected by the task demand and the individual's capacity, experience and knowledge. In addition, factors related to volition and societal expectations will also have an impact. Although all these factors (task demand, capacity, experience, knowledge, volition and societal expectations) are acknowledged as important, it can be very difficult to distinguish between them and to identify the point at which a change in performance is related to pathology. This is why normative data provided in standardised normative assessments (see Chapter 5) are useful when a therapist needs to conduct a discriminative assessment (see Chapter 3).

Hilko Culler (1993) cites the work of Chapparo (1979) describing how therapists, when undertaking initial assessments with people with neurological conditions, should select tasks with inverse cognitive and physical demands (that is a task with a high motor demand should have a low cognitive demand or vice versa) and explains how therapists should progress slowly to tasks with increasing levels of both motor and cognitive demands.

Some criterion-referenced assessments (see Chapter 5) take task demand into account and may present assessment items as a hierarchy from the simplest to the most complex task. For example, the Assessment of Motor Process Skills (AMPS; Fisher, 2003a) provides descriptions for a choice of instrumental activities of daily living (IADL) that have been calibrated through research to create a hierarchy from easiest to hardest task. Using hierarchies of task demand can save unnecessary testing time for both the therapist and client. For example, the Rivermead ADL Assessment (Whiting and Lincoln, 1980) is structured in terms of a hierarchy of items comprising increasingly demanding personal and household tasks. The therapist decides where on the hierarchy to begin testing, based on her hypothesis about which tasks the person may not be able to manage. If the person can perform the selected task, then the therapist ensures he can perform the three proceeding tasks and then progresses testing up the hierarchy until he fails to perform three consecutive tasks. Other assessments may be graded so that the person can be presented with progressively more demanding tasks as his ability increases, for example an assessment of meal preparation could be graded from using a pre-packaged cold meal to preparing a hot, three-course meal using raw ingredients (Hilko Culler, 1993).

THE IMPACT OF FAMILIARITY ON PERFORMANCE

Familiarity and practice influence performance. When a person practises a task over time, the demands of the task are learned and the person becomes more efficient in the use of his capabilities related to performing that task; the task becomes perceived as being easier. A good example is learning to drive a car. Two adults might have the same capacities, but the person who is familiar with driving a car will be better at driving than the person with no driving experience. Another example is that of cooking: 'it is less demanding for a person to cook a familiar recipe from memory than to follow a new recipe from a cookbook' (Hilko Culler, 1993, p. 218). Therefore, therapists need to be aware of how familiar or unfamiliar assessment tasks are to their clients. In addition, following a reduction in capacity, therapists can use practice and repetition to increase a person's task performance and use an ongoing reassessment of the task to monitor progress. When repeating an assessment in this way, the therapist must be able to differentiate between changes that result because the assessment is now familiar and changes that have resulted because of the person's capacity. Improvements in motor function are an example of this. Therefore, parallel forms of an assessment (see section on equivalent/parallel form reliability in Chapter 7, p. 199) might be used, where an unfamiliar task of the same demand and assessing the same capacity is given in place of the familiar assessment task.

THE INFLUENCE OF ENVIRONMENT ON PERFORMANCE

The environment in which an assessment is undertaken may also influence performance and can have an enabling or constraining effect on a person's function (Law *et al.*, 1996). The term *environment* usually makes people think about the physical elements (including accessibility, architectural barriers and structural adaptations) of a person's setting. However, therapists need to think about the environment in a broader context. The World Health Organization (WHO; 2002) states that 'disability and functioning are viewed as outcomes of interactions between health conditions (diseases, disorders and injuries) and contextual factors' (p. 10). Contextual factors include external environmental factors, which are defined as 'the physical, social and attitudinal environment in which people live and conduct their lives' (p. 10) and are subdivided into 'social attitudes, architectural characteristics, legal and social structures, as well as climate and terrain' (p. 10). The WHO definition of environment fits well with definitions from the therapy literature; for example, Cooper, Rigby and Letts (1995) state that environment is the 'physical, social, cultural, attitudinal, institutional, and organisational setting within which human function takes place' (p. 56) and several authors (for example Christiansen, 1991; Mosey, 1981) subdivide the environment into cultural, social and non-human/external/physical factors. The terms *external environment* and *non-human environment* have been used interchangeably in the therapy literature. Interacting with our environment facilitates the initial development, as well as maintenance of all, performance components (Mosey, 1981). Cultural and social factors need to be taken into account when selecting appropriate occupations for assessment and treatment. The non-human environment, in the form of setting and tools, needs to be carefully selected and structured during assessment in order to ensure meaning for the patient and fulfil the therapeutic purpose. An individual must interact with the non-human environment to engage in occupations. An activity (such as washing) occurs in a physical and social environment (washing may take place in a bathroom or by a river and the activity will be influenced by social and cultural norms). The performance of an activity may also involve the use of objects (washing may require the use of a washing bowl or basin, soap and towel). When a therapist uses the performance of ADLs as a method of assessment, she consciously structures an environment for this performance and selects specific tools for the client to interact with.

The Person-Environment-Occupation Model (Law *et al.*, 1996) provides a useful theoretical framework for considering the impact of the environment during therapy assessment. A person, his environment and his occupation (including activities and tasks) interact continually across time and space. The greater the overlap, or fit, between the person, environment and occupation, the more optimal will be the person's function. An intervention that increases the enabling aspect of the environment for an individual and thereby creates a compatible person-environment-occupation fit will increase, or with a progressive condition perhaps maintain, function. Therapists are involved with assessing and where necessary adapting a person's environment or teaching the person compensatory techniques to help them to cope with the challenges placed by negotiating the environment with a particular impairment. For example, if a therapist modifies a kitchen to increase accessibility for a person in a wheelchair, then the fit between the person's capacity, the kitchen environment and the activities of meal preparation, washing up and laundry will improve, leading to increased independence.

Familiarity with an environment may influence assessment results; the impact of familiarity does not just apply to the activity or task to be assessed but also to the familiarity of the environment in which the assessment is to be undertaken. For example, 'a familiar environment (e.g. kitchen at home) is less demanding than a new environment (e.g. clinic kitchen)' (Hilko Culler, 1993, p. 219), and a therapist could expect a client to be more independent within his own kitchen than in unfamiliar therapy-department kitchen areas. Even if the familiarity of an environment does not affect the final outcome of an assessment, it may affect the speed at which the task is completed. It is quicker, as we know, to make a cup of tea in your own kitchen because you know where everything is kept. You will still be able to make a cup of tea in a friend's kitchen but probably it will take you more time because you will be searching in the unfamiliar environment for the items and ingredients you need. The home environment does not always facilitate function; for example, people may be able to move better on the hard, flat surface of a physiotherapy department or hospital ward than on the different surface textures (for example carpet, floorboards, rugs, lino, tiles) in their own homes.

The WHO (2002) recommends that 'to assess the full ability of the individual, one would need to have a "standardised environment" to neutralize the varying impact of different environments on the ability of the individual' (p. 11). The WHO suggests that there are a number of environments that can be used for this purpose, such as:

a. 'an actual environment commonly used for capacity assessment in test settings
b. an assumed environment thought to have a uniform impact
c. an environment with precisely defined parameters based on extensive scientific research' (p. 11).

Therapists are often involved in conducting assessments in people's own home and work environments, as they need to evaluate both environmental barriers and environmental supports to performance. Assessment at home is considered useful because people are more likely to behave and communicate in their normal way in familiar surroundings. The therapist can build a more accurate picture of the person's needs during a home assessment. A home assessment can also facilitate access to the views and the needs of any carer. The environment selected for assessment is especially important for people with certain conditions. For example, it is essential to assess the influence of context and environment on the function of a person with dementia (Tullis and Nicol, 1999).

Where safety is a concern, it is critical to assess the person in the environment where he will be functioning to examine the relationship between potential environmental hazards and the person's ability. Once potential hazards have been identified, changes to the

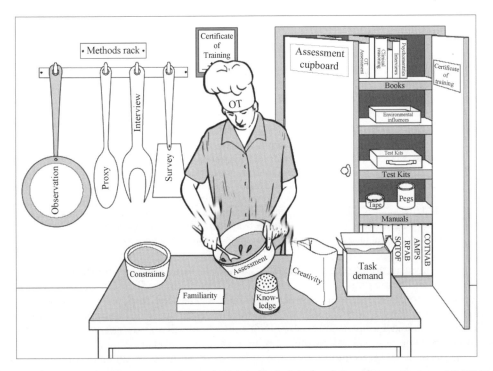

Figure 1.1 The therapist as a creative and expert chef. *Reprinted from Laver Fawcett AJ (2002) Assessment. In A Turner, M Foster and S Johnson (Eds) Occupational Therapy and Physical Dysfunction: Principles, Skills and Practice. London: Churchill Livingstone. Chapter 5, pp. 107–144. Copyright (2002), with permission from Elsevier.*

environment can be made to reduce the risks, for example a risk of falls. Some therapy assessments have been designed for use in the home environment. For example, the Safety Assessment of Function and the Environment for Rehabilitation (SAFER Tool; Letts *et al.*, 1998) was developed to assess people's abilities to manage functional activities safely within their homes, and the Home Falls and Accidents Screening Tool (Home Fast; Mackenzie, Byles and Higginbotham, 2000) was developed to identify hazards associated with falls in the home.

THE CONSTRAINTS OF THE PRACTICE SETTING

The practice setting will influence the therapist's choice of assessment and may serve to enhance or constrain her assessment practice. For example, if a therapist moves to a service that encourages standardised assessment and has a range of published tests available, then her knowledge of different tests and skills in standardised assessment may increase. Conversely, a therapist may be experienced with a particular standardised test but find that it is not available in a new practice setting or that with the demand of her new caseload there is not enough time to administer the test in its entirety. It may not be possible in some settings to assess the client at several different times in varying test environments and cover all the areas of interest within the assessment. Therefore, the therapist needs to use her clinical judgement to select the most effective assessment strategy within the physical and political boundaries of the therapy environment. She may only be able to conduct a brief assessment and will need to make decisions about the person's overall ability and prognosis from limited data projections (see section on predictive validity in Chapter 6, pp. 178–80). This is where the quality of the therapist's clinical reasoning can be critical.

CONCLUSION

The therapist needs to be like an experienced chef (see Figure 1.1): not following rigidly a set recipe but combining knowledge of different techniques and knowing what ingredients and flavours can be combined in a creative way for each particular situation.

> Evidence based medicine is not 'cookbook' medicine. Because it requires a bottom up approach that integrates the best external evidence with individual clinical expertise and patients' choice, it cannot result in slavish, cookbook approaches to individual patient care. External clinical evidence can inform, but can never replace, individual clinical expertise, and it is this expertise that decides whether the external evidence applies to the individual patient at all and, if so, how it should be integrated into a clinical decision. Similarly, any external guideline must be integrated with individual clinical expertise in deciding whether and how it matches the patient's clinical state, predicament, and preferences, and thus whether it should be applied. (Sackett *et al.*, 1996, p. 71)

Therapists 'need to adopt outcome measures which will document the efficacy of their interventions, and guide clinical decisions and treatment planning. These measures need to be clinically appropriate, functionally relevant, valid, reliable and responsive to change. In addition, they need to be user friendly so as to minimise the burden to therapists and patients' (Wright, Cross and Lamb, 1998, p. 216). Not only should therapists critique and implement valid and reliable assessments in their practice, they should also be prepared to add to the growing body of research into therapy measures. This might be by collaborating with a test developer to add to data on inter-rater reliability or by contributing their views on studies of clinical utility and aspects of validity.

Richards (2002) challenges therapists to contribute to the national political agenda: 'it behoves . . . therapists to contribute expert assessments which stand up to scrutiny, form a sound foundation for their intervention and link with valid outcome measures that clearly demonstrate the value of their contribution to efficient and effective service provision' (p. xviii).

We should not underestimate the responsibility we have to make sound judgements about our clients' abilities and dysfunction. The distance between theory and practice can sometimes feel like a wide chasm; we know that we should be using valid, reliable, standardised measures in our practice but the demands of the everyday practice settings in which therapists work (including limited time to review potential assessments and try them out and little money to purchase a new test even when there is strong evidence for its application) mean that sloppy – that is without a strong evidence or theoretical base – assessment processes are still occurring more often than we feel comfortable to admit. No matter how competent a therapist is at providing treatment, treatment will be useless if it is based on faulty evaluation and decision-making regarding the client's deficits and the resulting treatment plan. One of the best lessons I was taught as a basic grade occupational therapist was to take time out for continuing professional development (CPD). One time, I had agreed with my supervisor that I would allocate half a day that month to study the manual of a standardised test our department was considering using and would try out the test materials by role-playing the test administration with a colleague. Next supervision, I told her that I had booked my half-day CPD but had cancelled this time as I needed to do an urgent home visit assessment instead as the consultant was pushing to discharge a client. I was reprimanded, and she asked me to compare how many people had benefited from the home visit versus the number of potential people who would have benefited from a more accurate assessment. The next month, I did find time to review the test and found it to be relevant for our client group; within months all the therapists in the department were using this standardised assessment in their practice.

Therapists need to embrace evidence-based practice (EBP) as an opportunity rather than view it as a threat. It is about doing the very best we can for our clients. It also helps to further the development and standing of our professions, which will assist in ensuring ongoing and ideally increased funding for providing occupational therapy and physiotherapy to those people who would benefit from these services. Achieving EBP is a step-by-step process. This book aims to assist therapists to move towards a greater evidence base in their assessment and measurement practice. The first step is to raise a question or series of questions. Worksheets have been developed for each chapter to enable you to raise and answer questions related to different aspects of your assessment and measurement practice. Let us begin with a global question: 'How should I organise my assessment process in order to collect the right information, at the best time and in the most effective and efficient way to provide reliable, valid and responsive measurement in a manner that is acceptable to my clients?'

Once you have formulated a question as a focus for EBP, the second step is to search for evidence. Within the book, I have reviewed literature and research that will provide a sound knowledge base from which the student can start the journey of answering this question. As it is such a big question, it is helpful to break it down into a series of more specific questions. I have noted the main chapter or chapters that have been written to help you to answer each of these questions:

- *Who is the best source for this information?*
  - see Chapter 2
- *What is the best method for collecting this information?*
  - see Chapter 2
- *Why am I collecting assessment and measurement data?*
  - see Chapter 3
- *What level of measurement is required?*
  - see Chapter 4
- *How can I ensure my measurements are valid?*
  - see Chapter 6

- *How do I set about identifying appropriate standardised tests for my service?*
  ○ see Chapter 5 and Chapter 11
- *How do I evaluate whether my assessment process and the specific measures used are acceptable to my clients?*
  ○ see sections on face validity and clinical utility in Chapter 6 and the section on test critique in Chapter 11
- *How can I ensure my measurements are reliable?*
  ○ see Chapter 7 on reliability
- *How can I ensure my outcome measures are responsive to a clinically relevant degree of change?*
  ○ see Chapter 7 on reliability
- *How do I prepare for an efficient and effective test administration?*
  ○ see Chapter 8
- *How do I build rapport with my client?*
  ○ see Chapter 8
- *How do I ensure that my test administration remains standardised?*
  ○ see Chapter 8
- *How do I communicate the results of my assessment?*
  ○ see Chapter 8
- *What is the best way to collate and analyse the different types of data obtained through the assessment process to produce a coherent, meaningful picture of the person?*
  ○ see Chapter 9
- *How do I fit my assessment practice into the wider context of a multidisciplinary team and/or interagency approach?*
  ○ see Chapter 9
- *How do I combine the best available evidence, with my clinical experience and my knowledge of my client's preferences?*
  ○ see Chapter 10
- *How do I combine the best available evidence with my clinical experience and my knowledge of my client's preferences in order to implement the optimum assessment and measurement approach?*
  ○ see Chapter 11 and Chapter 12

I have included a number of worksheets in this book that can be used to focus your learning. If you are an undergraduate student, you might use the worksheets on clinical placement to explore the assessment processes being used by your supervisor and her colleagues. If you are a practising therapist, you could use the worksheet, alone or with colleagues, as a focus for your own CPD – remember to put a copy of any completed worksheet in your CPD portfolio as evidence of your work – or for your team's or department's service development activities.

2

Methods of Assessment and Sources of Assessment Data

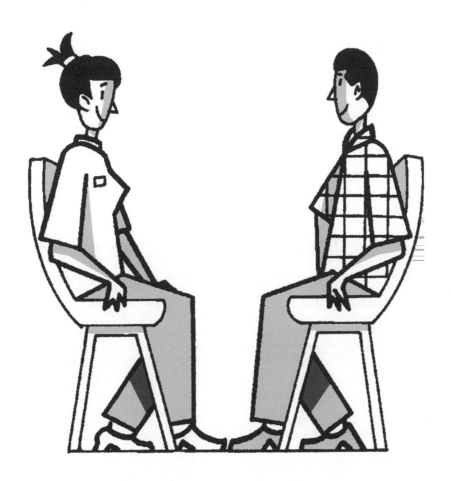

CHAPTER SUMMARY

This chapter discusses the merits of different methods of data collection. Methods used by therapists include interview, observation, survey, referral information, medical notes, letters, telephone calls and use of standardised tests. The sources of assessment data described will include client self-report, proxy sources, such as family members, friends, neighbours, home care workers, voluntary workers and other professionals involved with the client, and therapist observation and data collected by the therapist both formally, through standardised testing, and informally, through following a department checklist. Issues of culture, client age, technology, ethics and confidentiality will be discussed. Examples of published assessments for different methods and sources will be provided. The chapter concludes with a detailed case study that illustrates how these different methods and sources can be combined to provide a thorough assessment. It will also endeavour to answer the following question: 'What is the best method for collecting required assessment and measurement data and who will be the best source(s) of this information?'

In order to adequately assess a new client, the therapist must undertake a logical and well-planned assessment process. This process might require the therapist to:

1. determine what information is necessary to make sound clinical decisions and clarify what information is to be collected
2. identify relevant sources for this information
3. determine assessment methods to be used to collect this information from these sources
4. choose appropriate standardised tests to support informal assessment methods
5. undertake data-collection procedures such as record/referral review, interviews, observations and administration of standardised measures
6. score any standardised test data (this might involve converting raw scores or plotting scores on a normative graph)
7. analyse data
8. interpret data
9. report results (orally and in writing; it may be required to record summaries on a computer database).

This chapter will focus on steps 2 and 3 of this assessment process because therapists need to be able to identify good sources of information and select appropriate methods for obtaining assessment data from these sources.

METHODS OF DATA COLLECTION

A thorough assessment should involve a process that uses multiple methods for gathering and organising information required for making specific clinical decisions (Hayley, Coster and Ludlow, 1991). There are many different methods, both qualitative and quantitative, that can be used to help you collect, structure and analyse assessment data.

The College of Occupational Therapists (COT) outlines the assessment methods used by therapists in its position paper *Occupational Therapy Defined as a Complex Intervention* (College of Occupational Therapists, 2003a). The COT states that 'the therapist uses assessment methods which are appropriate to her/his own abilities and to the client's needs and situation. These include:

- interacting informally with the client
- observing activity in the client's own living, working or social environments or in the clinical setting

- setting the client specific tasks
- carrying out standardised tests
- interviewing clients and carers
- asking questions and discussing the situation informally' (p. 21).

The American Occupational Therapy Association (AOTA; 1984 and 1989) also provides a similar list of methods, including standardised tests, performance checklists, interviews, review of records, questionnaires and observations of activities and tasks designed to evaluate specific performance abilities.

The Chartered Society of Physiotherapy (CSP; 2001a) has also published a list of methods that are used by physiotherapists; this list includes:

- 'patient-completed self-report questionnaires
- clinician-completed observation scales
- task-specific activities/tests, e.g. sit to stand
- impairment tests, e.g. range of motion
- physiological tests' (p. 2).

Studies of therapist assessment practices have shown that therapists do use a variety of assessment methods; for example, results from a survey of 50 paediatric occupational therapists by Chia (1996) demonstrate that the following methods of assessment were used by the sample of therapists. These methods are listed below in the order of the frequency with which they were reported as a used method.

- interviewing (n = 49) used by 98% of the therapists
- standardised tests (n = 40) used by 80%
- structured observations (n = 36) used by 72%
- non-standardised tests (n = 35) used by 70%
- unstructured observations (n = 29) used by 58%

It is useful to combine qualitative and quantitative methods, to achieve a thorough assessment, because these have different functions and are designed to answer different questions (Eva and Paley, 2004). Qualitative data-collection methods include:

- informal observations (e.g. to look at the person's facial expression, quality of movement or social interactions with others)
- casual conversations with the client and their carers using open-ended questioning techniques
- the use of semi-structured interviews or questionnaires.

Qualitative information usually focuses on things like feelings, values and perceptions related to what has taken place or the significance of a problem.

The application of quantitative methods involves the administration of standardied or structured measurement, observational tests and interview schedules. The data collected focus on factual information and are often expressed in the form of numerical scores. For example, quantitative data might comprise:

- the raw or converted scores obtained administering a standardised outcome measure
- data collected from observation testing methods, such as the range of movement of a joint
- structured self-report or proxy report data, such as the number of times a particular daily-living problem occurs over a set time period.

Table 2.1 Examples of direct and indirect methods of data collection used by therapists

Direct methods	Indirect methods
Therapist observations	Referral information (written, faxed or via a letter or referral form)
Client self-report given direct to the therapist	Patient/client's previous records, such as medical records, therapy records, social services records; these might be accessed electronically, e.g. through a Single Assessment Process (SAP)
Administration of a standardised test to the client by the therapist	Proxy reports from formal sources, such as the patient's GP, doctor, other members of a multidisciplinary team, workers from other statutory services, teacher
Administration of a standardised test to the carer by the therapist to assess the carer him/herself (e.g. to examine level of carer burden or parental stress)	Proxy reports from informal sources, such as the patient's parent, spouse, children, neighbour, friend, voluntary worker or religious leader (e.g. priest)

In addition to categorising methods in terms of whether the method yields qualitative or quantitative data, methods can also be grouped in terms of whether they obtain direct or indirect data; examples of direct and indirect methods of data collection are provided in Table 2.1.

INTRODUCTION TO SOURCES OF ASSESSMENT INFORMATION

In the following sections, we will describe the three main sources of information used by therapists for assessment. These are client self-report (direct method), proxy report (indirect method) and therapist observational/collected data (direct method). I will describe the assessment methods used to collect data using each type of source and will provide examples of published assessments used by therapists to collect data from each of these sources.

SELF-REPORT

The World Health Organization (WHO) emphasises that all health professionals should pay attention to insider perspectives of people with a disability. The WHO states that 'disability and functioning are viewed as outcomes of interactions between health conditions (diseases, disorders and injuries) and contextual factors' (World Health Organization, 2002, p. 10). Contextual factors are divided, by the WHO, into external environmental factors and internal personal factors. Internal personal factors 'include gender, age, coping styles, social background, education, profession, past and current experiences, overall behaviour pattern, character and other factors that influence how disability is experienced by the individual' (p. 10). The therapist needs to engage the person in an assessment method that elicits information about these internal personal factors, and the person is usually the most reliable source for this information.

Clouston (2003) notes that 'involvement of the user in decisions about his or her own health and social care has become a key element of the changes encapsulated in the [British] Government's legislation. Listening to the service user and responding to his or her needs is an integral part of that change' (p. 136). This can be clearly seen in England, where the National Service Frameworks (NSFs) have put an emphasis on placing the client and his family at the centre of the health care process, not just as a service recipient. For example, Standard Two of the NSF for older people (Department of Health, 2001a) focuses on person-centred care and states: 'older people and their carers should receive person-centred care and services which respect them as individuals and which are arranged around their needs . . . Proper assessment of the range and complexity of older people's needs and prompt provision of care . . . can improve their ability to function independently . . . The views of patients and carers will be sought systematically' (p. 8). The introduction of a single assessment process (SAP) is a key component of the person-centred care standard of the NSF for older people (Department of Health, 2001a). In the Department of Health (DoH) guidance for the implementation of SAP (2002a, 2002c), explicit recommendations are made to professionals regarding the involvment of the older person in their assessment process.

> Agencies should encourage older people to contribute fully to their assessment, with due regard to individual circumstances . . . older people can be advised to think about the needs and issues they may wish to raise, and how this might be structured. Where appropriate, older people can be asked to complete customised forms or make written statements that can feed into the assessment process. Some older people might wish to complete self-assessment forms that mirror those used by agencies . . . the older person should be asked to describe their needs and expectations, and the strengths and abilities they can bring to addressing their needs, in their own words and on their own terms. This person-centred beginning should set the tone for the rest of the assessment and subsequent care planning, and due account of the user's perspective should remain to the fore throughout. (Department of Health, 2002c, p. 9)

Expert client programmes are being developed in a number of health care fields, and these expert clients are working together to enable people with long-term conditions to manage their own health with specialised support from health care professionals (Department of Health, 2001a).

Self-report assessment has been defined as 'a type of assessment approach where the patient reports on his or her level of function or performance' (Christiansen and Baum, 1991, p. 858). This is quite a narrow definition, as self-report is valuable in providing the therapist with a wide range of information, including:

- the person's description of his roles, occupations, routines and values
- his living situation (including the physical environment and sociocultural influences)
- his goals for the future
- the presenting condition and his experience of illness or disability and the symptoms associated with any current problems
- his opinion about his current and previous level of function and occupational performance.
- Self-report can also be used to help with the identification of available resources (financial, social and emotional) that might be used to support the client (Hilko Culler, 1993).

In addition to asking about level of function, it can be helpful to consider individuals' perceptions of how important different activities are to their lives and also how satisfied they are with their current level of performance (Law *et al.*, 1994). This information helps therapists to prioritise areas for further assessment and treatment. An example of this type of assessment is the Canadian Occupational Performance Measure (COPM; Law *et al.*, 1998), which is described briefly on p. 56 and applied in the case study at the end of this chapter.

Self-report can be very useful as it enables the therapist to access information that only the client knows. 'Self-report assesses what the client says about what he or she is thinking, feeling or doing. Self-report is important because it is our only measure of cognitive activity (such as obsessions or negative self-statements) or of subjective experience (such as pain. . .)' (Barlow, Hayes and Nelson, 1984, p. 124). In the past, particularly within a medical model, the use of objective (quantitative) data has been favoured over subjective (qualitative) data, and there was a 'belief that the patient's view was of no value in measurement' (Pynsent, 2004, p. 3). Nowadays, as therapists take a more explicit interest in client-centred practice, it is very relevant for them to collect assessment data from the person they seek to treat (Law *et al.*, 1994; Pollock and McColl, 1998). We have come to value that, although self-reports do not always coincide with observational or direct measures, 'it is not that self-report is an *inferior* measure, but rather that it is a *different* measure' (Barlow, Hayes and Nelson, 1984, p. 124). Carswell, *et al.* (2004) state that 'without some measure of the client's perspective, it is difficult to imagine how one might engage in client-centred therapy' (p. 219). This is echoed by Hammell (2003), who believes that 'we cannot claim allegiance to client-centred philosophy when we are not paying attention to what disabled people are saying' (p. 48), and by Clouston (2003), who emphasises the importance of 'listening to and valuing the voice of the user' and states that 'now, more than ever, . . . therapists have to show that this an integral part of their everyday practice' (p. 136).

An understanding of the client's perspective enables the therapist to find common ground from which to negotiate mutually agreed desired outcomes and treatment approaches, which are often referred to as *treatment goals*. Jette (1995) notes that 'physical therapists have always advocated and respected patient-level goals' (p. 967), and much of the client-centred literature in occupational therapy also emphasises that therapists should focus intervention on those areas of importance to the client. Partridge and Johnston (1989), in a study that examined perceived control of recovery and predicted recovery from a physical disability, found that a person was more likely to recover faster if he perceived himself to be in control of his rehabilitation. Using self-report as a significant component of the assessment processes engages the client and facilitates his involvement and sense of control in his rehabilitation process. So, self-report is a critical source of assessment data as it engages the person actively in the assessment process and elicits the client's own experiences, wishes, aspirations and beliefs. This assessment source provides subjective data, which help the therapist to obtain a picture of the person and how he views his life, illness or disability, problems and functioning. It is useful to try to engage a client in some form of self-report assessment whenever possible; even a client who is considered to have little insight (for example a person with severe dementia) will still have his perspective about what is problematic and may have ideas about what might help remedy the problem (Carswell *et al.*, 2004). Even if these ideas are incongruent with the therapist's knowledge and experience of what is safe and possible, it is very helpful to know the belief system and expectations that the client is bringing to the therapeutic relationship. Another group of clients who have previously been considered to have inadequate levels of insight to engage in self-report are children. In the past, paediatric assessment focused on the collection of observational data and information from proxy sources, such as parents and teachers. More recently, therapists have come to understand the benefits of collecting self-report data from children. Sturgess, Rodger and Ozanne (2002) cite three reasons for using self-report with young children:

> The first reason for using self-report with young children is that there is evidence that children hold a view about themselves which is unique, valid and stable over time. Secondly, increasingly sophisticated methods are being developed which provide ways for children to present this view reliably. Lastly, children have a right to be intimately involved in the decisions being made about them. These arguments for using self-report are being substantiated by research and emerging clinical frames of reference. (pp. 108–109)

Self-report data are critical when examining constructs such as pain. Pain is a very personal experience and is difficult to define and measure. In addition, research has indicated that carers overestimate pain relief following interventions compared with patients' reports. For example, see the study by Rundshagen *et al.* (1999), which examined patients' versus nurses' assessments of pain.

Self-report data can be collected using a range of methods, including:

- structured, semi-structured or informal interview, given either face to face or via telephone

- a written format provided by standardised and non-standardised questionnaires, check-lists and surveys, which can be given to the person or sent via mail, fax or email for completion
- self-ratings, e.g. on a visual analogue scale to rate pain
- self-monitoring through client journals, e.g. to record symptoms, feelings or activities undertaken
- card sorts (Barlow, Hayes and Nelson, 1984), e.g. the Activity Card Sort (ACS; Baum, 1993, 1995)
- narratives (e.g. see Clouston, 2003)
- play activities and the use of toys (e.g. dolls, dolls houses) for imaginary play and role play; joining children and participating actively in their play activities, particularly when the child is encouraged to direct the therapist and lead the play activity, can be very effective for opening up channels of communication (Swain, 2004)
- the arts, such as drawing, painting, sculpture, music to movement and improvised drama (e.g. see Dalton, 1994).

Many methods for collecting self-report data are cost-effective in terms of time and resources. Self-report is very flexible and, as only a few materials are required (a pen and paper or a test form if a standardised test is being applied), the data can be collected easily in various environments including the person's own home, day-care provider, outpatient clinic, ward, day hospital, workplace, school etc. The critical question is how best to ellicit what the person knows and feels and to distinguish between what they know and do not know and what they may or may not be prepared to share with you (Baldwin, 2000).

An example of a structured interview self-report schedule is the Functional Life Scale (Sarno, Sarno and Levita, 1973). An example of a self-report questionnaire is provided by the Satisfaction with Performance Scaled Questionnaire (Yerxa *et al.*, 1988).

Self-report data are crucial for developing intervention goals that will have relevance and meaning for the person and, provided the person is able to communicate in some manner, should be a key component of all assessments, no matter how brief. It can be used when the therapist does not have access to an environment suitable for observational testing or when the client refuses to undertake an observational assessment. In addition to being used as a baseline, descriptive form of assessment, self-report is being increasingly used in measures of outcome. Adams (2002) warns about the levels of reliability in some self-report measures and stresses that 'care should be taken to ensure that any self-report account can be integrated as a valid and reliable outcome measure' (p. 173).

INTERVIEWING AS A MEANS OF COLLECTING SELF-REPORT DATA

Borg and Bruce (1991) reviewed the literature on interviewing and conclude that: '(1) interviewing is a crucial component of any assessment used to plan treatment; and (2) there are multiple ways to conduct an interview and not any one method is correct' (p. 572). The interview is usually chosen, by both physiotherapists and occupational therapists, as the initial method of data collection and is a very useful method for collecting self-report data. Smith (1993) states: 'an initial interview serves several vital purposes. It provides for:

1. collection of information about the patient to help develop objectives and plans for treatment;
2. establishment of understanding on the part of the patient about the role of the therapist and the purposes of the . . . therapy process;
3. an opportunity for the patient to discuss the particular situation and think about plans for change' (p. 171).

In addition to collecting information for a baseline assessment, an initial interview forms the foundation for building rapport and forming the beginnings of an effective therapeutic relationship. Building good rapport is essential to obtaining a full history from the person, and so the therapist should consciously try to put the client at ease. Therapists need to be aware of how differences or similarities between themselves and their clients (for example age, gender and sociocultural background) can serve to either facilitate or hamper the development of rapport and the establishment of an effective therapeutic relationship (see p. 219).

It is important for the therapist to provide introductory information to set the scene for the first contact and for a potential therapeutic relationship. This information should include:

- introducing herself to the client
- outlining her role as an occupational therapist or physiotherapist
- explaining the purpose of the interview
- describing the type of occupational therapy or physiotherapy service that can be provided in that practice setting
- discussing the degree of confidentiality that applies by letting the client know with whom the therapist might share interview information.

When conducting an interview, therapists should check that the person is able to hear, comprehend and attend to the conversation. The nature of the assessment environment can serve to facilitate or disrupt the assessment process; so it is important that therapists provide a quiet, private interview environment that is free from interruptions and distractions. However, you should consider the nature of the referral when judging what the most appropriate environment will be. For example, Sturgess, Rodger and Ozanne (2002) note that for children who have experienced traumatic or stressful events removal to a separate room might make them feel isolated or trapped, and an environment where they are reassured by the presence of other children and therapists may make the child more relaxed and responsive. The environment should also be a comfortable temperature for the nature of the assessment – neither too hot and stuffy, which might make a client feel drowsy and could reduce concentration, nor cold and draughty, particularly if the person is being asked to undress for a physical assessment. Where possible, the person's usual environment should be selected, as the person is more likely to feel at ease in a familiar place. In addition, the person is likely to feel more empowered in their own environment, whereas in a therapy department the clinician needs to consciously consider that she is on her home territory and that her therapy environment may feel alien to her client.

It is important for the therapist to consider her body language. The therapist should choose carefully where she sits in relation to the person, for example a formal setup with the therapist sitting behind a desk might not be conducive to providing a relaxed atmosphere. Instead, set up two comfortable chairs at a 90-degree angle to each other; removing the barrier of the desk and the direct confrontation of sitting opposite the person can help facilitate the sharing of information. The chair selected needs to be of an appropriate height and style to facilitate safe transfers and ensure comfort, particularly during a long interview or test administration.

A number of authors have categorised factors that can influence the client, the therapist and/or the client–therapist interaction during an interview, and that may facilitate or impede successful data collection using the interview method. In the next section, two pieces of work that describe influential factors which therapists need to be mindful of while preparing for, during and reflecting upon an interview will be outlined. Fidler (1976, cited by Smith, 1993, p. 170) describes four *filters* that influence the interactions between people and can be significant in distorting the interview or observation process. These are:

1. 'Perceptual: how sensory stimuli (colour of clothing, perfume) affect the way the other person is perceived;
2. Conceptual: the knowledge base brought to the interaction;

3. Role: the way each person perceives the role he or she is to play in the interaction;
4. Self-esteem: the way each person feels about himself or herself.'

Therapists need to be aware of these four filters and how they may influence their objectivity during an assessment, and also how they may influence the response of the client to the therapist and affect the formation of an effective therapeutic relationship.

Borg and Bruce (1991) categorise factors that can influence an interview process in a slightly different way; they also identify four influences for the therapist to consider. These are:

1. the environmental factors, including the institution the therapist works for and the specific environment selected as the interview setting. Environmental issues have already been discussed above; in addition, Borg and Bruce (1991) recommend:
   a. selecting an atmosphere that conveys a feeling of warmth
   b. ensuring a minimum of distractions by putting a sign on the door indicating that an interview is in progress and by switching mobile/office phones to silent and letting the answerphone pick up messages during the course of the interview
   c. pre-planning so that any questionnaire, task or test materials that might be required during the interview are collected in advance and easily accessible during the interview.
2. the influence of the therapist, which includes 'the therapist's interview skills, personal values, beliefs and theoretical orientation' (p. 573), all of which can influence the interview's outcome. Good interviewing skills involve the therapist being an active listener who is aware of the impact of her verbal and non-verbal communication and understands how her facial expression, or a movement such as nodding her head, can convey acceptance or criticism of the client's comments or behaviour. When a therapist is able to actively listen, respect and identify with the client's viewpoint, while maintaining her own identity, she becomes empathetic. Clients who experience genuine empathy from their therapists are more likely to develop rapport and form effective therapeutic relationships. The therapist's theoretical orientation will shape the topics covered and the manner in which questions are asked; it will also influence the way in which the therapist analyses the information obtained and the nature of any hypotheses generated from this analysis.
3. client influences. As with the therapist, the client brings a unique set of values, beliefs and experiences to the assessment. As the person is presenting for therapy, he is likely to also come with needs, expectations and perhaps some anxiety. Borg and Bruce (1991) further describe clients' factors as: 'they may be fearful, wonder what is permissible to discuss, or may have a specific agenda they wish to share. Their previous therapy experiences may confirm their discomfort or support their investment in therapy' (p. 573). So it is important for the therapist to allow sufficient time for an initial interview to explore and understand any client-focused influences.
4. dynamic interactions between therapist and client. The fourth area is labelled by Borg and Bruce (1991) as 'patient symptoms and interviewer responses'. The dynamic interactions that occur while establishing the therapeutic relationship are affected by the nature of the client's presenting problem, therapist–client responses and time-pressure. The presenting problem can have a varying impact, depending upon its nature. For example, a therapist needs to be particularly mindful of therapist–client responses when interviewing clients with mental health problems. The therapist's verbal and non-verbal communication may be misinterpreted by the client, particularly if the client is experiencing paranoid or psychotic symptoms.

When interviewing young children, therapists are advised to ask questions in a clear, direct and unambiguous manner and to use concrete stimuli (such as objects, pictures or photographs) to support the self-report by clarifying both the therapist's question and the child's verbal response. Care must be taken when selecting stimuli to ensure they are not overstimulating, distracting or confusing (Sturgess, Rodger and Ozanne, 2002).

Benjamin (1974, cited by Smith, 1993) 'delineated three parts to an interview: initiation, development and closing' (p. 171). The initiation phase of an interview involves:

- the therapist explaining the purpose of the interview, including its parameters, how long it should take, the type of topics to be discussed and how the therapist plans to use the information
- the therapist describing her role in relation to the client in the clinical setting
- the therapist endeavouring to establish mutual understanding, respect and trust with the client in order to build rapport and set the foundations for an effective therapeutic relationship.

The development phase of an interview involves:

- the therapist, in the role of interviewer, poses a series of questions to elicit information and to explore issues with the client
- having a list of planned questions or an outline of topics to be covered to help focus the interview and ensure important information, vital to an accurate baseline assessment and identifying relevant treatment objectives, is not omitted
- the therapist asking open questions that elicit a descriptive response, as opposed to closed questions that produce a one-word (yes, no, maybe) answer
- while specifically providing guidance on communicating with people with speech deficits, Lewis (1989) makes many good points that can be applied to general interviewing techniques. These include asking one question at a time, focusing on one subject at a time (and so encouraging a client to do the same), using short, simple sentences, being an active and patient listener and being prepared to rephrase a question in order to clarify a respondent's answer.

The closing phase of an interview involves:

- the therapist identifying that either the questions/topics to be addressed have all been covered and that she has obtained the necessary information for this stage of the assessment process or that the allotted time has expired
- the therapist indicating to the client that the interview is coming to a close
- the therapist making clear that the interview is finishing and that there is no further opportunity at this time to bring up new issues
- identifying another time for continuing with the interview if there is further relevant information to be discussed
- the therapist summarising the key points that have been discussed to double-check that she has correctly understood and interpreted the information gained, if time allows.

COMMUNICATION, INSIGHT AND CAPACITY ISSUES

One disadvantage of self-report is that the information provided 'may not accurately reflect patient performance' and the person's report of his functioning 'may vary considerably from actual performance observed by the therapist' (Hilko Culler, 1993, p. 212). When selecting self-report as an assessment method, the therapist should be aware that a number of conditions might make the interview difficult to conduct and could reduce the reliability of the data collected. Prior to an initial interview, the therapist should check referral data to see whether there are any factors that might indicate difficulties using a self-report method. These could include communication problems, arising from speech problems such as aphasia or dysarthria or from hearing impairment. Cognitive capacity to provide a reliable self-report also should be considered. When the referral indicates a diagnosis such as dementia, acute confusional state, stroke or traumatic brain injury, the therapist should be alert to the possibility of a related cognitive deficit and should be prepared to explore the issue of cognitive capacity to self-report. Extremes in mood state, such as depression or mania, can also affect the person's ability to engage effectively in the interview process and may be associated with skewed responses, for example a person with depression might underestimate his opportunities, resources and abilities, while a person who is feeling elated during a period of mania might overestimate his opportunities, resources and abilities. While it is very important to gain insight to the person's viewpoint whatever his condition, in cases where the person's level of insight is questionable it is particularly useful to compare self-report data with therapist observations, standardised test results and proxy report.

CULTURAL ISSUES AND SELF-REPORT DATA COLLECTION

When conducting any assessment, and in particular interviews, therapists should take into account the person's cultural background. It can be more difficult to establish good rapport when dealing with language barriers and differences in accepted forms of verbal and non-verbal communication. When the therapist and client cannot communicate directly, a bilingual interpreter, volunteer or family member can be used as a translator. Where possible, try to obtain an outside interpreter. While family members can be very helpful, they might not always be the best interpreter 'since they may be uncomfortable interpreting intense personal feelings . . . or may distort what has been said due to their own interpretations' (McCormack, Lorens and Glogoski, 1991, p. 21). In addition, there might be some information that a person prefers to keep confidential and he may not want to discuss some things in front of family members. Therapists should try to use interpreters of the same sex and age as the person where possible, because generation and gender differences can affect the interview, particularly when the person is a first-generation immigrant. In addition to language barriers, the therapist should be aware of other factors that could impede the assessment process. These can occur when individuals' backgrounds lead to a distrust of health and social care providers and the health and social care system, or when people have a strong sense that these do not fit with their cultural traditions (McCormack, Lorens and Glogoski, 1991). The therapist's goals for assessment, rehabilitation and empowerment may need to be adapted if the person comes from a culture where a reliance upon family for care and support following an accident or illness exists, as opposed to an expectation to work towards maximising remaining skills in order to return to a maximum level of independence.

Although self-report is primarily used by therapists in the initial stages of assessment to form a picture of the person and the problems to be addressed through therapy, self-report can also be a useful method for monitoring progress during intervention. Used formally, self-monitoring is 'a process whereby the patient records specific behaviours or thoughts as they occur' (Christiansen and Baum, 1991, p. 858). Self-report is particularly useful for monitoring any side effects related to an intervention, for example increased pain following a series of prescribed physiotherapy exercises. Some standardised self-report tools have been developed as outcome measures that can be used to evaluate progress over time; the COPM (Law *et al.*, 1991), for example, provides a useful change score when used for reassessment. In addition, self-report data are an essential component of any service evaluation. An increased emphasis on clinical governance and best value is linked to a requirement for involving people not just in decisions about their own service provision but also in an evaluation of the strengths and weaknesses of that service and an involvement with the identification of changes that need to be made to modernise service provision. The NHS Modernisation Agency (2002c), for example, has produced a service improvement guide entitled *Involving Patients and Carers*.

EXAMPLES OF SELF-REPORT ASSESSMENTS

In this section, a few standardised tests will be shared as examples of self-report measures that can be used by physiotherapists and/or occupational therapists.

CANADIAN OCCUPATIONAL PERFORMANCE MEASURE (COPM)

The COPM is a good example of a robust self-report measure that can be used with a wide range of clients ranging from school-aged children up to older adults and with people who have a wide range of diagnoses, including both physical and mental health problems. Law *et al.* (1991) developed the COPM as a measure of performance, including the importance of performance problems and the client's level of satisfaction with performance. The COPM is a well-established standardised assessment and outcome measure, which is now published in its third edition (Law *et al.* 1998). The COPM 'has been officially translated into 20 languages' and is used 'by occupational therapists in over 35 countries throughout the world' (Carswell *et al.*, 2004, p. 210). In a recent review of the clinical and research literature published on the COPM, Carswell *et al.* (2004) identify 88 papers that mention the COPM in their title or abstract and report upon its psychometric properties, its contribution to research outcomes and its contribution to occupational therapy practice; this range of publication from a wide variety of authors indicates how widely the COPM has become accepted both in practice and research.

The COPM has a semi-structured interview format. It is usually first completed as an initial assessment so that therapy objectives can be based upon problems selected by the client. The assessment covers the domains of self-care, productivity and leisure. The client rates identified occupational performance issues in terms of importance on a scale of 1 to 10 (10 = extremely important; 1 = not important at all) and then rates the most important issues in terms of performance (10 = able to do it well; 1 = not able to do it) and satisfaction with that performance (10 = extremely satisfied; 1 = not satisfied at all). Following an agreed period of intervention, the COPM is administered again and the client rates the same problem activities for performance and satisfaction, and his scores are summed and averaged. The difference between the initial, baseline scores and the follow-up scores are calculated to provide a change score, which indicates outcome. Although the COPM was primarily developed as a self-report tool, it can also be used successfully as a proxy measure with a carer, such as a parent or spouse. (*Note:* for an example of the COPM applied in practice, please see the case study 'Scott' at the end of this chapter and especially pp. 76 and 87–88.)

CHRONIC RESPIRATORY DISEASE QUESTIONNAIRE (CRQ)

The CRQ (Guyatt *et al.*, 1987) is a self-report questionnaire used as a clinical measure of quality of life for people with chronic lung disease and has been used for planning and evaluating therapy and for research. It comprises 20 questions that are divided across four domains: dyspnoea, fatigue, emotional function and mastery (defined as the extent to which a person feels able to cope with his illness and in control). Items are scored on a seven-point Likert-type scale, with a score of 7 indicating best possible level of function and 1 indicating worst level of function.

LIFE EXPERIENCES CHECKLIST (LEC)

The LEC was developed by Ager (1990) as a quality-of-life measure designed to gauge 'the range and extent of life experiences enjoyed by an individual' (p. 5). It comprises a 50-item checklist, divided into five domains: home, leisure, relationships, freedom and opportunities. The LEC can be used 'with a wide range of client groups, including individuals with learning difficulties, the elderly and both mental health in-patients and out-patients' (p. 5). The LEC can be used as a self-rating tool or as a proxy measure. For clients/carers who have sufficient reading comprehension, the LEC is administered as a self-report checklist, and some services post it to the client and/or carer for completion. It can also be administered as an interview. The LEC has a dichotomous scoring system, in which either an item applies to the client or not; so each question has been written to elicit a clear yes or no response, and the client (or therapist if undertaking as an interview) simply ticks the items that apply. For example, an item from the leisure domain is: 'I visit friends or relatives for a meal at least once per month' (p. 2 of the LEC form).

VISUAL ANALOGUE PAIN SCALE (VAPS)

Visual analogue scales (VAS) have been used by therapists since the late 1960s. This form of measurement was introduced by Aiken (1969, cited by Cole *et al.*, 1995). A VAS comprises either a 100 mm or 30 cm line, drawn either horizontally or vertically, and labelled with two verbal expressions at the extreme ends to indicate the maximum and minimum points on a continuum of a sensation or feeling. A VAS is used for the assessment of intensity or magnitude of a subjective experience, such as pain, breathlessness or fatigue. The most commonly used VAS is the visual analogue pain scale (VAPS; Strong *et al.*, 1990), which is a widely used means for obtaining a self-report from clients on the intensity of their pain. The scale uses a horizontal line of 100 mm with ends labelled 'no pain' on the left and 'unbearable pain' on the right. The client is asked to mark or point to the position on the scale that represents the intensity of his pain, and the therapist then measures the distance from the left end to the client's mark (range 0 to 100). Therefore, a client must be able to conceptualise a sensory continuum and partition a closed range as an indication of their experience of pain on that continuum. Therapists find this simple to administer and easy to score (Pynsent, 1993). Chow (2001) used the VAPS with recipients of total hip replacement and as a proxy measure with carers who were asked to rate the perceived pain intensity that their care receiver was experiencing. Different versions of the VAS have also been used to rate other conditions, for example there is a visual analogue scale for dyspnoea (Gift, 1989), which has been used as a client's self-report of their difficulty breathing, in which the person chooses a point on the line that best represents their current degree of breathlessness, with the ends being marked with items such as 'not at all breathless' and 'worst possible breathlessness'.

OCCUPATIONAL PERFORMANCE HISTORY INTERVIEW (OPHI)

The OPHI was developed by Kielhofner and Henry (1988). It covers the domains of organisation of daily routines, life roles, interests, values and goals, perceptions of ability and responsibility, and environmental influences. The OPHI focuses on both the past and present for each area and comprises 39 questions. There is a Life History Narrative Form for summarising data. Scoring uses a five-point ordinal scale (5 = adaptive; 1 = maladaptive).

PROXY REPORT

In addition to seeking information directly from a client, information can be obtained from a number of other (proxy) sources. A *proxy* is defined as 'a person or agency of substitute recognized by law to act for, and in the best interest of, the patient' (Centre for Advanced Palliative Care, 2005). But in the context of therapy assessment, the term proxy is used more widely to refer to an informant (for example carer or professional) who has knowledge about the circumstances or condition of the client and who is able to share that knowledge with the person's permission or without breaking laws of confidentiality.

A proxy report is also sometimes referred to as an *informant interview* (Borg and Bruce, 1991). A proxy or informant report can be particularly helpful when a client has communication difficulties or lacks insight into his problems and level of ability, when therapists need to prioritise referrals prior to assessment, when the therapist wants to understand how a primary carer (such as a parent or spouse) is coping with their carer role or when the therapist wishes to check whether the client's perspectives and priorities are consistent with those of his family/teacher/ health care providers. Where the client has a condition that affects his ability to provide an adequate self-report, use of a proxy as translator to interpret sign language, symbol boards, facial expression and body language or as someone who knows the person's pronunciation and use of language sufficiently well to translate is very helpful. Also, where the client has communication difficulties the relevance of the perceptions and views of the family/carers becomes even more critical (Tullis and Nicol, 1999), such as when working with children, with people following a stroke and with people with dementia. Swain (2004), for example, states that 'though a physiotherapist working, for instance, with a person with learning difficulties may have difficulties understanding him or her, it is often the case that others, including members of a young person's family, other professions or an advocate, are "tuned in" to him or her' (p. 218).

Proxy sources may include:

- the person's primary carer (either an informal carer, e.g. a family member, neighbour or volunteer, or a formal carer – often referred to as a care-giver – e.g. a warden, nursing home staff or home help)
- other members of the therapist's multidisciplinary team (e.g. occupational therapist, physiotherapist, speech and language therapist, psychologist, social worker, nurse, doctor)
- other health professionals involved with the client's care (e.g. their GP, health visitor or district nurse)
- other professionals working with the client (e.g. a case manager, teacher or lawyer).

Proxy report is of great value because, in the majority of cases, other people will spend much more time than the therapist with the client and will have opportunities to see how the client is managing over a longer period and in a different and/or wider range of settings. For example, in an in-patient setting, nurses on the ward will be in greater contact with the person; in an outpatient setting, the parent or partner will have seen how the person is managing in the home environment, while a colleague, employer or teacher could share information about the person's abilities and problems in a work or school setting.

A proxy report may be obtained in person through interviewing the proxy face to face or over the telephone, through case conferences, ward rounds and team meetings or via written data. Written information from family members and neighbours might involve letters or the use of standardised or unstandardised checklists and questionnaires. Written information from other professionals might comprise referrals, letters, medical notes and assessment reports. Increasingly, much of this information is held in electronic formats and, depending on the clinical setting, might be accessible via a computer database, for example in a secondary care setting via the hospital's intranet. Reports and information from colleagues from other organisations and settings might be sent via internal mail, post, fax or email.

Proxy report is being increasingly used to help therapists screen referrals to help determine whether the referral is appropriate and/or to help prioritise referrals. Green *et al.* (2005) undertook a study that explored the value of parent and teacher reports using two standardised questionnaires in order to identify which referrals would require a full clinic-based observational assessment. They found that parent report was quite reliable in the identification of appropriate referrals. But they had a poor response rate from the teacher proxies and found that the increased time required by the therapists to chase schools to increase the return rate resulted in little cost benefit for their goal of better managing their waiting list.

The initial interaction with the person's family/carer can provide the foundation for building effective partnerships with carers. This can be critical to support the person and their carer to manage complex issues in the home/community environment and to integrate the intervention into the person's daily routines at home. An initial interview with a carer can serve several purposes, including the forming of a working relationship, the gathering of information about the client and his environment and the provision of information to the carer about the therapist's role, strategies for supporting the client, available services and carer support structures. In some practice settings (such as an acute, short-stay in-patient setting), the therapist may only have the opportunity to meet the carer on one or two occasions, for example when the family come onto a ward to visit or during a therapist's discharge assessment home visit. In this case, the therapist may need to interweave both the obtaining of data for assessment and intervention in the form of instruction, advice, support etc. A study by Clark, Corcoran and Gitlin (1995) identified four main types of interaction categories that occur between therapists and carers during assessment and treatment. These were:

1. *caring interactions* that focused on friendliness and support
2. *partnering interactions* that involved seeking and acknowledging input and reflective feedback to help carers make changes/modify behaviour or to affirm existing carer practices
3. *informing interactions* that involved gathering information, explaining information and clarifying information
4. *directing interactions* that involved the provision of instruction and advice.

The type of information provided by a proxy will vary considerably depending upon the amount of contact the proxy has with the person being assessed, their relationship and their degree of involvement. The therapist needs to be aware of these factors in order to evaluate the value and reliability of the proxy's report. In some instances, it can be useful to seek informal and/or standardised assessment data from more than one proxy, for example both a child's parents, a parent and teacher or all the children of a client. A mother and father might have different perceptions about a child's abilities and needs, as might children in relation to their parent's condition and problems. When interpreting discrepancies in viewpoints amongst multiple proxy reports, it is helpful to reflect on the amount of time a proxy spends with the client and also any cues that suggest the nature of the relationship between a proxy and a client. For example, Abidin (1995), author of the Parenting Stress Index (PSI), states that when the PSI is administered to both a child's parents 'spreads of up to 10 raw score points between mothers and fathers are to be expected' (p. 8). Abidin notes that where the mother is the primary carer of a child with a behavioural disorder therapists should expect the father's PSI scores to be lower and he explains that 'this does not indicate that fathers' perceptions are less clouded by their own situations, but [that] mothers' greater involvement with child care leaves them open to greater stress associated with their children's behaviour' (p. 8).

EXAMPLES OF ASSESSMENTS THAT USE INFORMATION FROM A PROXY

MEMORY AND BEHAVIOUR PROBLEM CHECKLIST (MBPC)

The MBPC is used with carers of people with dementia. The original version was published by Zarit, Todd and Zarit (1986) and a revised version has been reported by Teri *et al.* (1992). It can be administered by interview or by using a self-completion survey format. The MBPC covers items such as sleep disturbance, wandering, aggressive outbursts and help needed with self-care. Items are scored on a five-point ordinal scale that measures the frequency and intensity of observed problems (0 = problem has never been observed; 4 = indicates that problem occurs daily or more often).

PEDIATRIC EVALUATION OF DISABILITY INVENTORY (PEDI)

The PEDI was developed by Hayley *et al.* (1992) to assess the functioning of children aged six months to 7.5 years and covers the domains of self-care, mobility and social functioning. Proxy report can be gained from parents, or from teachers or rehabilitation professionals who are familiar with the child. The PEDI assesses capability using a functional skills scale and performance of functional activities using a carer assistance scale. A modifications scale records environmental modifications and equipment used by the child in routine activities of daily living (ADL) (also see pp. 75–76).

SCALE FOR ASSESSING COPING SKILLS

This assessment was developed by Whelan and Speake (1979) to assess adolescents and adults with learning difficulties. Proxy report can be obtained from either the parents or a professional who knows the client well. The Scale for Assessing Coping Skills covers three domains: self-help, social academic and interpersonal. The scale comprises 36 items that are described at five levels of difficulty (a = easiest level; e = most difficult level). Items are scored on two ordinal scales: a four-point scale of whether the particular ability exists (1 = can do without help or supervision, 2 = can do but only with help or supervision, 3 = cannot yet do, 4 = do not know whether he can do this) and a three-point scale (numbered 5 to 7) of whether the ability is adequately used or not (5 = uses this ability in an adequate amount, 6 = does not use this in an adequate amount, 7 = there is no opportunity to do this).

INFANT AND TODDLER SYMPTOM CHECKLIST

This is a proxy measure (developed by DeGangi *et al.*, 1995) for use with parents of seven- to 30-month-old infants and toddlers. The symptom checklist can be used as a stand-alone screen to identify infants and toddlers 'who are at risk for sensory-integrative disorders, attentional deficits, and emotional and behavioural problems' (p. 1). It can also be used alongside other observational developmental measures to aid diagnosis. The measure covers nine test domains: self-regulation; attention; sleep; eating or feeding; dressing, bathing and touch; movement; listening and language; looking and sight; and attachment/emotional functioning. It comprises five age-banded checklists (for seven to nine, 10 to 12, 13 to 18, 19 to 24 and 25 to 30 months) and a general screening version that can be used across a seven- to 30-month-old child population when it is not convenient to select an age-appropriate version, for example handed to parents to complete in an outpatient clinic's waiting room. The symptom checklist can either be given to parents to self-complete or as part of an interview. For parent self-completion, the authors provide an example cover sheet that explains the scoring and asks parents to record demographic information and details about the child's birth, delivery, medical problems etc. The manual states that it takes approximately ten minutes to complete and when I asked a parent to try completing a 25- to 30-month checklist for her toddler she said it was easy to do and took her five minutes. Most items are rated on a three-point ordinal scale: 'never or sometimes', if the child has never had this difficulty or has it infrequently or some of the time, 'most times', if this a difficulty the child experiences frequently or most of the time at present, and 'past', if this was a problem in the past but is no longer a problem.

CANADIAN OCCUPATIONAL PERFORMANCE MEASURE (COPM)

Although the COPM (Law *et al.*, 1991; see earlier summary on p. 56) was designed predominately as a self-report measure, it can also be used as a proxy report measure with a carer (such as a parent or spouse). Carswell *et al.* (2004) found a number of studies in their literature review that 'showed how the COPM could be used to gather information from proxy respondents on behalf of clients who cannot report reliably on their own occupational performance' (p. 216).

MEASURES THAT ASSESS THE PROXY

The main reason therapists choose to assess a carer is to explore levels of burden associated with the caring role and to evaluate the carer's ability to provide the required level of care. Within this type of assessment, therapists may measure physical burden and/or emotional burden; these domains include constructs, such as stress and quality of life. A couple of measures that assess the proxy are provided as examples below. More rarely, the therapist may assess a paid care provider (such as a home care worker, support worker, nursing home assistant or teaching assistant) in order to identify their knowledge, skills and level of confidence and to provide education to address any identified gaps in order to facilitate meeting the client's needs.

In some cases, where the proxy is an informal carer, such as a spouse, parent, sibling or child, the carer may also be the focus of part of the assessment. Where carer burden is identified, and intervention, such as respite, education and counselling, is called for, then the proxy also might become a service user in his or her own right.

LIFE SATISFACTION INDEX – PARENTS (LSI-P)

This is a self-report tool. The LSI-P (Renwick and Reid, 1992a) was developed as a research tool to explore the nature of quality of life for parents of a child with a disability. The LSI-P address five domains: general well-being, interpersonal relationships, personal development, personal fulfilment and leisure and recreation. The LSI-P is a 45-item index (nine items per domain) based on a series of statements that the parent rates on a Likert-type scale. Items are scored on a six-point scale: 1 = strongly disagree, 2 = disagree, 3 neither agree nor disagree, 4 = agree, 5 = strongly agree and 6 = not applicable. The LSI-P is a useful assessment to use with parents at the first appointment. They can be asked to complete it at home or it can be administered as an interview, which provides the therapist with the opportunity to discuss parents' responses to statements.

CAREGIVER STRAIN INDEX

Robinson's (1983) index comprises 13 items covering stressful aspects of caring, including demand on time, physical strain, emotional adjustment, changes in personal plans, work adjustment, sleep disturbance, inconvenience and upset related to changes in the cared-for person. Construct and predictive validity were established by the developer on a sample of 85 family carers of older people admitted to hospital owing to physical conditions (Robinson, 1983). The original version uses a dichotomous two-point scale. O'Brien (1993) revised the test and used a five-point Likert-type scale in a study to explore carer stress for people looking after someone with multiple sclerosis. The five-point-scale version was also used by Chow (2001) to investigate carers' burden before and after their family members had total hip replacements.

PARENTING STRESS INDEX (PSI)

The PSI (Abidin, 1995) is a proxy measure developed for use with parents of children aged one month to 12 years. The PSI is a normative assessment and original norms were based on 2633 mothers (age 16 to 61 years, mean age 30.9) of children aged one month to 12 years. References are provided for research using the PSI with a wide range of child populations, including birth defects (for example spina bifida, congenital heart disease), communication disorders (for example hearing impairment, speech deficits), attention deficit hyperactivity disorder (ADHD), autism, developmental disability, learning disabled, premature infants, at risk/abused children and other health problems (such as asthma, diabetes and otitis media). Originally developed in the US with norms mainly based on a white American population, the PSI has since been used in a number of cross-cultural studies and has been translated into Spanish, Chinese, Portuguese, Finnish, Japanese, Italian, Hebrew, Dutch and French. The manual states that the 'PSI was designed to be an instrument in which the primary value would be to identify parent-child systems that were under stress and at risk of the development of dysfunctional parenting behaviour or behaviour problems in the child involved' (Abidin, 1995, p. 6). The manual describes the PSI as a screening and diagnostic tool. The parent is given a seven-page reusable item booklet containing a front sheet with scoring instructions and 120 questions. The parent is given a separate answer sheet/profile form and is asked to circle his/her answer for each of the 101 PSI items and on the 19-item Life Stresses scale if required. The therapist then tears off the perforated edge and opens up the form, where inside answers are transformed to numerical scores that are summed and then plotted on the profile. For most items, an ordinal scale is used. The majority of items are scored on a five-point Likert-type scale: strongly agree, agree, not sure, disagree and strongly disagree. (*Note*: for more details on the PSI see a detailed test critique provided in Chapter 11, Table 11.2, pp. 354–9.)

OBSERVATIONAL ASSESSMENT METHODS

Therapists should not just rely upon self- and proxy report for the assessment, because some research studies have found discrepancies between reported and observed function. Some authors state that the most reliable form of functional assessment is considered to be direct observation (Law, 1993; Skruppy, 1993). For example, Skruppy (1993) conducted a study in which a sample of 30 subjects was interviewed and then observed performing ADL tasks using a standardised test. People without ADL limitations were able to report their abilities accurately. However, Skruppy found that patients with limitations in ADL functioning were aware of their difficulties but overestimated their abilities during the interview.

Although the term *observational methods* is used here, it refers more widely to methods in which the therapist directly uses her senses to assess some aspect of the client's problem or situation. Although visual observations and the use of verbal instructions/questions to elicit the client's response as a behaviour/reply will form the basis for a significant proportion of direct therapy assessment, the use of other senses can be very important. For example, some assessment methods use active listening (for example auscultation of lung sounds), smell (smells can help the therapist identify a problem with incontinence or the risk of the person consuming food that has gone off) or touch (where the therapist is assessing the degree of resistance in a muscle as an indication of stiffness or spasticity). Therapists are trained in direct observational skills, and many therapy assessments will involve some sort of observation. This method of assessment provides data about the person's level of ability performing specific tasks in specific environments and also yields useful information from the process used to attempt the assessment task and from the quality of the person's performance. Therapists, particularly physiotherapists, also use direct observational/auditory assessment to measure physiological processes, such as respiratory rate, blood pressure and heart rate using methods such as percussion, palpation and sphygmomanometers (Cole *et al.*, 1995).

Occupational therapists are trained in activity analysis, and a particular area of their expertise is considered to be 'in assessing clients and drawing inferences based on their direct observation of the client's performance' (Law, 1993, p. 234). Fisher (2003a) refers to this as a 'performance analysis', which she defines as 'the observational evaluation of the quality of a person's task performance to identify discrepancies between the demands of a task and the skill of the person' (p. 2). She recommends an assessment approach that involves the therapist observing and evaluating a client's skill as he 'engages in the course of actions that comprises the process of performing occupations' (p. 3).

There are several ways of observing clients, and therapists create opportunities to observe clients in a variety of formal, structured activities and informal, unstructured situations. For example, therapists may:

- administer a standardised test that requires the performance of test items which are observed and recorded
- set up an activity for the person to perform and then observe from the sidelines
- choose to be a participant-observer who will observe the client's performance while engaging in an activity or task with the person.

If the therapist can create opportunities to interact informally and spontaneously as a participant-observer in situations where role differentiation is less defined than in a formal testing situation, she can often obtain information (for example on roles, interests, values and functional ability) that might otherwise be difficult to assess accurately or might not come to light (Smith, 1993). Therefore, it is desirable to build opportunities for informal contact into the assessment if possible, particularly where an in-depth assessment is required and the therapeutic relationship is likely to last for some time (such as with a person with a serious mental illness who will have a therapist care coordinator from a community mental health team or a person with a stroke or head injury who will be treated in a rehabilitation unit over several weeks or months). Informal situations can be created even in more formal hospital environments, for example by escorting a person from the ward to the therapy department and seeing how they move, manage the lift or explore and purchase items in the hospital shop or restaurant. It can also be useful to allow a few minutes before or after a treatment session to interact informally with the person and their family or carer, for example in the waiting room or while family are visiting the person's bedside on the ward.

The ability of an individual to perform a set task to a specified standard is straightforward to observe. However, the underlying functions that affect task performance, such as the functioning of the sensory, perceptual and cognitive systems, cannot be observed directly. Within the therapy professions, it is accepted that therapists will draw inferences from observed behaviours about underlying functional status. The accuracy and value of observational assessment is dependent on the expertise of the therapist undertaking the observation and the thoroughness and objectivity with which observations are recorded.

> A key to successful evaluation lies in the therapist's skills in observation. The abilities to see and listen well must be accompanied by the abilities to sort through the mass of perceptual and conceptual data that may be presented and to focus on what is relevant to the process. (Smith, 1993, p. 170)

Therapists should be aware that there is a risk when making inferences from observed behaviour that their own, subjective, feelings will influence the behaviours which the therapist focuses upon during the observation and the way in which these behaviours are interpreted. Therapists construct inferences in the form of hypotheses, and this is linked to a process called diagnostic reasoning, which is explored later in Chapter 10.

There are some areas of assessment where it is particularly useful to use a formal or standardised assessment method rather than informal observation. For example, when measuring range of movement informal observational assessment has been found to be unreliable, and goniometric measurement has been found to be preferable (Atkins, 2004). Atkins also cites literature indicating 'that the visual inspection of gait is unsystematic, subjective and observer skill dependent' and states that 'even skilled observers miss subtle abnormalities and have difficulty quantifying simple parameters such as cadence, stride length and velocity' (p. 361). However, sometimes a therapist may be aware that a standardised measurement would be more reliable but might not have access to the relevant equipment or test, or be unable to apply it in her clinical setting. For example, gait analysis is often undertaken as a subjective observation in the client's own home or in a ward setting, but it can be measured more objectively when equipment is available in a physiotherapy department to undertake gait laboratory analysis, such as force and pressure measurements at the foot–ground interface and using electromyography to provide data on muscle action potentials.

A large proportion of therapy and rehabilitation assessments (both standardised and non-standardised) involve the observation of the performance of ADL. Examples include the:

- Functional Independence Measure (FIM; Granger *et al.*, 1993)
- Klein–Bell Activities of Daily Living Scale (Klein and Bell, 1982)

- Rivermead ADL Assessment (Whiting and Lincoln, 1980; Lincoln and Edmans, 1989)
- Rivermead Mobility Index (Collen *et al.*, 1991), which assesses a range of mobility tasks considered essential to basic ADL.

Another large group of assessments comprise batteries of observational tasks developed to assess functioning at an impairment level. Examples include the:

- Alberta Infant Motor Scale (AIMS; Piper *et al.*, 1992)
- Chedoke-McMaster Stroke Assessment (Gowland *et al.*, 1993)
- Chessington Occupational Therapy Neurological Assessment Battery (COTNAB; Tyerman *et al.*, 1986)
- Peabody Developmental Motor Scales (Folio and Fewell, 1983)
- Rivermead Perceptual Assessment Battery (RPAB; Whiting *et al.*, 1985).

A few observational assessments provide data across several levels of function. Examples of observational assessments that examine performance of ADL, at the disability level, and provide information about functional limitations and/or underlying impairment, such as motor and cognitive functioning, include the:

- Arnadottir OT-ADL Neurobehavioural Evaluation (A-ONE; Arnadottir, 1990)
- Assessment of Motor Process Skills (AMPS; Fisher, 2003a)
- Kitchen Task Assessment (KTA; Baum and Edwards, 1993)
- Structured Observational Test of Function (SOTOF; Laver and Powell, 1995).

EXAMPLES OF OBSERVATIONAL ASSESSMENT

GROSS MOTOR FUNCTION MEASURE (GMFM)

The GMFM (Russell *et al.*, 1993) is a criterion-referenced test that can be used to evaluate change in gross motor function over time with children with cerebral palsy (CP). The GMFM focuses assessment on how much of an activity the child can accomplish (as opposed to the quality of motor performance, that is how well a child can manage the motor activity). The test comprises 88 test items that assess motor activities in five dimensions: lying and rolling, sitting, crawling, standing, and walking. The items are scored on a four-point rating scale (0 = does not initiate, 1 = initiates, 2 = partially completes, 3 = completes). With most children, the whole test can be administered in 45 to 60 minutes. Some therapists choose to video the child performing items, and this can help the therapist, child and parent to observe changes in functioning on the items over time. It has been shown to be a reliable measure of change in motor function in children with CP (Russell *et al.*, 1993, 1989; Russell, 1987). The GMFM has been used as a means for structuring both therapists' and parents' judgements of children's motor function (Russell *et al.*, 1993; Russell, 1987); so in addition to being an observational measure it can also be used to collect proxy data.

CHESSINGTON OCCUPATIONAL THERAPY NEUROLOGICAL ASSESSMENT BATTERY (COTNAB)

The COTNAB (Tyerman *et al.*, 1986) was developed as an assessment of people with neurological conditions (studies focused on samples of people with head injury or stroke) and covers four domains: visual perception, constructional ability, sensory motor ability and ability to follow instructions. Each domain is examined through the observation of three tasks, giving a total of 12 observational test items. The test was originally standardised for people aged 16–65 years, but later studies, by Laver and Huchinson (1994) and Stanley *et al.* (1995), examined the performance of older people on the COTNAB and produced norms for an elderly population.

The COTNAB uses raw scores and time taken for each of the 12 subtests to produce derived scores, which are referred to as grades and are labelled ability, time and overall performance. The COTNAB is a normative test and the grading system is based on standard deviation (s.d.) and percentile equivalents, thus enabling the therapist to compare a person's test performance with that expected for a person of the same age and sex.

COMBINING METHODS

'The critical advice here is to obtain multiple measures to produce a complete assessment of the client's progress. It is especially important to use multiple measures, because the measures might produce different results' (Barlow, Hayes and Nelson, 1984, p. 124). The most comprehensive way in which to conduct an assessment is to collect data from several sources using a range of assessment methods and then compare the data, looking for similarities and differences in the findings. A major reason why therapists choose to interview people about their function rather than conduct an observational assessment is the time required (Skruppy, 1993). As it usually is not feasible to observe all areas of function relevant to the person, the most reliable method is to interview individuals and their proxies about their performance in the full range of their activities and then select a few key activities/areas of functioning for direct observation/testing. While self-report and proxy report can be useful adjuncts to observational data, they rarely replace observational assessment completely. Green *et al.* (2005) report that a parent report was valuable but that it did not replace the full clinical assessment undertaken by the therapist, as there were inadequate levels of specificity obtained from the proxy measure. Hammell (2004) warns that observational assessment cannot be a truly objective exercise because judgements made by a therapist reflect the particular values of that therapist which may not be shared by the client who is being assessed. Therefore, the most valid and reliable assessment will combine data-collection methods and compare and contrast the findings from each of the sources. The more significant the decisions that are to be made from the assessment, such as deciding who is fit to return home and who might require long-term institutional care, the more critical it is that the assessment fully represents all viewpoints.

Sturgess, Rodger and Ozanne (2002) describe the benefits of combining observational methods, such as videotape, with self-report and parent reports when assessing young children. They cite research which demonstrates that children's views are different from their parents'. They note that the parent can only provide an opinion about how they think a child feels and that this can be contaminated by the adult's view of how they think the child should feel or how they think they would have felt themselves in a similar situation.

Sometimes the therapist might obtain quite different, and even conflicting, information from different sources. When this happens, it is helpful for the therapist to develop a series of hypotheses about the client and his situation and then to examine these hypotheses using all the information available. When interpreting hypotheses using discrepant information from different sources, it is helpful to judge the data in the context of the motivations, fears and viewpoints of the people who provided the conflicting opinions. Factors that influence performance, such as pain, fatigue, medication and mood, can result in people forming different, yet valid, perceptions about a person's ability. What the therapist might observe a person do in a hospital environment on one occasion may be very different from what the person's family observe them doing regularly at home.

EXAMPLES OF HOW THERAPISTS COMBINE DIFFERENT ASSESSMENT METHODS

Examples of how therapists combine different assessment methods can be found in the literature. For example, in a study described by two senior physiotherapists and a research fellow in clinical gerontology (Wright, Cross and Lamb, 1998), the authors report collecting data of pre-morbid abilities by report from patients and their carers and selecting two standardised measures, the Rivermead Mobility Index (RMI; Collen *et al*., 1991), which can be scored by self-report or direct observation and the Barthel Index (BI; Mahoney and Barthel, 1965), which can also be scored by either self-report or observation. For their study, they report using observation by physiotherapists to collect data on the RMI and that data on the BI were collected from the medical and nursing assessments and had been recorded by direct observation of people's performance by the nursing staff.

DeGangi *et al*. (1995), authors of the Infant and Toddler Symptom Checklist (a proxy measure developed for use with parents of seven- to 30-month-old infants and toddlers), recommend that for screening purposes the symptom checklist should be combined with other observational tools and suggest the Test of Sensory Functions in Infants (DeGangi and Greenspan, 1989) 'a criterion-referenced instrument designed to measure sensory processing in infants from four to 18 months of age' (DeGangi *et al*., 1995, p. 4). If clinicians wish to use the Infant and Toddler Symptom Checklist for diagnostic purposes, the authors recommend that they should combine this parent proxy measure with 'traditional developmental tests . . . such as the Bayley Scales of Infant Development (Bayley, 1993) and observational tools that assess sustained attention . . . such as the Test of Attention in Infants (DeGangi, 1995), parent–child interactions, and sensory processing and reactivity. The Symptom Checklist helps validate clinical observations and provides an effective format for eliciting parent concerns' (DeGangi *et al*., 1995, p. 4).

Jacobs (1993) describes how therapists should combine methods to provide a thorough assessment of a person's ability to work. The suggested assessment process included:

1. 'Review of medical, educational and vocational records.
2. Interviews with the patient, family, employer, teachers and other personnel.
3. Observation.
4. Inventories and checklists.
5. Standardised and nonstandardised evaluations'. (p. 228)

An example of an assessment that combines methods is the Pediatric Evaluation of Disability Inventory (PEDI) (see pp. 59–60). The PEDI (Hayley *et al*., 1992) is a good example of a therapy assessment that combines data-collection methods within a standardised assessment. The PEDI requires the use of therapist observation, interview with the parent and judgement of professionals familiar with the child. The assessment covers three domains: self-care, mobility and social function. (*Note:* the PEDI is described in more detail in the case study 'Scott' at the end of this chapter, pp. 75–6.)

In this chapter, we have explored how therapists use a wide range of data-collection methods and sources of information in order to undertake a thorough assessment. These methods and sources are summarised in Figure 2.1 (below).

DOCUMENTATION

The therapist needs to find logical ways to structure and document the vast amount of information and observations that are obtained when she combines data-collection methods. One method commonly used is that of problem-orientated documentation (see Christiansen and Baum, 1991), which is a structured system of documentation that has four basic components:

1. a summary of subjective data (gathered from the client and any proxy)
2. a summary of any objective data (gathered from structured observations or the administration of standardised tests)
3. a problem list that is generated from both sources of data
4. a plan for treatment.

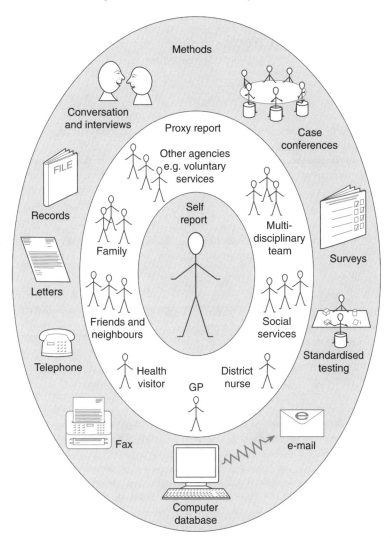

Figure 2.1 The wide range of data-collection used by therapists. *Figure reprinted from Laver Fawcett AJ (2002) Assessment. In A Turner, M Foster and S Johnson (Eds) Occupational Therapy and Physical Dysfunction: Principles, Skills and Practice. London, Churchill Livingstone. Ch. 5, pp. 107–144. Copyright (2002), with permission from Elsevier.*

These are sometimes referred to as SOAP notes (for an example SOAP entry, see Box 2.1 below), which stands for: subjective, objective, assessment (the analysis of data to formulate an understanding of the client's problems) and plan (for intervention/management/treatment). Identified problems are numbers. Each subsequent entry in the notes can refer to one or more problems, with the related problem number written in the margin. Entries are only made when there is something of significance to report, such as new information or a change in functioning. So the last entry for a numbered problem should be the most up to date, regardless of when it was written. Not every SOAP heading has to be used for each entry, for example the therapist may record something said by the client and her assessment of what this meant but have not undertaken any related direct measurement (nor would she need to take action at this point); in this case entries will be made under the headings S and A only.

Box 2.1 Example SOAP notes

S = Subjective This includes relevant comments, feelings or opinions made by the client/carer about a specific problem.

Examples

- Mr Brown says he doesn't know why he had to come today (refusing to join reminiscence group).
- Spoke to wife on the telephone: Mrs Brown reports her husband was very agitated this morning and didn't want to get on the ambulance to come to the day hospital.

O = Objective This is what the therapist does, observes or measures, and should be repeatable had it been undertaken by another therapist. Treatment/interventions given can also be recorded here, in addition to assessment information.

Examples

- Reassessed Mr Brown on the six-item Cognitive Impairment Test (6-CIT) to see if there was further decline in mental state. Scored 21/28. Previous score from GP referral undertaken two months ago was 14/28, indicating an increased level of impairment.
- Tried reality-orientation techniques with Mr Brown in a one-to-one session for 30 minutes, orientating him to where he was, why his GP had referred him to the day hospital, day, date, time and looked at the newspaper together.

A = Analysis This is a statement of the therapist's professional opinion based on the information recorded under S and O. Hypotheses with therapist's rationale can be written here.

Examples

- Mr Brown's 6-CIT scores indicate increased level of cognitive impairment and Mr Brown appeared more disorientated and agitated today; this may be related to multi-infarct dementia and Mr Brown may have suffered from another infarct. He might also have an infection that is causing the sudden deterioration in function.
- Mr Brown appeared to respond well to the one-to-one attention and reality-orientation approach.

P = Plan This is what the therapist plans to do about the problem, in the short or long term.

Examples

- Ask duty psychiatrist to undertake a physical examination today and check for a chest infection, urinary tract infection etc.
- Report to consultant psychiatrist at the next multidisciplinary team meeting the change in 6-CIT scores.
- Involve Mr Brown in a reality-orientation group each morning on arrival to day hospital.
- Train Mrs Brown in the reality-orientation approach for her to use with Mr Brown at home.

Therapists need to be scrupulous about their documentation and record keeping to prevent being exposed to claims of negligence or breach of confidentiality laws. Therapists must make their records carefully and avoid abbreviated or ambiguous notes and ensure any handwritten notes are legible. All documentation should not be open to misinterpretation as therapists may have to rely on them should their practice face a legal challenge, which could occur several years later. Therefore, notes should be accurate, contemporaneous, concise, legible, logical in sequence and signed after each entry.

CONFIDENTIALITY

When considering the collection of information about a client and his carer, confidentiality is critically important. Occupational therapists and physiotherapists are both ethically and legally obliged to safeguard confidential information relating to a client (College of Occupational Therapists, 2000; Chartered Society of Physiotherapy, 2002c, 2002d). These documents provide clear guidelines related to confidentiality. The CSP *Rules of Professional Conduct* (Chartered Society of Physiotherapy, 2002c) Rule 3 pertains to confidentiality and is divided into four sections:

1. confidentiality within the context of a multiprofessional team (p. 23)
2. how to handle requests for information (p. 23)
3. how to handle extraneous information, such as knowledge of criminal activities, evidence of abuse or environmental issues (e.g. an infestation by fleas or structural damage to a patient's home) (pp. 23–24)
4. security of patient information (p. 24).

In addition, the CSP's (2001b) Rule 4 (p. 13) relates to confidentiality and states: 'Physiotherapy assistants shall ensure the confidentiality and security of information acquired in a professional capacity.'

The *Code of Ethics and Professional Conduct for Occupational Therapists* (College of Occupational Therapists, 2005f, p. 6) states that a therapist may only disclose information (such as the client's diagnosis, treatment, prognosis, personal circumstances or future requirements) under one of three conditions:

1. the client has given consent
2. there is legal justification (e.g. by statute or court order)
3. it is considered to be in the public interest in order to prevent serious harm, injury or damage to the client, carer or any other person.

A good example of the third point is provided by the *Physiotherapy Assistants Code of Conduct* (Chartered Society of Physiotherapy, 2002d), Rule 4, which provides some examples and offers guidance as to how to deal with some of the complex situations that arise in respect of confidentiality.

> A patient is proposing to undertake an activity which because of their clinical and/or other condition could be harmful to themselves and/or others, e.g. driving or operating potentially dangerous machinery. The assistant must discuss this with the supervising physiotherapist who should take appropriate action. (Chartered Society of Physiotherapy, 2002d, Rule 4)

Therapists are obliged to keep all information secure and only release records to people who have a legitimate right and need to access them. Therapists should be aware of local and national policies on electronic notes (which include emails, computerised records, letters and faxes) and should adhere to these policies. They should also be aware of other codes of practice, policies and law relating to confidentiality issues, such as the Data Protection Act 1998, Human Rights Act 1998, Access to Personal Files Act 1987, Access to Medical Records Act 1988, Access to Health Records Act 1990 and the Patient's Charter 1994 (College of Occupational Therapists, 2000).

The security of information and records is very important. The CSP recommends that:

> Patients' clinical records, whether they are held in paper format or electronic format, must be stored in a secure manner. The holding of electronic records must comply with local Trust protocols, usually administered by Caldicott guardians and in conjunction with the Data Protection Act (1998). When passing sensitive and confidential information via email, it must be transmitted by a secure server or encrypted. If a fax is used, ensure the person who requires the information is available to receive it directly, usually by making immediate contact before transmitting the information. (Chartered Society of Physiotherapy, 2002d)

FURTHER READING

For students, the process of selecting and pulling together the results of a number of different methods of assessment may feel daunting. Case histories/studies/scenarios can be an excellent way of understanding how theory translates into practice and of illustrating an approach in a clinical setting. In addition to the detailed case study presented below, the following references may also be of interest.

- Baum, Perlmutter and Edwards (2000) in their article on 'Measuring function in Alzheimer's disease'. The paper describes a range of measures including self-report, proxy and observational measures and illustrates how these can be applied to an assessment process through the case of a 62-year-old man with dementia cared for by his wife.
- Unsworth's (1999) text *Cognitive and Perceptual Dysfunction: A Clinical Reasoning Approach to Evaluation and Intervention* contains a number of detailed case studies; for example, Laver and Unsworth (1999) have written a case study about a 29-year-old man who experiences cerebral bleeding leading to stroke, in which an assessment process using standardised self-report, proxy report and observational measures is applied.

CASE STUDY: 'SCOTT'

By Sally Payne, Claire Howell and Alison Laver Fawcett

This case study illustrates how staff at a new therapy service developed a thorough assessment process by assembling a toolkit of standardised assessments that could be used to obtain information from a range of sources using a number of different methods. The first part of this study describes the service and the rationale for the measures that therapists have selected to use within this service. The second part of this study shows how these assessments are applied in a clinical setting through the case of a teenage boy, who we will refer to as Scott.

ABOUT THE OCCUPATIONAL THERAPIST

Sarah qualified as an occupational therapist 15 years ago and for 14 of these years has worked with children, both as an independent practitioner and for the NHS. She has worked as a member of two multidisciplinary pre-school child development teams and with a variety of agencies when working with school-aged children in the community. Currently, Sarah leads a small community paediatric occupational therapy service (one part-time Head III therapist and a full-time Senior I) in an urban area on the edge of a large city with a population of 212 000.

THE SETTING

The community paediatric occupational therapy service was established two years ago, and the Person-Environment-Occupation (PEO) model of practice (Law *et al.*, 1996) was selected to guide the development, delivery and evaluation of services to children, young people and their families. The PEO model encourages a top-down approach to occupational therapy referral, assessment, intervention and evaluation, with improved occupational performance being the aim of therapy. The PEO is a 'trans-active' model of occupational behaviour in which occupational performance is considered to be the product of a dynamic relationship between people, occupations or roles and their environment (Law *et al.*, 1996). The occupational therapist facilitates change in the person, environment and/or occupational dimensions to improve occupational performance.

Children and young people are referred to the occupational therapy service by any adult who knows the child well, and who has a concern about their occupational performance. Occupational therapy is usually provided within the child's own environment, at their home, school or nursery, and involves developing collaborative relationships with the child or young person and his or her parents/carers, teachers and other professionals. Assessment and intervention plans are developed to meet the needs of the individual.

As this was a new service, the therapy team was able to develop an assessment process based on current best practice as evidenced within occupational therapy literature (for example Burtner *et al.*, 1997; Case-Smith, 2001; Coster, 1998; Dunn, 2000) and the therapists' experience of what has worked best in the past. It includes both standardised and non-standardised assessments in order to gain both qualitative and quantitative information. While quantitative data are useful for help with the diagnosis and for providing evidence when applying for additional resources for the child, the qualitative data are most useful in helping to identify the impact of the young person's difficulties on their daily life, their priorities for intervention and for guiding intervention planning.

ASSESSMENT PROCESS

The assessment tools were selected to be congruent with the chosen model of practice. Selected assessments that are occupation-focused include the:

- Assessment of Motor and Process Skills (AMPS; Fisher, 2003a and b)
- School Assessment of Motor and Process Skills (School AMPS; Fisher, Bryze and Hume, 2002)
- School Function Assessment (SFA; Coster *et al.*, 1998)
- Pediatric Evaluation of Disability Inventory (PEDI; Hayley *et al.*, 1992)
- Canadian Occupational Performance Measure (COPM; Law *et al.*, 1991).

A number of component-based assessments are also used by the therapists, including the:

- Movement Assessment Battery for Children (Movement ABC; Henderson and Sugden, 1992)
- Developmental Test of Visual Motor Integration (VMI; Beery, 1997)
- Test of Visual Perceptual Skills (TVPS; Gardner, 1996).

These tools are used to support the information gained from informal interviews with the child/young person and parents/carers, and general observations made by the therapist. A thorough assessment can take three to four sessions, and usually starts with a telephone call to the parents/carers to clarify the assessment aims and parents' concerns.

SUMMARY OF THE STRENGTHS AND LIMITATIONS OF SELECTED ASSESSMENT TOOLS

Observational Assessments

The Assessment of Motor Process Skills (AMPS) The AMPS (Fisher, 2003a and b) is a standardised observational assessment that allows the therapist to simultaneously assess a person's ability to perform activities of daily living (ADL) (domestic and personal) and the quality of their motor and process skills. Motor skills are the observed actions that the person uses to move himself or objects during the tasks performed, and include walking, reaching, manipulating and lifting. Process skills are how a person sensibly organises himself, his tools and his actions over time, and reflects how effective he is at overcoming or compensating for any problems that he encounters.

The AMPS assessment is usually undertaken in the individual's home. Individuals (from three years of age) select two or more familiar activities that they are willing to demonstrate. Tasks frequently chosen by young people include preparing a bowl of cereal and a cold drink, making a jam sandwich and dressing. The therapist observes the person performing his activities and rates his motor and process abilities. The results are computer-analysed. This test was selected for use in this community paediatric occupational therapy service for the following reasons.

- The AMPS has been standardised internationally and cross-culturally on more than 46 000 subjects (AMPS International).
- It is a standardised test of occupational performance that clearly demonstrates to parents and others the link between skills and occupational performance.
- It can be used with children, young people and adults.
- It is very popular with children and young people, who enjoy choosing their activities and carrying them out. Tasks chosen are meaningful to the individual, and are culturally appropriate.
- It is a sensitive tool that demonstrates why a person has difficulty performing daily tasks.
- The test is carried out in the young person's own environment, and so demonstrates the interaction of the person, the environment and the activity.
- It helps with intervention planning and reflects an individual's own circumstances.
- It can be used to objectively measure therapy outcomes.

Disadvantages Therapists have to attend a five-day training course to qualify to use the tool and must use it regularly to maintain standardisation. Although the AMPS is increasingly being used with paediatric populations, published evidence of its use with children is limited as yet.

The School AMPS The School AMPS (Fisher, Bryze and Hume, 2002) is a modified version of the AMPS and is a standardised assessment tool for measuring a young person's schoolwork task performance within their own classrooms and routines. The therapist observes the young person in class and assesses the motor and process skills used to perform school activities as chosen by the class teacher. The therapist develops a collaborative relationship with the class teacher to understand the teacher's expectations of the individual and the class, the class routine and the tools that the child is expected to use at school. Assessment results are computer-analysed and can be used to demonstrate the young person's motor and process skills in comparison to other children of the same age. This test was chosen for use in this service for the following reasons.

- The School AMPS is a valid, reliable assessment tool.
- It is a sensitive measure of occupational performance and demonstrates the interaction between the young person, his environment and his schoolwork activity.
- It clearly demonstrates to teachers the role of the occupational therapist and facilitates collaborative working between therapists and teachers.
- It takes account of the roles and role expectations of the young person within a particular class environment.
- Interventions arising from the assessment are relevant to the individual.
- It can be used as an objective measure of change following intervention.

Disadvantages In order to use the School AMPS, therapists must have completed their AMPS training and undertake a further three-day course (*Note*: there are currently plans to develop a five-day training for the School AMPS alone.) As this is a relatively new assessment, there is limited published evidence of its clinical use.

The Movement Assessment Battery for Children The Movement ABC (Henderson and Sugden, 1992) is a standardised norm-referenced assessment for children from four to 12 years of age. It provides objective quantitative data on children's motor performance in the areas of manual dexterity, ball skills and balance. Children's scores are compared to a norm sample to indicate whether the child falls below the level of his age peers. Additional qualitative data are collected to indicate how the child performs each task.

This assessment was chosen for use in the community paediatric occupational therapy service for the following reasons.

- The Movement ABC is a valid, reliable assessment of impairments of motor function.
- It has been standardised on over 1200 children from America and Europe (as stated in the Movement ABC Manual; Henderson and Sugden, 1992).
- It has been used extensively for research and clinical purposes (e.g. Rodger *et al.*, 2003; Smyth and Mason, 1998).
- With practice, it is fairly quick to administer (taking between 30 minutes to one hour).
- It is useful for helping to diagnose developmental coordination disorders.

Limitations Although this assessment is extensively used by occupational therapists in the UK (Payne, 2002), it is also used by educationalists and other health professionals. It can, therefore, be difficult to explain the unique contribution of occupational therapy if this is the only assessment used. It is a measure of component skills and does not take account of contextual factors: it cannot be assumed that the child who scores well on the Movement ABC does not have difficulty performing ADL in the classroom or at home. It can be difficult to use this test to monitor change over time as the test activities vary between age bands. This test seems to emphasise children's difficulties as it is often obvious to them when they have 'failed'. It also requires a certain amount of preparation and space to administer. It is only standardised for children up to 12 years of age.

The Developmental Test of Visual Motor Integration (VMI) The VMI (Beery, 1997) is a standardised test of visual motor integration for people aged three years and over. Individuals copy a series of increasingly complex geometric forms, and an individual's score is calculated as the number of patterns that have been successfully copied, prior to three consecutive failures. Two supplemental tests examine visual perception and motor coordination using the same stimulus patterns as the VMI. Raw scores are converted to standard scores and scaled scores to give an indication of how the person has performed in comparison to other people of the same age.

This assessment was chosen for use in this community paediatric service for the following reasons.

• The VMI has been standardised on 2512 individuals (Beery, 1997).
• It is useful for identifying children who may have difficulty integrating the visual and motor skills required for writing and drawing.
• It can suggest to the therapist that further assessment of motor or visual skills is required.
• It is quick to administer and can be used with individuals or groups.
• It can provide evidence that a child is not yet ready to learn formal pencil and paper writing (Beery, 1997, p. 126).
• This assessment can be used to evaluate change in visual motor integration after intervention that has focused on this area.

Limitations The VMI was standardised on an American population and the authors recommend that local norms be developed, but this is impractical for a small therapy service. Although scoring criteria are given, scoring can still be quite subjective. The VMI is used by a range of professionals, particularly those in education, and so it can be difficult to demonstrate the unique role of the occupational therapist if this is the only test used. Children who perform well on the VMI may still have difficulty with visual perceptual or motor skills within a classroom context.

The Test of Visual Perceptual Skills (TVPS) The TVPS (Gardner, 1996) is a standardised assessment of seven distinct areas of visual perception: visual memory, visual discrimination, visual form constancy, visual sequential memory, visual closure, visual figure/ground discrimination and visual–spatial relationships. Children look at the patterns on a test plate and indicate which of the stimulus patterns are the same or different (according to the subtest). Choices are indicated verbally or by pointing: no motor skills are required. There are two versions of this test, one for children aged four to 13 years and one for those aged 12 to 17 years. Test scores are converted into perceptual ages, scaled scores and percentiles for each subtest, and into perceptual quotients, percentiles and median perceptual ages for the combined scores.

This assessment was chosen for use in this paediatric community service for the following reasons.

• This is a standardised test of children's visual perceptual strengths and weaknesses.
• The standardisation sample included more than 1000 students (Gardner, 1996).
• It can be used with children who have poor motor or verbal skills.
• It can be useful in helping to explore why children may have functional problems, for example when copying from the board, finding clothes in a drawer etc.

Limitations The TVPS was standardised on an American population. It can be quite lengthy to administer, depending on the age of the child, and it can be difficult for children to maintain their levels of attention throughout. Although reliability is acceptable for the combined test score (reliability coefficients 8.3–9.1), it is less reliable for individual subtests

(0.27–0.8). This assessment looks at skills in isolation: a child can score well on the TVPS but still struggle with classroom activities because of environmental factors.

ASSESSMENTS USING REPORTS FROM A PROXY (PARENT, TEACHER)

The School Function Assessment (SFA) The SFA (Coster *et al.*, 1998) is a criterion-referenced assessment that uses a questionnaire format. The questionnaire is completed by a member of the school team who knows the young person well. The SFA comprises three parts:

1. *Participation* is used to measure the person's level of participation in six major school settings (the classroom, playground, transportation to and from school, bathroom and toileting activities, transitions to and from class, lunchtime).
2. *Task supports* covers the support currently provided to the student when he or she performs school-related tasks. These include adult assistance and adaptations (modifications to the environment or activity).
3. *Activity performance* examines the person's performance of specific school-related activities, including moving around the classroom, using school materials, interacting with others and following school rules.

This test was chosen for use in this service for the following reasons.

- The SFA has been standardised on 678 students (Coster *et al.*, 1998).
- It is a top-down measure of social participation, tasks and activity performance rather than component skills and, therefore, reflects the occupational nature of the therapist's work.
- The test examines the non-academic activities that often present a challenge to young people with special needs at school.
- It records the effects on performance of both personal and environmental factors.
- It is useful for identifying areas of need for intervention planning.
- It facilitates collaborative planning with school staff.
- The tool can be used to measure change.

Limitations The SFA can be quite lengthy to administer. It may be easier to use the questionnaire as the basis for a structured interview with the young person and his main support assistants or teachers at school. Although no special training is required to administer the SFA, the therapist must have a good understanding of the terms and performance rating scales used.

The Pediatric Evaluation of Disability Inventory (PEDI) The PEDI (Hayley *et al.*, 1992) was designed to describe the functional performance of children aged six months to seven years. It is usually administered through a structured interview and measures capability and performance in three areas: self-care, mobility and social function. Parents or carers indicate whether a child is able to consistently perform functional skills (capability), and how much carer assistance is required. The test also enables the therapist to identify what environmental modifications or equipment are used by the child during his daily activities. Normative standard scores and scaled performance scores are used to develop a profile of the child's performance across the three areas; this can be computer-generated.

This test was selected for use in this service for the following reasons.

- The PEDI is a valid, reliable, standardised test of functional capability and performance.
- It has been used extensively in research (e.g. Knox and Evans, 2002; Ostensjo, Carlberg and Vollestad, 2004).
- It was developed in part by an occupational therapist and reflects the occupational nature of the therapist's work.
- It measures functional performance rather than component skills.
- The child's profile can be used to monitor change over time.

Limitations   The PEDI can be lengthy to administer and relies on accurate reporting by the parent/carer in order to develop a realistic profile of skills. The mobility and social function sections may be best completed by other members of the multidisciplinary team. This assessment is norm-referenced for children up to seven years of age; there is no equivalent assessment for older children. The therapists in this community-based paediatric service have, therefore, developed a checklist based on the PEDI areas; this home-grown checklist is used as a criterion-referenced assessment tool to help indicate significant areas of concern for the young person aged eight and above and his family.

SELF-REPORT ASSESSMENTS

The Canadian Occupational Performance Measure (COPM)   The COPM (Law *et al.*, 1998) has already been mentioned as a good example of a self-report assessment earlier in this chapter. The COPM is an individualised outcome measure that is used for assessing and evaluating the child's self-perception in occupational performance and covers the domains of self-care, productivity and leisure. The area of self-care includes personal care, functional mobility and community management. The area of productivity includes paid or unpaid work, household management and school or play. Leisure includes quiet recreation, active recreation and socialisation. Function is rated in terms of importance, performance and satisfaction on three 10-point scales. The COPM can be administered separately to the child and his parent or carer. It takes between 20 to 40 minutes to administer. This test has been selected for use in this service for the following reasons.

- The test has acceptable levels of test–retest reliability (Law *et al.*, 1998).
- The test has good clinical utility (Law *et al.*, 1994).
- It encompasses the occupational performance areas of self-care, productivity and leisure.
- It incorporates the roles and role expectations of the child.
- It considers the importance of performance areas to the child and the parent.
- It considers the child's and parent's satisfaction with present performance.
- It focuses on the child's own environment, thereby ensuring the relevance of the problems to the child.
- It allows for input from members of the child's social environment (e.g. parent, teacher) if the child is unable to answer on his own behalf.
- The test has been used for previous research in child populations (e.g. studies with children with cerebral palsy: Pollock and Stewart, 1998; Law *et al.*, 1995; Wilcox, 1994).
- The test is useful for measuring the outcomes of intervention, from the client's perspective.

Limitations   This test is easier to use with older children who are able to understand the concepts of performance and satisfaction. With younger children it is helpful to use pictures and visual scales to help the children identify their priority areas and satisfaction with these areas; at present pictorial scales have to be developed locally.

The Perceived Efficacy and Goal Setting System (PEGS) The PEGS (Missiuna, Pollock and Law, 2004) is a new assessment tool that helps children to identify challenging tasks and priorities for intervention using picture cards that illustrate 24 tasks essential for daily living and participation in school. Parents and teachers complete an additional questionnaire regarding the child's ability to perform daily tasks and to outline their priorities. This is a new tool, which promises to be very useful but has yet to be tested within the clinical setting.

CASE STUDY: SCOTT'S REFERRAL INFORMATION

Thirteen-year-old Scott was referred for the advice of an occupational therapist by his mother. She indicated on the referral form (Figure 2.2 below) that school activities were the main area of concern, closely followed by ADL and leisure activities. Specific difficulties were identified with using a knife and fork, tying shoelaces, managing buttons and other fine-motor tasks. At school, Scott's writing was very laboured and required great concentration, and his hand hurt after a period of writing. In physical education classes (PE) he found slow movements difficult and appeared clumsy when moving quickly. Scott's mother felt he had general difficulties with perceptual tasks. Other information on the referral form indicated that Scott had a diagnosis of verbal dyspraxia and that he attended a mainstream secondary school with support from a specialist language resource centre. He was receiving speech and language therapy at school. Scott had seen an occupational therapist previously (when he was seven years old), who, his mother reported, had provided useful advice and help with tying shoelaces.

INFORMATION GATHERING: PROXY REPORT FROM SCOTT'S PARENT AND TEACHER

A letter was written to Scott's parents acknowledging the referral and enclosing two questionnaires: one for parents/carers (Figure 2.3 below) and the other to be passed on to Scott's teachers (Figure 2.4 below). These questionnaires have been developed by the occupational therapy service and the school questionnaire is based on the occupational therapy referral form and behaviour checklist (Dunn, 2000). Information provided through the questionnaires is used to help prioritise the referrals. Very occasionally, parents indicate that they do not wish the school to be contacted. This request is respected, and if the primary area of concern relates to self-care activities, then the occupational therapist focuses on this area for assessment and intervention. If, however, there are concerns relating to school issues, then this is discussed with the parents in person, and an appropriate plan is agreed with them.

Questionnaires were completed and returned to the occupational therapist. Additional information provided by Scott's parents (Figure 2.3) indicated concerns regarding dressing, following instructions, a poor sense of danger and difficulty accessing mainstream leisure opportunities. Scott's mother was concerned that Scott had developed many avoidance strategies and that his current good level of self-esteem might suffer as he struggled to succeed at increasingly challenging activities.

The school questionnaire was completed and returned by his teacher (Figure 2.4). It indicated that Scott had a statement of educational needs and was supported by specialist teaching from the language resource centre. The difficulties identified by school included that Scott seemed weaker than other children and had problems running, he avoided drawing and had an awkward pencil grip, he found it difficult to manage tools such as a ruler and set of compasses, he found it generally difficult to produce written work and worked slowly and he was easily distracted in class. No sensory-processing issues were identified. Scott's teachers forwarded an example of his written work. The occupational therapist noted that this was difficult to read, letters were poorly formed and squashed together and he seemed to have pressed hard.

Family name: ......*Jones*............   **Child's name**: ......*Scott*............
Address: ....   Tel: ....
....   DOB ....
          Post code ....

Parent/Carer's names   **Relationship**
Mary Jones...................................   *Mother*..................................
Steve Jones...................................   *Father*..................................

GP's name *Dr Smith*...............   **Consultant** *Dr Black*...............
Address ....   Base ....
....

Other professionals involved   **Diagnosis** *Verbal Dyspraxia*...........
Jane Sykes, SaLT...........................

School/Nursery attended   **Teacher** *Mrs B*...................
....   Tel: ....

- Please indicate if you are making a referral for the following reasons:
  o The child has an acute/deteriorating/life-limiting condition
     (please circle)
  o Malfunction/breakdown of essential equipment putting
     child/carer at risk

- Please circle the main performance area of concern:

Activities of daily living   (**School nursery**)   **Play/leisure**

Reason for referral: *Scott still has difficulty using a knife and fork. Tying shoelaces, doing up buttons, any fine-motor control tasks. School: writing is very laboured, needs great concentration and his hand hurts after a few minutes. Sports/PE: finds slow movements hard but performs fast movements clumsily. Experiences general difficulties with perceptual skills.*

                              Date of referral:

Parent/Carer: *I agree for this referral to be made to occupational therapy.*

Signed: *Mary Jones*   Print: *MARY JONES*

Referrer: *Mary Jones*   Signed: *Mary Jones*

Designation: *Parent*   Contact no:

Please return this form to: Occupational Therapy, 41 Old Street, Anytown
                    Tel:

Figure 2.2 Completed referral form for Scott.

Child's name: *Scott Jones*   DoB:

Date sent:

Scott has been referred for an occupational therapy assessment. To help with the evaluation, we would be grateful if you could complete the questionnaire and return it to the occupational therapy department by:...............

- The information that you provide will remain confidential.

Family
Mum's name:............*Mary Jones*....................   Dad's name: *Steve Jones*........

Siblings: ....*Susie*...........................   ....

          ....

With whom does the child live?   *Family*..

Tel:

School/Nursery
School/Nursery   ....
Tel: ....
Address: ....

- We are enclosing a questionnaire for you to pass to your child's school/nursery teacher. If you do not wish us to contact the school/nursery please tick here: ☐

Listed below are some of the areas in which an occupational therapist may be able to help a child. Please tick the areas that your child finds difficult and comment if appropriate

Activities of daily living
- ✓ Dressing   *buttons, zips, laces, doing a tie*

- ✓ Eating and drinking   *using a knife, opening tins, spreading anything on bread*

- ✓ Toileting

- Washing/bathing

- Seating at home

Figure 2.3 Completed parent questionnaire for Scott.

School/Nursery
- ✓ Using a pencil/writing   *Writing very laborious, can only manage for short periods*

- • Using computer equipment

- • Concentration/attention

- ✓ Following instructions   *If too much information is given*

- • Moving around the school

- • Organisation

Play/Leisure
- ✓ Avoids activities such as *Lego, jigsaws*

- • Dislikes playground equipment e.g. slide, roundabout
  The opposite, does not see potential dangers and throws himself at every activity

- • Prefers sedentary (quiet) play

- • Always seems very active

- ✓ Has difficulty accessing leisure opportunities   *Attends leisure opportunities organised by local support group, but mainstream sports have not been successful due to competition, teasing, misunderstanding of coach.*

Please comment on any other concerns that you have about your child in the space below
Scott has learned various strategies to avoid certain activities. As he gets older his difficulties become more apparent to peer group. We are concerned that this will affect his self-esteem.

Thank you for your help!

Signature of person completing the form: *Mary Jones*

Date: Name (print): *MARY JONES*

Relationship to the child: *Mother*

Please return this form to: Occupational Therapy
                             41 Old Street
                             Anytown
                             Tel:

(continued)

Scott Jones (DOB) has been referred for an occupational therapy assessment. To help with the evaluation we would be grateful if you could complete the questionnaire and return it to the occupational therapy department by...........

Thank you very much for your help!

Date questionnaire sent:............ Sent to: *Parents*.........

Formal evaluations
- Cognitive tests e.g. IQ

Name of test:...

Full score:..

Verbal:...

Performance:..

- Academic levels

Reading *<6.01*........................Date of assessment: ....

Spelling *<6.00*........................Date of assessment: ....

Maths ....Date of assessment: ....

- Other pertinent evaluations

.... Date of assessment:........

.... Date of assessment:........

.... Date of assessment:........

When is the child due to change school? *N/A – at secondary*.............

What stage of the SEN Code of Practice is the child at? *5 – Statemented*

Please tick the statements that are pertinent to this child
Gross motor
- ✓ Seems weaker than other children his/her age
- ✓ Does not have the endurance other children his/her age have for an activity
- ✓ Difficulty with hopping, jumping, skipping or running compared to others his/her age
- ✓ Appears stiff and awkward in his/her movement
- ✓ Clumsy, does not appear to know how body works, bumps into others or objects, never quite sits in chair correctly
- Does not seem to understand concepts such as right, left, front or back as it relates to his/her body
- Shies away from playground equipment. May only play on one particular item
- Poor posture (always seems to be leaning against something, shoulders slump forward)
- Has difficulty with transitions between activities and locations

Figure 2.4 Completed teacher questionnaire for Scott.

✓ Requires adaptation of the physical environment to access educational opportunities (e.g. seating, positioning, modified PE equipment etc.)

Fine motor
- ✓ Difficulty with drawing, colouring, tracing
- ✓ Performs these activities quickly and result is usually sloppy
- ✓ Avoids fine-motor activities
- ✓ Problem holding pencil, grasp may be very loose or very tight
- ✓ Printing is too dark, too light, too large, too small
- • Does not seem to have a dominant hand
- ✓ Has difficulty manipulating school tools such as ruler, paintbrush, compass
- ✓ Has difficulty or is unable to produce handwritten work

Academic
- ✓ Easily distracted
- • Restless
- ✓ Slow worker
- • Disorganised, messy desk
- • Short attention span
- • Hyperactive
- • Can't follow directions
- • Never completes assignments

Sensory processing
- • Withdraws from touch
- • Touches everything
- • Avoids being close to others
- • Fearful of being off the ground
- • Doesn't like playground equipment such as slide, swing
- • Can't seem to stop moving, craves swinging, rocking
- • Trouble discriminating shapes, letters or numbers
- • Cannot complete puzzles appropriate for age
- • Difficulty copying designs, letters or numbers
- • Difficulty tracking (e.g. reading or following teacher's arm movements)

Emotional and behavioural responses
- • Does not like to have routine changed
- • Is easily frustrated
- • Cannot get along with others
- ✓ Accident prone
- • Copes better 1:1 or in a small group

Personal care
- • Needs assistance with toileting
- • Needs assistance or extra supervision with meals/drinks/snacks

Please attach a typical example of the child's writing or a drawing, and their most recent Individual Education Plan.
Signature of person completing the form:
Date:

(continued)

Given the information on the referral form, Scott was put onto a waiting list for children who attend a secondary school and where there is a significant difference between their performance and their potential.

THERAPIST'S REFLECTIONS UPON INITIAL DATA

The referral information suggested that Scott's mother had a good understanding of occupational therapy and what it might have to offer her son. It gave clear indications of the functional areas of difficulty and also demonstrated a concern for Scott's self-esteem. Sarah, the occupational therapist, also recognised that Scott, at 13 years old, would have his own ideas about what was important to him and that is was possible that Scott's priorities would be different from those of his parents. At 13, Scott would also have developed his own strategies and ways of managing.

The school questionnaire indicated that Scott was attending a mainstream school, which suggested that his cognitive levels were comparable to his age peers. However, he received extra professional support for language. Despite this, he continued to have difficulty demonstrating his potential in the written form.

Sarah was aware that people with verbal dyspraxia also have difficulties with coordination, and this was reflected in the information provided by parents and school. Previous experience and research evidence also suggests that people may have perceptual and organisational difficulties (for example Schoemaker *et al.*, 2001; Wilson and McKenzie, 1998). The therapist was aware that these areas would need to be considered when assessing Scott's performance problems.

INITIAL ASSESSMENT: PROXY REPORT FROM SCOTT'S MOTHER

Because of the huge demand for occupational therapy services, there was a delay of nine months before it was possible to offer Scott an assessment. This is the cause of huge frustration for therapists, who believe that their desire to offer client-centred, timely services is being compromised as a result of limited resources. At this point, Sarah telephoned Scott's mother to let her know that she could now meet with Scott, and to update the information that she had gathered. This telephone conversation continued the information-gathering process and formed part of the initial assessment. It also enabled the therapist and parent/carer to prioritise the young person's needs in order to focus the assessment appropriately.

Scott's mother explained that Scott spent some time each day in the language resource centre for small group work to develop reading and writing skills. He also had speech therapy input at school on a weekly basis. Scott was supported by a number of different learning support assistants in several mainstream classes where there was a large written component. Scott's mother was frustrated that Scott often did not note down his homework accurately and she felt that with the level of support that Scott received his homework should be recorded precisely. She reported that she provided a lot of support for Scott at home by scribing and helping him to organise his work. The family had purchased a 'Read out loud' computer system and site licences to use the software at school and at home. Scott used this frequently at home, for example to read back his work and when researching using the Internet, but his mother felt that more use could be made of this system at school.

Scott's mother explained that she was a member of the local aphasic support group and had been a member of the local dyspraxia support group when it was active some years ago. She regularly acted as the parent contact for local authority consultations on educational issues for children with speech and language needs. Sarah recognised that this mother was very supportive and understanding of Scott's needs. Sarah hypothesised that Scott's mother would actively engage in the assessment and intervention process and may have additional experience and insights that would help the therapist to develop a family-centred intervention.

Sarah asked Scott's mother if she could provide some information about Scott's perform-ance of self-care activities. She then asked questions about dressing, eating, washing and so on, using a prompt sheet based on the PEDI (Hayley *et al.*, 1992). This has been adapted by the therapists to cover children over the age of seven years and ensures that information is gathered on all aspects of self-care. It also helps to clarify areas of concern and informs the therapist of any compensations that the young person and family are already using.

At the end of this conversation, Sarah suggested to Scott's mother that the current areas of concern seemed to be:

- difficulty producing legible, timely written work at school
- a need to help Scott develop independence skills at home
- a need to maintain and promote self-esteem.

Sarah and Scott's mother agreed that it would be useful to meet with Scott at home to iden-tify his concerns, strengths and priorities and to observe Scott as he participated in some activities, to gain a clearer picture of any underlying difficulties. Sarah was concerned to in-volve Scott in the assessment process to engage him in identifying and prioritising interven-tion areas. She felt that there was more chance of a positive outcome if this were the case.

THE HOME ASSESSMENT VISIT: SELF-REPORT AND OBSERVATIONAL ASSESSMENT

A visit was arranged for the therapist to meet Scott at home after school with his mother. Sarah was concerned that Scott should not be withdrawn from school as he was already experiencing difficulties keeping up with schoolwork. She also felt it was important to meet Scott on his own territory as this helps young people to feel more comfortable about sharing the challenges they face. Sarah explained to Scott that an occupational therapist is interested in finding out how a person manages their daily occupations and which of these are difficult or challenging. The therapist explained that she was interested to know whether there were any activities that Scott would like to participate in but felt unable to do so at present, and also what activities he enjoyed and what he considered to be his strengths. Scott told the therapist that he was good at swimming, riding a bike and organising himself. Sarah was a bit surprised at the last comment, but, on reflection, hypothesised that Scott was referring to the strategies he and his mother had put in place to accommodate his organisational dif-ficulties. Scott said that he had difficulty with writing and spelling and that his hand ached at times. He couldn't tie his shoelaces or his school tie (his mother had adapted his tie so that it fastened at the back with Velcro), and he didn't enjoy ball games. Scott shared that he enjoyed being in the Scouts and had participated in many weekend activities with them. He was currently having individual swimming lessons and had recently achieved an adult swimmer certificate. He attended dance club at school and was the only boy in his year to do so.

Scott showed Sarah some of his schoolbooks and explained that he was often provided with handouts to reduce the amount of writing. He felt his drawings were not as good as those of his peers. Sarah asked Scott about using a computer; Scott said he liked to use the computer at home but was not able to use it much at school.

DIRECT OBSERVATIONAL ASSESSMENT USING A STANDARDISED TOOL

Sarah decided to use the AMPS (Fisher, 2003a and b). The therapist had found that young people enjoy choosing and participating in the assessment activities and, unlike some of the component-based assessment tools, it is unusual for a person to feel that they have failed the test, because the activities they have chosen are familiar to them. At 13, Scott was also too old for the Movement ABC. The AMPS would provide good information about the effect of any motor and process difficulties on Scott's performance of self-care activities.

Sarah was able to identify several activities that Scott might like to perform from information he had provided. Scott decided to prepare a bowl of cereal and a cold drink, and to change the covers on his duvet. The therapist invited Scott's mother to watch Scott perform the tasks – as long as she did not say anything.

After Scott had completed the activities, Sarah suggested to Scott and his mother the areas that she thought he had found difficult. These included:

- positioning himself effectively in front of his workspace
- managing tasks that require the use of both hands together
- manipulating objects
- maintaining smooth, fluent arm movements
- holding objects securely
- handling objects
- organising equipment.

Scott seemed to have difficulty accommodating his difficulties and so they persisted throughout the activities. Scott and his mother agreed that this was a true reflection of the difficulties he experienced in other ADL tasks at home and at school.

At the end of this visit, Sarah agreed to contact Scott's teachers to discuss school issues with them. A further home visit was arranged to discuss the assessment findings and to make a plan for future intervention.

THE SCHOOL VISIT: PROXY REPORT AND DIRECT OBSERVATIONAL ASSESSMENT

Sarah arranged to meet with the head of the resource centre, Mrs B., and Scott's speech therapist at school, and to observe Scott in a science lesson. This lesson was chosen because it would have a written component and Scott would be using some small equipment. Mrs B. described Scott as having a very positive attitude towards school. However, he had difficulty organising his ideas and writing these down. He had support to help him with reading and spelling. It was not always possible to read his work, but he was allowed to use a computer to write up his work 'in best'. Technology lessons were identified as challenging; Scott had various teachers who did not all understand his needs. Scott had in the past injured himself when using some equipment and was felt to be at risk of harm. Support was provided in these lessons. The resource centre had provided all teaching staff with a student profile explaining Scott's difficulties and the accommodations they could make. This included the recommendation that Scott be provided with handouts enlarged to A3 size and gapped worksheets where possible to reduce the amount of writing.

Scott was observed in a science lesson using a School AMPS format (Fisher, Bryze and Hume, 2002). An assistant supported Scott during this lesson. The assistant sat to his left and provided help to understand the task, to move on to the next stage, to sequence the activity and to support the ruler when drawing lines. The assistant also glued Scott's worksheet into his book and helped him to pack his bag at the end of the lesson. Scott participated in the lesson by putting up his hand to answer questions. However, Sarah observed that he did not sit squarely in front of the desk, compromising the fluency of arm movements to control his pen. His workspace was cluttered and Scott appeared to be distracted by objects around him, such as his eraser. He had difficulty drawing lines with the ruler and organising his graph on the page so that it was not too squashed. The lesson ended with an activity that Scott completed on a worksheet rather than copy from the board.

At the end of the lesson, the teacher reported that Scott's behaviour had not been affected by Sarah's presence in the class. She informed the therapist that Scott enjoyed science but it was difficult for him to record his work in a way that could be assessed to accurately reflect his ability. The therapist felt that the assistant had provided too much help at times, for example she believed that Scott could have managed to glue in his own worksheet. The therapist decided that she would suggest a session with the assistant, during which she could advise her about appropriate prompts and cues to help to improve Scott's independence skills in the classroom.

NEEDS IDENTIFICATION: ASSESSMENT REPORT

Sarah then wrote a detailed assessment report for Scott and his family that could be shared with his speech and language therapist and school staff. This included a summary of the assessment process and performance analysis and the identification of the difficulties affecting Scott's performance of everyday activities at home and at school. Strengths and needs were organised under the person/environment/occupation headings.

Person Level Issues

For Scott, these could be divided into those that related to motor or to process aspects. Motor difficulties included balance and the ability to position himself appropriately in relation to his workspace. Scott used increased effort to perform activities and had difficulty with activities that required the use of two hands together or the manipulation of small objects. He tired quickly. Process difficulties included organising his work and materials (he sometimes knocked them over), organising his work on the page and sequencing activities. He had difficulty moving on to the next part of the activity and sometimes stopped too soon or during an action to do something else. This interrupted the flow of his work. However, despite these difficulties, Scott appeared to be very determined and was willing to participate in class discussions. He had taken on board many strategies that he and his mother had developed and seemed pleased to be in control of implementing these strategies to help himself. He had a wide range of after-school activities and achieved success in these pursuits.

Environmental Level Issues

These were different for home and school. At home, Scott could be quite focused. Scott and his family had accommodated many of his needs and structured their routines and physical environment to help promote Scott's independence and self-esteem. They made good use of timetables and colour coding. Scott was accepted for himself and his interests were encouraged. At home, Scott was seen as a person first and as someone with a disability second.

At school, Scott received good support from the resource centre and the therapist was encouraged to see the accommodations that the science teacher had made by providing a worksheet. In lessons, Scott was encouraged to speak out, despite his language difficulties. The use of support assistants enabled Scott to participate in the learning experience and to demonstrate his learning on paper. Despite this support, Scott still found it difficult to remain focused, particularly towards the end of the lesson when he typically did not record his homework.

Occupational Level Issues

These are defined as the occupations, tasks or activities that a person performs during his daily life, and for Scott included:

- production of written work at school: this difficulty was a consequence of the inter-action between language difficulties, physical and process difficulties and the school environment
- dressing: Scott was not independent in the more complex activities of tying shoe laces and a school tie
- snack preparation: Scott had difficulty with the organisation of the activity and the handling of tools and equipment.

GOAL SETTING, ACTION PLANNING AND SETTING A BASELINE FOR OUTCOME MEASUREMENT

Sarah took the assessment report back to Scott and his parents, who all agreed that this painted a good picture of Scott, his strengths and difficulties. Scott and his mother agreed that a referral could be made to the community physiotherapy department for advice with regard to balance and stability. The physiotherapists accepted the referral and, following a physiotherapy assessment, organised shoe inserts to correct his foot position.

Sarah explained that she could offer some time-limited intervention to work on some specific skills. Sarah used the COPM (Law *et al.*, 1991) as a self-report assessment to help her prioritise and measure some relevant, client-centred treatment goals for Scott. Using the COPM, Scott identified handwriting, tying shoelaces and tying a tie as being his priorities for intervention. His baseline performance and satisfaction ratings are provided in Table 2.2 below.

Table 2.2 Scott's COPM identified problems and baseline scores

Performance problems	Performance (out of 10)	Satisfaction (out of 10)
Tying shoe laces	2	3
Tying a tie	2	1
Handwriting	2	2

Sarah then calculated a total performance score (sum of the scores divided by number of areas scored, that is 6/3) and a total satisfaction score; these are provided in Table 2.3.

Table 2.3 Scott's COPM baseline total scores

Total Performance Score	2
Total Satisfaction Score	2

A series of after-school visits were arranged to work on these areas with Scott at home. A further school visit was arranged to discuss the assessment findings and their implications with Scott's teachers.

INTERVENTIONS

Scott had identified developing neater writing as a priority for intervention. However, Sarah felt that the time was right for considering alternative methods of written communication at school. She raised this issue with Scott and his parents, who were very keen to explore this idea further. Sarah forwarded to Scott's parents some information about a national initiative for helping children with communication difficulties through the provision of assistive technology. Sarah also discussed this possibility with Scott's teachers. The necessary paperwork was completed by school staff, with encouragement from Scott's parents, and an assessment requested to identify and supply the appropriate equipment.

While at the school, Sarah also suggested that Scott might benefit from using a sloping work surface when working on literacy skills in the resource centre. The resource centre staff were keen on this idea, and Sarah provided a wooden slope for Scott to try. The head of the centre decided to ask the technology department to produce some similar slopes for several of the children to use while in the centre. Meanwhile, Sarah and Scott worked on tying his shoe laces and school tie during five home visits. A cognitive, task-specific approach was adopted in which Sarah encouraged Scott to develop the skills to complete the tasks independently. Strategies used included the therapist breaking down the task into each component and modelling these and Scott developing his own verbal prompts to remind himself of the actions to be taken. Each week, the strategies were modified and amended. After eight weeks, Scott was able to complete both activities independently.

MEASURING THE OUTCOME

At the first home visit during the intervention stage, Sarah videoed Scott attempting to tie his laces and tie. Consent was given by Scott and his parents for the video to be used for therapeutic and professional training purposes. At the last home visit, another video was taken of Scott successfully performing the tasks. Scott also repeated the COPM and re-rated his performance and satisfaction (Tables 2.4 and 2.5). Scott was not asked to re-rate his performance and satisfaction with the third activity, handwriting, as this area was not targeted for intervention while alternatives were being explored.

Table 2.4 Scott's COPM identified problems and follow-up scores

Performance problems	Performance (out of 10)	Satisfaction (out of 10)
Tying shoe laces	8	8
Tying a tie	7	8

Table 2.5 Scott's COPM follow-up total scores

Total Performance Score	7.5
Total Satisfaction Score	8

Sarah calculated COPM change scores to evaluate overall improvement. Scott's scores gave an overall performance score of 7.5 at follow-up. Sarah deducted the baseline score of 2, which gave a change in performance score of 5.5. Scott's scores gave an overall satisfaction score of 8 at follow-up; minus the baseline score of 2, this gave a change in satisfaction score of 6 points. Validity studies conducted on the COPM have indicated that a change score of 2 or more represents an outcome that is considered clinically important by the client, family and therapist (Carswell *et al.*, 2004; Law *et al.*, 1998). Scott's change scores were above 2 for both performance and satisfaction, indicating clinically important change following intervention.

DISCHARGE

At the last home visit, Scott's parents indicated how pleased they were with the progress that he had made. Sarah explained that, although she was not going to offer a formal review or further intervention at this stage, she would be happy to see Scott again in the future if other issues arose.

Scott's mother regularly attends the new local support group for parents of children with coordination disorders. Sarah has also invited Scott's mother to share her experiences as the parent of a young person with a coordination disorder at secondary school at meetings for parents of children who are due to transfer to secondary school. This information has been well received by both therapists and parents.

REFLECTING ON THE DATA-COLLECTION METHODS
YOU USE IN YOUR PRACTICE

At the back of this book, you will find templates for a series of worksheets designed to assist you in applying principles of assessment and outcome measurement to your own practice. Please now turn to Worksheet 2 (p. 397).

STUDY QUESTIONS

Reflecting on the questions below will help you to check you have understood the content of this chapter. If you are unsure, go back and re-read the relevant section or follow up on any of the publications referenced to explore an area in further depth.

2.1 Give examples of direct and indirect assessment methods.
2.2 What are the three categories of sources for gathering assessment data?
2.3 What methods could you use for collecting self-report data?
2.4 List the types of informants/proxies a therapist might use.
2.5 What methods could you use for collecting proxy/informant report data?
2.6 What are the three main phases of an interview?
2.7 What factors might influence the outcome of an interview?
2.8 Give an advantage and a disadvantage for using self-report data.

You will find brief answers to these questions at the back of this book (p. 389).

3

Purposes of Assessment and Measurement

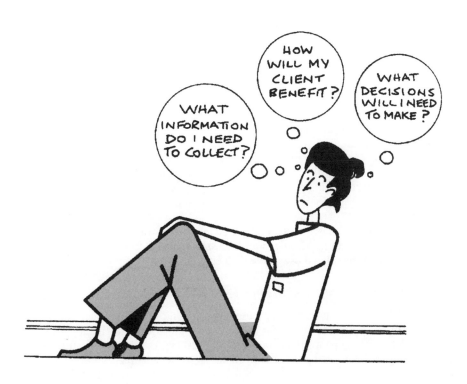

CHAPTER SUMMARY

This chapter will present the main reasons why therapists need or are required to assess clients and categorise these reasons in terms of the different timings of assessment throughout a therapy process. In this chapter, we will explore four distinct purposes of assessment: descriptive, discriminative, evaluative and predictive. Examples of published assessments that address these different purposes will be provided and a case vignette will be presented to demonstrate how these different purposes can be addressed. This chapter will also present the need for service review (which is also referred to as programme evaluation in some parts of the world) and will consider service inputs, processes and outcomes and briefly present how these might be evaluated. A case study is provided at the end of the chapter as an example of how two therapists started a new intervention and thought about how this could be evaluated. It will also endeavour to answer the following question: 'Why am I collecting assessment and measurement data?'

The purpose of conducting an assessment needs to be conscious and articulated. Before you start an assessment process, you need to be able to answer some basic questions.

- Why am I doing this assessment?
- What information do I need to collect?
- What decisions will I need to reach from this information?
- What will be the benefit to the client (and where relevant the carer) from undertaking this assessment?

Articulating the answers to these questions enables the therapist to select an effective and efficient assessment approach. The Chartered Society of Physiotherapy (CSP) in its guidance document on outcome measures (2001a) highlights the importance of considering the purpose of assessment.

> There is a wide choice of measures, systems, and means for capturing the outcome of clinical care. However, if you have carefully considered the purpose for evaluation, whom the information is for, and what the aim of intervention is, choosing, appraising and rejecting a measure should be less complicated. (Chartered Society of Physiotherapy, 2001, p. 4)

The therapist must not only understand the purpose of the assessment for herself. She must also be able to educate the client, and where appropriate the carer, about the purposes and procedures involved in the assessment process. She must be able to explain the specific rationale for using any standardised measures as part of this assessment process. The requirement to explain the purpose of an assessment to the client has been identified as a standard for practice for occupational therapists by the American Occupational Therapy Association (AOTA; 1992, cited in Hopkins and Smith, 1993a, p. 883). So being able to answer the questions asked at the start of this chapter helps the therapist to provide a clear explanation to the client and carer about why the assessment is necessary and why the particular assessment approach has been selected.

Purposes for assessment may be categorised in a number of ways, the most frequent of which are categorisation in terms of the timing of an assessment and categorisation based on the reason for the assessment and the related use of the data collected.

TIMING OF ASSESSMENT IN THE THERAPY PROCESS

It is useful to think about the therapy process when planning an assessment approach and to consider carefully the optimum timing for the assessment(s) within the therapy process. For example, the College of Occupational Therapists (COT; 2003a) outlines the occupational therapy process as a complex intervention that has 11 major steps, which are:

1. referral or reason for contact
2. information gathering
3. initial assessment
4. reason for intervention/needs identification/problem formulation
5. goal setting
6. action planning
7. action
8. ongoing assessment and revision of action
9. outcome and outcome measurement
10. end of intervention or discharge
11. review.

Steps 2, 3, 4, 8 and 9 explicitly relate to assessment; as this is not a strictly linear process, steps may be taken more than once.

The physiotherapy process also has assessment embedded throughout. The World Confederation for Physical Therapy (WCPT; 2006b) describes the following process.

1. *Assessment* includes both the examination of individuals or groups with actual or potential impairments, functional limitations, disabilities or other conditions of health by history taking, screening and the use of specific tests and measures and evaluation of the results of the examination through analysis and synthesis within a process of clinical reasoning.
2. *Diagnosis* arises from examination and evaluation and represents the outcome of the process of clinical reasoning.
3. *Planning* begins with determination of the need for intervention and normally leads to the development of a plan of intervention, including measurable outcome goals negotiated in collaboration with the patient/client, family or carer.
4. *Intervention* is implemented and modified in order to reach agreed goals. Intervention may also be aimed at prevention of impairments, functional limitations, disability and injury including the promotion and maintenance of health, quality of life and fitness in all ages and populations.
5. *Evaluation* necessitates re-examination for the purpose of evaluating outcomes.

REFERRAL

This is the process during which a therapist comes into contact with a potential client. Referrals are made in a variety of ways depending on the service specification and policy and may be received in written format, as a letter, completed referral proforma, fax or email. Other referrals may be made verbally, either via telephone (such as to a fast-response service where a written referral would delay the initiation of the service and thus cause a potential crisis) or in a ward round or multidisciplinary team meeting. The amount of information provided in a referral can also vary greatly, both in terms of what the service specifies as the minimum information required for a referral to be accepted and also because referrers vary greatly in the level of information they provide. At the end of the therapy process, the therapist may also make a referral to put the client and/or carer in contact with another required agency or professional (College of Occupational Therapists, 2003a).

INFORMATION GATHERING

The information provided in a referral is not always sufficient. Therapists, therefore, choose to gather more information about the person, the reason for the referral and the presenting problem prior to conducting the initial assessment. At this stage, the therapist often engages in a screening process. This is a review of referral and other available information to determine whether the referral is appropriate and therapy services are relevant and necessary. Where a service operates a waiting list, the referral might also be prioritised in terms of urgency in order to categorise the referral and place the person on the appropriate waiting list. For example, some services use three categories for sorting referrals, which are:

1. crisis: contact to be made within four hours and client to be see within one working day, e.g. to prevent an admission to hospital
2. urgent: client to be see within seven working days
3. non-urgent: client to be seen when service has capacity.

INITIAL ASSESSMENT

On referral, the therapist will need to conduct an initial (or *screening*) assessment. The purpose of this level of assessment is to identify potential problem areas for further in-depth assessment. *Initial assessment* has been defined as:

Definition of initial assessment

'The first step in the . . . therapy process following referral; the art of gathering relevant information in order to define the problem to be tackled, or identify the goal to be attained, and to establish a baseline for treatment planning' (College of Occupational Therapists, 2003a, p. 54).

Some services triage referrals at this stage to either prioritise referrals for a waiting list system or to signpost the client to the most relevant service/team member/therapist. Screening is an investigative process used by therapists to determine the need for a comprehensive assessment and potential intervention. The initial assessment is used to provide a baseline for treatment planning. An initial or screening assessment may be short and take only one session (for example the assessment of an in-patient being referred for a total hip replacement or in an intermediate care team). In some settings, the initial assessment may require several sessions, perhaps comprising an initial interview, an informal observation of aspects of function and the administration of a standardised assessment battery (for example when deciding the appropriateness of a referral to a community mental health team or a referral for a period of intensive rehabilitation in a stroke unit).

ONGOING EVALUATIVE ASSESSMENT

Assessment should not stop with the initial assessment but be an integral part of the treatment and assist the therapist's clinical reasoning process as she considers the way in which the person is responding to the treatment plan. Ongoing assessment helps with examining progress and monitoring the effects of the intervention. Government policy now articulates the need for continuing assessment in a number of clinical areas, for example the White Paper *Reforming the Mental Health Act* (Department of Health, 2000, 3.19) states that there will be a 'continuing assessment of patients' care and treatment needs by the clinical team, with or without medical treatment'. *Ongoing assessment* has been defined as:

Definition of ongoing assessment

'An integral part of the process of intervention in which information is collected and used to examine the client's progress or lack of progress, to monitor the effects of intervention and to assist the therapist's clinical reasoning process' (College of Occupational Therapists, 2003a, p. 56).

The frequency of evaluative assessment to monitor progress will be related to the anticipated length of contact and the predicted rate of progress. The person's contact with occupational therapy and physiotherapy services might last as little as a couple of days, for example during a short hospital admission for a planned operation, or might last years, for example with a child who is born with cerebral palsy. Where the therapist is involved over several years and where progress is expected to be gradual, a monitoring assessment may be carried out at monthly or even biannual intervals. Where contact is brief, such as when a client is referred to a crisis intervention or rapid response service, or frequent changes are anticipated, then regular evaluation (every couple of days or weekly) may be required (Foster, 2002). When an assessment is re-administered following a short time period, it is essential that any learning effect related to test items is accounted for when interpreting test results. Therapists should examine the test–retest reliability data for the measure and will find some assessments, which are influenced by a learning effect, will have parallel forms of the test for evaluation (see the section on parallel form/equivalent form reliability in Chapter 7, p. 199).

There is a trend towards shorter lengths of stay in hospital, especially in acute care, and therapists play an important role in pre-discharge assessment. A pre-discharge assessment provides information about the person's readiness for discharge (including safety and risk factors), the necessary and available physical and social supports and any requirements for follow-up therapy (Laliberte Rudman *et al.*, 1998).

OUTCOME AND OUTCOME MEASUREMENT

The therapist also should conduct a final outcome assessment when the person is discharged from the therapy service. The final assessment serves to provide an evaluation of the effectiveness of intervention to date and may also provide new baseline data to be passed on to other colleagues if the person is being referred to another service provider.

REVIEW

Some therapists offer a review post discharge from the service. This is particularly helpful for clients suffering from a long-term condition. Therapists may decide to book a review where continued improvement, or the maintenance of improvement, is anticipated following a period of rehabilitation. Some clients experience deterioration in functioning once the support of the therapist is removed, and so a therapist may want to check that the client's function has not reached a plateau or declined post discharge, for example because the client has not continued with an exercise programme or is not using aids and adaptations effectively. A good example is with a service for older people with a history of falls. The client attends a time-limited rehabilitation programme for falls. On discharge from the programme, a number of home modifications are recommended to reduce hazards and an exercise programme is taught to improve strength, range of movement and balance. In this case, the therapist reviews the client at home one, three and six months post discharge from the falls programme to:

- check the modifications have been made and that no additional hazards are present
- observe the exercise routine and ensure that the client continues to do exercises correctly and regularly, and to assess whether the exercises can be upgraded (if function has continued to improve) or modified (if the client finds them too challenging or tiring)
- monitor the outcome in terms of taking a history of any falls that have occurred since discharge or the last review.

Review is also helpful when the person has a condition where a decline in functioning is anticipated over time, such as with dementia or Parkinson's disease, and where the therapist/multidisciplinary team wishes to monitor the rate of decline in order to change the medication and/or care package accordingly. The timing of any reviews will vary depending on the nature of the person's condition and the purpose of the service.

INTRODUCTION TO PURPOSES OF ASSESSMENT

When selecting a specific assessment or an overall assessment strategy for a person, it is essential that the therapist considers the purpose for which the assessment information is gathered and how the results or the assessment might be interpreted and used. When undertaking a critique of potential assessments, it is vital to consider the intended purpose of the assessments under review, because the content, methods, psychometric properties and clinical utility of an assessment should be evaluated against its intended purpose. In terms of client assessment, assessments can be grouped into four main purposes: evaluative, descriptive, predictive and discriminative (Hayley, Coster and Ludlow, 1991; Law, 1993). Some assessments are developed to address just one of these four purposes. However, there are many assessments that can be used for a combination of purposes. Later in this chapter, we will also consider another purpose, that of the evaluation of a therapy service.

DESCRIPTIVE ASSESSMENTS

Most therapy assessments provide some sort of descriptive data. Descriptive assessments are the most frequent type of assessments used by therapists in day-to-day clinical practice. For the purposes of this book, *descriptive assessment* will be defined as:

Definition of descriptive assessment

A descriptive assessment is an assessment that provides information which describes the person's current functional status, problems, needs and/or circumstances.

Descriptive assessments mostly provide information that describes the person's current functional status, such as their ability to perform activities of daily living (ADL), the range of movement (ROM) of a particular joint or their mobility and transferring. Descriptive assessments often focus on identifying strengths and limitations. They provide a snapshot of the person's function, circumstances and needs at one point in time only and are often used to provide baseline (see definition below) data for treatment planning and clinical decision-making. Descriptive assessments may also be used to identify symptoms and problems to help aid diagnosis. In terms of underlying psychometrics, standardised descriptive assessments should have established and adequate content and construct validity (see Chapter 6). For the purposes of this book, *baseline assessment* will be defined as:

Definition of baseline assessment

A baseline assessment is the initial data gathered at the start of therapeutic intervention. Baseline data can be used to guide the nature of the required intervention. A baseline forms the basis for comparison when measuring outcomes to evaluate the effects of intervention.

An issue to consider when selecting a descriptive assessment is the level of data obtained related to the requirements for accurate treatment planning. For example, ADL assessment might describe the person's function on a four-point independence scale; however, a score of 'unable to perform' or 'dependent' does not provide data on the limiting factors in the person's performance within an activity or the reason for any observed deficits. The treatment plan will need to be different for a person dependent in dressing because of a motor deficit from a person who is dependent because of apraxia, or visual field deficit or problems within initiation. Most therapists require more information than a simple description of what the person can and cannot do; they need data that help them to problem-solve and hypothesise about the reasons behind observed dysfunction. Therefore, when selecting a descriptive assessment, the therapist needs to think about what behaviours/circumstances she needs to describe and may need to use more than one descriptive assessment to answer all the questions that need answers to form an accurate baseline for treatment planning. For example, she may need a description of the person's home environment and social supports at a societal limitation level, a description of the person's ability to mobilise, transfer and perform ADL at a disability level and also a description of the person's motor and sensory functioning at an impairment level (see Chapter 9).

Many assessments focus on the person's ability to carry out a test item or his degree of independence, but there are other more qualitative aspects of performance that therapists may want to describe as the basis for treatment planning. These include:

- the physical effort that the client exerts to perform the assessment, which indicates the magnitude of physical difficulty or fatigue
- the efficiency with which the client carries out the assessment, which indicates the extent of any unnecessary use of time, space or objects or evidence of disorganisation
- safety issues, as therapists often need to consider the risk of personal injury or environmental damage (Fisher, 2003a).

An example of an assessment that provides descriptive data at different levels of function is the Structured Observational Test of Function (SOTOF; Laver and Powell, 1995). The SOTOF is a standardised, valid and reliable measure with established clinical utility and face validity (Laver, 1994) that enables the therapist to describe the person's ability to perform four basic self-care tasks (washing, dressing, eating, pouring a drink and drinking). Each ADL scale is broken down into small subcomponents, and so the therapist also obtains detailed descriptive data about the aspects of the task the person finds difficult. For example, the SOTOF enables the therapist to answer questions about how the different components of the task are undertaken. These questions are:

- Can he recognise the objects required for the task?
- Does the client accurately reach for the item of clothing?
- Can he organise the garment to put on?
- Does he sequence the task correctly?
- Has he the fine-motor skills to do up the buttons?

From data collected about how the person attempted each task, the therapist is then guided through a diagnostic reasoning process to hypothesise about the underlying impairment level deficits (see Chapter 10). Some test items are also included to directly assess impairment level functioning, such as sensory functioning (for example tactile, taste and temperature discrimination), perceptual functioning (for example colour recognition, right/left discrimination, figure/ground discrimination, depth and distance perception) and visual functioning (visual acuity, field loss, neglect, scanning) and motor functioning (muscle tone, dexterity, bilateral integration, ideomotor apraxia).

DISCRIMINATIVE ASSESSMENTS

Therapists use discriminative assessments to distinguish between individuals or groups. For this purpose, comparisons are usually made against a normative group or another diagnostic group. Comparisons may be made for reasons such as making a diagnosis, matching a client against referral criteria or for prioritising referrals, deciding on appropriate placement or evaluating a person's level of dysfunction in relation to expectations of performance of other healthy people of that age (for example to see if a child is developing skills at the expected stage versus has a developmental delay). For the purposes of this book, *discriminative assessment* will be defined as:

Definition of discriminative assessment

A discriminative assessment is a measure that has been developed to 'distinguish between individuals or groups on an underlying dimension when no external criterion or gold standard is available for validating these measures' (Law, 2001, p. 287).

Depending on their precise purposes, both descriptive and discriminative assessments can be labelled as *diagnostic indices*, which are used to assist clinical diagnosis and to detect impairment and/or disability in a diagnostic group. Therapists, often working in a multidisciplinary team setting, use discriminative assessments to help with accurate diagnosis, for example to assess whether a person has dementia versus depression, or dementia versus cognitive decline associated with the normal ageing process, or to diagnose a specific type of dementia, such as Lewy Body dementia (Saxton *et al.*, 1993). In an ageing population, changes occur as a result of normal ageing, for example in the cognitive-perceptual system. Therefore, comprehensive normative data for older populations are required so that therapists can evaluate assessment results in the context of normal ageing processes to discriminate pathology from expected change.

When selecting standardised tests for discriminative assessment, the value of the test is dependent on the adequacy of, and the ability to generalise from, the normative sample or client population used to obtain reference data. The lack of normative or comparative test standardisation with a population similar to the specific client restricts the therapist's ability to make accurate and valid comparisons. An example of this is where assessments initially developed and standardised for child populations have been used with adult populations or where tests developed in another country for a different cultural group are used without consideration to potential differences. In addition, test developers should undertake validity studies to explore the value of test items for discriminating between groups of interest. *Discriminative validity* relates to whether a test provides a valid measure to distinguish between individuals or groups (see Chapter 6).

An example of a test that has a discriminative purpose is the Infant and Toddler Symptom Checklist (DeGangi *et al.*, 1995). This is a proxy measure developed for use with parents of seven- to 30-month-old infants and toddlers. The Symptom Checklist can be used to discriminate between infants and toddlers who are developing normally and those who have sensory-integrative disorders, attentional deficits and emotional and behavioural problems. The Symptom Checklist is provided in five age bands (7–9, 10–12, 13–18, 19–24 and 25–30 months) and normative data giving expected score ranges and a cut-off to discriminate an expected from a deficit score are provided for each age band.

At a time when many therapy departments are struggling to deal with waiting lists and have more demands placed on their service than capacity to deliver a service promptly to all referrals, therapists should consider the use of discriminative assessments as screening tools to help identify the appropriateness of referrals and prioritise referrals. In order to prioritise their referrals and offer a prompt service to those children in greatest need, Green *et al.* (2005) carried out a study to explore whether two questionnaire-based screening tools could differentiate between children with a developmental coordination disorder (DCD) who needed a full therapy assessment and children with only a low risk of DCD. They compared the results of a parent-completed assessment (the Development Coordination Disorder Questionnaire (DCDQ; Wilson *et al.*, 2000) and a teacher-completed checklist for the Movement Assessment Battery for Children (Movement ABC; Henderson and Sugden, 1992) with the results of the therapist's observational assessment. The therapist assessment comprised standardised tools including the Assessment of Motor Process Skills (AMPS; Fisher, 2003a and b) and the Movement ABC. The researchers found that there was a strong relationship between the parent report using the DCDQ and the therapist's classification of a child as having, or being at risk of, DCD following observational assessment. Green *et al.* (2005) conclude: 'the sensitivity of the DCDQ in this instance suggests that it performs well in screening those children most likely to have coordination difficulties' (p. 7). However, the checklist version of the Movement ABC used with teachers was found to have 'poor discriminative ability . . . as a screening measure for a clinically referred population' (p. 8).

PREDICTIVE ASSESSMENTS

Predictive tests are also sometimes labelled as *prognostic measures*. For the purposes of this book, *predictive assessment* will be defined as:

Definition of predictive assessment

Predictive assessment is undertaken by therapists to predict the future ability or state of a client or to predict a specific outcome in the future (Adams, 2002).

Therapists use predictive assessments to classify people into pre-defined categories of interest in an attempt to predict an event or functional status in another situation on the basis of the person's performance on the assessment. For example, a kitchen assessment in a therapy department might be used to predict whether the person should be independent and safe in meal preparation once discharged home, or a work assessment may be used to predict current and future employment potential. A predictive test is a measure that has been designed to 'classify individuals into a set of predefined measurement categories, either concurrently or prospectively, to determine whether individuals have been classified correctly' (Law, 2001, p. 287). It is critical that a test used for predictive purposes has established predictive validity (see Chapter 6). *Predictive validity* has been defined as 'the accuracy with which a measurement predicts some future event' (McDowell and Newell, 1987, p. 329).

Predictive assessments can be used to identify patients at risk of a particular factor, such as suicide, abuse or falling. In premature or young infants, a predictive assessment may be used to identify those children at risk of developing a problem such as a developmental delay or emotional and behavioural problems; this can enable therapists to channel limited resources to those children most at risk and most likely to benefit from an early intervention. For example, in addition to meeting a discriminative purpose, the Infant and Toddler Symptom Checklist (DeGangi *et al.*, 1995) also aims to predict infants and toddlers 'who are at risk for sensory-integrative disorders, attentional deficits, and emotional and behavioural problems' (p. 1). In a study of 14 infants, 12 were assessed on the Symptom Checklist as falling within the risk range, and the authors report that all 12 had demonstrated regulatory problems when tested on standardised measures, with nine having sensory-processing deficits, three having attentional deficits and one child showing both sensory and attentional problems.

Lewis and Bottomley (1994) give an example of how a standardised test can be used to make predictions by interpreting scores from the Barthel Index:

> A score of 60 or above means that the person can be discharged home but will require at least 2 hours of assistance in ADLs. If they score 80 or above, it means that the person can be discharged home but will require assistance of up to 2 hours in self-care! (Lewis and Bottomley, 1994, p. 150)

EVALUATIVE ASSESSMENT

For the purposes of this book, *evaluative assessment* will be defined as:

Definition of evaluative assessment

Evaluative assessment is used to detect change in functioning over time and is undertaken to monitor a client's progress during rehabilitation and to determine the effectiveness of the intervention.

Evaluative tests are commonly known as *outcome measures*. When measuring outcomes, the therapist explores whether any change in the client has occurred as a result of a specific therapy intervention. An evaluative assessment is a measure that can detect and measure the amount of change of the desired outcome over time (Adams, 2002). Evaluative tests are used 'to measure the magnitude of longitudinal change in an individual or group on the dimension of interest' (Law, 2001, p. 287). Evaluative tests should have established test–retest and inter-rater reliability (see Chapter 7).

Responsiveness to change refers to the measure of efficiency with which a test detects clinical change (Wright, Cross and Lamb, 1998). When selecting an evaluative measure, therapists should consider how responsive the test is to detecting the type of clinical change they wish to measure. Therapists should look for reference to psychometric studies that demonstrate responsiveness, specificity and sensitivity as an evaluative measure needs to be a specific and sensitive measure that can pick up the type and degree of change in function that is anticipated (for more information on responsiveness, sensitivity and specificity see Chapter 7). Improvements in function may be small and slow, and many assessments lack sensitivity because they do not have sufficient graduations to measure change or because they do not include test items that are the focus of rehabilitation. There is also a paucity of test–retest reliability (see Chapter 7) data for many current assessments. It is critical to use objective and sensitive measures because 'any subjective estimate, especially if made by the clinician who has invested time, effort and perhaps more in treating the client, is likely to be unreliable' (de Clive-Lowe, 1996, p. 359).

The CSP offers the following advice for selecting appropriate measures of outcome.

> Consider this question: What am I attempting to change? In general the answer might be to speed up recovery or maintain functional status. However, to help choose a measure, consider the question in more depth; what is it about recovery or functional status that you want to speed up or maintain? This could be a patient's ability to cope, their self-esteem, confidence, sleep patterns, an impairment, improved ability to do something, or to participate in day to day life . . . Once you have identified your aims of treatment it will be easier to decide how you will record whether you succeed or not. (Chartered Society of Physiotherapy, 2001a, p. 4)

Enderby (1998, cited in Adams, 2002, p. 173), in a book on therapy outcome measures, groups the aims of therapy into four categories, which are:

1. improvement or remediation of any underlying impairment
2. extension of functional performance
3. improvement of social integration
4. alleviation of emotional distress.

It is critical to identify the aim of your intervention because, if your goal is the improved performance of an ADL, measurement of an underlying component would not measure your outcome. You might learn that the person had increased in strength or ROM but you would not know if these improvements at an impairment level had resulted in improvements in function in the person's daily activities (see Chapter 9 for further exploration of levels of function). In the same way, a measure of level of independence in ADLs would not enable you to measure the person's level of social inclusion or their experience of emotional distress.

An outcome measure should be used at the start of intervention to provide a baseline and then re-administered when intervention ceases in order to ascertain the effects of the intervention. The process for measuring outcomes has been described by the COT (2003a, p. 25) as:

- establishing a baseline from which to measure change
- agreeing realistic, desired outcomes
- defining those outcomes as observable and measurable items of performance
- implementing treatment for an agreed period
- carrying out the same assessment again
- reviewing goals and, if appropriate, revising desired outcomes.

An example of an evaluative test is the Therapy Outcomes Measure (TOM; Enderby and John, 1997). This measure was developed in the UK, initially as a measure of speech therapy outcomes. It was adapted for use by occupational therapists, physiotherapists and rehabilitation nurses by Enderby, John and Petherham (1998). The TOM provides a global measure of health outcomes and can be used with clients of different ages and with a wide variety of diagnoses. The conceptual foundation of the TOM was based on the World Health Organization's (WHO; 1980) International Classification of Impairments, Disabilities and Handicaps (ICIDH-1) (see Chapter 9 for a description of the ICIDH model). The therapist records baseline and post-test scores for four test domains: impairment, disability, handicap and distress/well-being. Scoring is undertaken using an 11-point ordinal scale (see Chapter 4 for a definition of an ordinal scale). Recently, research has been conducted in Australia to develop outcome measures based on the revised WHO model (2002) International Classification of Functioning, Disability and Health (ICF; see Chapter 9 for more details of the ICF model), which provides a greater focus on health rather than disease. Commonwealth Government funding has enabled researchers to adapt the TOM to be compatible with the ICF and to produce separate scales for occupational therapy, physiotherapy and speech pathology (Perry *et al.*, 2004).

The occupational therapy version, Australian Therapy Outcome Measures for Occupational Therapy (AusTOMs-OT; Unsworth and Duncombe, 2004), now comprises four domains, with the first three drawn from the ICF model: impairment, activity limitation, participation restriction and distress/well-being. It is made up of 12 scales (for a list of these scale items see Chapter 9) of which the therapist selects only those that relate to agreed therapy outcomes; in practice this tends to range between one to five outcome scales being used per client (see Figure 3.1).

Initial reliability studies for the AusTOMs-OT look favourable, with acceptable levels of inter-rater reliability (over 70% agreement) demonstrated (Unsworth, 2005). Thirty-three of the 48 test items (12 scales by four domains in the total test) were found to have test–retest reliability levels of at least 70% agreement, with the lowest level for the remaining items being 50%. A further reliability study that just focused on the self-care scale (found to be the most frequently applied scale) showed better levels of reliability (Wiseman, 2004, cited by Unsworth, 2005), with 'inter-rater interclass correlation coefficients (ICCs) over 0.79 for the three domains of activity limitation, participation restriction and distress/wellbeing, and over 0.70 for impairment. Test–retest reliability was also reported to be quite high, with ICCs of 0.88 for activity limitation, 0.81 for participation restriction, 0.94 for distress/wellbeing and 0.74 for impairment' (p. 356). Unsworth (2005) also reports on a study to examine the sensitivity of the AusTOMs-OT to detect change in client status over time. A large sample of 466 clients was assessed across 12 health facilities and results indicated 'that all scales were successful in demonstrating statistically significant client change over time' (p. 354).

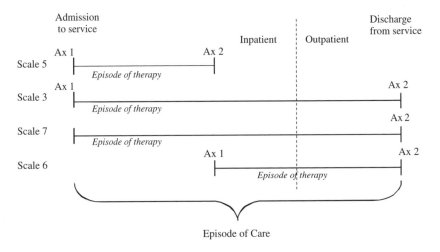

Key

Ax1 – Assessment 1
Ax2 – Assessment 2
Scale 5 – Transfers
Scale 3 – Upper limb use
Scale 7 – Self care
Scale 6 – Using transport

Figure 3.1 Scoring AusTOM-OT scales with Josef. *Reprinted with permission from Unsworth, CA and Duncombe D (2004) AusTOMs for Occupational Therapy. La Trobe University, Melbourne, and as published in Unsworth (2005) in the British Journal of Occupational Therapy.*

ASSESSMENT FOR PARTICULAR PURPOSES

SINGLE ASSESSMENT PROCESS

An interesting example of how policymakers for health and social care have thought explicitly about the purposes of assessment is provided by the single assessment process (SAP). The introduction of a single assessment process is a key component of the person-centred care standard of the *National Service Framework for Older People* published by the Department of Health (DoH; 2001a). The SAP aims to make sure older people's care needs are assessed thoroughly and accurately, but without procedures being needlessly duplicated by different agencies. The DoH states: 'the purpose of SAP is to ensure that older people receive appropriate, effective and timely responses to their health and social care needs, and that professional resources are used effectively. In pursuit of these aims, the SAP should ensure that:

- Individuals are placed at the heart of assessment and care planning, and these processes are timely and in proportion to individuals' needs.
- Professionals are willing, able and confident to use their judgement.
- Care plans or statements of service delivery are routinely produced and service users receive a copy.
- Professionals contribute to assessments in the most effective way, and care co-ordinators are agreed in individual cases when necessary.
- Information is collected, stored and shared as effectively as possible and subject to consent.
- Professionals and agencies do not duplicate each other's assessments'(Department of Health, 2006b).

Both physiotherapists and occupational therapists have key roles to play in the development and implementation of a SAP. The DoH issued statements for a number of different professional groups including one concerning the single assessment process and its key implications for therapists. This acknowledges that:

> Physiotherapists [and] occupational therapists, . . . as part of allied health professionals, play a critical role in assessing the needs of older people, and all have expertise and experience working with older people who are experiencing health and social care difficulties. Too often this contribution is under-recognised. However, . . . therapists will contribute to all types of assessment described in the detailed single assessment process guidance. (Department of Health, 2002b, p. 1)

A significant number of therapists have already been involved with pilot SAP projects and SAP tool development. The domains described for SAP assessment are domains frequently assessed by occupational therapists and physiotherapists (see Box 3.1 below and pp. 263–79).

Earlier in this chapter, we looked at a therapy process and considered where assessment fitted within this process, both in terms of timing and purpose. The DoH recommends that a clear process should be established with well-defined stages of assessment care planning, review and other aspects of care management. This process has some overlap with a therapy intervention process. The DoH (2002a, p. 4) recommends a SAP process should cover:

- publishing information about services
- completing assessment
  - contact assessment, including the collection of basic personal information
  - overview assessment
  - specialist assessment
  - comprehensive assessment
- evaluating assessment information
- deciding what help should be offered, including eligibility decisions
- care planning
- monitoring
- review.

As this chapter is focused on the purpose of assessment, it is useful to briefly present the way in which the DoH has identified four different purposes of assessment for a SAP. The first type of assessment has been labelled a *contact assessment*. This has been defined as:

Definition of a SAP contact assessment

A contact assessment 'refers to a contact between an older person and health and social services where significant needs are first described or suspected . . . At contact assessment basic personal information is collected and the nature of the presenting problem is established and the potential presence of wider health and social care needs is explored . . . where:

- presenting needs are not clear cut; or
- other potential needs are identified; or
- requests for more intensive forms of support or treatment have been made' (Department of Health, 2002c, p. 4).

A formal contact assessment does not have to be undertaken for every contact. In some cases, a therapist could be the first point of contact. The following guidance is helpful in enabling a therapist to judge when a contact assessment should be recorded.

Where presenting needs or requests are straightforward and people have indicated there are no other needs or issues, it would usually be inappropriate for professionals to prolong the assessment or even to regard every such contact as amounting to contact assessment as defined here . . . Some people may only request pieces of assistive equipment such as grab rails, helping hands or bath mats. These requests can be dealt with promptly, provided there are no other needs, the equipment is appropriate to the assessed or eligible need, and its safe use is explained. (Department of Health, 2002c, p. 3–4)

Box 3.1 SAP assessment domains

User's perspective

- Needs and issues in the user's own words and service user's expectations, strengths, abilities and motivation

Clinical background

- History of medical conditions and diagnoses, history of falls, medication use and ability to self-medicate

Disease prevention

- Under this section the most relevant domain for therapists relates to assessing the person's exercise and nutritional patterns and smoking and drinking habits.

Personal care and physical well-being

- Personal hygiene, including washing, bathing, toileting and grooming, dressing, oral health and foot-care
- Pain
- Tissue viability
- Mobility
- Continence and other aspects of elimination
- Sleeping patterns

Senses

- Sight
- Hearing
- Communication

Mental health

- Cognition and dementia, including orientation and memory
- Mental health, including depression, reactions to loss and emotional difficulties

Relationships

- Social contacts, relationships and involvement in leisure, hobbies, work and learning
- Carer support and strength of caring arrangements, including the carer's perspective

Safety issues

- Abuse and neglect, other aspects of personal safety and public safety

Immediate environment and resources

- Care of the home and managing daily tasks, such as food preparation, cleaning and shopping, housing (location, access, amenities, heating), access to local facilities and services
- Level and management of finances

As part of a contact assessment, seven key issues are identified, which should be explored when identifying needs (Department of Health, 2002c, p. 3):

1. The nature of the presenting need.
2. The significance of the need for the older person.
3. The length of time the need has been experienced.
4. Potential solutions identified by the older person.
5. Other needs experienced by the older person.
6. Recent life events or changes relevant to the problem(s).
7. The perceptions of family members and carers.

The second type of assessment has been labelled an *overview assessment.* The purpose of an overview assessment is to provide a broad, contextual assessment of the person's situation and problems. For the purposes of this book, *overview assessment* will be defined as:

Definition of overview assessment

An overview assessment is required if the presenting problem is not clear-cut or if there is evidence of potential wider health and/or social care needs. An overview assessment is undertaken by a health or social care professional who undertakes a broad assessment of some or all of the SAP domains.

'Professionals carry out an overview assessment if, in their judgement, the individual's needs are such that a more rounded assessment should be undertaken' (Department of Health, 2002c, p. 4). For an overview assessment, all or some of the SAP domains (see Box 3.1) are assessed. The DoH states that an overview assessment should be completed by a single professional from either health or social services; this professional could be an occupational therapist or physiotherapist as the domains covered for SAP are domains frequently assessed by therapists. An overview assessment may identify domains that require a more in-depth specialist assessment. While the DoH (2002b) notes that therapists 'may do their fair share of overview assessment', it states that 'therapists will contribute greatly to specialist and comprehensive assessments' (p. 1).

The third type of SAP assessment is labelled *specialist assessment,* which will be defined as:

Definition of SAP specialist assessment

A specialist assessment is 'an assessment undertaken by a clinician or other professional who specialises in a branch of medicine or care, e.g. stroke, cardiac care, bereavement counselling' (Department of Health, 2001a, p. 160).

Specialist assessment is undertaken when a SAP domain needs to be explored in detail. The DoH (2002c) states: 'as a result of a specialist assessment, professionals should be able to confirm the presence, extent, cause and likely development of a health condition or problem or social care need, and establish links to other conditions, problems and needs' (p. 7).

Both occupational therapists and physiotherapists are seen to play an important role in providing specialist level assessments as part of the SAP. The DoH names therapists as appropriate professionals who can provide specialist assessments.

> At all times, specialist assessments will rely for their quality on the involvement and judgement of appropriately qualified and competent professionals, such as occupational therapists, physiotherapists . . . (Department of Health, 2002c, p. 7)

In particular, the DoH (2002b) notes that therapists 'can offer a specialist contribution to the assessment of mobility, transfers . . . eating, drinking, and functional capacity, and the impact of the home and wider environment on assessed needs' and goes on to acknowledge that 'in particular therapists are skilled in the assessment of potential for rehabilitation and independence' (p. 1).

The use of standardised assessments is of particular importance for both specialist and comprehensive assessments. Therapists are advised that 'they should ensure that assessment scales to identify physical and personal care problems have a prominent role in assessment procedures' (Department of Health, 2002b, p. 1). However, the value of professional judgement is also highlighted 'but these scales [should] not predominate and are used to support professional judgement' (p. 1).

The fourth, and final, type of SAP assessment is labelled a comprehensive assessment. A comprehensive assessment may be required for several reasons. For the purposes of this book, *comprehensive assessment* will be defined as:

Definition of SAP comprehensive assessment

A comprehensive assessment provides an assessment that is both broad and deep and involves specialist assessments of all or most of the domains of the single assessment process. A comprehensive assessment 'should be completed for people where the level of support and treatment likely to be offered is intensive or prolonged, including permanent admission to a care home, intermediate care services, or substantial packages of care at home' (Department of Health, 2002c, p. 8).

As stated earlier, therapists have a key role to play in providing comprehensive assessment. This will often be as part of a specialist geriatric or elderly psychiatry multidisciplinary team. A coordinated multidisciplinary approach is seen to be 'crucial for accurate and timely diagnoses of treatable and other health conditions, without which wider assessment and subsequent care planning is likely to be flawed' (Department of Health, 2002c, p. 8). For a comprehensive assessment, it is also critical that any specialist assessments, particularly if these have been conducted by a number of different professionals, are coordinated, compared and interpreted.

These four types of assessment should not be considered as sequential. The four types are distinguished by the breadth and depth of information collected. Therapists involved with SAP have to use their judgement as to how broad (number of domains covered) and how specific (the depth to which a particular domain is assessed) the assessment should be for each client. The purposes and timing of these four types of assessment are summarised in Table 3.1 (below).

Reviews related to SAP

The DoH provides guidance related to the review of older people in terms of the SAP.

> Reviews of care plans should be scheduled and undertaken on a routine basis. According to 'Better care, higher standards' there should be an initial review within three months of health, housing and social services first being provided or major changes in service provision being effected. Thereafter, reviews should be scheduled at least annually, or more often if necessary. From time to time, unscheduled reviews will be required when unexpected major changes occur. (Department of Health, 2002c, p. 15)

The DoH goes on to recommended that 'one-off pieces of assistive equipment do not need reviewing after initial confirmation of suitability and safety when used' (p. 15). However, it

Table 3.1 SAP: Summary of the four types of assessment

Type	Summary of purpose	When used?	Who can undertake?
Contact	• basic personal data • identify the nature of presenting problem • establish presence of wider health/social care needs	At first contact between an older person and health/social services where significant needs are first described or suspected.	Trained person, but does not have to be a professionally qualified staff member
Overview	• explores all or some of the SAP domains • professional judges which domains to assess • scales used	Conducted if presenting problems are not clear and/or undertaken if there is an indication of a wider/other need identified in the contact assessment.	A single professional from health or social care
Specialist	• all or some domains • professional judges which domains to assess • specific needs examined in detail • standardised tests used	To confirm the presence, extent, cause and prognosis of a health condition or social care problem. To establish links to other problems, conditions or needs.	Appropriately qualified professional(s)
Comprehensive	• includes specialist assessment of all/most domains and sub-domains • involves coordination and collating of assessments and interpretation of test results • scales used	If the person is likely to require intensive or prolonged support/treatment (e.g. substantial packages of care, intermediate care, longer-term rehabilitation or need permanent admission to a care home).	A range of appropriate professionals and/or specialist teams

advises that 'major items of equipment should be reviewed as to their suitability and safety on an annual basis' (p. 15). The DoH summarises the purpose of reviews for older people as being to:

• establish how far the support and treatment have achieved the outcomes set out in the care plan
• re-assess the needs and issues of individual service users
• help determine users' continued eligibility for support and treatment
• confirm or amend the current care plan or lead to closure
• comment on how individuals are managing direct payments [payments received to purchase support direct from providers], where appropriate. (Department of Health, 2002c, p. 15)

CAPACITY ASSESSMENT

Therapists may need to consider capacity issues. First, does the client have the capacity to consent to the proposed physiotherapy and/or occupational therapy intervention. Second, a therapist might be asked to contribute to an assessment of the person's capacity in a particular situation, for example to assess whether someone remains competent to drive following a stroke or the onset of dementia.

The COT's position statement on consent for occupational therapy (1993, 4.4) considers the issue of capacity.

> Whilst no-one can consent on behalf of an adult, in relation to the consumer who lacks capacity, at common law, the occupational therapist in common with other health professionals owes a duty to act in the consumer's best interests. Such action may include substantial treatment to preserve the life and health of the individual, but may also include routine matters to preserve the consumers' general well-being. (College of Occupational Therapists, 1993, 4.4)

Therapists may be asked to make an informed judgement about a person's capacity or incapacity. *Incapacity* is defined by the DoH as:

> He or she is unable to understand or retain the information to the decision, including information about the reasonably foreseeable consequences of deciding one way or another or failing to make the decision. He or she is unable to make a decision based on the information relevant to the decision, including information about the reasonably foreseeable consequences of deciding one way or another or failing to make the decision. (Department of Health, 1999a, p. 89)

More recently, the Mental Capacity Act 2005 (Department of Health, 2006a) provides a detailed consideration of capacity issues. This is a very important Act and therapists should be aware of its implications. The Act is underpinned by a set of five key principles stated in Section 1:

- 'A presumption of capacity: every adult has the right to make his or her own decisions and must be assumed to have capacity to do so unless it is proved otherwise;
- The right for individuals to be supported to make their own decisions: people must be given all appropriate help before anyone concludes that they cannot make their own decisions;
- That individuals must retain the right to make what might be seen as eccentric or unwise decisions;
- Best interests: anything done for or on behalf of people without capacity must be in their best interests; and
- Least restrictive intervention: anything done for or on behalf of people without capacity should be the least restrictive of their basic rights and freedoms' (Department of Health, 2006a).

The Act discusses the assessment of a person's capacity and acts by carers of those who lack capacity. In relation to assessing lack of capacity the *Mental Capacity Act – summary* states:

> The Act sets out a single clear test for assessing whether a person lacks capacity to take a particular decision at a particular time. It is a 'decision-specific' test. No one can be labelled 'incapable' as a result of a particular medical condition or diagnosis. Section 2 of the Act makes it clear that a lack of capacity cannot be established merely by reference to a person's age, appearance, or any condition or aspect of a person's behaviour which might lead others to make unjustified assumptions about capacity. (Department of Health, 2006a)

The Mental Capacity Act states factors that decision-makers must explore when deciding what is in a person's best interests. Therapists will need to explore whether the person has made an 'advanced wishes' statement and must consider any written statement in which the person has articulated his wishes and feelings when making a determination about the person's best interests. Carers and family members also have a right to be consulted. Section 5 of the Mental Capacity Act 2005 clarifies that, where a person is providing care or treatment for someone who lacks capacity, the person can provide the care without incurring legal liability. The key will be proper assessment of capacity and best interests; so therapists must ensure that a thorough assessment of capacity has been undertaken and that the process and descision made from this assessment are clearly and thoroughly documented. This assessment and documentation serves to cover any actions that would otherwise result in a civil wrong or crime if someone has interfered with the person's body or property in the ordinary course of caring.

The Mental Capacity Act 2005 also introduces a new role in the appointment of a independent mental capacity advocate (IMCA). An IMCA is seen as 'someone appointed to support a person who lacks capacity but has no one to speak for them. The IMCA makes representations about the person's wishes, feelings, beliefs and values, at the same time as bringing to the attention of the decision-maker all factors that are relevant to the decision. The IMCA can challenge the decision-maker on behalf of the person lacking capacity if necessary' (Department of Health, 2006a). In future, therapists may need to consult with an appointed IMCA when assessing and treating a person who has been found to lack capacity to consent to the therapy intervention.

ASSESSMENT FOR TRIBUNALS

Occupational therapists and physiotherapists (for example as members of the care team) may be required to provide information for tribunals that includes baseline assessment data, treatment plans, evaluation of the effectiveness of the treatment, plans for continuing care/review post discharge. Therapists may be involved in providing information that enables a tribunal to judge whether the criteria for compulsory powers are met, the proposed care plan is consistent with the principles set out in the law and the interventions are appropriate to the treatment of the person's disorder/diagnosis (Carr, 2001).

RISK ASSESSMENT

Assessment of risk is a very big part of occupational therapists' and physiotherapists' clinical work. It can range from a small and fairly straightforward risk decision, for example: 'What is the risk that this elderly person will trip on their loose mat and should I advise that it is taken up before their discharge home?' to decisions that relate to potentially life threatening events, such as: 'What is the risk that this person will become violent and hurt another person?', 'What is the risk that this child is being physically abused by his parent?' and 'What is the risk that this person will forget to turn the gas cooker off?'

Systematic risk assessment is defined as a 'systematic approach to the identification and assessment of risks using explicit risk management techniques' (Department of Health, 2004, p. 22). More tools are now available to assess aspects of risk. For example, guidance related to SAP explicitly addresses the assessment of risk. (*Note:* we looked at the SAP earlier in this chapter.)

> As needs are fully described and explored, the individual and professional should consider and evaluate the risks to independence that result from the needs. This evaluation should take full account of the likely outcome if help were not to be provided. In considering how needs and risks might change over time, professionals should focus on the impact of needs on people's independence both in the immediate and longer term and consequent risks to independence. (Department of Health, 2002c, p. 11)

The DoH also lists the following factors as particular areas to be considered as part of a risk assessment.

- autonomy and freedom to make choices
- health and safety, including freedom from harm, abuse and neglect, and taking wider issues of housing circumstances and community safety into account

- the ability to manage personal and other daily routines
- involvement in family and wider community life, including leisure, hobbies, unpaid and paid work, learning and volunteering (Department of Health, 2002c, p. 11).

Therapists are also instructed to consider risks faced by people close to their clients, such as carers. Therapists need to identify 'which risks cause serious concern, and which risks may be acceptable or viewed as a natural and healthy part of independent living' (p. 11) and discuss these with clients and carers so that informed choices can be made.

In response to SAP guidance, a number of tools have been developed. One test that is being implemented in the older people's mental health service in which I work is the Functional Assessment of Care Environment (FACE) Risk Profile. This is one scale in the FACE Assessment and Outcome System (Clifford, 2002). Clifford's PhD work (2003) provides the foundation for the FACE. His thesis presents 'the development and testing of a new approach to outcome measurement referred to as the "infometric approach". The key principles behind this approach are that it follows the naturally occurring clinical process, integrates recording and measurement functions and is based on a multi-axial representation of a person' (p. 2). Clifford details the development of the FACE, which has been designed to measure health and social functioning and risk. His study draws upon outcomes data collected on more than 1000 patients. In the analysis, Clifford describes the psychometric properties of FACE and examines broader issues, including: 'the relationship between global clinical judgements of impact upon quality of life and clinical assessment at the item and axial level; the relationship between judgments of risk and the observation of risk factors and warning signs; the prediction of risk behaviour; the relationship between practitioner perception of severity of problems and patient perceptions of quality of life; and the relationship between practitioner and patient perceptions of risk' (p. 2). He concludes that the FACE can be used to represent accurately patient characteristics and to measure change.

Two of the most important areas of risk that a therapist might need to assess are risk of harm to self and risk of harm to others. Blank (2001) undertook a systematic review of 10 studies related to the assessment of risk of violence in a community mental health setting. She focused on both clinical and contextual factors in the prediction of violence risk. This is an area where the predictive validity (see Chapter 6) of any measure of risk is very important. Blank explored two main approaches to the assessment of risk of violence. The first approach involves clinical judgement and the therapist's assessment of the person's predisposition to violence based on available data about the person and his background, diagnosis, history and social situation. The second approach is called 'actuarial prediction of violence' and 'involves the assigning of a numerical value to factors known to contribute to being violent. For example, being male, falling within a certain age-group or having a coexisting diagnosis of substance misuse would all attract certain scores. Risk is then calculated by the overall score' (Blank, 2001, p. 585).

Blank found very little literature in therapy journals but review of the 10 studies, identified by her literature search, did yield information of relevance to therapists, and she concludes that:

> therapists are well placed to assess factors . . . it appears from the four studies looking at the context of violence risk that factors such as social support, the environment in which a person lives and family dynamics are significant when predicting risk of violence (Blank, 2001, p. 587)

These factors are areas of assessment that are routinely considered by therapists.

One measure used for the assessment of suicidal ideation is the Beck Scale for Suicide Ideation (BBS; Beck and Steer, 1991). This is a 21-item self-report assessment that is used with adolescents and adults to detect and measure the severity of suicidal ideation. Therapists might presume that such a test would provide a predictive assessment of suicide but should look carefully at any predictive validity data to justify this presumption. The authors originally developed other scales in this field, including the Scale for Suicide Ideation (SSI; Beck, Kovacs and Weissman, 1979) and the Beck Hopelessness Scale (BHS; Beck and Steer, 1988). In the current BSS manual, the authors refer to a predictive validity study of the SSI and BHS that was a longitudinal study with 207 people who had been identified as suicide ideators (Beck *et al.*, 1985). They found that the SSI did not predict eventual suicide but that the BHS did (Beck and Steer, 1991, p. 21). In a further study, they found that the predictive validity for the SSI improved if people were asked to rate the items in terms of 'their feelings at the worst period in their psychiatric illness' (p. 21). In this study of 72 outpatients, the eight people who went on to commit suicide had a mean SSI score of 21.75 (s.d. = 10.43) compared to the remaining 64 patients, who had a mean SSI score of only 9.7 (s.d. = 9.98); this was found to be a significant difference (p < 0.01). The BSS was built upon earlier studies and is a self-report version of the SSI that has been developed to be used either alone or with the clinical (interview/observational) rating version. At the beginning of the BSS, the authors note a number of cautions and limitations of the measure, including:

1. 'The BSS scores are best regarded as indicators of suicide risk rather than as predictors of eventual suicide in a given case' (p. 1).

So therapists need to be aware that the BSS does not actually predict who will go on to commit suicide, but it may help them identify people at risk of committing suicide.

2. 'The BSS systematically covers a broad spectrum of attitudes and behaviors that clinicians routinely consider in judging suicidal intention. The BSS measures suicide ideation: as such, it should not be used as a sole source of information in the assessment of suicide risk. Any endorsement of any BSS item may reflect the presence of suicide intention and should be investigated by the clinician' (p. 1).

Therapists should use the test as a starting point and should undertake more detailed assessment of those areas of suicidal ideation that are shown up on the BSS. The 21 BSS items comprise 19 items that measure facets of suicide and two items that relate to the number of previous suicide attempts and the seriousness of the person's intention to die when the last suicide attempt was made.

3. 'The BSS is a self-report instrument and contains no mechanism to detect dissimulation or confusion. Suicidal patients may deliberately conceal their intentions from others and may distort their BSS responses' (p. 1).

A person who is very serious in his intention to commit suicide may not want help and may deliberately underrate himself on the self-report scale. In Chapter 2, we considered the value of obtaining assessment data from three different sources (self-report, proxy report and therapist observation) and then triangulating data to explore consistencies and inconsistencies in the results obtained from each source. For the assessment of risk of suicide, such an approach is very valuable, and a measure, such as the BSS, would form just one part of your total assessment.

Another more common area of therapy risk assessment involves the assessment of the person's home environment, such as at a pre-discharge home visit. The DoH (2001a) defines a *home safety check* as 'a check made, for example, by an occupational therapist to ensure that an individual is safe and can manage in their own home' (p. 155). There are a number of standardised assessments that can make such an assessment more rigorous, for example the Safety Assessment of Function and the Environment for Rehabilitation (SAFER Tool) developed by the Community Occupational Therapists and Associates (COTA; 1991).

NEEDS ASSESSMENT: CONSIDERING WIDER POPULATIONS

Therapists have an important role to play as advocates and lobbyists for people with disabilities. For example, therapists may be asked to undertake an assessment to evaluate the accessibility of their local community. Even if we are not asked, as professionals embracing the health promotion and inclusion agendas, we should put ourselves forward with this assessment purpose. Many communities still pose severe challenges for people with disabilities, and even the simplest of needs, such as an accessible toilet, is sadly lacking in many environments. We are being encouraged by people with disabilities to help in this fight. Bonnie Sherr Klein, who suffered a stroke, writes:

> We demand a right to pee! writes disability activist Joan Meister. Lack of accessible washrooms limits the lives of many disabled people. It's amazing how many public places will tell you that they're wheelchair accessible and it turns out their toilet is down a flight of stairs. Or the washroom is too narrow to fit a wheelchair. Or there's no grab-bar. Or the grab-bar is installed too high. I have a friend who drinks no liquids all day if she's planning to go out in the evening. I have other friends who just don't go out. Unholy details can determine where we live, work or go to school, not just whether we go out for an occasional movie. (Sherr Klein, 1997, p. 235)

SHARING YOUR PURPOSE

It is critical that you not only clarify the purpose(s) of your assessment for yourself but that you also share the purpose with the client and, where appropriate, his family/carer and the multi-disciplinary team. In sharing your assessment purposes with the client, it is also essential that you ask what he wants to gain from therapy in general and what he would like to learn from any assessment. An excerpt from Bonnie Sherr Klein's book *Slow Dance*, in which she describes her experience of having a stroke, helps to illustrate the pitfalls of not sharing our purpose or seeking that of our client.

> The [physiotherapist] spent weeks 'assessing' me: measuring every minute angle of movement; testing and timing my reactions to hot and cold, sharp and dull. The testing seemed irritatingly pointless to me, but it was also tiring, and I needed many rest stops when I would just lie still on the mattress, which seemed irritatingly pointless to the [therapist]. At the very end of our time she'd stretch my arms and legs, and do some passive range-of-motion exercises. After a few weeks of this and a few awkward weekends in bed at home, I asked her if she could stretch my groin so it would be possible to have intercourse. She pretended not to hear me. No one ever talked to me about sex: no physio, no doctor, no OT, no psychologist. Michael [her husband] and I figured it out for ourselves, not without pain. (Sherr Klein, 1997, p. 220)

CASE VIGNETTE: 'Mr SMITH'

This case vignette is based on my experience of working for a couple of years as a therapist in a geriatric day hospital setting and on my (Laver Fawcett) research experience with people with stroke. It is not based on one particular case but rather an imaginary case developed to illustrate the application of explicit thinking about purposes of assessment to a clinical setting.

Mr Smith is a 66-year-old man who has been discharged home from a stroke rehabilitation unit (SRU) at his local district hospital. He was admitted to the SRU five weeks previously with a right parietal infarct. The therapist in this scenario is a senior occupational therapist working as a member of a community-based intermediate care team. Mr Smith has been referred for continuing occupational therapy and physiotherapy for up to six weeks to help him adjust to community living post-stroke. The referral information states that Mr Smith has a mild hemiplegia of his left upper and lower limbs and can transfer and move with the assistance of one person. He also has some unilateral neglect. The therapist plans her assessment process by reflecting on the following questions.

Why am I Doing This Assessment?

I need to understand the impact of the diagnosis (stroke) and impairment (left-sided hemiplegia and unilateral neglect) on Mr Smith's functioning in everyday tasks in his home environment so I can develop a client-centred treatment plan and to provide baseline information so I can monitor the effects of my intervention. I also want to assess the couple's affect and coping skills, as clients often fully realise the impact of the stroke when they return home and try to function outside an in-patient environment, and they can become depressed at this stage. For family members, also, the full impact of their loved one's stroke is realised on discharge home and the change of role to a carer becomes apparent; so I need to consider carer burden.

What Information Do I Need to Collect?

I will need information about Mr Smith's lifestyle prior to his stroke. I want to know what were his roles and interests, and what kind of lifestyle does he want to create post stroke? I need to know his pre-stroke and current level of independence in personal and domestic ADL, leisure and productive activities. I need his viewpoint on which activities are most important to him to achieve independently and what his priorities are for improving his function. I require information about his mood. I should seek information about how his wife is coping in her new role as a carer and about her priorities.

What Decisions will I Need to Make from This Information?

I will use the information to identify problem areas relevant to occupational therapy intervention and then to negotiate treatment goals with the client in order to prioritise areas for intervention and develop a treatment plan.

What Will Be the Benefit to the Client (And, Where Relevant, the Carer) from Undertaking This Assessment?

Accurate assessment will enable a realistic and effective intervention to be implemented. As self-report and proxy data-collection methods will be implemented, the couple will become active partners in the therapeutic process as their views and priorities will be taken into account when identifying problems, setting outcome goals and prioritising the treatment plan. By undertaking a re-assessment, I will be able to demonstrate any changes in function following my intervention – this helps the client and family to see improvements and should help boost morale and confidence. If I identify carer burden, I will direct Mrs Smith to supporting agencies, such as the Carers' Resource.

Articulating the answers to these questions enables me to focus my assessment and to select an effective and efficient assessment approach, in summary:

- To collect the necessary information, I will have to use several data-collection methods, including the informal and standardised use of client self-report, carer proxy report and observation, and I plan to triangulate assessment data to get a comprehensive picture.
- I require a descriptive assessment of functioning in everyday tasks, but I also need this to be an outcome measure as I want to be able to evaluate outcomes to monitor the effects of my intervention.
- I also need to understand what problems are most significant for the client and his carer so that we can select relevant, mutually agreed, outcome goals for intervention.
- I want to assess his mood in order to identify any depression. This will need to be an evaluative test so that I can monitor any depression over time.
- I want to assess whether Mrs Smith is experiencing any carer burden and monitor the degree of burden over time.

There are quite a few standardised tests that I could use but I do not want to waste too much intervention time as my intermediate care service is only for six weeks and I do not want to over assess the client, which might lead to fatigue or him disengaging from the therapeutic process. So I need to select assessments that will meet more than one purpose wherever possible.

I will start the assessment with an informal interview. I find this helps to build rapport and establish a therapeutic relationship. I will explain my role and the purpose of this first assessment home visit; for example, I might say:

> I want to get to know about your previous lifestyle so I can help you work towards regaining as much of that lifestyle as possible, and I need to understand any problems you are experiencing now you're back home so that we can develop strategies to try to overcome these problems.

During the informal interview, I would ask how the couple have been managing since discharge and about their lifestyle prior to his stroke, what his roles and interests are and what kind of lifestyle they want to lead in the future.

On the first visit, I plan to use the Canadian Occupational Performance Measure (COPM; Law *et al.*, 1994), which is a self-report assessment that provides an individualised measure of a client's self-perception in occupational performance and covers the domains of self-care, productivity and leisure. The domain of self-care includes personal care, functional mobility and community management. The area of productivity includes paid or unpaid work, household management and school or play. Leisure includes quiet recreation, active recreation and socialisation. Function is rated in terms of importance, performance and satisfaction on three 10-point scales. I selected this as my first standardised assessment because:

- the COPM identifies information about the activities from across a person's lifestyle (personal ADL, domestic ADL, transportation, shopping and leisure) and incorporates the roles and role expectations of the client
- it is a person-centred tool that considers the importance of activities to the person and his level of satisfaction with current ability, as well as how well he can do each of the activities discussed; this will help me to prioritise client-centred areas for treatment
- the COPM focuses on the client's own environment, thereby ensuring the relevance of the problems to the client; this is relevant because Mr Smith has now been discharged home and previous assessments were undertaken in an in-patient setting
- it is a well-researched measure with published psychometric properties (Carswell *et al.*, 2004)
- it is good for evaluating clinical change and has acceptable levels of test–retest reliability so that I will be able to re-assess using the COPM and measure the effectiveness of my intervention
- it can be used as a self-report or proxy report measure and allows for input from members of the client's social environment if the client is unable to answer on his own behalf. This will be useful if Mr Smith is unable to comprehend the assessment. I could use the tool with both Mr and Mrs Smith, as his wife may have different perspectives about his level of performance and about importance.

On the home visit, I explain the purpose of the COPM to the couple and describe how we will do the assessment. I clarify that I need their independent viewpoints initially and that then we will discuss the results together. I then administer the COPM to Mr Smith in the living room as an interview as I anticipate that he will need extra explanation and prompting to complete the test, while Mrs Smith completes the COPM individually in the kitchen (I ask her to pop back to me in the living room if anything is unclear or if she has any questions). I then review the two sets of data while Mrs Smith makes us all a cup of tea and the three of us sit down to discuss the results and identify similarities and differences in their scores to negotiate the mutually agreed priority areas for treatment.

In order to examine carer burden, I decide to use a self-report measure, the Zarit Burden Interview (Zarit, Reever and Bach-Peterson, 1980). The Zarit Burden Interview was developed to report the burden experienced by the carer in managing the person with cognitive impairment. Factor analysis revealed two important variables: emotion-focused stress and demand stress. The assessment can be completed in an interview or a survey format by the carer. The test is scored on a five-point scale according to how the carer feels about the item presented. The score 0 = indicates no feeling, 1 = a little, 2 = feel moderately, 3 = feel quite a bit and 4 = feel extremely. I selected this tool because:

- it was developed to report the burden experienced by the carer and considers both emotion-focused stress and demands placed by the physical tasks associated with caregiving
- it can be administered either as an interview or as a survey
- it is quick to complete
- it is easy to score.

I decide to use the survey version and leave it with Mrs Smith at the end of the first home visit for her to complete in her own time and return to me when I visit two days later.

From the COPM, Mr and Mrs Smith both identify that feeding, washing and dressing are areas where he cannot manage without her help. Mr Smith feels very strongly that he does not want to be dependent on his wife for these self-care tasks. When I question the couple further about what kind of help he needs, it sounds like the unilateral neglect might be more problematic than the hemiplegia. I feel I need to observe Mr Smith doing these tasks to identify the main problems, assess the level of physical help and cueing he requires and select appropriate treatment strategies. I therefore decide to administer a standardised observational test, the Structured Observational Test of Function (SOTOF; Laver and Powell, 1995), on my next home visit. The SOTOF gives data about the level of independence, the behavioural skill components of the tasks and about underlying motor, sensory, cognitive and perceptual functioning. This is a standardised assessment that can be used for both descriptive and evaluative purposes. I selected this measure because:

- it provides a structured diagnostic reasoning tool that involves the observation of feeding, pouring and drinking, hand-washing and dressing tasks, the kind of personal ADL tasks identified as problematic and important by Mr Smith and his wife
- it provides a simultaneous assessment of both self-care function, residual and deficit skills and abilities within ADL performance (e.g. reaching, scanning, grasping and sequencing) and of underlying neurological deficit, thus eliminating the necessity to administer two separate tests and showing the explicit relationship between functional performance dysfunction and underlying neurological deficit
- it allows the therapist to prompt the person and observe responses to those prompts
- the test has good face validity with clients who have a primary diagnosis of stroke
- it has been shown to have good clinical utility and is age-appropriate and quick and simple to administer
- it has acceptable levels of test–retest reliability and so can be used as an evaluative measure
- the SOTOF self-care tasks are broken down into discrete skill components, making the test very sensitive to small changes in function within the task performance (e.g. if the subject does not change from dependent to independent feeding but can complete some aspects of the feeding task more easily this will be shown); this is important because progress following a stroke can be slow and my intervention period is short (usually about six weeks) when working in an intermediate care setting.

The SOTOF allows me to simultaneously address four related assessment questions; these are:

- How well does Mr Smith perform basic personal ADL tasks, independently or dependently, and how much help and prompting does he need?
- What skills and abilities does Mr Smith have intact, and what skills and abilities have been affected by the neurological damage caused by his stroke?
- Which of the perceptual, cognitive, motor and sensory performance components have been affected by the neurological damage? (Based on referral information I am anticipating that the motor and perceptual components are impaired.)
- Why is function impaired? (I will be able to identify the cause through the naming of the specific neurological deficits and underlying pathology; in this case, I am expecting unilateral neglect to be one of these deficits.)

The SOTOF was administered on the second home visit and the results formed the basis of the treatment approach for two agreed intervention goals, which were:

- To get dressed independently (he agreed that to begin with his wife would lay out clothes ready on their bed).
- To eat independently using adapted cutlery and crockery to enable one-handed feeding (Mr Smith conceded his wife would need to cut up some food for him and agreed to work on strategies to overcome his neglect).

At the beginning of the third visit, the results of the carer burden measure were discussed with Mrs Smith and she agreed to referral to Carers' Resource for advice on benefits and to attend a carers' support group. At the end of the six-week intervention, Mr Smith was re-evaluated on the COPM for the agreed dressing and feeding goals and the two SOTOF scales related to feeding and dressing were re-administered.

SERVICE EVALUATION

So far this chapter has focused on purposes of assessment related to an individual client or group of clients. Evaluation should become not just an essential component of clients' assessments but should also be regularly undertaken to monitor and review your service. According to Corr (2003), evaluation should be undertaken to 'assess the effects and effectiveness of a policy, practice or service' and to 'establish whether the effects of a service can really be attributable to the service or whether they result from some other factors' (p. 235). Undertaking a service evaluation can lead to 'recommendations for change, which ultimately shape and focus a service' (p. 235). In addition to using measurement to explore individual client outcomes, therapists can apply the same or different measures to explore group outcomes and evaluate various aspects of their service. Functional outcome measures can be used to address important questions related to service provision, funding issues and health care policy. For example, functional outcomes may be used to determine eligibility criteria for a particular service or to evaluate the performance of a service to decide upon future service provision. For an example, see the 'Carol' case study in Chapter 12 (pp. 387–8) in which the COPM is used as both an individual client measure and as a measure for a wider evaluation of three pain management group programmes. If therapy services are to be well funded, therapists must carefully select appropriate outcome measures for evaluating and demonstrating the effectiveness of their services. Unless we evaluate our services, we cannot know whether we are truly meeting our aims and objectives. Even if we can demonstrate we are meeting the clinical aims and objectives outlined in our service specification, we might be unable to demonstrate that our service is efficient and offering best value for money.

The British government is now placing a much greater emphasis on evaluating the performance of health care providers. 'Pursuing Perfection' is a philosophy described by the National Health

Service Modernisation Agency and is prompted by the belief that 'it is necessary to aim for perfect care because aiming for anything less implies that it is acceptable for some people to receive care that is below the agreed standards' and 'that while ambition and leadership are necessary, they are not sufficient and need to be accompanied by focused improvement activity' (NHS Modernisation Agency website, www.modern.nhs.uk, accessed 26.03.05). Performance assessment frameworks have been developed and are designed to give a general picture of NHS and social care performance. The NHS evaluation approach focuses on areas like: 'health improvement; fair access to services; effective delivery of healthcare; efficiency; patients and carer experience and health outcomes' and in social care evaluation focuses on 'cost and efficiency; effectiveness of service delivery and outcomes; quality of services for service users and carers; and fair access' (Department of Health, 2001a, p. 157). Performance measures (often referred to as indicators) are used to compare performance between similar services or organisations and are usually expressed as rates or percentages to enable comparison (Department of Health, 2001a). Collecting data from service users and carers is an important aspect of service review and something that health care providers have been instructed to embrace. For example, Standard Two of the *National Service Framework for Older People* (Department of Health, 2001a) focuses on person-centred care and states 'that the views of patients and carers will be sought systematically' (p. 8).

The COT (2003a) recommends that therapists review and evaluate their service in order to 'safeguard good standards of practice' (p. 26). It suggests that service evaluation is undertaken using the following methods:

- self-appraisal and reflection
- supervision and peer review
- client feedback via discussion, an evaluation form or a consumer questionnaire
- audit.

The framework of quality (Donabedian, 1980) considers the structure, process and outcome of a service. Other authors (for example Colborn and Robertson, 1997) focus on the inputs, processes and outcomes of a therapy programme/service/intervention, while the NHS Modernisation Agency (2004) talks about the analysis of structures, process and patterns. In the next section, we shall explore what is meant by these terms and discuss briefly how they might be measured as part of an evaluation of your service.

KEY COMPONENTS OF A SERVICE EVALUATION

Service structures

Refer to the 'layout of equipment, facilities and departments as well as organisational structures such as maps showing roles, committees, working groups etc.' (NHS Modernisation Agency, 2004, p. 12).

Patterns

Refer to 'patterns of behaviour, patterns of conversations, patterns of clinical outcomes or the patterns of anything that can be counted such as waiting lists, prescribing or demand' (NHS Modernisation Agency, 2004, p. 12).

Process

To evaluate therapy services, we need to measure both process and service outcomes (also called programme outcomes). *Process outcomes* is a term used to describe measures of the therapeutic intervention itself (Colborn and Robertson, 1997, p. 36). In a wider sense, the NHS Modernisation Agency (2004) refers to processes as 'the patient pathways and journeys and any supporting parallel processes' (p. 12). A process transforms inputs (such as materials, staff and equipment) into outputs (also called outcomes). Every process has at least one output. For example, this could be an assessment report, or the client could have a set of new skills or could be provided with a new piece of equipment. The COT (2003a) defines a *process goal* as 'what the therapist hopes to achieve during the process of intervention. This may be action by the therapist or a change in the therapist's knowledge, skills or attitudes' (p. 57). Therapeutic factors are the elements of an intervention that act, separately or together, to bring about change in the recipient of the intervention (MRC, 2000, cited in College of Occupational Therapists, 2003a, p. 60).

Process outcomes are based on:

- feelings
- client and therapist perspectives
- reactions to doing tasks
- analysis of what facilitated function (Colborn and Robertson, 1997, p. 37).

But these constructs are complex to measure. Research that focuses on clinical reasoning is helping therapists to understand the process of assessment and intervention (see Chapter 10).

It is useful to examine our process outcomes for a number of reasons, namely:

- to understand what we are currently achieving
- to understand how the client, and if appropriate the carer, experiences the process
- to understand what causes staff to be frustrated
- to understand what we need to improve.

Process measurement can include the examination of:

- process time or cycle times
- satisfaction
- errors
- utilisation.

Service outcomes

This is a term applied to measures of the overall occupational therapy or physiotherapy service's efficiency and effectiveness. If you are undertaking a service evaluation exercise, it is vital to define the global service outcomes and the range of individual client outcomes that the service aims to achieve. The outcome measures you select for the service evaluation must be matched by the intended goals of your service. The service level pre-determined outcome(s) may be articulated in your service specification and/or in clinical guidelines, protocols or standards. Individual client/therapist outcome goals are negotiated within the framework of the above for each client and should be documented in the client's notes. Service outcomes provide information about the overall therapy service, and quantitative data about your service can include:

- number and patterns (e.g. referral sources) of referrals during a defined period
- length (range, mean, standard deviation) of waiting times during a defined period
- caseload numbers (range, mean, standard deviation) for therapists and therapy support staff during a defined period
- some therapy services operate a maximum caseload and use a caseload weighting system to decide on an optimum and maximum caseload: factors used to calculate caseload weighting can be analysed

- frequency and duration of contact with clients
- how many treatments were provided
- therapists' client-contact/treatment hours versus non-client contact hours
- how many clients were discharged to independent living situations
- how many clients were able to return to work following intervention
- delayed transfers of care, e.g. how many patients were ready for discharge but were awaiting aids and adaptations or the start of another service before they could be discharged safely from your service
- discharge destinations.

Measures of service outcome are useful because they can serve to (Austin and Clark, 1993, p. 21):

- show that the intervention offered by the service is appropriate and effective
- indicate areas where service development might be required or additional resources deployed
- enable changes that lead to an improvement in consumer satisfaction
- show that a contracted service has been provided
- indicate effective use of health resources.

Service inputs

These are the factors that are required to deliver the entire service, including staffing costs, the service environment, equipment, materials and other overheads (such as mileage costs for travelling to home visits and outreach clinics). If you wish to measure service inputs, you could consider:

- staff input requirements, including professional staff, assistants/technician/support staff and administrative staff (e.g. receptionist, secretary)
- service environment department/service accommodation and overheads, such as clinic space rented from other service providers (e.g. to run a pain assessment and management clinic at a health centre)
- equipment needed to perform a test (e.g. standardised test materials, tape measure, stop watch, goniometer) or used to assess the client's potential improvement using a piece of equipment (e.g. walking frame or stick or a raised toilet seat)
- materials: these are often consumable and may need replacing (e.g. stationery, test forms, food for a kitchen assessment, disposable gloves).

Financial data are often analysed as part of a service evaluation. This might include analysis of the cost of service inputs (such as staffing costs, mileage for making home assessment visits, cost of equipment and materials). Financial analysis might also involve the comparison of costs and outcomes of different models of service delivery. For example, you might compare the cost of a proxy report of the home environment versus a therapist observational assessment undertaken at a home visit with an outcome of re-admission rates following discharge. The hypothesis might be that although the observational assessment is more expensive (therapist's time and travel costs) it leads to a more accurate assessment of risk and requirements for aids and adaptations to ensure a safe discharge.

Where possible, combine methods of measurement and/or sources of data and triangulate results to increase the reliability and validity of your findings. In Chapter 2, we looked at how self-report, proxy and observational data can be triangulated to provide a comprehensive assessment of an individual client. This same process can be applied to service evaluation. To do this you could divide the outcomes you evaluate into categories. These might be related to the stakeholder focus (Table 3.2).

Table 3.2 Concepts of outcome and outcome measurement: the different perspectives of stakeholders. Adapted from Austin and Clark, 1993, p. 21

Stakeholder	Perspective related to service outcomes
Client, Carer	• relief of distress and discomfort • reduced disability • increase satisfaction with their health and abilities • appropriate and timely information about their condition and the assessment and intervention process • redress when the initial outcome is unsatisfactory • safety during care • value for money in terms of any charges paid (e.g. for aids and adaptations) and a return on taxes paid towards the NHS • equity and a personalised service • to be treated as a whole person
Therapist, Clinician	• to measure the direct results of their interventions with individual clients (e.g. achieving a cure for an illness or relief from symptoms) • achieving an optimal level of functioning for the client • the client's satisfaction with the process of assessment and intervention
Manager	• resources used to provide an effective and efficient service • referral rates, waiting times, discharges, throughput of clients through the service within a specific time frame • caseload numbers and weighting • staff skill mix • sickness, vacancies and use of agency staff • number and nature of complaints and compliments about the service received from clients and carers
Commissioner, Funding agency	• achieving the highest improvement to the collective health status of the population • population-wide indicators of the level of service (e.g. as mortality rates, morbidity indicators, waiting times, re-admission rates) • number and nature of complaints and compliments received from clients, population, MPs etc.
Consumer groups, Charities, Voluntary sector	• advocate for better service provision • provide information to clients on rights, services and benefits available • identify unmet and ill-met needs and may provide services to supplement statutory provision
Wider population	• that people should be treated as individuals and given choice, respect and dignity • access to possible services if they were to need them

Another way to categorise is by source of data, for example client-focused measures versus staff-focused measures. Client-focused measures might include:

• the number of handoffs a client experiences between therapists, members of the multi-disciplinary teams or between qualified and unqualified staff members
• waiting times and delays experienced
• use of expert, professional versus assistant, staff time.

Staff-focused measures could be used with therapists, managers, admin staff, support staff and members of the multidisciplinary team and might include:

* a staff-satisfaction questionnaire
* sickness and absence data
* staffing levels, unfilled vacancies and the use of agency staff.

Measures can also be categorised in terms of direct and indirect service outcomes. Direct measures of service outcome will include data from standardised tests, questionnaires and client/patient records. 'Indirect measures are measures which, by inference, should indicate performance' (Austin and Clark, 1993, p. 23). They include data such as 'weekly/monthly work analysis surveys, records of staff turnover, client throughput, waiting lists and readmission rates' (p. 23) and less easily measured variables such as 'opportunity for staff to become involved in continuing education and research, the cooperation of staff with outside agencies, professional identity and confidence. These reflect aspects of a working environment which one assumes to be conducive to the delivery of a quality service' (p. 23). Caution needs to be taken in supposing a direct relationship between these measures and the quality of a service. For example, one therapist might see more clients than another therapist. This provides a valid measure of throughput during a given period and might be used to consider efficiency, but it will not provide any indication of whether the first or second therapist is providing a more effective service. A direct measure to evaluate whether clients were achieving their pre-defined/desired outcomes would be needed to measure the effectiveness of the service.

BEGINNING A SERVICE EVALUATION

First you need to define the service you wish to evaluate. It helps to have a service specification. If you do not have a specification for your service, Table 3.3 (below) provides guidelines for the content of a service specification. In the table, I have provided examples from several teams/services from within the Mental Health Directorate I work in. In many instances, several statements will be required to adequately describe each section, but I have only included one statement in each area as an example.

Once you have a clear description of the service or the part of a service (for example a time-limited treatment group, such as a falls prevention programme, pain management programme, anxiety management group or reminiscence group) to be evaluated, you need to clearly outline the parameters of the evaluation by answering the following questions.

* What do we want/need to know/measure about this service?
* In order to obtain this information/measurement, what information do we need to collect?
* What decisions will be made from this information (e.g. whether to continue with a pilot intervention approach, or might this form the evidence for a bid for additional funding to spread the treatment programme to another part of the service or for funding for an additional therapist)?
* What will be the benefit to the stakeholders (e.g. clients, therapists, referral sources, managers, funding agencies) of undertaking this service evaluation?

When setting objectives for service improvement, it is helpful to write these using a SMART format (Griffiths and Schell, 2002, p. 232):

> S = Specific
> M = Measurable
> A = Achievable
> R = Realistic
> T = Time bound

Table 3.3 Key headings and example content for a service specification

Heading	Intention	Example
Objective(s)	State the main purpose of your service.	The Intensive Home Treatment Team (IHTT) will provide a needs-led home treatment service, as an alternative to hospital admission, for people who are experiencing an acute mental health crisis.
Aims	State how you intend to meet the service objective.	The team will assess all referrals where hospital admission is thought necessary in order to formulate an alternative treatment plan where appropriate.
Principles	List the principles on which the service is based.	User and carer involvement will be integral to the process of assessment, care planning, treatment and evaluation.
Services provided	Overview of what the service provides. State when the service is provided and how many people can access the service at any one time.	Comprehensive, multidisciplinary needs and risk assessment will be provided in a day hospital setting for up to 10 clients per day and between 9.30 a.m. and 4 p.m. five days per week between Monday and Friday. Clients will usually attend twice per week for up to eight weeks.
Referral criteria, sources and process	Describe the criteria for referrals to your service, the process for making and receiving referrals and the types of people who can be referred to this service.	Referral criteria: the service is for older people with a mental health problem who would benefit from further outpatient assessment and intervention related to their problem. Referral sources: consultant psychiatrist or CMHT professionals. Referral process: verbal referrals will be accepted for urgent cases (e.g. to prevent an admission to hospital) and should be followed up by a written referral within seven working days.
	Explain whether you operate a waiting list and describe any process for prioritising referrals.	The day hospital operates a waiting list; referrals are prioritised by the team into 3 categories (high, medium, low).
Staffing, skill mix and skills required	State professional qualifications required, number of staff in each category and time per week of required input into the service.	The CMHT will comprise 1 FTE senior I occupational therapist, 1 FTE F grade community psychiatric nurse, 0.5 FTE-approved social worker, 2 FTE health care assistants (NVQ level 3).
	State any specialised skills required and related training needs	The occupational therapist needs to be qualified to administer the AMPS, which requires attendance at a five-day AMPS course and the completion and submission of 10 assessments to be calibrated.
Assessment	State screening, assessment process and standardised outcome measures used.	Initial multidisciplinary screening to ensure provision is appropriate to service user. Comprehensive multidisciplinary needs assessment will include standardised measures such as the AMPS, physical health assessment where appropriate, risk and psychological assessment using the FACE Risk Profile.

Table 3.3 (*continued*)

Heading	Intention	Example
Interventions	State treatment techniques used and methods of delivery.	Individual and group-based therapeutic interventions (e.g. reminiscence, reality orientation, memory strategies, relaxation and groups based on ADLs (such as cooking), leisure pursuits (gardening, woodwork) or crafts (art)).
Locations	State where assessment and intervention will take place.	Most assessment and intervention will be provided at the client's place of residence.
Facilities, equipment and materials required	Describe the clinical environment(s) required and any specialist equipment that needs to be provided and materials that are used on a recurring basis.	A hoist, specific types of bed, bath or chair.
Discharge/ discontinuation criteria and process	State criteria for discontinuation of intervention or discharge from the service.	Patients who have completed a short-term treatment programme or who need no other service offered by the day hospital will be prepared for discharge.
Service evaluation	Describe the process to be undertaken to evaluate the service and describe specific measures to be used.	The IHTT will be evaluated annually using the IHTT Service User and Carer evaluation questionnaire. An audit of client records will be made annually as part of a regular care programme approach audit process. The evaluation and audit findings will be fed back to the Sector Manager, an action plan developed and progress monitored through the Governance Board.
References	Include references for any published assessments and for any evidence upon which aspects of your assessment and intervention are based.	Reference for a standardised test: Fisher AG (2003a) *Assessment of Motor and Process Skills Volume 1: Development, Standardization and Administration Manual.* Fort Collins, CO, Three Star Press, Inc.

When undertaking a service evaluation, try not to re-invent the wheel: where possible use available data collected routinely as part of your normal service process. Review all the current information you have about your service, for example:

- referral criteria
- any printed information for clients, carers, referral sources (e.g. service users' leaflet about the service, information about how to use a piece of equipment, instructions for exercises)
- forms used for assessment, care planning, documenting client notes
- standardised tests used, especially outcome measures
- any data that are routinely recorded (e.g. waiting list numbers, referral and discharge rates per month, patient contacts, caseload sizes).

You can also use data from national standards, beacon site examples of good practice and public health data to help provide a benchmark for comparison. In the absence of ongoing continuous data about an aspect of your service, do a snapshot data-gathering exercise to provide you with a baseline. Then, in future, ensure that measuring is an ongoing part of the new process.

Once you have identified your service evaluation parameters, formulate some specific questions. The nature of the question will lead you towards your evaluation method. Weigh up the pros and cons of the possible methods.

Service evaluation should lead to plans for improvement, which in turn should be evaluated following implementation, thus leading to a continuous cycle of service improvement.

A useful paper on therapy service evaluation is provided by Heaton and Bamford (2001). They review the literature to consider the best approach for assessing the outcomes of the provision of equipment and adaptations. In their paper, they consider the outcomes that could and should be measured and review a number of standardised tests that provide measures of functional status, wider health status and quality of life. They also consider user satisfaction and discuss how this can be evaluated in this clinical area. A specific example of a review of the provision of equipment is given by Chamberlain *et al.* (2001). These therapists undertook a service evaluation with a retrospective sample of 100 service users who had received equipment, and obtained a sample of 57 telephone interviews. Their objective was to obtain data to 'determine whether or not the provision of equipment/adaptations [had] enabled clients/carers to cope better with daily living tasks in the longer-term' (p. 600). For their evaluation, they used a qualitative, self-report data-collection method. They found that 83 per cent of the equipment issued between 18 months to two years prior to their evaluation was still being used when the service users were interviewed and 69 per cent of equipment was still being used on a daily basis. They found that service users' satisfaction was higher with equipment and adaptations being used independently, compared to satisfaction levels with equipment and adaptations that were used with help from others. They conclude that 'the equipment and adaptations provided were being used as an integral part of daily life and that they had been prescribed appropriately' (p. 595). The paper includes a brief review of literature related to the evaluation of equipment prescription and also a copy of their telephone interview schedule.

A good resource for therapists involved with evaluating their service and planning service improvements is provided by Iles and Sutherland (2001), and is available free of charge. I downloaded this publication off their website. Their book is a good introductory guide and aims to provide a resource and reference tool to health care practitioners and managers on change management literature and to consider the evidence available on different approaches to change. In terms of service evaluation, 'Part 2: Tools, models and approaches' is a good starting point. The *Improvement Leaders' Guides* published by the NHS Modernisation Agency, and particularly the guides on process mapping, analysis and redesign (2002a) and measurement for improvement

(2002b), also provide useful information and ideas for embarking on a service evaluation. These are also available free of charge as pdf files from the NHS Modernisation Agency's website.

(*Note:* for more ideas about undertaking a service evaluation, see Chapter 11, particularly the sections on SWOT and mapping, pp. 339–42.)

Another good reference is by Letts *et al.* (1999), which I think will be equally valuable to physiotherapists as well as the occupational therapy audience for whom it was written.

CASE STUDY: SERVICE EVALUATION – THE MEMORY ACTIVITY AND SELF HELP GROUP

By Karen Innes and Alison Laver Fawcett

This provides a very good example of how a team started thinking about and trying to undertake service evaluation. Karen provides a very genuine account of the problems they encountered and their plans for improvement in their service evaluation attempts in future. In real clinical settings, service evaluation does not always follow a smooth path and therapists cannot always obtain the perfect samples of pre- and post-intervention data anticipated when a more controlled research study is undertaken. The important thing is to make service evaluation an explicit part of your planning, to reflect on problems encountered and to continue to learn from your experiences for the benefit of clients.

ABOUT THE OCCUPATIONAL THERAPIST

Karen is a Senior I occupational therapist working in an older people's mental health (OPMH) service. She has provided this case study as an illustration of how an occupational therapist and physiotherapist, collaborating to develop a new service, began thinking about joint assessment and treatment in a group-intervention situation and also how they planned to evaluate their new service.

THE SETTING

The Memory Activity and Self Help Group (known as the MASH group) was developed as a result of two separate discussions that the occupational therapist in the community mental health team (CMHT) had with two other professionals; the first discussion was with a psychology assistant involved with a memory clinic service, which provided assessment, diagnosis and intervention for people with suspected dementias. Owing to financial limitations, time restrictions and a predominantly medical-model focus, the occupational therapist's and psychology assistant's roles had focused primarily on assessment rather than treatment. The professionals were frustrated that, once diagnosis was given to the clients, follow-up support came from voluntary agencies and medical staffed outpatient clinics rather than from an integrated multidisciplinary treatment process looking at maintenance of skills.

ASSESSMENT PROCESS

The occupational therapist was using the Assessment of Motor and Process Skills (AMPS; Fisher, 2003a) for functional assessment in the memory clinic service. The AMPS was selected for use in the memory assessment service to identify what impact any deterioration in the client's cognitive function has on his functional abilities. The psychology assistant was using the Cambridge Neuropsychological Test Automated Battery (CANTAB; Cambridge Cognition, 2006), which is a measure that is sensitive to identifying cognitive changes caused by a wide range of central nervous system disorders and medication effects. It was administered on a laptop computer using touch-screen technology and was selected as it gives a rapid and non-invasive evaluative assessment. CANTAB has been developed over a 15-year period and is well accepted in clinical practice (see http://www.camcog.com for more information).

Staff and service user evaluation of the memory clinic service indicated that clients and carers often requested simple advice on keeping themselves active and independent and on maintaining their memory function. The occupational therapist and psychology assistant undertook a review of best practice in working with clients newly diagnosed with dementia. Information was found through a literature search, through the Dementia Services Collaborative (DSC) network and from some abstracts from the World Federation of Occupational Therapy's (WFOT; WFOT Congress, June 2002, Stockholm, Sweden) conference, which were passed on by a colleague who had attended it. This review formed the basis for the content of an advice leaflet, which they developed to hand out to clients attending the memory clinic. Further discussions took place between the therapist and psychology assistant about possible hands-on treatment strategies that could be utilised to support the advice provided in the leaflet, such as the use of group work.

Around the same time, the occupational therapist and the CMHT physiotherapist were also talking about the needs of people in the early stages of dementia. Some clients were referred from the memory clinic to the CMHT. These clients generally presented similar patterns of deficits, as highlighted by the AMPS assessment. These deficits included motor process skill problems, which often prompted a referral to the physiotherapist. The clients also tended to experience a general awareness of their increasing memory problems and complained of word-finding difficulties and episodes of minor short-term forgetfulness, which frequently adversely affected their confidence in social situations. Many of the clients were becoming socially isolated, as they often felt embarrassed about their poor memory.

The physiotherapist identified an increased risk of falls amongst the early-onset dementia client group. Both the occupational therapist and physiotherapist agreed that these clients required some therapeutic input in the form of falls prevention work, memory maintenance strategies, building the therapeutic relationship for future involvement and also monitoring the clients' mental health status. However, the clients did not usually need regular intensive involvement or support of a CMHT professional or health care assistant. It was decided that the way to effectively use CMHT time and staff resources would be to devise a community-based intervention programme to provide some evaluated, evidence-based therapeutic intervention through short-term group work.

Over a period of a few weeks, meetings with the rest of the multidisciplinary team were set up to identify the way forward. All members of the CMHT (that is psychiatrist, community psychiatric nurse, social worker, occupational therapist, physiotherapist) were included in the discussion as well as consultation with the Alzheimer's Society, who agreed to provide refreshments for the group, and the Royal British Legion, who allowed the CMHT regular weekly use of a room in one of their residential homes. The provision of purpose-built accommodation run by the Royal British Legion meant that the logistics of running the group (that is health and safety regulations, access, refreshment facilities) were dealt with as well as the overhead costs associated with gathering people in community resources, such as insurance and rental costs. The process of setting up the group was also a means of getting organisations from the statutory and voluntary sectors talking and working together constructively.

AIMS OF THE MEMORY ACTIVITY AND SELF HELP GROUP

The initial aims for the MASH group were:

- to provide information and advice for clients and carers on memory maintenance
- to introduce activities to reinforce and promote memory maintenance and independence
- to reduce the risk of falls and encourage clients to remain physically active
- to increase confidence in skills and improve self-esteem

- to encourage concentration and motivation
- to raise mood
- to give a structured activity in the clients' week
- to provide social support and have fun
- to offer a safe environment to allow clients and carers to share worries and fears about memory problems
- to encourage communication through creativity
- to reinforce and validate past experiences
- to improve the range and quality and activities of daily living (ADL) undertaken by clients
- to utilise staff time effectively and efficiently
- to build the therapeutic relationship with clients
- to start to monitor clients' progression through their organic illness
- to address the lack of therapy intervention following memory clinic appointments.

CRITERIA FOR REFERRAL TO THE MASH GROUP

These were set and included:

- group members (clients) should have a similar level of cognitive impairment
- referral was through the memory clinic or via the CMHT
- individuals should be ambulant
- clients should not be involved with any other NHS group
- group members (clients and their carers) should have adequate ability to hear and communicate
- clients should be insightful of their memory problems
- clients, and where relevant their carers, should consent to attend the group
- as funding was not available for transport costs, another criteria for the first pilot group was that the client/carer could organise their own transport to and from the group.

CHOOSING APPROPRIATE MEASURES

It was agreed that there should be some method for monitoring the effectiveness of the intervention. As this was a pilot intervention, it was particularly important that there should be some baseline measures and outcome data collected. The team began by reviewing the aims of the group. Some of these were quite vague and hard to measure. Also the list of aims was very long and it was felt that it would be overly tiring and stressful to submit this client group to a long battery of tests at the beginning and end of the group intervention. It was felt that over assessment might work against the aims of offering social support, having fun and developing rapport. Therefore, the group decided to use a qualitative method for evaluating a number of the aims and planned to interview the clients and carers at the end of the intervention. They also decided to select just a few constructs/domains that could be measured and identified measures that were familiar to members of the team and were relatively quick and easy to administer. These are summarised in Table 3.4 (below).

The Six-item Cognitive Impairment Test (6-CIT; Brooke, 2000; Brooke and Bullock, 1999; see Figure 3.2) and the Four-item Geriatric Depression Scale (4-GDS; Brooke, 2000) had been recommended in the service's dementia primary care protocol for use by GPs as screening tools for identifying people who should be referred for memory clinic assessment. The tests were also used by staff in the memory clinics and CMHTs and were very quick and easy to administer. The purpose of using these tests was to provide a baseline of cognitive function and mood at the start of MASH and to monitor any changes at the end of intervention. The 6-CIT is an administered test, and the 4-GDS has a self-report interview

Table 3.4 Aims of the MASH group and selected evaluation measures

Aim of MASH group	Domain or construct to be measured	Possible measure
Prevent falls	Balance History of falls	Berg Balance Scale (Berg *et al.*, 1992) Get Up and Go Test (Mathias, Nayak and Isaacs, 1986)
Prevent depression	Mood state	4-item Geriatric Depression Scale (Brooke, 2000)
Maintain cognitive function	Cognitive functioning	6-item Cognitive Impairment Test (Brooke, 2000; Brooke and Bullock, 1999) Clinical Dementia Rating (Berg, 1988)
Maintain independence in ADL	Level of independence in specified ADL	Assessment of Motor Process Skills (Fisher, 2003)
Maintain engagement in meaningful activities	Personal and domestic ADL, productivity and leisure	Mayers' Lifestyle Questionnaire 2 (Mayers, 2003)
Improve quality of life	Quality of life	Mayers' Lifestyle Questionnaire 2 (Mayers, 2003)
Reduce carers' perception of burden	Carer burden	Zarit Care Giver Burden Scale (Zarit, Todd and Zarit, 1986)

format. The tests were, therefore, to be used both as baseline descriptive tests and evaluative tests.

In addition, the team wanted to group people together who had similar levels of cognitive impairment. This assessment purpose can be categorised as discriminative. As the 6-CIT is primarily used as a GP screening tool, the three-part staging on the test (0–7 cognitive impairment = not significant; 8–9 = probably significant, referral is advised; 10–28 = significant – refer) meant that in order to have been referred into the memory service the clients would already fall into the middle two categories, and the third category represented all levels of impairment above the score of 10 threshold and was too gross a measure. As the MASH group was being aimed at people with mild cognitive impairment in the early stages of dementia, the team wanted to discriminate between people with dementia in terms of mild, moderate or severe cognitive impairment and/or in terms of the disease process (early, middle, late). The team selected the Clinical Dementia Rating (CDR; Berg, 1988), which is a global rating of dementia that takes 'into account both the results of clinician testing of cognitive performance and a rating of cognitive behaviour in everyday activities' (Berg, 1988, p. 637). This is used to place the person into one of five categories: none, questionable, mild, moderate or severe dementia.

Another MASH aim related to supporting carers to reduce their experience of burden. The team decided that they needed a measure of carer burden to assess this outcome. They chose the Zarit Caregiver Burden Scale (Zarit, Todd and Zarit, 1986), which was one of two burden measures that had been piloted within the memory clinic service. It is a carer self-report

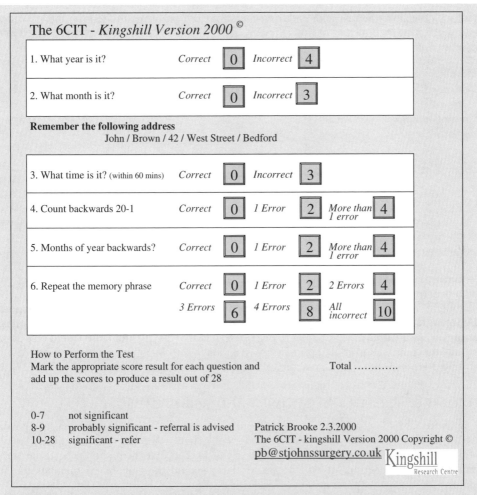

The 6CIT - *Kingshill Version 2000* ©

1. What year is it?	*Correct*	0	*Incorrect*	4	
2. What month is it?	*Correct*	0	*Incorrect*	3	

Remember the following address
John / Brown / 42 / West Street / Bedford

3. What time is it? (within 60 mins)	*Correct*	0	*Incorrect*	3			
4. Count backwards 20-1	*Correct*	0	*1 Error*	2	*More than 1 error*	4	
5. Months of year backwards?	*Correct*	0	*1 Error*	2	*More than 1 error*	4	
6. Repeat the memory phrase	*Correct*	0	*1 Error*	2	*2 Errors*	4	
	3 Errors	6	*4 Errors*	8	*All incorrect*	10	

How to Perform the Test
Mark the appropriate score result for each question and   Total ....
add up the scores to produce a result out of 28

0-7   not significant
8-9   probably significant - referral is advised   Patrick Brooke 2.3.2000
10-28   significant - refer   The 6CIT - kingshill Version 2000 Copyright ©
        pb@stjohnssurgery.co.uk Kingshill
        Research Centre

Figure 3.2 The Six-item Cognitive Impairment Test (6-CIT). *Brooke P (2000) The 6-CIT Kingshill version 2000. For further information see www.kingshill-research.org. Reprinted with permission of Patrick Brooke, Kingshill Research Centre.*

measure that the team used as a prompt list to encourage conversation with the carer to find out whether they were having difficulties in caring for the client and their experience of both physical and emotional burden.

The physiotherapist selected two observational measures to look at the aim related to falls prevention; these were the Berg Balance Scale (Berg *et al.*, 1992 and 1989) and the 'Get Up and Go' Test (Mathias, Nayak and Isaacs, 1986) as screening measures to identify people with poor balance, either sedentary or dynamic, who are at risk of falling.

In terms of assessing meaningful engagement in ADL, productivity and leisure activities and evaluating any impact on the person's quality of life, the team reviewed the Mayers' Lifestyle Questionnaire. The team considered the literature on the original Mayers tool (Mayers, 1995 and 1998) and also the work that looked at the application of the Lifestyle Questionnaire for people with mental health problems (Mayers, 2000 and 2003). The Mayers' Lifestyle Questionnaire is a self-report measure that the author describes as 'a client-centred tool which enables people with enduring mental health problems to identify and prioritise issues affecting their quality of life' (Mayers, 2003, p. 388). The questionnaire is divided into nine sections (see Box 3.2).

Box 3.2 The domains addressed by the Mayers' Lifestyle Questionnaire
(Mayers, 2003, p. 390)

Section number	Domains
1	Looking after yourself
2	Living situation
3	Looking after others
4	Being with others
5	Being in or out of work/attending college
6	Your beliefs and values
7	Choices
8	Finances
9	Activities you enjoy doing/want to do

The Lifestyle Questionnaire items can be reviewed together with the therapist as an interview or left with clients for them to complete on their own, which involves placing ticks in columns next to each item and then putting a * against the areas that matter to them most. The team felt that the literature (Mayers 1998 and 2003) indicated the tool had good clinical utility and face validity (see Chapter 6, pp. 187–9) and that the questionnaire would be a good prompt for conversation around priority areas, although they hypothesised that it might be too abstract for people who have moderate to severe cognitive impairment.

FORMAT OF THE MEMORY ACTIVITY AND SELF HELP GROUP

The entire CMHT agreed to be involved with the project. It was decided that the group would meet for two and a half hours on a weekly basis. A team rota was drawn up to allocate staff attendance and involvement. It was agreed that there should be three staff present at each meeting, of which one of these should be a qualified member of the team.

The team looked at the pros and cons of inviting clients and carers to attend MASH together. The team considered how joint attendance would affect both the client and carer and wondered whether the clients might feel unable to open up in front of their carers. They also hypothesised that carers might want the group to be a form of respite care. On balance, the team felt that the potential advantages of including both clients and carers in the group outweighed potential disadvantages. In particular, the team's consensus was that advice and intervention strategies, passed on during the group, could be reinforced by carers in the home environment and that carers may also be supported in the MASH group situation. The team's approach was to see this as a flexible programme development project, to have both informal reviews of each group session as well as more formal service evaluation in order to measure outcomes and identify any limitations as they arose. In this way, problems could be discussed and improvements made as the group developed. Baseline assessment was to be undertaken at the start of the group, with follow-up evaluation being done at six- and 12-week intervals. The staff decided that both clients and carers should be involved in the service evaluation process.

The group was a closed one, and so the same attendees remained together for the duration of the programme. MASH groups started with an informal welcome over a cup of tea and chat, clients then had 15 to 30 minutes exercise and t'ai chi followed by another cup of tea and this was followed by either a speaker or an activity session. Speakers included an Age Concern worker, Alzheimer's Society worker, pharmacist, speech and language therapist and a drama therapist. Activities ranged from quizzes, creative crafts, reminiscence and lots of practical tips. The work of Molly Burnham (1999) was used as the template for the practical sessions; however, fun was the emphasis of the session.

Two consistent activities were used in all sessions. These were:

- t'ai chi and gentle exercise, as good evidence suggests that improvements are seen in balance, confidence, strength and general well-being
- use of life story sessions to allow people to discuss episodes of their lives that they wanted to remember and to give them a chance to compile an album about their lives, past experiences and validation of life skills.

GROUP REVIEW

Owing to the pressure new referrals placed upon the capacity of the team, the six-week review did not occur as planned; however, the final review included a focus group that two qualified team members ran with the carers and clients, and elicited valuable qualitative feedback on how clients and their carers felt about the MASH group, their needs and expectations.

The main disadvantage identified from the pilot group was the low number of attendees. Ideally, the optimum number of participants identified for the group was 12 (six clients and six carers). However, from the 21 people invited to attend the group, only seven attended regularly. The low numbers of attendees affected the group dynamics in two ways: there was limited interaction and what interaction occurred was rich and genuine owing to the open and honest expression of feelings and experiences shared. Also, the small numbers of attendees had a big impact on analysing the significance of any change in group scores on the selected outcomes.

The qualitative feedback from the focus group review was generally positive from both the clients and carers, who reported that the main benefit from the group was that they all had enjoyed the opportunity of being able to openly share problems and socialise with others who understood. The feeling was so positive about this that the group wanted to meet up after the scheme had ended. Staff supported attendees to set up their own support group on discharge from MASH, and this continues to be run with help from the team's health care assistants.

The practical tips given during the sessions were found to be implemented better, and had therefore been more useful, when clients had the continual support from carers who prompted them to implement the advice at home. Opportunities to be creative and use drama therapy as a means of letting go and playing together met with mixed feelings; some people admitted they had forgotten to allow themselves time to engage in creative pastimes that were perceived to be 'less productive'.

From a negative perspective, the use of the life story book activity was less successful as the clients viewed this as homework: the suggestion was subsequently made that this be used as a practical session within the group situation as most people found it hard to start the project off in their own time and required prompts as to what to put in it.

The application of outcome measures did not go as smoothly as staff anticipated as several clients were not enthusiastic about being measured and refused to be re-tested at the 12-week evaluation. The only measure that had a reasonable sample of post-test scores was the Berg Balance Scale. The results from this were very positive, but as previously mentioned the sample was too small to yield conclusive results about the relationship between the t'ai chi and exercise sessions and balance.

The team decided that the initial review data, albeit patchy, were positive enough to merit running another MASH programme. They decided that service evaluation would be prioritised for this second group as a lot of teething problems associated with setting up a new intervention programme had been overcome. Evaluation was also very important because other teams were interested in the MASH group and the mangers needed to decide whether this programme should be spread to other parts of the older people's mental health service. Future groups are to be evaluated with outcome measures embedded as part of the whole process, and the team noted that this needed to be sold to the clients and carers as they start the group. Currently, the team is also reviewing whether different measures might have better face validity and clinical utility (see Chapter 6). One of the outcome measures under consideration is the Bradford Well Being Profile (University of Bradford, 2002; Bruce, 2000), an observational assessment that subtly identifies small changes in a person's well-being (MacRae, 2005). This profile may seem less threatening to the clients but it would provide more of a qualitative subjective indication of how clients are benefiting from attending the group, rather than gaining a quantitative measure. A disadvantage to using it is the length of time needed for administration and the availability of staff time in the CMHT setting. Time would need to be designated specifically in the weekly rota.

Another aspect for consideration, and one of the aims of the group, is the effective use of staff time. The low numbers of clients attending was accepted as this was a pilot intervention group. However, an analysis of the inputs required to run the MASH programme compared to the outputs (number of clients and carers attending and benefits demonstrated by both qualitative data and quantitative outcomes) is essential to justify continuing the group and disseminating the treatment approach across the service. The frequency with which the group can be offered needs to reflect the numbers of referrals received. One area for review is the initial criteria set. A number of clients with dementia with moderate levels of cognitive impairment are not receiving any other intervention except for periodic outpatient reviews; this population might also benefit from the MASH approach. If this group is to be included, the type of activities provided may need to be adapted to accommodate clients with greater cognitive impairment.

Usually, the team works with individual clients but the experience of developing and reviewing the MASH programme allowed the team to get to know each other better and to work closely together. This was an unanticipated positive outcome of the development of MASH.

REFLECTING ON PURPOSES OF ASSESSMENT IN YOUR OWN PRACTICE

At the back of this book, you will find templates for a series of worksheets designed to assist you in applying principles of assessment and outcome measurement to your own practice.

Please now turn to Worksheet 3 (p. 398). For this reflection you will need to review the range of unstandardised and standardised data-collection methods and outcome measures used within an occupational therapy or physiotherapy service or by a multidisciplinary team. If you are a student, reflect on the range of assessments and outcome measures that you have seen used on one of your clinical placements. The worksheet takes you through a series of questions that are related to each of the four main assessment purposes: descriptive, evaluative, predictive and discriminative. There is also a section related to service evaluation. You will be asked to think about the data currently collected for each purpose and to reflect on how these data are used (for example to make decisions about the client's problems, symptoms and need for further intervention). There is then space to list the standardised and unstandardised assessments that currently provide data for this purpose and to reflect upon whether these are adequate. Finally, there is space to list other potential measures that can yield data for a specific purpose.

STUDY QUESTIONS

3.1 What factors should you consider when selecting a discriminative assessment for your service?

3.2 Define *predictive assessment*.

3.3 Why do therapists undertake evaluative assessment and why should they use standardised outcome measures for this purpose?

3.4 Why should therapists evaluate their service?

You will find brief answers to these questions at the back of this book (p. 390).

4

Levels of Measurement

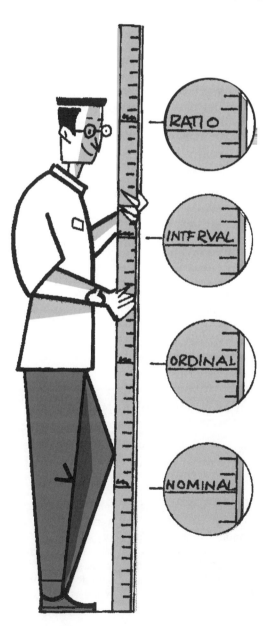

CHAPTER SUMMARY

This chapter will define and describe four levels of measurement: nominal, ordinal, interval and ratio and present the conditions for using data obtained from these different levels of measurement. It will also cite a few examples of everyday measurements and therapy tests that provide data at each level of measurement and discuss the pitfalls of using data from some levels of measurement incorrectly, for example summing scores from ordinal level data. Lastly, a brief introduction to Guttman scaling and Rasch analysis will be given. It will also endeavour to answer the following question: 'What level of measurement is required?'

WHAT IS MEASUREMENT?

In the introduction, *measurement* was defined as the data obtained by measuring. Measuring is undertaken by therapists to ascertain the dimensions (size), quantity (amount) or capacity of a trait, attribute or characteristic of a person that is required by the therapist to develop an accurate picture of the person's needs and problems to form a baseline for therapeutic intervention and/or to provide a measure of outcome. A measurement is obtained by applying a standard scale to variables, thus translating direct observations or patient/proxy reports to a numerical scoring system.

Sarle (1997) provides a simple example to explain the concept of measurement.

> Suppose we have a collection of straight sticks of various sizes and we assign a number to each stick by measuring its length using a ruler. If the number assigned to one stick is greater than the number assigned to another stick, we can conclude that the first stick is longer than the second. Thus a relationship among the numbers (greater than) corresponds to a relationship among the sticks (longer than).

Sarle goes on to use the same example of measuring sticks to show how more complex measurements can be made:

> If we lay two sticks end-to-end in a straight line and measure their combined length, then the number we assign to the concatenated sticks will equal the sum of the numbers assigned to the individual sticks (within measurement error). Thus another relationship among the numbers (addition) corresponds to a relationship among the sticks (concatenation). These relationships among the sticks must be empirically verified for the measurements to be valid.

WHAT IS MEASUREMENT THEORY?

A basic understanding of measurement theory (sometimes referred to as test theory) is important for all therapists. There are a number of problems that clinicians have to grapple with when measuring human behaviour, particularly when they are attempting to measure psychological attributes (referred to as constructs) that cannot be observed directly.

- Measurements obtained are always subject to some degree of error (Crocker and Algina, 1986, p. 6). This error may occur for a wide variety of reasons, e.g. errors may occur because the person is more fatigued than usual or is feeling anxious about being tested or is having to perform in a strange environment instead of his own home. A big problem for therapists is how to establish the amount of error that is present in the person's test results.
- Measurements are usually based on limited samples of behaviour (p. 6). Therapists often have a limited amount of time in which to undertake assessment. So measurement

may only be taken at one point in time or functional ability may have to be judged on a limited observation of performance.

- No single approach to the measurement of any construct is universally accepted (p. 6). Therapists are faced by a wide range of published tests all purporting to measure the same thing, such as depression or pain or independence in activities of daily living (ADL).
- There is a lack of well-defined units on a measurement scale (p. 6). Many therapy scales use labels like 'independent', 'severe' or 'frequently', but what do these labels really mean and do they mean the same thing to each person rating the test?
- When measuring a psychological construct, such as memory, 'the construct cannot be defined only in terms of operational definitions but must also have demonstrated relationships to other constructs or observations' (p. 7). To understand processes that we cannot directly observe, we turn to theoretical explanations. Such theories will postulate relationships between different observed behaviours and the construct of interest (such as attention) and also between different constructs (such as attention and short-term memory).

Measurement theory can help therapists to understand and reduce the impact of such problems. It encourages therapists to reflect on the meaning of the data they obtain through testing and supports a critical examination of the assumptions behind the analysis of test data. Sarle (1997) provides the following definition of *measurement theory*.

> Measurement theory is a branch of applied mathematics that is useful in measurement and data analysis. The fundamental idea of measurement theory is that measurements are not the same as the attribute being measured. Hence, if you want to draw conclusions about the attribute, you must take into account the nature of the correspondence between the attribute and the measurements . . . Mathematical statistics is concerned with the connection between inference and data. Measurement theory is concerned with the connection between data and reality. Both statistical theory and measurement theory are necessary to make inferences about reality.

There are three types of measurement theories discussed in the literature. These are generally referred to as:

- representational measurement theory
- operational measurement theory
- classical measurement theory, also sometimes referred to as traditional measurement theory (see Crocker and Algina, 1986).

Sarle (1997) distinguishes between these three approaches to measurement in the following way.

> The representational theory assumes that there exists a 'reality' that is being measured, and that scientific theories are about this reality. The operational theory avoids the assumption of an underlying reality, requiring only that measurement consist of precisely specified operations; scientific theories concern only relationships among measurements. The classical theory, like the representational theory, assumes an objective reality, but, unlike the representational theory, holds that only quantitative attributes are measurable, and measurement involves the discovery of the magnitudes of these attributes. In the classical theory, like the operational theory, meaningfulness comes from empirical support for scientific theories describing the interrelationships of various measurements.

THE ASSIGNMENT OF NUMBERS FOR THE PURPOSES OF ASSESSMENT

We have seen in Chapter 2 that there are many different methods, both qualitative and quantitative, that can be used to collect and record assessment data. Using numbers adds to the range of evidence at a therapist's disposal (Eva and Paley, 2004). Numbers are a tool therapists can use to aid their understanding and documentation of their client's problems, functioning and situation. Lord Kelvin (one of the founders of modern physics and considered to be one of the great applied scientists of the Victorian era and a very talented scientific instrument designer) talked about the usefulness of using numbers to define a construct: 'When you can measure what you are speaking about, and express it in numbers, then you know something about it, and when you cannot express it in numbers, then your knowledge is of a meagre and unsatisfactory kind' (Hunter, 1997, pp. 87–88). However, in some health care disciplines, there is considerable distrust of quantification. Many therapists are wary of using numbers to quantify aspects of human function, because they believe that there is something limiting about numbers and that numbers cannot adequately describe the psychological, social and spiritual dimensions of human life (Eva and Paley, 2004). The therapist must 'select the most relevant permutation of facts and figures in any given situation, where relevance is determined by the specific purpose that we have or the specific question that we are trying to answer' (p. 48). While it is true that assigning numbers will not offer a complete description of function, and cannot illustrate every aspect of a client that is of interest, numerical scoring systems offer a useful permutation in assessment, particularly in the measurement of outcome in order to evaluate whether intervention has achieved the desired results. Numbers are used in very different, and not always appropriate, ways in therapy assessments. In order to be able to interpret and handle appropriately any numerical scores, it is critical that you are able to determine and understand the type of numerical scale and level of measurement being used.

Many standardised and non-standardised assessments score the person's performance on some sort of scale. Scaling methods vary in complexity, and the therapist needs to judge whether the scaling method used provides at least an adequate measurement system and at best the ideal level of measurement for the construct or behaviour being measured.

WHAT ARE LEVELS OF MEASUREMENT?

When numbers are applied to a measurement tool in order to evaluate something, they are sometimes nothing more than labels (and therefore are devoid of any quantifiable value). When numbers are used to replace labels in this way, they will not contain any mathematical properties at all. It is really important to understand how much information can be gained from a number in a particular scale. Many measures involve scoring systems that include summing or manipulating scores to obtain a total score or subtest scores. Therapists need to be sure that they are using numbering on a scale in a valid and meaningful way. The different ways in which numbers are applied for measurement has been categorised. These categories are perceived to fall in a hierarchy of four levels of measurement. We can undertake different mathematical procedures or statistical tests depending on the level of measurement. It is, therefore, critically important that you understand the differences between these four levels of measurement. You need to be able to look at the scoring system of a measure and identify its level of measurement. Once you know the level of measurement, you need to understand what you can and cannot do with numerical scores obtained on the test.

Fundamental to all scaling methods is a distinction between four ways of applying numbers in measurement. These four applications of numbers to scales 'lie in a hierarchy of mathematical adequacy' (McDowell and Newell, 1987, p. 19). Stanley Smith Stevens (1946) described this model of four levels of measurement scales back in the 1940s, and his model is still widely used today to classify scoring systems. Stevens' system identified scales that differ in the extent to which their scale values retain the properties of the real number line. The four levels are called nominal, ordinal, interval and ratio scales. These four levels will now be defined and described in turn.

NOMINAL SCALES

At the lowest level of measurement lie nominal scales. In fact, the nominal level does not provide a system of measurement at all but rather a system of classification. A nominal scale simply uses numbers to classify a characteristic and is used to identify differences without quantifying or ordering those differences. This means that no inferences can be drawn from the numbers used; whether one category is allocated a higher or lower number than another is arbitrary. These scales are sometimes referred to as categorical scales because numbers are used simply as labels for categories (McDowell and Newell, 1987). Nominal scales can be used for any information that contains mutually exclusive categories. Numbers are assigned to nominal scales to either aid data entry, for example when medical and therapy records are entered onto a computer database, or to aid analysis for research. In research literature, you may see the terms *categorical data* or *nominal data* used. Stevens (1946) described a nominal scale as a scale in which:

- numbers are used purely as labels for the elements in the data system
- numbers assigned to a nominal scale do *not* have meaningful mathematical qualities; this means numerical scores do not have the properties of meaningful order within the scale, items within the scale do not have equal distances between them and there is no fixed origin or zero point
- any set of numbers may be used
- each unique object or response in the data system must be assigned a different number
- any other set of numbers could be substituted as long as one-to-one correspondence between members of the sets is maintained; this is called isomorphic transformation.

Nominal level information provides us with some descriptive information, but has no hierarchical value (Lewis and Bottomley, 1994). In a nominal scale, numbers are assigned to mutually exclusive categories (Polgar, 1998). Numbers used in a nominal scale are not meaningful in a quantitative sense (Polgar, 1998) and do not have any meaning except in the context in which they are being used (Hunter, 1997). There are no *less than* or *greater than* relations among nominal scores, and operations such as addition or subtraction are not possible. Nominal scales are useful if the frequencies or proportions of a particular characteristic within a sample need to be recorded (Hunter, 1997). The scores indicate that qualitative differences between categories exist and the scores serve as shorthand labels. This can be useful when entering information into a computer database. When data are collected using a nominal scale, non-parametric statistical techniques (for example chi square) are used if statistical analysis is needed (Hunter, 1997).

EVERYDAY EXAMPLES OF NOMINAL SCALES

Lewis and Bottomley (1994) state that 'something is nominal if it is naming something, such as the months of the year' (p. 604). Traditionally, we assign numbers to represent months as a shorthand dating system, that is 1 = January, 6 = June and 12 = December. An example of a nominal scale is where gender is coded 1 for female and 2 for male, even though no quantitative distinction between the two genders is implied. Many variables used to describe populations when collecting normative data (discussed in Chapter 5) are measured at a nominal level, in addition to gender these include race, place of residence and birthplace. Other examples of nominal scales include the numbers assigned as international telephone codes for different countries, the numbers selected for players in a sports team, such as football, to wear on their shirts or the numbers chosen for different routes taken by different buses and shown on the front of a bus.

HEALTH CARE EXAMPLE OF A NOMINAL SCALE

The *International Classifications of Disease* produced by the World Health Organization (WHO) uses numbers as a code for classification of health disorders and to aid reliability of diagnosis.

The ICD system of nominal labels uses a numeric or alphanumeric code that represents a clinical description and diagnostic guideline for a wide range of disorders for clinical, educational, research or service use worldwide. For example, *ICD-10 Classification of Mental and Behavioural Disorders* (World Health Organization, 1992) uses an alphanumeric code involving a single letter followed by two numbers at the three-character level, for example: F00 is used to label Dementia, F00.0 = Dementia in Alzheimer's Disease with early onset, F00.1 = Dementia in Alzheimer's Disease with late onset, while F06.0 = organic hallucinations. The *ICD-9* uses numeric codes only ranging from 000–999.

EXAMPLE NOMINAL SCALES USED BY THERAPISTS

Some scales used in occupational therapy and physiotherapy assessments are nominal scales. Nominal scores can be applied to categories such as diagnosis, type of living accommodation, equipment provided and discharge destination. For example, discharge destination of service users might be recorded as follows:

1 = discharged to own home
2 = discharged to a relative/friend's home
3 = discharged to an intermediate care setting for further rehabilitation
4 = discharged to long-term residential care
5 = discharged to long-term nursing home care
6 = transferred to another unit/ward
7 = died while undergoing treatment/during admission

ORDINAL SCALES

An ordinal scale can be applied when data contain information that has relative magnitude or a rank order (1st, 2nd, 3rd etc). Numbers are allocated depending on the ordering of the property assessed, from *more to less* or *first to last,* and so they have real meaning beyond being used simply as labels (Lichtman *et al.,* 1989). This means that the numbers allocated reflect the ascending order of the characteristic being measured (McDowell and Newell, 1987). Numbers indicating position in a series or order are called ordinals. The ordinal numbers are first (1st), second (2nd), third (3rd) and so on. Variables measured using an ordinal scale are called ordinal variables or rank variables.

Stevens (1946) describes an ordinal scale as a scale in which:

• the elements in the scale can be ordered on the amount of the property being measured
• the scaling rule requires that values from the real number system must be assigned in the same order
• scores may be converted to other values, as long as the original information about the rank order is preserved; this is called monotonic transformation.

So, like a nominal scale, an ordinal scale does *not* have the properties of equal distance between units or a fixed origin.

EVERYDAY EXAMPLE OF AN ORDINAL SCORE

An everyday example of an ordinal score is placing runners in a race. Lichtman *et al.* (1989) give the example of a horse race: 'we can assign the rank of "one" to the horse who comes first, "two" to the horse who comes second, and "three" to the third place finisher' (p. 6), and we could go on assigning numbers to the whole field of horses based on their finishing order. This information might be used to describe the 'form' of horses and is often summarised in a race guide and used by racegoers thinking of placing a bet. The order of winners, though useful, tells

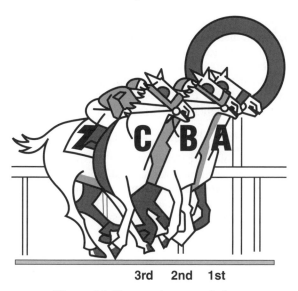

3rd   2nd   1st

Figure 4.1 Horse racing example 1.

us nothing about the distance between the runners. The first three horses could have finished so close together that a photograph was required to judge their order or they could have crossed the finish line with considerable distance between them. If you were thinking of placing a bet, the interval (or distance) a horse came behind others in the field would also be helpful information, but would not be provided by an ordinal scale. See Figures 4.1 and 4.2. Figure 4.1 shows a close finish: the horses A, B and C finish in the same order as those in Figure 4.2 below but the distance between the horses at the finishing post is much shorter.

In Figure 4.2 the horses finish in the same order but the distance between them is more spaced out and there is not an equal distance between the 1st and 2nd and between the 2nd and 3rd horses.

From this example, we can see that an ordinal scale is used to rank the order of the scores assigned to the characteristics being measured. The numbers represent values relative to each other (Lewis and Bottomley, 1994). The order of scores indicates that the parameter being measured is either greater (better) or less (worse) than the other scores, but the therapist cannot

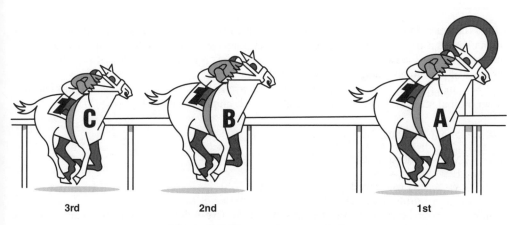

3rd   2nd   1st

Figure 4.2 Horse racing example 2.

make inferences about the magnitude of the difference between scores (Hunter, 1997; Polgar, 1998). Non-parametric techniques are used if statistical analysis of ordinal level data is needed. Willcoxon or Mann–Whitney U tests are used if groups are being compared. To examine hypotheses, correlation coefficients (such as Spearman or Kendall rank correlations) are used (Hunter, 1997). Hunter also states that it is 'more appropriate to compare the median values of scores, rather than their mean, since this reflects the number of recordings above and below, rather than their mathematical weight' (p. 89).

EXAMPLES OF ORDINAL SCALES USED BY THERAPISTS

Many assessments used by therapists are based on ordinal scales. Fisher (1993) states that 'virtually all functional assessments, even timed tests, yield ordinal raw scores' (p. 322). Lewis and Bottomley (1994) explain that ordinal level information is provided by scales indicating a continuum, such as stronger to weaker or faster to slower. A frequently used example of an ordinal scale is where scores are assigned to describe the levels of independence or amount of assistance required to complete an activity:

    1 = independent
    2 = needs verbal prompting
    3 = needs physical assistance
    4 = dependent and unable to perform activity

Another example is the assessment of severity of a symptom (Hunter, 1997), for example:

    1 = none
    2 = mild
    3 = moderate
    4 = marked
    5 = severe

Ordinal scales are also used for the measurement of pain and pain relief (McQuay, 2004), for example:

    4 = complete relief
    3 = good relief
    2 = moderate relief
    1 = slight relief
    0 = no relief

Likert (numerical rating scales) are also used frequently for the measurement of pain. These are often given as a 100 mm line and give seven or 11 points along the line to choose on a continuum that is defined at the two ends, for example between least possible pain to worst possible pain or no relief of pain to complete relief of pain (McQuay, 2004).

When undertaking work assessment, levels of strength/endurance have also been measured on an ordinal scale (US Department of Labor, 1981, cited in Hill, 1993):

    S: sedentary
    L: light work
    M: medium work
    H: heavy work
    V: very heavy work

A more complex example of an ordinal scale is the five-point scale used for manual muscle testing (MMT) as described by Smith (1993). This scale has a number of subdivisions that can aid sensitivity and the responsiveness of the measure to small amounts of change (providing there is good inter-rater and intra-rater reliability amongst the therapists using the scale) but is still basically an ordinal scale:

0   0   *Zero:* no evidence of contractility
1   T   *Trace:* evidence of contractility on palpation; no joint motion
    P − *Poor minus:* less than complete range of movement (ROM) with gravity eliminated
2   P   *Poor:* complete ROM with gravity eliminated
    P + *Poor plus:* complete ROM with gravity eliminated, takes minimal resistance
    F − *Fair minus:* less than full ROM against gravity
3   F   *Fair:* complete ROM against gravity
    F + *Fair plus:* complete ROM against gravity with minimal resistance
    G − *Good minus:* complete ROM against gravity with less than moderate resistance
4   G   *Good:* complete ROM against gravity with moderate resistance
5   N   *Normal:* Complete ROM against gravity with full resistance

Therapists should be aware that some ordinal rating scales (used widely in both occupational therapy and physiotherapy) are open to a considerable degree of subjectivity. People use the same adverbs, such as *frequently*, in different ways. This means that therapists should not assume that what frequently means to one client or carer or colleague is the same for all the people who may be using that assessment. This means that the term frequently cannot indicate the same frequency for the occurrence of a symptom or behaviour of interest to the therapist (McDowell and Newell, 1987). Fisher (2003a) warns therapists that:

> There is a general misconception that scales which describe a client's ADL task performance in terms of level of independence are objective . . . in actual practice, any rating scale that relies on professional judgement of a client's ADL performance is subjective. While the use of scales that reflect a client's level of independence is common and widely accepted as 'objective', it is likely that we have confused familiarity and common usage with objectivity. (p. 136)

The issue of subjectivity is illustrated by the common assessment of the level of assistance required for ADL. For example, when assessing the level of independence a person demonstrates for transfers and mobility, the level of assistance might be rated in terms of the type of assistance required (for example a three-point scale: standby, verbal prompts, physical assistance) or the level of assistance needed (for example a three-point scale: minimal, moderate, maximum) or the amount of assistance (for example given as a percentage: 10 per cent of the time, 25 per cent of the time, 50 per cent of the time). Subjectivity can influence the assessment as different therapists may have varying judgements as to what behaviour represents each definition of assistance, for example rating minimum versus moderate assistance. Evidence of strong inter-rater reliability is, therefore, particularly important when using assessments with these types of scales.

INTERVAL SCALES

An interval scale is the level where the scale is truly quantitative (as opposed to numbers being used as codes to categorise qualitative data). From a purist's point of view, this is the level of data at which measurements can be taken. Wright and Linacre (1989), for example, argue that measurements must be taken at least at an interval level, whereas observational assessments produce ordinal level data. The interval level of measurement goes beyond either nominal or ordinal scaling as interval scores are classified by both order and by a known and equal interval between points (Lichtman *et al.*, 1989). Stevens (1946) describes an interval scale:

Principles of Assessment and Outcome Measurement

- An interval scale has rank order and the distances between the numbers have meaning with respect to the property being measured.
- If two scores at the low end of an interval scale are one unit apart, then two scores at the high end are also one unit apart and the difference between these two high scores and two low scores represents the same amount of the property.
- Transformation of values in an interval scale is restricted and must contain the information in the values of the original scale.

An interval scale describes, provides a hierarchy and ascribes a numerical difference (Lewis and Bottomley, 1994). Interval scales have a constant, common unit of measurement and the gap, or interval, between each position on the scale is kept the same. However, the units of measurement and the zero point on an interval scale are arbitrary (Hunter, 1997). Statistical analysis of data collected using interval scales can be undertaken with parametric statistics, including mean, standard deviation and Pearson correlation coefficients. Statistical tests of significance, such as a t-test, can be used if the data are normally distributed (Hunter, 1997).

EVERYDAY EXAMPLES OF INTERVAL SCALES

The measurement of temperature is a good example of an interval scale. Equal units, known as degrees, are used to measure temperature and these can be added or subtracted to examine increases or decreases in temperature. On the Fahrenheit temperature scale (Figure 4.3) zero does not represent an absence of heat; in fact 32 degrees is given as the freezing point on the Fahrenheit scale. A good example of an interval scale is the IQ test. 'A score of zero on an intelligence test does not mean the examinee had no intelligence; it only means that on that specific sampling of intelligence, no score was achieved. The zero point was set arbitrarily by the test developer' (Lichtman *et al.*, 1989, p. 7).

The measurement of temperature on the centigrade scale is also an interval scale as the zero point on this scale is also arbitrary. Both scales, however, 'contain the same amount and the

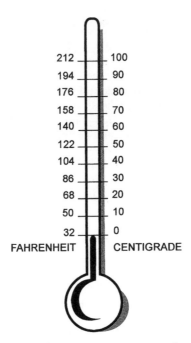

Figure 4.3 Measurement of temperature as an example of an interval scale.

same kind of information . . . because they are linearly related. That is, a reading on one scale can be transformed to the equivalent reading on the other by the linear transformation $F = \frac{9}{5}$ C + 32 where F = number of degrees on Fahrenheit scale, C = number degrees on centigrade scale' (Siegel, 1956, p. 27, i.e. multiply by 9, divide by 5 and add 32).

The year date on many calendars is also an interval measurement. For example, the Gregorian calendar is the calendar that is used in many places in the world. This calendar does not have an absolute zero as people have not been able to establish a precise starting point for the beginning of time. Rather, with the Gregorian calendar the years are numbered using the perceived birth date of Jesus Christ.

In rehabilitation, some therapists have tried to convert ordinal scales to interval scales by weighting the value attached to particular scores. McDowell and Newell (1987) describe the equal-appearing interval scaling method, which is used by some test developers:

> In this approach a sample of people is asked to judge the relative severity . . . of each of the items used in the health index. Verbal descriptions of the response categories, such as 'severe pain' and 'mild pain', are sorted by each person into ten to fifteen ordered categories to reflect the relative severity of the problem implied by each statement. For each description a score is derived from the median of the category numbers to which the statement is assigned by the raters. Transformations may be applied, and the resulting score is used as a numerical indicator of the judged severity of that response. This approach has been used in scales such as the Sickness Impact Profile. (pp. 20–21)

The Sickness Impact Profile (SIP; Bergner *et al.*, 1981) was developed to assess perceived health status to provide a descriptive measure of changes in a person's behaviour that have resulted owing to sickness. The test developers wanted to provide a measure that could be used with a broad population of people experiencing a wide range of illnesses of varying degrees of severity. The SIP has a number of purposes, including evaluating a patient's progress and measuring outcomes of health care to inform service planning and policy development (for a critique of SIP, see McDowell and Newell, 1987, pp. 290–295).

RATIO SCALES

A ratio scale is also a truly quantitative scale; it has a constant unit of measurement, a uniform interval between points on the scale and a true zero at its origin (Hunter, 1997). Stevens (1946) describes a ratio scale:

- A ratio scale has the properties of order, equal distance between units and a fixed origin or absolute zero point.
- Once the location of the absolute zero is known, non-zero measurements can be expressed as ratios of one another.
- Transformation of values is very restricted.
- Parametric statistics can be used to analyse ratio scales.

EVERYDAY EXAMPLES OF RATIO SCALES

Everyday examples of ratio scales include length or height measured in inches or centimetres, distance measured in kilometres or miles, weight measured in pounds or kilograms, time measured in seconds, minutes, hours, days, months or years and age measured in days, months or years since birth. Volume is also measured using ratio scales with a score of zero indicating an absence of liquid regardless of whether the volume is being measured in litres or pints. Other everyday examples include income, price, costs, sales revenue, sales volume and market share.

EXAMPLES OF RATIO SCALES USED BY THERAPISTS

When evaluating a therapy service, many measures used in health economics, such as cost per case, are ratio scales. Lewis and Bottomley (1994) also give the examples of timed scores and goniometric measurements. In physiotherapy, speed (measured as distance over time) is a useful ratio scale. An example of a ratio scale used by both occupational therapists and physiotherapists is joint ROM assessment using a goniometer. A goniometer has a scale from zero to 180 degrees with zero indicating a total absence of movement around the joint (for instructions on measuring using a goniometer, see Smith, 1993). As a ratio scale can be used to provide a quantitative measure of change, meaningful comparisons can be made between people, and between individual measurements taken over time, using measurement tools like a goniometer. For example, if a person improves from 40 degrees to 80 degrees of shoulder movement, he can be said to have twice as much movement at the shoulder joint than before. Grip strength can also be measured using a ratio scale.

McDowell and Newell (1987) describe a method called magnitude estimation, which is used by some test developers to produce a ratio scale estimate: 'a more sophisticated approach to scaling statements about health . . . has people judge the relative severity implied by each statement on scales with no limits placed on the values' (p. 21). With the equal-appearing interval scaling method (described earlier in the section on interval scales), the raters sort verbal descriptions of the construct or behaviour being measured into a defined number of categories. There have been objections to category scaling, derived from this application of a fixed number of categories, because it is thought that people are able to make more refined and accurate judgements of relative magnitude than the fixed categories method permits. An example of a test that has been developed following magnitude estimation procedures is the Pain Perception Profile (Tursky, Jamner and Friedman, 1982). For a description and critique of the Pain Perception Profile, see McDowell and Newell (1987, pp. 264–267).

APPLICATION OF DIFFERENT LEVELS OF MEASUREMENT

The four levels of measurement form a hierarchy of sophistication, with nominal scales being the least and ratio scales being the most sophisticated level of measurement. In this hierarchy, the scale above contains the properties of the scale below, that is values meeting the requirements of a ratio scale may be regarded as meeting the requirements for an interval scale and data collected on an interval scale may be regarded as providing ordinal level information. To summarise, 'nominal measurement shows difference in type, ordinal in rank, and interval or ratio in amount' (Kovacs, 1985, cited in Lichtman *et al.*, 1989, p. 9). Hunter (1997) provides a useful summary of the ways in which each level of scale may be used:

- 'a nominal scale is sufficient to measure the proportion of a population in achieving a particular outcome
- an ordinal scale can describe how x compares with y
- an interval scale defines how x differs from y
- while a ratio scale tells us how proportionally different x is from y' (p. 89).

Lichtman *et al.* (1989) report that usually the first three levels of measurement are used to measure abilities, attitudes or intelligence. Most variables can only be measured at one of the four levels of measurement. However, some common types of scales, such as Likert scales, can be found in the literature as examples of both ordinal and interval scales. Lichtman *et al.* (1989) found disagreement about 'whether Likert distributions fall within the realm of ordinal or interval measurements because of the inability to assume equal distances between values. The distance from "strongly disagree" to "disagree" may be different than the distance from "disagree" to "agree", thus raising the question of whether or not it is appropriate to classify these kind of measures at the interval level' (pp. 7–8). In my opinion, in the majority of cases the constructs measured by therapists using Likert scales do not have equal intervals between properties and should be treated as ordinal scales. This is particularly important when conducting clinical research as different statistical analyses can be applied to interval scales that are not appropriate for ordinal scales. When you are in doubt about the level of measurement being used, it is wise to assume the lower level of measurement until you have sought clarification.

Another debate with Likert-type scales centres around how many points the scale should have in order to achieve the best levels of sensitivity and reliability. There is no one best solution, and factors, such as the age of the client group, need to be taken into consideration. For example, Sturgess, Rodger and Ozanne (2002) found that three categories/scale points were most frequently used on self-report scales designed for young children. They acknowledge that statistical analysis of three-point scales cannot produce the same power as five-, seven- or 10-point scales and that three-point scales are less likely to be sensitive to small clinical changes. However, test developers for paediatric populations have found that young children can only discriminate between a few responses, making three-point scales more reliable for children, whose cognitive functioning is predominately at a level of dichotomous thought; therefore, if you are seeking a measure for a children's service, you may decide to compromise statistical power and responsiveness for reliability.

It is very important that therapists do not handle scores in a manner that is inconsistent with the level of measurement used. This is a particular problem with ordinal scales. As the value of numbers used in an ordinal scale, and the numerical distance between each point in an ordinal scale, hold no intrinsic meaning, a change between scale points at one level in the scale (such as from 1 to 2) is not necessarily equivalent to a change between to other neighbouring scale points (such as 5 to 6 or 8 to 9) elsewhere in the scale. McDowell and Newell (1987) make it clear that mathematical calculations using such scores cannot be meaningfully undertaken and should be used with caution.

> Strictly speaking, it is not appropriate to calculate differences between ordinal scores by subtraction, or to combine them by addition, because resulting scores cannot be meaningfully compared: differences of a certain number of points between scores may not represent equivalent contrasts at different points on the scale. This is not to say that adding ordinal scores to make an overall score cannot be done – it is frequently done. Whilst purists may criticise . . . pragmatists argue that the errors produced are small . . . Although many health indices do calculate overall scores on the basis of adding ordinal scales, the reader should be aware that this may lead to incorrect conclusions. (p. 20)

Fisher (1993) agrees that the summing of ordinal scores to provide a total score 'does not result in a number that is a valid means of making quantitative comparisons of performances, whether it be between two different persons or the same person on different occasions' (p. 319). So summed ordinal scores just result in numerical values that are 'assigned to qualitative differences in ability' (p. 319). Despite these limitations, a significant number of therapy assessments are based on ordinal level data and sum item or subscale scores to provide an overall score. The Barthel Index (BI; Mahoney and Barthel, 1965) is a well-known measure that has an ordinal level scale that requires the addition of scores to provide a total score from the test items. Summing scores is possible with interval level scales where the unit of measurement between each scale item is known and equal. Letts and Bosch (2001), in their critique of the BI, note as a weakness of the measure that 'the Barthel's ordinal scale has not been validated or shown to produce interval level measurements' (p. 131). Hunter (1997) states that the practice of summating scores awarded to the items which comprise an ordinal scale compromises the scale and cites both the BI and the Functional Independence Measure

(FIM; Granger *et al.*, 1993) as examples of problematic ordinal scales with a summed total score. Summating scores is dubious because to be independent in one activity, such as in making a cup of tea, does not equal the same level of function as being independent in another activity, such as cooking a meal. McAvoy (1991) states that one reason why therapists may not use existing standardised assessments is that therapists find 'a global score is difficult to interpret; a patient may achieve a "totally independent" score, that is, 100 with the Barthel Index, but still be unable to live independently at home because, for example, he/she is unable to cook for himself or is unsafe or unsteady, or independence may not be the ideal aim where energy conservation or safety are important' (p. 385). Several other authors (for example Hogan and Orme, 2000; Murdock, 1992) argue against the use of the BI because the total score has no real meaning and the same total score does not carry the same meaning for all people with that particular score. In addition, two people might show equal increases in their total scores when re-tested following treatment but their gains in functional status might be very different (Eakina, 1989).

Another practice to avoid when implementing an ordinal level scale is presuming that an increase in function indicated by moving from needing verbal prompting (score 2) to being independent (score 1) equals the same amount of change as moving from dependence (score 4) to physical assistance (score 3). The presumption of equal change occurring between two scores can be made only when using interval or ratio level scales.

Addition and subtraction are permissible at the top two levels of measurement (interval and ratio scales) because the unit of change between each item in the scale remains constant across the whole scale. With this level of measurement, it is possible to calculate differences in scores and to calculate averages. Because a ratio scale has a zero point, it is only at this highest level of measurement that you can calculate how many times greater one score is compared to another score (McDowell and Newell, 1987).

Therapists need to identify the level of measurement used when critiquing a potential measure for use in their service or when reading journal articles describing research to explore the psychometric properties of potential therapy assessments. For example, in a study examining the responsiveness to change of the Rivermead Mobility Index (RMI) and the BI the authors (Wright, Cross and Lamb, 1998) explore the pros and cons of different statistical procedures for calculating responsiveness to change related to the level of measurement used in the two tests.

> Disadvantages of using effect sizes to estimate the responsiveness of ordinal scales like the RMI and BI are that they assume that each successive point on the score represents an equal amount of change (which is not strictly the case for the BI and RMI) and that the data are normally distributed (referred to as parametric assumptions) . . . to overcome these difficulties both parametric and non-parametric methods of calculations were used. (p. 217)

Such a transparent discussion related to limitations in statistical analyses of nominal and ordinal data is rare in therapy literature and so therapists need to be discerning readers when critiquing a research article and deciding whether the results reported should lead to changes in clinical practice.

When a therapist undertakes an assessment, she does not want to bore the client by presenting him with lots of very easy items or disillusion the client by forcing him to attempt test items that are too demanding. (*Note:* the influence of the demands of the assessment task has already been discussed in Chapter 1.) Some assessments do provide scales where the level of difficulty of a task is taken into account and provide a hierarchy that represents level of difficulty/demand, for example the Assessment of Motor Process Skills (AMPS; Fisher, 2003a). Two methods have been applied to therapy and health measures to provide these types of scales. The first method is Guttman scaling and the second is Rasch analysis.

GUTTMAN SCALING

Guttman scales can be helpful because they are constructed in a way that enables the therapist to just administer those items which fall at the outer boundaries of the client's ability and provide a useful indicator of the maximum level of difficulty that the person can master. Guttman (1941, cited in Crocker and Algina, 1986) describes a response-scaling method called scalogram analysis. Items are worded so as to increase in strength/severity/demand so that once a respondent agrees with one item statement he should also agree with all the statements that express weaker/less severe/less demanding items. In a Guttman scale, if the client passes an item high up on the scale the implication is that he will also be able to pass less demanding items lower down on the scale (McDowell and Newell, 1987). On these types of scales, the therapist will often be directed to start testing at the test items level she hypothesises the client can manage. She will test up the scale items until the person has three consecutive failures and will test down the scale to achieve three consecutive passes. Therapists have been using Guttman scaling methods for many years. The Physical Self-maintenance Scale (PSMS), developed by Lawton and Brody back in 1969, was founded on the theory that a person's functional ability could be ordered in a hierarchy ranging from physical self-maintenance, instrumental ADL to behaviours related to motivation and social interaction (Lawton and Brody, 1969). The PSMS comprises five-point scales, which range from total dependence to total independence and are used to rate six test items that fall on a Guttman scale. The six domains are toileting, feeding, dressing, grooming, physical ambulation and bathing (see McDowell and Newell, 1987, pp. 66–68, for test items and a critique of the measure, and Letts and Bosch, 2001, p. 151, for a more recent critique).

Another example of a Guttman scale is the Arthritis Impact Measurement Scale (AIMS; Meenan, Gertman and Mason, 1980; Meenan *et al.*, 1982), which is a client self-report measure that covers the domains of physical, social and emotional well-being and was developed as an outcome measure for intervention with people with arthritis. The AIMS comprises 45 items grouped into nine scales (mobility, physical activity, dexterity, household activity, social activity, ADL, pain, depression and anxiety) comprising five items each. Items for each scale were selected using Guttman analyses and internal consistency correlations. For each of the nine scales, items are listed in hierarchical order of difficulty, as experienced by people with arthritis and based on the Guttman order; so a person indicating disability on one question would also be expected to indicate disability on the items below it (see McDowell and Newell, 1987, pp. 271–276, for the test items and a critique of the AIMS).

RASCH ANALYSIS

A big limitation of many therapy observational assessments is that they produce ordinal level raw scores. The unit of measurement needs to be at an interval level so that comparisons of how much more or less the person exhibits of the construct or behaviour can be made (Hayley *et al.*, 1998). In the past decade or so, therapist researchers have turned to Rasch analysis to help develop a more robust form of functional measurement. The Rasch measurement model enables a test developer to produce a uni-dimensional linear measure that is based on additive numbers. It can be applied to convert ordinal scores into linear (also referred to as additive) level measures and is useful for developing criterion-referenced hierarchical scales (Fisher 1993, 2003a). Test developers use Rasch analysis 'to convert observed counts of ordinal data (raw scores) into an approximately equal-interval number line (linear continuum or scale representing the variable)' (Fisher, 1993, p. 320). Rasch analysis provides goodness-of-fit statistics that are used to undertake construct validity analyses of a scale by, first, exploring hypotheses about what should occur when a particular sample is given the test and, second, confirming whether or not the test items fit the hypothesised model (Fisher, 1993). In this approach, the test developer begins by defining the construct or performance variable to be measured as a continuous, uni-dimensional construct or behaviour. This should be a construct of which people possess varying degrees.

The construct should have the potential to be visualised as falling along a line. A measurement developed to evaluate this construct should cover the full range. For example, a measure of some domain of function, such as mobility, should encompass all levels of that function from minimal through moderate to maximal level of performance. Different people measured against this construct would be placed at various points along the line depending on how much or little they demonstrated the trait/ability/behaviour being measured. Fisher (1993) explains that the 'length of the line determines the range of the test and the range is delimited by the easiest item (base) and the hardest item (ceiling)' (p. 320). The greater the person's level of ability, the more test items he should pass. So, when test items are ordered in terms of difficulty, we are able to hypothesise where a person will be positioned along the line and then to determine their exact location after they have been rated on all the test items. For a more detailed presentation of Rasch analysis, refer to Wright and Masters (1982).

One of the best-known examples of a therapy measure that has been developed using the Rasch measurement model is the AMPS (Fisher, 2003a). Its test developer, Anne Fisher, was one of the first therapists to recommend this approach to scaling. The AMPS is based on two linear scales: the AMPS motor skill scale and the AMPS process skill scale. Rasch analysis has been used to calibrate the challenge presented by the ADL that are observed for the test, the difficulty of the skill items on the linear scales and also the severity of the therapist raters who administer the test.

Another example is the Pediatric Evaluation of Disability Inventory (PEDI; Hayley *et al.*, 1998). The authors report that the Rasch model was used to assist the development of the PEDI and scale construction in three ways: '1) content specification and scale validation, 2) summary score development, and 3) goodness-of-fit analysis between individual child profiles and the overall hierarchical structure intended for each scale' (p. 19).

APPLYING CONCEPTS OF LEVELS OF MEASUREMENT TO YOUR OWN PRACTICE

At the back of this book, you will find templates for a series of worksheets designed to assist you in applying principles of assessment and outcome measurement to your own practice. Please now turn to Worksheet 4: Reflecting on levels of measurement (p. 399).

The first column of this worksheet lists the four levels of measurement (nominal, ordinal, interval and ratio). In the second column you are asked to consider the level of measurement that is provided by each of the assessments (standardised and unstandardised) that you are using in your clinical practice or which you observe being used by therapists while on clinical placement. List the tests/assessment methods you identify in the row for that level of measurement. The third column is used to reflect on whether you are using data in an appropriate way for the level of measurement. Look at the way raw scores are used and identify any issues or limitations in current assessment practice. In the last column, you are encouraged to list potential assessments that you could use to collect data at the different levels of measurement. This is particularly important if the majority of your assessment data is collected at the lower nominal and ordinal levels.

STUDY QUESTIONS

4.1 Describe the similarities and differences between nominal and ordinal scales.

4.2 What property does a ratio scale have that is not present in the other three types of scale?

4.3 Define an *interval scale*.

4.4 What would be the benefit of applying Rasch analysis to an observational ordinal scoring system?

You will find brief answers to these questions at the back of this book (p. 390).

5

Standardisation and Test Development

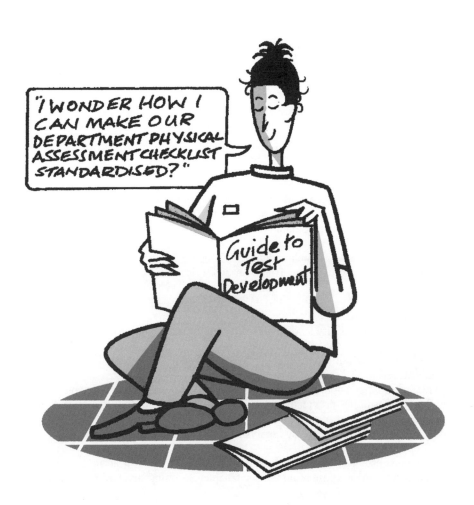

CHAPTER SUMMARY

This chapter discusses what is meant by standardisation and outlines the properties that should be provided by a rigorously standardised test. The process for developing and standardising an assessment for use in occupational therapy or physiotherapy practice is outlined. The chapter also explores the differences between criterion-referenced tests and norm-referenced tests. The process for undertaking a norming study is summarised and definitions for key terms, including normal distribution, percentile ranks, standard deviation and mean, are provided. It will also endeavour to answer the following question: 'How can I make the assessment we developed for our service standardised?'

STANDARDISED ASSESSMENTS

Therapists need reliable, valid and sensitive outcome measures in order to obtain an accurate baseline for intervention and to examine whether that intervention has been effective. Quantifiable data are required in order to undertake the statistical analyses required to demonstrate that results obtained from an intervention are significant and not just owing to chance factors (de Clive-Lowe, 1996). As discussed in Chapter 1, the requirement to demonstrate the effectiveness of therapeutic interventions has led to an increase in the development and use of standardised assessments within both the occupational therapy and physiotherapy professions.

WHY SHOULD THERAPISTS USE STANDARDISED TESTS?

Most testing errors occur when the therapist has done one or more of the following (Vitale and Nugent, 1996).

- collected insufficient data
- collected inaccurate data
- used unsystematic data-collection methods
- obtained irrelevant data
- failed to verify data collected
- obtained data that have been contaminated by bias or prejudice (e.g. either by the person completing the self-report or proxy survey or by the therapist)
- not accurately communicated data collected

The use of standardised tests can help reduce the chances of errors resulting from such practices. A rigorously developed and psychometrically robust test will:

- involve the collection of sufficient data for the purpose of the test (e.g. to screen for a specific impairment)
- have established reliability so data are collected accurately
- use a systematic data-collection method
- have established validity so that data obtained are related to the stated purpose and focus of the test
- provide information about confidence intervals so the therapist can judge how likely it is that this test result has provided a true picture of the person's ability and/or deficits
- reduce the influence of bias or prejudice on test results
- have a record form for recording, analysing and communicating scores.

The therapist must establish that the assessment she plans to use will accurately provide the information needed for the purpose required (see Chapter 3). Using standardised tests can facilitate objectivity, and this is very important because when assessing human functioning it is virtually impossible to obtain complete accuracy and objectivity. Bartram (1990b) states that 'the major advantage of a statistically-based assessment – and it is crucial to professional effectiveness and quality of decision making – is that it provides an objective source of data, unbiased by subjective feeling' (p. 3). The American Occupational Therapy Association (AOTA; 1984) defines *objective* and *subjective* in terms of therapy assessment.

Definition of objective

'Facts or findings which are clearly observable to and verifiable by others, as reflecting reality.'

Definition of subjective

'An observation not rigidly reflecting measurable reality; may imply observer bias; may not be verifiable by others in the same situation.'

(American Occupational Therapy Association, 1984, cited by Hopkins and Smith, 1993a, p. 914)

WHAT IS A STANDARDISED TEST?

Therapists may refer to a published tool used for data collection as a standardised test, standardised assessment, standardised evaluation, standardised measure/outcome measure, standardised instrument or standardised scale. (*Note*: definitions of assessment, outcome measure, scale and instrument and discussion about the use of these terms in therapy has been provided in the Introduction.)

So what do we mean by *standardised*? The word standard has been defined as a 'weight or measure to which others conform or by which the accuracy or quality of others is judged' or 'a degree of excellence etc. required for a particular purpose' and the verb to standardise means to 'make conform to a standard; determine properties of by comparison with a standard' (Sykes, 1983). In the context of therapy, the AOTA defines the word standardised as 'made standard or uniform; to be used without variation; suggests an invariable way in which a test is to be used, as well as denoting the extent to which the results of the test may be considered to be both valid and reliable' (American Occupational Therapy Association, 1984, cited by Hopkins and Smith, 1993b, p. 914). Standardisation, therefore, 'implies uniformity of procedure in administering and scoring [a] test' (Anastasi, 1988, p. 25).

Cole *et al.* (1995) describe a standardised test as a measurement tool that is published and has been designed for a specific purpose for use with a particular population. They state that a standardised test should have detailed instructions explaining how and when it should be administered and scored and how to interpret scores. It should also present the results of investigations to evaluate the measure's psychometric properties. These instructions are usually contained in a test protocol, which describes the specific procedures that must be followed when assessing a client (Christiansen and Baum, 1991). Details of any investigations of reliability and validity should also be given. In order to maintain standardisation, the assessment must be administered according to the testing protocol. The conditions under which standardised tests are administered have to be exactly the same if the results recorded from different clients by different therapists, or from the same person by the same therapist on different occasions, are to be comparable.

Being standardised does not necessarily mean that the test is an objective measure of externally observable data. Therapists also develop standardised tools that enable clinicians to record internal, unobservable constructs, for example a person's self-report of feelings, such as pain, sadness or anxiety. However, any standardised test, whether of observable behaviours or psychological constructs, should be structured so that the method of data collection will yield the same responses for a person at a specific moment in time and the same responses for the person being tested regardless of which therapist is administering the test.

Some standardised tests are referred to as a *battery*. This is an 'assessment approach or instrument with several parts' (Christiansen and Baum, 1991, p. 848). For example, the Rivermead Perceptual Assessment Battery (RPAB; Whiting *et al.*, 1985) comprises 16 subtests covering several domains of perception: form constancy, colour constancy, sequencing, object completion, figure/ground discrimination, body image, inattention and spatial awareness.

WHAT IS AN UN-STANDARDISED ASSESSMENT?

The terms *non-standardised* and *un-standardised* are used interchangeably in the literature. These are assessments that provide the therapist with information but have no precise comparison to a norm or a criterion. Some un-standardised tests are structured assessments that are constructed and organised to provide guidelines for the content and process of the assessment, but their psychometric properties have not been researched and documented.

STANDARDISATION

Standardisation is a process of taking an assessment and developing a fixed protocol for its administration and scoring and then conducting psychometric studies to evaluate whether the resultant assessment has acceptable levels of validity and reliability. There are two ways in which assessments can be standardised: either in terms of procedures, materials and scoring or in terms of normative standardisation (de Clive-Lowe, 1996). The first method of standardisation involves the provision of detailed descriptions and directions for the test materials, method of administration, instructions for administration, scoring and interpretation of scores (Jones, 1991). Standardisation 'extends to the exact materials employed, time limits, oral instructions, preliminary demonstrations, ways of handling queries from test takers, and every other detail of the testing situation' (Anastasi, 1988, p. 25). This information should be provided in the test manual or, if a test is published in its entirety in a professional journal, should be included in the description of the test.

To standardise the test materials, the exact test materials should be listed or included. Some tests provide materials as part of a standardised test battery. If the therapist has to collect the materials together for the test, then precise details of how to construct the test (with exact sizes, colours, fabric of materials etc.) are required. A good example of clear, detailed instructions of test materials is provided by Baum and Edwards (1993) for their Kitchen Task Assessment (KTA). They list the following materials for the test.

> 2 or 3 flavours of pudding mix (the type that requires cooking, not instant); a 1–1½ quart saucepan with a heat-resistant handle; a wooden spoon; a rubber scraper; a 2 cup glass measuring cup; 4 small dishes (paper cups will do); have a quart of milk in the refrigerator; print instructions on a piece of paper and mount the instructions where the person can read them, use the same instructions that are on the box, except add 'pour into cups'; have hand soap and paper towels near the sink. (pp. 435–6)

To standardise the method of administration, the test conditions should be described in detail. The number of people tested at any one time should be specified (for example individual or group assessment, size of group). Information about time required for administration should be given.

In order to produce standardised instructions for administration, detailed written instructions for the therapist should be provided. Exact wording for any instructions to be given to the test taker are required. To maintain standardisation, therapists should be told to follow all instructions exactly. An example of test instructions is taken from the Gross Motor Function Measure (GMFM; Russell *et al.*, 1993, pp. 41–42).

Example test instructions from the GMFM

Lying and rolling
This dimension includes 17 items in the prone and supine positions.
These items include the child's ability to:

* roll from prone or supine
* perform specific tasks while maintaining supine or some variation of prone.

Item 1. Supine, head in midline: turns head with extremities symmetrical

0. does not maintain head in midline
1. maintains head in midline 1 to 3 seconds
2. maintains head in midline, turns head with extremities asymmetrical
3. turns head with extremities symmetrical

Starting position
Position the child with head in midline and, if possible, the arms at rest and symmetrical (but not necessarily at the side). This will make it easier to determine the appropriate score.

Instructions
Instruct the child to turn the head from side to side or follow an object from one side to the other.
   The child can be instructed to keep the arms still, or, in the case of a younger child who may try to reach for the object, observe whether the upper extremity movements are 'symmetrical' or 'asymmetrical'.
   For a score of 2 (extremities 'asymmetrical'), there should be very obvious asymmetry that is dominated by head position.

To standardise the scoring system, clear guidelines need to be provided for scoring. The person's performance on the test should be evaluated on the basis of empirical data. Scoring methods vary from test to test and may include the use of raw scores that may then be converted to another type of score. If scores are being added, deducted, divided or multiplied, make sure the level of measurement allows the numbers to be handled in that way (see Chapter 4 for more information). Information should be included to guide the therapist in the interpretation of scores. Therapists should be aware that a number of factors may influence the person's performance on the test, including test anxiety, fatigue, interruptions and distractions.

   In addition to basic administration details, other subtle factors might affect a person's test performance. For example, when giving oral instructions, 'rate of speaking, tone of voice, inflection, pauses, and facial expression' (Anastasi, 1988, pp. 25–26), all may influence how a person responds.

CONSTRUCTING A STANDARDISED TEST

As therapists often find that they cannot obtain a published measure which measures exactly what they want, with the group of clients they treat and in the setting that they practice, they sometimes decide to design their own measure. The College of Occupational Therapists (COT) warns therapists against developing a 'home-grown' measure.

> There is a temptation to think that 'home-grown' measures will be more easily integrated into practice but designing measurement tools is a very complex procedure, which requires extensive piloting and testing for validity and reliability. This technical complexity is often under-rated and as a result many home made measures are of very poor quality. Developing a good quality measure is something that takes several years and extensive research. This is the same for standardised measures that have been adapted or altered to fit a particular service or client group. (Clarke, Sealey-Lapes and Kotsch, 2001, p. 11).

Test development is a time-consuming, complex and iterative process of construction, evaluation, revision and re-evaluation. As the process of rigorous test construction is complex, it is not the intention to provide detailed guidance in this text. Several authors describe and discuss the process of test construction and would provide a sensible starting point for any therapist considering embarking on test development, for example see Anastasi (1988); Benson and Clark (1982); Crocker and Algina (1986); and Kline (1990 and 1986). In particular, I found Chapter 4 of Crocker and Algina's book very useful when embarking on the development of the Structured Observational Test of Function (SOTOF) for my doctoral studies (Laver, 1994; Laver and Powell, 1995).

Pynsent (2004) also advises 'that designing a new instrument is a complex task not to be undertaken lightly' (p. 2). He provides a 'design pathway' for the process of developing an outcome measure (Figure 5.1).

Even if you have no intention of attempting to develop a test yourself, it is useful for any student or clinician to have a basic understanding of the test development process so that they can establish whether a potential measure for their service has been rigorously developed. Crocker and Algina (1986, p. 66) summarise the test construction process as a series of ten steps:

A 10-step test construction process

1. Identify the primary purpose(s) for which test scores will be used.
2. Identify behaviours that represent the construct or define the domain.
3. Prepare a set of test specifications, delineating the proportion of items that should focus on each type of behaviour identified in step two.
4. Construct an initial pool of items.
5. Have items reviewed (and revise as necessary).
6. Hold preliminary tryouts (and revise as necessary).
7. Field-test the items on a large sample representative of the examinee population for whom the test is intended.
8. Determine statistical properties of item scores and, when appropriate, eliminate items that do not meet pre-established criteria.
9. Design and construct reliability and validity studies for the final form of the test.
10. Develop guidelines for test administration, scoring and for the interpretation of test scores (e.g. prepare norm tables, suggest recommended cutting scores or standards for performance etc.).

The psychometric literature focuses on the scientific aspects of test construction, such as item analysis and factor analysis. Other aspects, such as item writing, have 'remained private, informal, and largely undocumented . . . typically the test developer will conceptualize one or more incidents, direct observations, expert judgement and the development of instruction objectives' (Crocker and Algina, 1986, p. 67). Identifying the primary purpose and then defining relevant content and selecting specific test items for a measure is a critical part of test development that

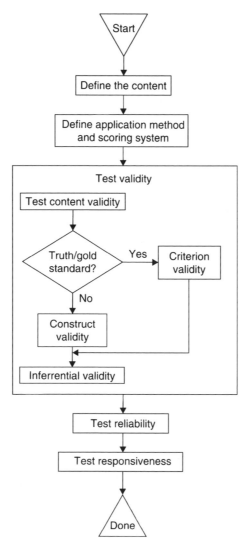

Figure 5.1 A flow diagram showing the requirements for the design of an outcome measure. *Pynsent (2004) Choosing an outcome measure. In P Pysent, J Fairbank, A Carr (eds). Outcome Measures in Orthopaedics and Orthopaedic Trauma (2nd edn.). London: Arnold. © Arnold. Reproduced with permission of Edward Arnold (Publishers) Ltd.*

(*Note:* Definitions for some of the psychometric terms in this figure are provided in Chapter 6 and Chapter 7.)

will help ensure that a clinically useful measure is produced; 'clarifying the major purposes for which test scores will be used and establishing priorities among these probable uses greatly increases the likelihood that this final form of the test will be useful for the most important purpose it is to serve' (p. 67). This is more challenging when the focus of the measure is a psychological construct, as opposed to an observable behaviour or functional ability. In this case, a very thorough understanding of the theory underlying the construct is the starting point for test development. Stanley and Hopkins (1972, cited by Royeen, 1989, p. 57) describe a four-step process for developing a measure of a construct and then establishing the measure's validity:

1. Develop a set of tasks or items based on the rational analysis of the construct.
2. Derive testable predictions regarding the relationship between the construct and other variables (e.g. if the test measures anxiety, we should expect to find some relationship between test scores and clinical ratings of anxiety).
3. Conduct empirical studies of these theoretical predictions.
4. Eliminate items or tasks that operate contrary to theory (or revise the theory) and proceed again with steps 2 and 3.

Crocker and Algina (1986, p. 68) suggest that 'to broaden, refine, or verify the view of the construct to be measured, the test developer should engage in one or more of the following activities:

1. *Content analysis:* with this method, open-ended questions are posed to subjects about the construct of interest, and their responses are sorted into topical categories . . .
2. *Review of research:* the behaviors that have been most frequently studied by others are used to define the construct of interest . . .
3. *Critical incidents:* a list of behaviors is identified that characterises extremes of the performance continuum for the construct of interest . . .
4. *Direct observations:* the test developer identifies the behaviors by direct observation . . .
5. *Expert judgement:* the test developer obtains input from one or more individuals who have first-hand experience with the construct . . .
4. *Instruction objectives:* experts in a subject are asked to review instructional materials and develop a set of instructional objectives when an achievement test is being developed. An instructional objective specifies an observable behavior that [people] should be able to exhibit after a course of instruction . . .'

If you do decide to attempt to develop a test yourself, then for a comprehensive and detailed breakdown of the procedures and sequence of content validation needed for robust test development see Haynes, Richard and Kubany (1995, Appendix A). They state that content validation is a multi-method, quantitative and qualitative process that is applicable to all elements of a test. The reason test developers need to focus on content validation during initial test development is 'to minimize potential error variance associated with an assessment instrument and to increase the probability of obtaining supportive construct validity indices in later studies' (p. 10 of the pdf version).

When developing an assessment that will be used to measure outcomes, the test developer needs to consider a number of issues. The sensitivity of an outcome measure to the type and amount of change anticipated to occur during a therapeutic intervention is one of the most important considerations. Many functional assessments measure a narrow range of functions with scales that have large increments between each recorded ability level. Such scales produce summary scores that often do not have the sensitivity to detect small improvements in function (Fisher, 2003a). A scale that comprises more increments of change is likely to be more sensitive, and longer scales make it easier to measure change over a wider range of functional ability (Fisher, 2003a).

When developing a test, there are a number of decisions to be made because the type of information collected and the proposed purpose of the new test can influence its construction. The elements of a test 'are all the aspects of the measurement process that can affect the obtained data. For example, the elements of questionnaires include individual items, response formats and instructions. The elements of behavioural observation include observation codes, time sampling parameters, and the situations in which observation occurs' (Haynes, Richard and Kubany, 1995, p. 2 of pdf version). When a test is being developed, all these elements need to be considered. This means that lots of decisions have to be made during a test development process.

TEST CONSTRUCTION DECISIONS

This list is based on answers.com (http://www.answers.com/topic/scale-social-sciences, accessed 27.12.06).

- What level of data is involved (nominal, ordinal, interval or ratio)? (*Note:* see Chapter 4 for definitions and descriptions of data at each of these measurement levels.)
- What will the results be used for? (*Note:* see Chapter 3 for a discussion about the different requirements therapists have for making measurements.)
- Should you use a scale, index or typology? (*Note:* see the Introduction for definitions of scale, index and typology.)
- What types of statistical analysis would be useful?
- Should you use a comparative scale or a non-comparative scale?
- How many scale divisions or categories should be used (e.g. 1 to 10, 1 to 7, -3 to $+3$)?
- Should there be an odd or even number of scale divisions? (An odd number of divisions gives a neutral centre value, while an even number of divisions forces respondents to take a non-neutral position.)
- What should the nature and descriptiveness of the scale labels be?
- What should the physical form or layout of the scale be? For example: graphic, simple linear, vertical or horizontal.
- Should a response to each item be forced or be left optional? For example, by providing a not-applicable or not-tested option.

Examples of comparative scaling techniques used in some therapy assessments include:

- paired comparison scale: the client is presented with two items at a time and asked to select one (e.g. 'Do you prefer to be alone or to socialise with friends?')
- rank order scale: the client is presented with several items simultaneously and asked to rank them (e.g. 'Rate the following leisure activities from 1 to 10 with 1 = the activity that you enjoy doing the most and 10 = the activity that you enjoy the least'). This is an ordinal level scaling technique.

Examples of non-comparative scaling techniques used in some therapy assessments include:

- continuous rating scale (also called the graphic rating scale): the client is asked to rate the test item (e.g. the degree of pain experience when undertaking a particular movement) by placing a mark on a line. The line is usually labelled at each end (e.g. 'no pain' at one end and 'unbearable pain' at the other). There are sometimes a series of numbers, called scale points (e.g. 0 to 10) under the line.
- Likert scale: with this type of scaling, people are asked to specify their level of agreement to each of a list of statements. This form of scale was named after Rensis Likert, who invented the scale in 1932. Clients have to indicate the amount of agreement or disagreement they have with each test item statement (from strongly agree to strongly disagree). This is usually presented on a five- or seven-point scale. The same format is used for multiple test items, e.g. in a measure of carer burden carers might be asked to rate the following type of item: 'Owing to the amount of time spent caring for my loved one, I do not have enough time to socialise with other family members.' They would then answer this by circling one of the following responses:

1. Strongly disagree
2. Disagree
3. Neither agree nor disagree
4. Agree
5. Strongly agree

Royeen (1989) provides a checklist for instrument development; this takes the form of a series of questions related to different psychometric properties. Validation is undertaken by a test developer to collect evidence to support the types of inferences that are to be drawn from the results of an assessment (Crocker and Algina, 1986). Although validity can be quantified, it can be related to the robustness of the theoretical underpinnings of a test and, therefore, an evaluation of test validity may involve qualitative and subjective methods. Cronbach (1960s) suggests that test developers do not validate their test but should rather explore validity in terms of an interpretation of data arising from a specified procedure.

Royeen (1989) notes that 'the validity question is always specific: how well does this instrument assess the characteristic, construct, or behaviour the user desires to measure?' (p. 55). Royeen (1989, p. 54) suggests that to establish whether a measure has acceptable levels of validity, the following questions should be addressed. (*Note:* information pertaining to these areas should be provided by test developers in a test manual and/or in research articles in professional journals.)

If **content validity** is claimed, answers are needed to these questions:

- Source(s) of items?
- Panel of content experts used?
- Statistical techniques(s) used (e.g. factor analysis)?
- Item–total correlation (r and N)?

If **criterion validity** is claimed, answers are needed to these questions:

- Outside criterion used?
- Standardisation (validity) group used? (Describe characteristics, size etc.)
- Correlation with criterion?

If **construct validity** is claimed, answers are needed to these questions:

- Theoretical basis? (Describe)
- Source(s) of items?
- Panel of experts used?
- Statistical technique(s) used (e.g. convergent-divergent)?
- Item–total correlation (r and N)?

(*Note:* for definitions of the different types of validity see Chapter 6. In terms of the abbreviations used by Royeen, *r* refers to *Pearson r coefficient* of correlation (p. 61) and *N* is traditionally the abbreviation used to represent the total *number* of items.)

Standardised assessments provide for measurement against a criterion or norm and can be divided into two main types: norm-referenced or criterion-referenced tests. The following sections will describe each of these types.

CRITERION-REFERENCED TESTS

A criterion-referenced test is a test that examines performance against pre-defined criteria and produces raw scores that are intended to have a direct, interpretable meaning (Crocker and Algina, 1986). The person's score on this type of test is interpreted by comparing the score with a pre-specified standard of performance or against specific content and/or skills. The therapist uses this type of test to judge whether the person has mastered the required standard (for example to judge whether the person has sufficient independence to be safely discharged from hospital to live alone at home). The person's performance is not compared to the ability of other people; it is evaluated only against the defined criteria (whereas norm-referenced assessments evaluate performance against the scores of a normative sample, see below).

Criterion-referenced tests usually have one of two main purposes, which are:

- estimation of the domain score (i.e. the proportion of items in the domain that the subject can pass correctly
- mastery allocation.

In mastery allocation, the domain score is divided into a number of mutually exclusive mastery categories that are defined by cut scores. The observed test results are used to classify people into the mastery categories. 'The most commonly cited example has one cut score and two categories, master and non-master' (Crocker and Algina, 1986, p. 193). This is useful for therapists who are often involved with examining a person's competence or level of mastery. Criterion-referenced tests are important because therapists are concerned with desired outcomes, such as specified levels of ability in activities of daily living (ADL) tasks, range of movement (ROM) or mobility. In a therapy assessment a score representing *master* might be labelled *able* or *independent* or *observed*, while a score representing *non-master* might be labelled *unable* or *dependent* or *not observed*.

With a criterion-referenced test, it is essential to have a detailed and unambiguous definition of the criteria against which the person is to be judged. For example, if the desired outcome is independence in getting dressed, then the test should describe exactly what the person should be able to do in order to be assessed as being competent in dressing. Depending on the activity to be assessed, different criteria might be necessary for people of different gender, age or cultural backgrounds. In some cases, a time limit might form part of the criteria.

An example of a criterion-referenced test is the Severe Impairment Battery (SIB; Saxton *et al.*, 1993). This test was developed to evaluate severe cognitive deficits. The test has 40 items, 38 of which use mastery scoring with a three-point scale (Saxton *et al.*, 1993, p. 5):

2 = correct
1 = partially correct, an approximate or closely related answer
0 = incorrect

The test developers state 'there is, of course, no cut off for normal as the test should only be used with patients known to be severely impaired' (p. 5).

NORM-REFERENCED TESTS

In the literature, the terms *norm-referenced test* and *normative test* are used interchangeably; in this book, we shall be using the term norm-referenced test. The second method of standardisation involves conducting a norming study, and so the second type of standardised measure to be discussed is the norm-referenced test. Sometimes it is difficult to make useful inferences from raw scores alone; the scores need to be considered within a context. A person's performance can be considered in the light of expected, or 'normal', performance by comparing it to the range of scores obtained by a representative group of people; this is known as a normative sample or normative group. The COT (2005c) states that when a test has been 'normatively standardised' this means it 'has been used with a very large group of similar people, giving an average or range of expected scores that the tester and service user can use to compare their own results' (p. 1).

The scores obtained from a normative group provide the normative data, also known as norms, for the test. *Norms* have been defined as 'sets of scores from clearly defined samples' of a population (Kline, 1990, p. 17). While not intrinsic to the test, comprehensive norms from a representative sample are an important characteristic of a robust test. Norms indicate the average performance on the test and the varying degrees of performance above and below average. Norms should be based on a large, representative sample of people for whom the test was designed. The normative sample should reflect the attributes of the client population (for example geographical, socioeconomic, ethnic, age, sex, level of education). The size of the sample used for normative data will vary depending on the nature of the test, the number of test items and the variability in test scores, but in general the larger the sample the more useful the normative data. Since norms vary over time and across societies, therapists should remember that it is impossible to define or label behaviour in absolute terms. If normative data were collected some years ago, there is a risk that it may have become outdated and will not be representative of the current client group.

CRITERIA FOR JUDGING NORMS

These criteria are based on notes by Linda Gottfredson, available from the University of Delaware website at: http://www.udel.edu/educ/gottfredson/451/unit10-chap19.htm (accessed 10.06.06).

1. Norms should be relevant to your area of practice:
   • Is this particular norm group appropriate for (a) the clinical decision you need to make and (b) the group of clients involved?
2. The normative sample should be representative of your client group:
   • Was the norm group created with a random sample or stratified random sample?
   • Does it match census figures (by race, sex, age, location etc.) for the client population being considered?
3. Norms should be up to date:
   • Read the manual to see how old the norms are; do not rely on the copyright date of the test manual as the manual may report research conducted significantly before publication.
4. Comparable:
   • If you want to compare scores on tests with different norm groups, check the test manuals to evaluate how comparable those groups are.
5. Norms should be adequately described; to ensure this check for details of the:
   • method of sampling
   • number and distribution of people in the norming sample
   • age, race, sex, geography etc. of norm sample
   • extent to which standardised conditions were maintained during the testing of the norm sample.

The normative sample is usually tested before the test is published and the results are often provided in the test manual in the form of tables that give the distribution, or spread, of scores that the normative group obtained (de Clive-Lowe, 1996). Crocker and Algina (1986) describe nine basic steps for conducting a norming study, which they state are recommended whether norms are intended for local or wider use:

1. Identify the population of interest (e.g. people with a particular diagnosis or service users eligible for a particular health service, or people of a specified age, geographical or socio-economic background).
2. Identify which statistics are to be produced on the normative sample data (e.g. mean, standard deviation and percentile ranks).
3. Decide what amount of sampling error can be tolerated for any of the statistics identified (a common example is the sampling error associated with the mean).
4. Develop a method for sampling from the population of interest (this might involve random sampling, stratified sampling or seeking volunteers).

5. Estimate the minimum sample size needed to keep the sampling error within the specified limits.
6. Obtain the sample, administer the test and collect data. The test developers should record any reasons for attrition; if a substantial number of people pull out of the sample, it may be necessary to continue to implement the sampling method to obtain additional people from the population to ensure the desired sample size.
7. Calculate all the statistics of interest.
8. Identify the normative scores that are needed from the data and develop normative score conversion tables for the test.
9. Write up the norming procedure in the test manual and prepare guidelines for the interpretation of the normative scores.

Normative data provide a numerical description of the test performance of a defined and well-described sample group (known as the normative group or normative sample or reference group) that then serves as a reference from which therapists can evaluate the performance of the other people who take the test. Most norms tables provide, in descending order, the range of test scores and the percentage of people in the normative sample who scored below each score level. By obtaining a client's score, the therapist can then determine how he compares with the normative group. Statistical analyses are undertaken to give technical information about the distribution of the normative group's test scores, such as the average score. These statistics may be presented as a labelled normal curve with specified values attached to standard deviations above and below the mean (Anastasi, 1988). Therapists should understand statistical concepts such as mean, standard deviation and normal distribution. The definitions presented below have been developed following an examination of some measurement literature, for example Anastasi (1988) and Crocker and Algina (1986), and also from a Web-based search that was undertaken to check these older texts still provide accepted definitions. Sources included http://www.answers.com, http://www.thefreedictionary.com, http://en.wikipedia.org/ and http://www.collegeboard.com/about/news_info/sat/glossary.html (all accessed 3.06.06). Another key source was the HyperStat Online Statistics Textbook (Lane, 2006), which is available online at: http://davidmlane.com/hyperstat/index.html (accessed 4.06.06).

TERMINOLOGY RELATED TO NORM-REFERENCED TESTS

OBTAINED SCORE

The score achieved by a person taking a test.

RAW SCORE

A raw score is the original numerical score that has not been transformed. In therapy measurement the raw score is the original result obtained by a client on a test (for example the number of correctly answered items) as opposed to that score after transformation to a standard score or percentile rank.

FREQUENCY DISTRIBUTION

A frequency distribution is a table of scores (either presented from high to low, or low to high scores) providing the number of people who obtain each score or whose scores fall in each score interval. Frequency distributions are used to determine tables of percentile ranks.

MEAN

The mean (μ) is a measure of central tendency. It is the arithmetic average: the sum divided by the number of cases. Therefore, in testing the mean score is the average score obtained by a group of people on a test. The mean score is calculated by adding the scores obtained by all people taking the test and then dividing this total by the number of obtained scores. For normal distributions, the mean is the most efficient and, therefore, the least subject to sample fluctuations of all measures of central tendency (Lane, 2006). The mean can be affected by a few extremely high or low values.

MEDIAN

The median is the value above and below which half the cases fall. If there is an even number of cases, the median is the average of the two middle cases when they are sorted in ascending or descending order. With test scores the median is the score below which 50 per cent of people's scores fall. Like the mean, the median is a measure of central tendency. But, unlike the mean, the median is not sensitive to outlying scores. Therefore, if the distribution of scores is distorted by a few atypical scores (that are considered to have little clinical relevance), then the median may be a better summary description of the group's performance than the mean. If the distribution is symmetric, then the median and mean will be almost identical. The median is also by definition the 50th percentile.

NORMAL DISTRIBUTION

The normal distribution is a theoretical frequency distribution for a set of variable data, usually represented by a bell-shaped curve symmetrical about the mean. The normal distribution is also known as the *Gaussian distribution* (after the nineteenth-century German mathematician Karl Friedrich Gauss). It is used to represent a normal or statistically probable outcome. Normal distributions are symmetric with scores more concentrated in the middle than in the tails. They are defined by two parameters: the mean (μ) and the standard deviation (σ). The normal distribution curve is symmetrical and bell-shaped, showing that scores will usually fall near the mean value, but will occasionally deviate by large amounts. The normal distribution curve has a line representing its mean at the centre (see Figure 5.2 below).

Test developers frequently discover that the results for a group of people who have taken their test match a normal distribution curve (bell curve). This means that they find a large number of people perform moderately well on their test (that is their results fall in the middle of the bell), some people do worse than average and some do better than average on the test (that is their results fall in the sloping sides of the bell) and a very small number of people achieve very high or very low scores (that is their results fall in the rim of the bell) (Lane, 2006).

Normal distribution is important to therapists because many psychological and behavioural constructs are distributed approximately normally. For example, Lane (2006) reports that measures of reading ability, introversion, job satisfaction and memory are among the many psychological variables approximately normally distributed. Although the distributions are only

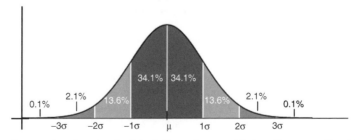

Figure 5.2 A normal curve showing standard deviations above and below the mean. Graph by Beirne, created 5.01.06 for Wikipedia, a free online encyclopaedia at: http://upload.wikimedia.org/wikipedia/en/4/4f/Standard_deviation_diagram.png, accessed 23.06.06.

approximately normal, they are usually quite close. Normal distribution is also important for test developers and for therapists undertaking research, because many statistical tests can be applied to normally distributed data. If the mean and standard deviation of a normal distribution are known, it is easy to convert back and forth from raw scores to percentiles (Lane, 2006).

STANDARD DEVIATION

The standard deviation (σ) is a measure of the spread or extent of variability of a set of scores around their mean. It is the average amount a score varies from the average score in a series of scores. The standard deviation reflects the degree of homogeneity of the group with respect to the test item in question, that is the less the scores are spread across the range of possible scores, the smaller will be the standard deviation. Therefore, a large standard deviation indicates that the scores obtained are scattered far from the mean, while a small standard deviation indicates that the obtained scores are clustered closely around the mean. 'Standard deviation is defined as the square root of the variance. This means it is the root mean square (RMS) deviation from the average. The standard deviation is always a positive number (or zero) and is always measured in the same units as the original data. For example, if the data are distance measurements in meters, the standard deviation will also be measured in meters' (answers.com, 2006b).

Standard deviation is the most commonly used measure of spread. An important attribute of the standard deviation as a measure of spread is that, if the mean and standard deviation of a normal distribution are known, it is possible to compute the percentile rank associated with any given score. In a normal distribution, about 68 per cent of the scores are within one standard deviation of the mean and about 95 per cent of the scores are within two standard deviations of the mean (Lane, 2006).

The standard deviations from the mean indicate the degree to which a person's performance on the test is above or below average. It is helpful to think about these as 'deviations from assumptions of normality' in order to emphasise that the concept of both norm and deviance are constructed either by society and/or the application of statistics (Hammell, 2004, p. 409).

- One standard deviation either side of the mean represents 34.13 per cent of the population (decimal points are often not used and this is represented as 34 per cent of scores, or is given with only one decimal point as 34.1 per cent – see Figure 5.2). So a score falling between minus one or plus one standard deviation from the mean represents a score obtained by 68.26 per cent (or roughly 68 per cent) of the population (Anastasi, 1988).
- The percentage population that falls between one and two standard deviations above the mean is 13.59 per cent, and as the curve is symmetrical the percentage population that falls between one and two standard deviations below the mean is also 13.59 per cent. So scores falling between minus two or plus two standard deviations above the mean represent those of 95.44 per cent of the population (Anastasi, 1988).
- The percentage population that falls between two and three standard deviations above the mean is 2.14 per cent, and as the curve is symmetrical the percentage population that falls between two and three standard deviations below the mean is also 2.14 per cent. So scores falling between minus two or plus three standard deviations above the mean represent those of 99.72 per cent of the population (Anastasi, 1988).

Some tests use standard deviations to provide a cut-off point at which a person's performance is said to be dysfunctional or at which a specific deficit is considered to be present. For example, the RPAB (Whiting *et al.*, 1985) provides a graph that profiles scores in relation to expected levels for people of average intelligence and sets a cut-off level of three standard deviations below the mean to indicate a level below which perceptual deficit is presumed. For many tests of dysfunction, the cut-off point for identifying a deficit falls one standard deviation below the mean.

PERCENTILE VALUES

Percentile values are values of a quantitative variable (for example numerical test scores) that divide the ordered data into groups so that a certain percentage is above and another percentage is below. Quartiles (the 25th, 50th and 75th percentiles) are used to divide the obtained scores into four groups of equal size.

PERCENTILE RANK

The percentage of people in the norm group scoring below a particular raw score is called the percentile rank. It indicates a person's relative position in the group for the ability/characteristic tested. Percentile rank is widely used (for example for infant growth charts) and is quite easily understood. With a percentile rank, the remaining scores are at the same level (equal scores) or are higher/greater scores. For instance, if a physiotherapy student received a score of 95 on a test and this score were greater than or equal to the scores of 88 per cent of the other physiotherapy students taking the test on that course, then the student's percentile rank would be 88 and she would be in the 88th percentile. Percentiles provide a useful way of comparing people and identifying when a person's attributes (such as height, weight and head circumference) or performance is significantly below a level expected for his age and background.

A norm-referenced test, therefore, determines a person's placement on a normal distribution curve. It is used often in education, and students compete against each other on this type of test. This is sometimes referred to as *grading on a curve*. In therapy, it is a test that is used to evaluate the performance of an individual client against the scores of a peer group whose performance has been described using a normative sample. Types of scoring on normative tests can include developmental norms, within-group norms, (standard scores, percentiles) and fixed-reference group norms.

A good example of a norm-referenced test, whose test manual clearly explains the application of the normal curve, is provided by Dunn (2002) in the Infant and Toddler Sensory Profile manual. In Figure 5.3 below, the normal curve is shown and indicates that typical performance of infants from birth to six months is found to fall in the range of −1 standard deviation (s.d.) to +1 s.d. from the mean. Scores falling outside this range are either more or less than the majority of other infants of this age, and the therapist is recommended to follow up these babies. As the Infant and Toddler Sensory Profile assesses responsiveness to sensory stimuli, scores representing both under-responsiveness and over-responsiveness are of concern to a therapist. In many other normative assessments, the therapist would focus on scores below the mean that equated to a dysfunction and would not concern herself with people who showed a greater-than-average ability on the test:

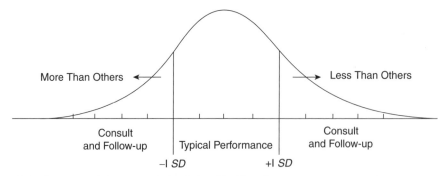

Figure 5.3 The Normal Curve and the Infant/Toddler Sensory Profile Classification System for children aged birth to six months. *Infant/Toddler Sensory Profile. Copyright © 2002 by Harcourt Assessment, Inc. Reproduced with permission. All rights reserved.*

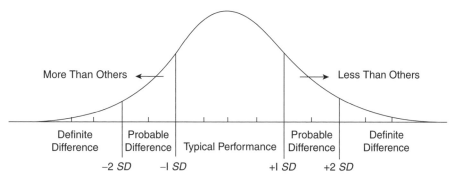

Figure 5.4 The Normal Curve and the Infant/Toddler Sensory Profile Classification System for children aged seven to 36 months. *Infant/Toddler Sensory Profile. Copyright © 2002 by Harcourt Assessment, Inc. Reproduced with permission. All rights reserved.*

Figure 5.4 shows how the normal curve is used to identify children exhibiting typical performance for their age from children with a probable difference (whose scores fall within the 1 to 2 s.d. range) and a definite difference (whose scores fall + or −2 s.d. from the mean).

The standard against which a person is assessed should be what typically is seen for a person of the same age, and the process through which the person accomplishes the assessment task must be evaluated against the process for that age and cultural background. It is, therefore, critical for therapists to understand normal human development, from birth to old age, and to understand the impact of cultural and environmental factors upon performance. In order to be sure that the data from the normative sample can be generalised to their clients, therapists should review the representativeness and sample sizes of the normative data upon which assessments have been standardised. To do this, the therapist must consider the characteristics of her clients (such as age, sex, education, sociocultural background) and compare these to the characteristics of the normative sample. The importance of these factors will vary depending on the construct measured. The therapist should consider which characteristics are likely to be relevant to the skills or constructs that the test is designed to measure (de Clive-Lowe, 1996). For example, with a paediatric developmental assessment a child's age will have a profound effect on the motor, language, cognitive and perceptual skills that a therapist would expect a child to have mastered. With an older client group assessed on an instrumental activities of daily living (IADL) scale, the sex and sociocultural background of the client and normative sample might have an effect on people's prior experience and performance of specific IADL items, for example an older woman might not have dealt with the family's finances and an older man might not have dealt with laundry.

Norms are not 'universal truths' but are based upon 'cultural judgements' (Hammell, 2004, p. 409). Therefore, norms in any society can be fluid and may change in response to changes in other aspects of society, such as value systems. Therefore, depending on the construct being tested, some normative data should be updated at regular intervals.

TRAINING AND INTERPRETING STANDARDISED TEST SCORES

It is important to check whether the therapist administering the test has the appropriate knowledge and skill to administer, score and interpret the results of the test correctly. Most published tests require that the person administering the test has obtained certain qualifications and expertise. Some tests require that the test administrator has undertaken specific training on the administration and scoring of the test (de Clive-Lowe, 1996). For example, to be calibrated to administer the Assessment of Motor and Process Skills (AMPS; Fisher, 2003a), therapists have to attend a one-week training course.

Most standardised assessments provide raw or standard scores. These scores are not sufficient alone and must be interpreted within the wider context of the specific testing situation and influences of the test environment and the client's current situation and personal idiosyncrasies (de Clive-Lowe, 1996). For more information on interpreting test scores see Chapter 8.

PSYCHOMETRIC PROPERTIES

Therapists often want to use test scores to draw inferences about the person's functioning in situations that are beyond the scope of the assessment session. For example, a therapist might need to use the person's test scores on a mobility assessment to predict his mobility in the community. In order to do this, the therapist must be able to justify any inferences drawn by having a coherent rationale for using the test score in this way. Therapists also need clear reasons for selecting a particular test instead of other available assessments. An essential part of such justification involves an understanding of the validity and reliability of test scores (Crocker and Algina, 1986). It is particularly important that students and clinicians establish whether a measure has acceptable levels of validity and reliability, and so these two areas are covered in some depth in Chapter 6 and Chapter 7.

When reviewing potential assessments for practice, therapists should examine the original work on the development of the measure and consider the following aspects: standardisation, validity, reliability and, if it is to be used as an outcome measure, sensitivity to the desired outcome (Jeffrey, 1993). Some assessments have been used and evaluated by other authors, and additional useful information may be found in journal articles that describe further exploration of the psychometric properties of a measure or its use with other client populations or cultures; for example, Sewell and Singh (2001) conducted a study in England to evaluate the reliability of the Canadian Occupational Performance Measure (COPM; Law *et al.*, 1991) with clients with chronic obstructive pulmonary disease. Chapter 11 provides further advice on test critique and on how to locate and select appropriate standardised tests for therapy service.

WORKSHEETS

At the back of this book, you will find templates for a series of worksheets designed to assist you in applying principles of assessment and outcome measurement to your own practice. Please now turn to Worksheet 5 (p. 400). The worksheet takes you through a series of questions to help you establish whether a test has been standardised. Identify at least one standardised criterion-referenced test and one norm-referenced test suitable for use with your caseload. If you are a student therapist, identify an example of each type of test for a client group you are working with on placement. Use a separate copy of Worksheet 5 to examine each of your selected tests. Examine all the test materials available to you and try to answer as many of the questions as possible.

If you wish to undertake a detailed evaluation of the strengths and limitations of the tests you have selected, use Worksheet 12 (pp. 414–7). For assistance completing Worksheet 12, turn to Chapter 11 and find the section headed 'Test critique'. This provides details on how to undertake a test critique. For an example of a completed critique see Table 11.2 (pp. 354–9).

STUDY QUESTIONS

5.1 What makes a test standardised?
5.2 What is a criterion-referenced test?
5.3 What is a norm-referenced test?
5.4 What is standard deviation and how is it used in measurement?

You will find brief answers to these questions at the back of this book (pp. 390–1).

6

Validity and Clinical Utility

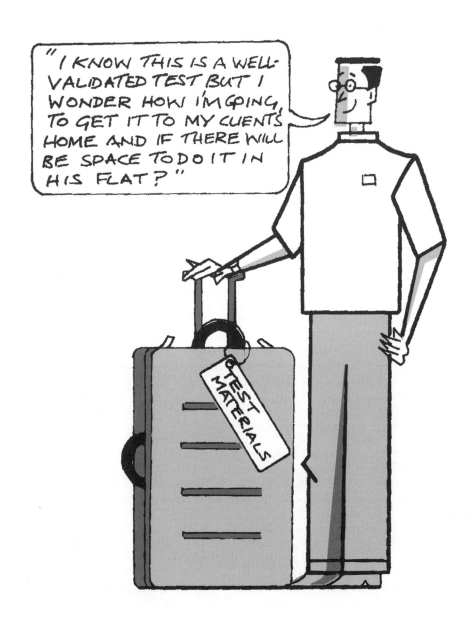

CHAPTER SUMMARY

This chapter will define the main types of validity of relevance to therapists. This will include definitions of content, construct and criterion-related validity as well as descriptions of subtypes of these three main validation studies, such as predictive validity, discriminative validity and concurrent validity. External validity and face validity are also discussed. The chapter ends by considering the concept of clinical utility. It will also endeavour to answer the following questions: 'How do I ensure my measurements are valid?', 'How do I evaluate whether the measures I use are acceptable to my clients?' and 'How do I identify whether an assessment will be clinically useful in my practice setting?'

In order for any measurement to be clinically useful, it should meet two essential requirements. First, it should measure what it intends or is supposed to measure. Second, it should make this measurement with a minimum of error (Pynsent, 2004). The first type of requirement is called validity and is explained in this chapter. The second type of requirement is known as reliability and will be explored in Chapter 7.

DEFINITION OF VALIDITY

A test is considered valid when research demonstrates that it succeeds in measuring what it purports to measure. When a test is developed, the researcher needs to define the domain to be assessed in order to construct relevant test items. This definition of the domain specifies what the test is supposed to measure, but is no guarantee that the resultant test will actually assess this intended domain (Bartram, 1990a). Therapists need to know whether the items contained in a measure, both individually and as a whole, adequately represent the performance domains and/or constructs they are supposed to measure, and whether the assessment items address these domains and/or constructs in the correct proportions (Asher, 1996). Therefore, therapists need some evidence of the test as an indicator of what it was designed to measure. This is known as validity.

Definition of validity

Validity relates to the appropriateness and justifiability of the things supposed about the person's scores on a test and the rationale therapists have for making inferences from such scores to wider areas of functioning (Bartram, 1990a).

Validation is undertaken by a test developer to collect evidence to support the types of inferences that are to be drawn from the results of an assessment (Crocker and Algina, 1986). Bartram (1990a) states that the evidence used to establish validity, and justify inferences made from test scores, ranges from 'appeals to common sense at one extreme to quantifiable empirical evidence at the other' (p. 76). There are several types of validity that therapists should be able to understand in order to critically review test manuals to identify whether psychometric studies have shown the test has appropriate levels of validity. Three types of validation studies, known as content, construct and criterion-related validation, are traditionally performed during test development (Crocker and Algina, 1986). These areas of validation can be further subdivided into specific validity study areas exploring aspects such as predictive validity, discriminative validity, factorial validity and concurrent (also referred to as congruent or convergent) validity. External validity is relevant when we want to generalise findings. Face validity is also considered by some researchers and has a strong link to clinical utility. An examination of validity should be built into a test development process from the outset, and the development of a valid test will involve several, sequential processes undertaken throughout test development. This is particularly true for content and construct validity, whereas criterion-related validity studies are more often conducted towards the end of test development (Anastasi, 1988).

CONTENT VALIDITY

Content validity (also sometimes called content relevance or content coverage) refers to the degree to which an assessment measures what it is supposed to measure judged on the appropriateness of its content.

Definition of content validity

Law (1997) defines content validity as 'the comprehensiveness of an assessment and its inclusion of items that fully represent the attribute being measured' (p. 431).

Content validation examines the components of a test and examines each test item as to its representativeness of the entire sample of potential items representing the domain to be measured. Content validity, therefore, relates to the rigour with which items for a test have been gathered, examined and selected. Content validation is needed when the therapist wants to draw inferences from the test scores about the person's ability on a larger domain of activities similar to those used on the test itself (Crocker and Algina, 1986). For example, if you want to measure balance and have 10 different items related to aspects of balance, you would need to examine each item separately to see if it really did relate to the domain of balance (Lewis and Bottomley, 1994). Content validity relates to the relevance of the person's individual responses to the assessment items, rather than to the apparent relevance of the assessment item content. Asher (1996) notes that content validity is descriptive rather than statistically determined. Because of this, it is sometimes considered a weaker form of validity compared to other types of validity, such as predictive or discriminative validity.

Crocker and Algina (1986) state that a content validation study should as a minimum involve:

- a definition of the performance domain being measured; in achievement tests this is often defined by a list of instructional objectives
- the use of a panel of qualified experts in the content domain
- the development of a structured framework for the process of matching test items to the overall performance domain
- the collection and summarising of data collected by the expert panel when undertaking this matching process.

When matching test items to the performance domain to be measured, experts can either make a dichotomous decision (that is the item either is or is not an aspect of the performance to be assessed) or experts rate the degree of match between the test item and the performance domain (for example using a five-point scale where 5 = an excellent match and 1 = no match).

One issue that should be considered during content validation is whether aspects of the performance domain to be measured should be weighted to reflect their importance. Sometimes all aspects of the performance domain are of equal value. However, in therapy assessments, sometimes some aspects of performance are more critical than others. For example, if undertaking an assessment of the person's functioning to assess readiness for discharge home, the assessment of items related to risk (ability to manage the gas, likelihood of falling or wandering, ability to self-medicate etc.) is more important than other areas that are more easily addressed (for example inability to cook meals can be addressed by the provision of meals on wheels). In a content validation study where weighting importance is required, the researcher needs to provide the panel of experts with a definition of importance and may use a scale to identify the importance of different test items to the critical aspects of the performance domain.

A good example of a content validity study, and one that provides clear details of the methodology followed, is provided by Clemson, Fitzgerald and Heard (1999). They describe a series of studies that contributed to the content validity of the Westmead Home Safety Assessment (WeHSA), a test developed to identify fall hazards in a client's home environment. The first study they undertook to ensure content validity involved a content analysis of literature that studied falls and the home environment. They followed a process outlined by Babbie (1992, cited in Clemson, Fitzgerald and Heard, 1999, p. 173) that outlines four steps for this type of analysis, which are:

1. develop operational definitions of the key variables
2. decide what to include in the analysis
3. classify and record data
4. analyse data.

Their literature search identified 26 relevant studies that were analysed during WeHSA test development. The test developers used their initial version of the WeHSA 'as an organising framework for the content analysis and the types of home environmental hazard reported in each study were tallied' (p. 173). If a new hazard was identified in the literature, this was added. Frequencies for each hazard cited across the 26 studies were calculated and tables summarising this analysis included in the test manual (Clemson, 1997).

The second study completed to evaluate the content validity of the WeHSA involved an expert panel review. They followed a methodology outlined by Popham (1978, cited in Clemson, Fitzgerald and Heard, 1999) to construct test specifications for a criterion-referenced assessment. This involved the writing of a 'descriptive scheme' (p. 173), which provided:

- a general description of the tool's purpose that gives a brief overview of what is being assessed and a description of the purpose of the test
- a list of stimulus attributes to define the assessment's attributes (instrument specifications); this includes all the factors that influence the composition of test items, for example:
  - 'the assessment needs to be in a form manageable on a home visit and able to be completed in a home situation, or soon afterwards.
  - Items must identify features of the environment that may impact on the risk of falling' (p. 178); four features are then listed, such as:
    - 'design and condition of objects (for example, equipment, furniture, footwear' (p. 178).
- specification of eligible content.

The expert review process used for the WeHSA study comprised 'assessment users, developers and beneficiaries, medical and interdisciplinary workers in falls speciality areas and care of older people, and those with expertise in the areas of geriatric home assessment, falls, older people and disability issues and architecture' (p. 174). The expert panel also included some lay people to represent the views of clients and carers. The panel comprised 14 expert reviewers, of which 13 completed stage one, 12 completed stage two and eight responded to the final review. Clemson, Fitzgerald and Heard (1999) used a Delphi panel approach for their review that involved 'anonymous gathering of responses, feedback from respondents and the opportunity to alter responses based on their feedback' (p. 174). For stage one of the content validity study, an open-ended questionnaire was used to record the expert panel's examination of the stimulus attributes, coverage domain and completeness.

For stage two of the expert review, the panel were asked to rate the degree of relevance of the WeHSA items using a five-point scale of 'relevance-taxonomy' (p. 174), which is made up of:

1. Essential: defined as 'item is essential and must be included in the home assessment for falls risk assessment. It would be a hazard for any elderly person who is at risk of falling.'

2. Important
3. Acceptable
4. Marginally relevant
5. Not relevant: defined as 'This item would never be a hazard for falls.'

The test developers decided to quantify the level of content validity of the WeHSA by calculating the percentage agreement of experts using a content validity index (Waltz and Bausell, 1981, cited in Clemson, Fitzgerald and Heard, 1999). This content validity index (CVI) is calculated by dividing the proportion of items judged by an expert panel to have content validity by the total number of items in a test. They also drew from the work of Lynn (1986, cited in Clemson, Fitzgerald and Heard, 1999) and examined the content validity of each item on the test by calculating the proportion of expert judges who rated each item as valid. The article by Clemson, Fitzgerald and Heard provides a clear summary of results for each part of their content validity study. The expert panel were asked to review 250 WeHSA items and 98 per cent of these (n = 245 items) were judged relevant. The test developers used an individual item cut off of CVI > 0.78, which is the level recommended when using a panel of 10 or more judges (Lynn, 1986 cited in Clemson, Fitzgerald and Heard, 1999). Comments from the expert panel also 'led to rewording or subsuming of some items, for example *Lighting* and *Dark/dim* were combined into *Poor illumination*' (p. 176). Clemson, Fitzgerald and Heard cite an overall CVI of 0.80. This represented 'the proportion of items that was rated as having acceptable relevancy or higher by *all* the experts (that is, a CVI = 1.00) was 0.80' (p. 176).

For a detailed review of the definition, importance, conceptual basis and functional nature of content validity, along with quantitative and qualitative methods of content validation, see Haynes, Richard and Kubany (1995).

CONSTRUCT VALIDITY

A construct can be described as an idea or mental representation or conceptual structure that is generated from informed scientific imagination in order to categorise and describe behaviour and assist thinking about the factors underlying observed behaviour (Christiansen and Baum, 1991). It is an abstract quality or phenomenon that is thought to account for behaviour. Construct validation is necessary if the therapist wants to draw inferences from the person's performance on an assessment to performances that can be grouped under the labels of a particular construct (Crocker and Algina, 1986), for example generalising from the score on an item testing an aspect of short-term memory to the overall construct of short-term memory.

Definition of construct validity

Construct validity involves the extent to which an assessment can be said to measure a theoretical construct or constructs.

Construct validity has also been described as relating to 'the ability of an assessment to perform as hypothesized (e.g. individuals discharged to an independent living situation should score higher on a self-care assessment than individuals discharged to a long-term care living situation' (Law, 1997, p. 431). Any assessment that uses observed behaviour as an indicator of functioning related to theoretical constructs about unobservable areas of function should clearly state the underlying assumptions regarding the relationships between observed behaviour and related concepts of function. Fitzpatrick (2004) regards construct validity as a more quantitative form of validity (as compared to content and face validity) and states that, as no single correlation provides sufficient support for construct validity, a test developer or therapist should look for a cumulative pattern of evidence. For example, the construct of disability 'is expected to have a set of quantitative relationships with other constructs such as age, disease status and recent use of healthcare facilities' (p. 55).

Crocker and Algina (1986) describe a four-step process for establishing construct validity:

1. Formulate one or more hypotheses (based on an articulated theory) about how people who will vary on the construct are expected to differ on other variables, such as: observable behaviours measured as performance criteria, demographic characteristics (e.g. age, sex, ethnicity, occupation, level of education) or performance on another measure of the same construct that has already been validated.
2. Select a test that has items covering behaviours that are considered manifestations of the construct.
3. Collect data related to the hypothesised relationship(s) to be tested.
4. Establish whether the data collected supports the hypothesis and determines the extent to which the data could be explained by alternative explanations or theories. If data could be explained by a rival hypothesis, try to eliminate these if possible: this might require more data collection.

An example of a construct validity study is provided by a group of five occupational therapists (Letts *et al.*, 1998) who examined the construct validity of the Safety Assessment of Function and the Environment for Rehabilitation (SAFER Tool). They thought that clients 'who were more independent in completing self-care and instrumental activities would be less likely to have problems related to their ability to function safely in their homes' (p. 128). They also thought that for people 'with cognitive impairments, it would be expected that the number of safety concerns would be greater due to their impaired judgement' (p. 128). For the study, they set a hypothesis that stated: 'lower scores on the SAFER Tool (meaning fewer problems) would be associated with:

1. Subjects who were more independent in activities of daily living (ADL) and instrumental activities of daily living (IADL)
2. Subjects who had mild to no cognitive impairment' (p. 128).

To examine these hypotheses, the therapists administered a battery of tests to a sample of 38 subjects recruited from across five therapy sites in Ontario and British Columbia, Canada. All subjects were 65 years old or older, able to communicate in English and were living in the community. The sample had a mean age of 77.3 years and standard deviation (s.d.) was 6.5 years and comprised 11 men and 27 women. The tests used were:

- the SAFER Tool (Community Occupational Therapists and Associates, 1991)
- the Physical Self-maintenance Scale (PSMS; Lawton and Brody, 1969)
- the Instrumental Activities of Daily Living Scale (IADL Scale; Lawton and Brody, 1969)
- the Standardised Mini-mental State Examination (SMMSE; Molloy, Alemayehu and Roberts, 1991).

For the analysis, three hypotheses were explored and three correlation coefficients (for more information about correlation coefficients see Chapter 7) were calculated to examine these. The researchers set a level of Pearson correlation coefficients of 0.40 or greater as the acceptable level for construct validity and quoted the work of Kramer and Feinstein (1981, cited in Letts *et al.*, 1998) in justifying that 'this value is high enough to demonstrate a medium to large effect size' (p. 129). The first hypothesis looked at the relationship between SAFER Tool and PSMS scores. A negative correlation was expected, in which people with fewer safety problems as measured by the SAFER Tool would be more independent in ADL and higher PSMS scores.

However, the researchers report that 'the correlation was slightly positive and did not meet the criterion of 0.40' (p. 131). In discussing this result, they note that the range of scores on the PSMS for their sample was very small and the samples 'were quite independent in ADL' and wonder whether 'the lack of range of PSMS scores may have contributed to this finding' (p. 131). In terms of the second hypothesis, scores on the SAFER Tool were correlated with the IADL Scale. In this case, the correlation was negative, as hypothesised, and the Pearson correlation coefficient was −0.2471 and did not meet their 0.40 criterion. The final hypothesis was supported by the results with a negative correlation of −0.41 found between SAFER scores and SMMSE scores. While construct validity of the SAFER Tool was partly supported through the demonstration of a relationship between cognitive impairment and safety functioning, further construct validity studies are required to examine the relationship between the SAFER Tool and other measures of ADL and IADL.

FACTORIAL VALIDITY

Asher (1996) reports that 'factorial validity may be considered with construct validity because it can identify the underlying structure and theoretical construct' (p. xxxi).

Definition of factorial validity

Factorial validity relates to the factorial composition of a test. It is the correlation between a test and the identified major factors that determine test scores (Anastasi, 1988).

Test developers use factor analysis to explore this type of validity. Factor analysis was developed to isolate psychological traits and is a statistical technique that is used for analysing the inter-relationships between data that record behaviours. Anastasi (1988) considers it to be 'particularly relevant to construct validation' (p. 154). Through the process of factor analysis, a number of variables (which could be total scores from different tests or items from the same test) that describe some aspect of a person's performance/behaviour are reduced to a smaller number of common traits, which are labelled *factors*. Anastasi states 'a major purpose of factor analysis is to simplify the description of behaviour by reducing the number of categories from an initial multiplicity of test variables to a few common factors, or traits' (p. 155). For example, Baum and Edwards (1993) used factor analysis 'to explore the component structure of the variables' (p. 434) and 'identify common relationships among the variables' (p. 432) in their Kitchen Task Assessment (KTA). The KTA has been developed as a functional measure that assesses the level of cognitive support needed by a client with senile dementia of the Alzheimer's type (SDAT) to undertake a cooking task successfully. The test looks at practical organisation, planning and judgement skills (Baum, 1993). Baum and Edwards (1993) performed an analysis to 'determine the internal structure of the variables and to establish the KTA as a unidimensional instrument' (p. 434) using data from a sample of 106 people diagnosed with SDAT. They report that only one major factor was identified and that this accounted for 84 per cent of the variance. Another example of a factor analysis study, used in test development, is provided by Dunn (2002). During the development of the Infant/Toddler Sensory Profile, the test developers 'conducted several principal components factor analyses to determine whether items clustered meaningfully into independent groupings' (p. 19). The first analysis was undertaken using data from a sample of 150 infants aged from birth to six months who did not have disabilities. Dunn reports that 'the initial factor analysis yielded 6 factors . . . that accounted for 48.19% of the variance (i.e., 40% of the variation among the scores of the children could be accounted for by these factors)' (p. 19). The six factors identified were labelled as: low threshold (self) = 9.29 per cent, low registration = 9.18 per cent, seeking = 9.06 per cent, avoiding/high noticing = 8.37 per cent, low threshold (regulation) = 7.79 per cent and context awareness = 5.11 per cent. In a second study, the researchers undertook principal components factor analyses on a sample of 659 children aged seven to 36 months who did not have disabilities. In this study, the factor analysis yielded 10 factors accounting for 40.5 per cent of the variance. Further analysis 'using a varimax rotation' found 'that a 6 factor solution was the most interpretable' and accounted for 44.3 per cent of the variance (p. 22). Further factor analyses were conducted on samples of children with diagnosed disabilities. Dunn concludes that the results of all the factor analyses appeared to fit with constructs she had described in her Model of Sensory Processing and notes that items on the Infant/Toddler Sensory Profile had not loaded according to related sensory systems but according to their sensory processing characteristic. Each analysis had included 'factors in which items cluster based on thresholds and behavioural responses (i.e. Low Registration and Sensation Seeking, which are the high threshold components of Dunn's Model of Sensory Processing, and Sensory Sensitivity and Sensation Avoiding, which reflect low threshold components)' of Dunn's model (p. 22). She found that, in general, the same constructs had emerged from these factor analyses as had emerged during the development of other versions of the Sensory Profile for adolescents/adults and for children aged three to 10 years.

DISCRIMINATIVE VALIDITY

A discriminative test is a measure that has been developed to 'distinguish between individuals or groups on an underlying dimension when no external criterion or gold standard is available for validating these measures' (Law, 2001, p. 287).

Definition of discriminative validity

Discriminative validity relates to whether a test provides a valid measure to distinguish between individuals or groups.

Discriminative validity is explored when a test is developed to measure a construct in order to distinguish between individuals or groups. For example, a test might be developed to measure the construct of memory in order to discriminate between people with dementia versus people with memory deficits associated with normal ageing processes, or between people exhibiting temporary memory problems associated with depression as opposed to people with permanent memory impairment related to organic problems, such as dementia. Test developers obtain samples of the groups of interest and then compare their scores on test items to see whether the clinical group, for example people with dementia, do in fact obtain scores indicating higher levels of deficit on the construct of interest, such as showing a greater degree of memory deficit, than the group of matched norms. In this type of study, the clinical groups and normative samples should be comparable in terms of significant or potentially significant factors (confounding variables), such as age, sex, educational level and socio-economic background.

An example of a discriminative validity study is provided by DeGangi *et al.* (1995), who examined the discriminative validity of the Infant and Toddler Symptom Checklist by testing samples of infants assessed by other measures as either developing normally or as having regulatory problems. They then computed the mean scores for the norm and clinical groups for each item in their draft version of the checklist. They evaluated mean differences to provide a discrimination index and calculated t-test values to look at level of significance. They reported that only items with a medium (0.5 to 0.8 difference in means) to a large ($>$ 0.8 difference in means) were included in the final version of the Infant and Toddler Symptom Checklist. As a result of their discriminative validity study, they discarded 14 items on the draft test version because they did not significantly discriminate between normally developing infants and infants known to have regulatory disorders.

CRITERION-RELATED VALIDITY

As discussed in Chapter 5, a criterion-referenced test is a test that examines performance against pre-defined criteria and produces raw scores that are intended to have a direct, interpretable meaning (Crocker and Algina, 1986).

Definition of criterion-related validity

Criterion-related validity looks at the effectiveness of a test in predicting an individual's performance in specific activities. This is measured by comparing performance on the test with a criterion, which is a direct and independent measure of what the assessment is designed to predict.

Criterion-related validity 'can best be characterized as the practical validity of a test for a specified purpose' (Anastasi, 1988, p. 151). Criterion-related validation is needed when therapists want to draw an inference from the person's test score to other behaviours of practical relevance (Crocker and Algina, 1986). Both predictive and concurrent measures can be used to determine criterion-related validity. The most frequent analysis used to explore criterion-related validity is the correlation coefficient. Crocker and Algina (1986, p. 224) describe a five-step process for undertaking a criterion-related validation study:

1. 'Identify a suitable criterion behaviour and a method for measuring it.
2. Identify an appropriate sample of examinees representative of those for whom the test will ultimately be used.
3. Administer the test and keep a record of each examinee's score.
4. When the criterion data are available, obtain a measure of performance on the criterion for each examinee.
5. Determine the strength of relationship between test scores and criterion performance.'

CONCURRENT VALIDITY

Concurrent validity studies enable researchers to correlate the test of interest with other test variables. Concurrent validity is also sometimes referred to as congruent or convergent validity or diagnostic utility.

Definition of concurrent validity

Concurrent validity is 'the extent to which the test results agree with other measures of the same or similar traits and behaviours' (Asher, 1996, p. xxx).

Concurrent validation is undertaken by comparing two or more measures that have been designed to measure the same or similar content or constructs. Lewis and Bottomley (1994) give the example of correlating a manual muscle test with mechanical tests, or correlating a balance assessment developed by therapists within their own physiotherapy department with a standardised and accepted balance measure used within the field of physiotherapy. With concurrent validity, the test developer is hoping to find sufficient correlation with an established and recognised measure of the same trait or behaviour to indicate that the same trait/behaviour is being measured by their new test. However, if their new test correlates too highly, and does not have the added advantage of improved clinical utility (for example it is shorter or easier to administer), then it will be perceived as simply reinventing the wheel and having no extra clinical advantage over the already established measure (Anastasi, 1988).

Concurrent validity studies are one of the most frequent types of validity study reported in therapy literature. An example of a concurrent validity study is reported by Wright, Cross and Lamb (1998), who correlated three sets of scores on the Rivermead Mobility Index (RMI) and the Barthel Index (BI) obtained by a physiotherapy client sample. They report that 'scores on the BI and RMI were highly correlated prior to admission, and at admission and discharge (Spearman's rank 0.74, 0.78, 0.87 respectively p < 0.001 for all comparisons)' (p. 219). Another good example of a concurrent validity study is provided by Scudds, Fishbain and Scudds (2003), who examined the concurrent validity of an Electronic Descriptive Pain Scale (EDPS), which they describe as a pain scale built into a transcutaneous electrical nerve stimulation device, compared to three other recognised measures of pain in a sample of 100 physiotherapy outpatient clients. The three concurrent measures selected were a visual analogue scale (VAS), a numerical pain rating scale and the McGill Pain Questionnaire's Present Pain Intensity (MPQ PPI; Melzack, 1987). The authors used Spearman's rank correlation coefficients to test for concurrent validity, and statistics were calculated for the EDPS and the other three measures before and after physiotherapy treatment. Scudds, Fishbain and Scudds (2003) report: 'correlation coefficients ranged from 0.76 to 0.80 before treatment and from 0.84 to 0.88 after treatment' (p. 207). They conclude: 'the EDPS has a reasonably high level of concurrent validity when compared with three scales that are routinely used in clinical practice' (p. 207).

In addition to using a concurrent validity study to show that a new test measures content or constructs as well as or better than some accepted gold standard of measurement, concurrent validity studies can also be used to show that a new test is offering measurement of some distinct content or construct compared to available measures. DeGangi *et al.* (1995) examined the discriminative validity of the Infant and Toddler Symptom Checklist by calculating inter-correlations among Symptom Checklist scores and test scores obtained for samples of 157 normal and 67 regulatory-disordered infants on the Bayley Scales of Infant Development – Mental Scale (Bayley, 1993), the Test of Sensory Functions in Infants (DeGangi and Greenspan, 1989) and the Test of Attention in Infants (DeGangi, 1995). They found that none of the inter-correlations were significant for the regulatory-disordered sample and that only a few correlations were significant for the normal sample. They conclude that the findings 'suggest that, for the most part, the Symptom Checklist provides information that is distinct from that obtained by other diagnostic measures (such as sensory processing, attention), particularly for 10 to 30-month-olds'(p. 44).

PREDICTIVE VALIDITY

A critically important type of criterion-related validity is predictive validity. A predictive test is designed to 'classify individuals into a set of predefined measurement categories, either concurrently or prospectively, to determine whether individuals have been classified correctly' (Law, 2001, p. 287).

Definition of predictive validity

Predictive validity is 'the accuracy with which a measurement predicts some future event, such as mortality' (McDowell and Newell, 1987, p. 329).

Predictive validity refers broadly to the prediction from the test to any criterion performance, or specifically to prediction over a time interval (Anastasi, 1988). Crocker and Algina (1986) define predictive validity as 'the degree to which test scores predict criterion measurements that will be made at some point in the future' (p. 224). Predictive validity is also sometimes referred to as predictive utility (Anastasi, 1988). This is critical to therapists because in clinical practice they often need to make predictions. For example, therapists may need to predict a client's function in a wide range of activities from observation of just a few activities. Therapists frequently have to predict functioning in the future, such as upon discharge. They often need to predict the client's function in a different environment, such as predicting meal preparation ability from a kitchen assessment undertaken in an occupational therapy department to how the client should manage in his own kitchen when discharged home or predicting mobility from a mobility assessment undertaken on a flat, lino surface in a ward or therapy department to how the person should be able to move in a home environment containing a range of flooring including carpet, rugs, laminate and tiles. Therefore, therapists need to be careful that the predictions made from specific test results to other areas of function really are valid. For example, Donnelly (2002) explored whether the Rivermead Perceptual Assessment Battery (RPAB; Whiting *et al.*, 1985) could predict functional performance. The aims of her study were 'to determine if a relationship exists between RPAB and functional performance and to ascertain if the RPAB could predict discharge functional performance' (p. 71). She assessed 46 adults with stroke on the RPAB and a functional measure, the Functional Independence Measure (FIM), over an 18-month period. She found 'little relationship between the RPAB results and functional performance on admission to rehabilitation' and concludes:

> the RPAB results may not be useful to clinicians when attempting to ascertain if the functional problems experienced by some people on admission to rehabilitation are perceptually based. Also, if the prediction of functional outcome is desired, the RPAB may be seen as far too time consuming and therefore not cost-effective when age of the subject can be included into the predictive equation with the same degree of confidence (Donelly, 2002, p. 79).

A useful example of a study that demonstrated good levels of predictive validity is provided by Duncan *et al.* (1992). They examined the predictive validity of the functional reach in identifying elderly people at risk of falls. The functional reach measure is the 'maximal distance one can reach forward beyond arm's length whilst maintaining a fixed base of support in the standing position' (p. M93). A sample of 217 older men living in the community were given baseline screening, including a functional reach test, and were then followed up for six months. One of the challenges of predictive studies is the follow-up of subjects, particularly where the construct of interest cannot be measured directly by the researcher, as in the case of falls. These researchers used a rigorous method for supporting subjects to accurately report falls. Each subject was given six calendars each covering a 30-day period. They were asked to mark any falls on the calendar and were given stamped addressed envelopes to encourage return. The subjects were telephoned once a month by the researcher to ask about any falls and any changes in health or medication. They also gave subjects stamped addressed postcards to post to the researchers as soon as they had a fall, and any person sending in a postcard was contacted straight away for a telephone interview to record the details of the fall, including any injuries sustained. Two members of the research team, who were blinded to all other subject data, then reviewed the falls records and classified the falls as either counting or not counting as a fall for the purpose of this study; if these two researchers did not agree, a third researcher reviewed the falls record. Subjects were then classified as being either fallers or non-fallers at the end of the six months, and any older person who had fallen two or more times was classified as a recurrent faller. The authors undertook a logistic regression and examined the relationship between the history of falls and functional reach baseline data, as well as exploring a number of other variables measured at baseline (including mental state, mood, vision and blood pressure). They report that 'the association between functional reach and recurrent falls was not confounded by age, depression, or cognition' and conclude 'that functional reach is a simple and easy to use clinical measure that has predictive validity in identifying recurrent falls' (p. M93). (*Note:* this paper by Duncan *et al.* (1992) also provides a succinct table comparing the established psychometric properties (inter-observer and test–retest reliability, criterion and construct validity, and sensitivity to change) of 14 measures of balance as part of their literature review.)

Another example of a predictive validity study is found described in the manual for the Infant and Toddler Symptom Checklist (DeGangi *et al.*, 1995), which is used with parents of seven- to 30-month-old babies to predict infants and toddlers 'who are at risk for sensory-integrative disorders, attentional deficits, and emotional and behavioural problems' (p. 1). In a study of 14 infants from paediatric practices in the Washington DC area, 12 subjects were assessed on the Symptom Checklist as falling within the risk range. These 12 infants were then assessed on a number of standardised, observational tests. The authors report that all 12 infants 'demonstrated regulatory problems when tested . . . nine had sensory-processing deficits as determined by the Test of Sensory Functions in Infants (DeGangi and Greenspan, 1989), three had attentional deficits as determined by the Test of Attention in Infants (DeGangi, 1995) and one child had both sensory and attentional problems' (p. 42).

One issue identified by Anastasi (1988) is that of sample size: 'samples available for test validation are generally too small to yield a stable estimate of the correlation between predictor and criterion . . . the obtained coefficients may be too low to reach statistical significance in the sample employed and may thus fail to provide evidence of the test's validity' (p. 152). Therapists, therefore, need to pay particular attention to sample sizes when examining validity data in journal articles or test manuals.

Validity is more than just the matching of what a test actually measures with that which it was designed to measure. Sometimes there can be uncertainty about what a test really measures, yet it may still be a good predictor of an outcome of concern because we have evidence that scores on the test are related to that outcome (Bartram, 1990a). Therefore, if therapists need to make predictions about future performance (for example safety at home alone), the predictive validity of a test could be more important than its content validity.

OTHER TYPES OF VALIDITY

There are some other types of validity of relevance to therapists, but these are less frequently mentioned or addressed in therapy/rehabilitation literature and test manuals. These include ecological and external validity, which are very closely related.

Definition of ecological validity

Ecological validity addresses the relevance of the test content, structure and environment to the population with whom the test is used (Laver, 1994).

External validity is also sometimes referred to as validity generalisation and has been defined as:

Definition of external validity

External validity is 'the extent to which findings can be generalised to other settings in the real world' (Lewis and Bottomley, 1994, p. 602).

Lewis and Bottomley give the following example: 'the results of a study testing muscle strengths on aging rats has external validity to a rat population but lacks external validity in humans' (p. 602). External and ecological validity are relevant to therapists for a few reasons. Individual therapy departments may develop criterion-referenced tests for a specific service; external validity explores the generalisability of test validity to different situations outside of the original service where the test was developed (Anastasi, 1988). For example, Wolf (1997) reports that 'ADL scales often used in rehabilitation are not valid and reliable measures of outcome for clients of community services' (p. 364). Many tests are originally developed as research tools and are administered to research subjects in highly controlled formal testing environments. A client's home environment or the assessment space available in an outpatient department or on a ward may have many more potential distractions. There are pros and cons to both situations. In a highly controlled testing environment removed from the client's home or hospital ward setting, the formality and unfamiliarity of the testing environment could lead to test anxiety, which could affect performance and, hence, the reliability of results. However, the background noises and possible interruptions that occur in home and therapy/ward environments can affect the client's concentration and may, therefore, also negatively affect performance.

ESTABLISHING THE OVERALL VALIDITY OF A TEST

If a test is to be used for a range of purposes, then several types of validity may need to be examined. Anastasi (1988, p. 162) provides an excellent example of how an arithmetic test could be used for four different purposes, each of which would require a different validity study:

1. If the test was to be used as a maths test in a primary school and the purpose was to identify how much a pupil had learnt about maths up to this point, then the validity study required would be a content validity study.
2. If the arithmetic test was being used as an aptitude test to predict which pupils would be good at maths at secondary school and the purpose was to judge how well a pupil might learn maths in future, then criterion-related validity is required and evidence of predictive validity will be needed.
3. If this same arithmetic test is also to be used for diagnosing people with learning disability by identifying specific areas where a person is not performing at maths to a level expected for his age, then again criterion-related validity will be required, but this time concurrent validity and discriminant validity studies will be undertaken.
4. Finally, if the arithmetic test is to be used as a measure of quantitative reasoning and the therapist wishes to assess a person's cognitive processes, then construct-related validity would be required.

As there is no one recognised measure of validity, it is usual for researchers to conduct a range of studies to examine its different aspects (Bartram, 1990a). For example, Baum and Edwards (1993) undertook four analyses to examine aspects of the validity of the KTA:

1. Correlation analysis was used to examine the relationship among the six variables in the measure; correlation coefficients of 0.72–0.84 'suggested that one dimension might exist . . . and that the cognitive domains selected for the KTA all contribute to the measurement of the cognitive performance of the task' (p. 433).
2. As mentioned earlier in this chapter, factor analysis was undertaken to identify common relationships among the variables to determine the internal structure of the variables and to establish the KTA as a uni-dimensional instrument.
3. Correlation analysis was undertaken with other published valid and reliable tests, three neuropsychological and two functional assessments, to determine the construct validity of the KTA. Results indicated that 'the KTA, as a test of practical cognitive skills, is related to the cognitive skills measured by [the other three] neuropsychological tests' (Baum and Edwards, p. 435).
4. The fourth investigation involved an analysis of variance to examine performance of subjects on the KTA compared to stages of SDAT. Results showed that 'the KTA differentiates performance across all stages of the disease' (p. 435).

The developers of the Life Satisfaction Index – Parents (LSI-P; Renwick and Reid, 1992a) have undertaken several studies to examine different aspects of the validity of their test. Studies have been conducted to examine the construct validity, concurrent validity and discriminant validity of the LSI-P (Renwick and Reid, 1992b). The LSI-P was developed through several processes, including: 'literature review, results of an interview study on stress and coping of children with DMD [Duchenne muscular dystrophy]' (Jones, 1988, cited by Renwick and Reid, 1992b) 'and interviews with clinicians treating adolescents with DMD and other chronic disorders and their families' (p. 299). The initial version consisted of 18 items for each of the five domains. These items went through two review processes. First, items were reviewed by three occupational therapy clinical experts. Second, a four-item criterion for review was used by 23 reviewers across five Canadian provinces to examine the content validity of each item. A criterion level of reviewer agreement was set for the inclusion of items in the final version of the test. The discriminant and concurrent validity of the LSI-P were examined with a sample comprising 17 parents of a child with DMD and 39 parents of children without physical disabilities. The LSI-P was administered to both groups of parents in their own homes. Parents also completed a concurrent measure (the Satisfaction with Life Scale and the Questionnaire on Resources and Stress).

FACE VALIDITY

In simple terms, face validity is whether a test *seems* to measure what it is intended to measure (Asher, 1996).

Definition of face validity

Face validity is 'the dimension of a test by which it appears to test what it purports to test' (Christiansen and Baum, 1991, p. 851).

The concepts of content and face validity are similar but should not be confused (Anastasi, 1988). 'The difference is that face validity concerns the acceptability of a test to the test-taker, while content validity concerns the appropriateness of the content of the test as judged by professionals' (Bartram, 1990a, p. 77). For example, if you are a therapy student taking an end-of-module exam on assessment and you believe that the exam questions are about assessment and are measuring your understanding of therapy assessment, then that exam has face validity. Lewis and Bottomley (1994) provide the following example: 'If you are looking for the components of gait and you are doing a gait analysis on the face of it, you are measuring gait' (p. 602).

All definitions of face validity agree that the test should be acceptable to the test-taker (client). However, within the literature, definitions of face validity vary in terms of who else the test should appear to be acceptable to. For example, Bartram (1990a) defines face validity as solely the 'degree to which the test-taker sees a test as being reasonable and appropriate' (p. 76). However, Crocker and Algina (1986) broaden this definition to include 'laypersons or typical examiners' (p. 223). While Anastasi (1988) perceives face validity as pertaining to 'whether the test "looks valid" to the examinees that take it, the administrative personnel who decide on its use, and other technically untrained observers' (p. 144). Lewis and Bottomley (1994) state 'face validity is usually measured through professional judgement as to whether or not it is face valid' (p. 602). Therapists need to consider the scope of their service when deciding on the best definition of face validity for their own purpose.

Face validity is not validity in a technical sense and so it has little direct psychometric importance. However, its evaluation is significant for occupational therapists and physiotherapists because if therapists are to be client-centred in their practice then the client's perception of any assessment as being relevant and meaningful is critical. Therapist authors have criticised the use of tests based on items that have little meaning and relevance for the test-taker. For example,

Law (1993) notes that 'the client's perspectives, values and efforts are not considered'. She also found that assessments 'tend to score performance and emphasize quantity rather than quality of function', that 'few instruments consider client satisfaction' and that 'with most evaluations clients' culture, roles, developmental stages and the environment in which they live are not considered' (p. 235). In a study of ADL and IADL used by community-based occupational therapists working with people who had physical disabilities, Wolf (1997) concludes: 'respondents in this study thought that published ADL scales did not generally reflect their own priorities or those of their service users' (p. 363).

Bartram (1990a) has presented several arguments for ensuring good face validity. First, good face validity can have indirect effects on the outcome of a person's performance 'by facilitating rapport between the test and the test-taker which may, in turn, increase reliability' (p. 76). Secondly, engaging a person's motivation to engage in an assessment to the best of his ability is critical to obtaining valid and reliable test results and 'people are more likely to take seriously activities which seem reasonable and which they feel they understand'(p. 76).

Face validity is particularly important when a test developed for one population is used with a different client group. For example, many neuropsychological tests were originally developed for child populations. Some of these tests were later standardised for an older adult population; however, the content of the tests often remained unchanged. Thus, the test content was not necessarily meaningful and relevant for older adults who might perceive test materials as childish and demeaning. A person's perception of the relevance of test materials affects his motivation to undertake the test and, therefore, affects the reliability of test results. If the tasks selected as the basis of a neuropsychological test do not relate to the tasks the person would be undertaking in everyday life, then the client may not understand the relevance of a test to his own life and situation. For example, an older adult will rarely need to construct a three-dimensional block design from a diagram or model, or be required to copy geometric shapes as part of his everyday activities. The more contrived a test content is from the everyday activities of the person being tested, the more important it is to consider face validity. Therapists should always explain the purpose of an assessment procedure to the client prior to testing, but this is especially important where face validity is not strong.

When reviewing potential tests, therapists may have to conduct their own face validity studies because there is a 'paucity of available research on face validity, despite its probable contribution to prevalent attitudes towards tests' (Anastasi, 1988, p. 145). Face validity studies are critical to client-centred practice and clients and their carers must be engaged to 'play an active and integral part in the validation process' if measures are 'to be truly valid' (Wolf, 1997, p. 364). An example of a face validity study is provided by Laver (1994), who demonstrated that the Structured Observational Test of Function (SOTOF; Laver and Powell, 1995) had high levels of face validity with a sample of 40 clients with stroke. Following the administration of SOTOF, people were given a structured interview that comprised both open and closed questions. For example, clients were asked:

- 'What did you think this assessment was for?'
- 'Were these tasks something you would normally do?'
- 'Did you mind being asked to do these tasks?'
- 'What did you think of the assessment?'

Clients were also given questions related to their experience of being tested:

- 'Did you find the assessment . . . easy, upsetting, enjoyable, difficult, boring, stressful, useful, interesting, relaxing, irrelevant?'

This question format presented the possibility of a negative testing experience and enabled subjects to give an affirmative answer to a negative concept; this is particularly important when conducting research with older populations, who tend to be acquiescent, polite and affirmative in their responses. When seeking feedback from clients on their experience of a test or conducting a face validity study, it is preferable to have the client interviewed by a different therapist than the one who undertook the assessment as some clients find it more difficult to provide negative feedback to the person who has given the test.

CLINICAL UTILITY

Just because a test is well standardised, valid and reliable does not mean it automatically will be useful in the clinical environment. Many an expensive test gathers dust in occupational therapy and physiotherapy departments for practical reasons, such as the therapists discovering after purchase that it was too lengthy to administer or too cumbersome to move around. Therefore, it is critical to consider the clinical utility of potential assessments for your service to ensure that the selected assessment can be easily and economically administered (Jeffrey, 1993).

Definition of clinical utility

Clinical utility is 'the overall usefulness of an assessment in a clinical situation' (Law, 1997, p. 431) and covers aspects of a test such as reasonable cost, acceptability, training requirements, administration time, interpretation of scores, portability and ease of use (Jones, 1991; Law, 1997; Law and Letts, 1989).

COST

When estimating the overall cost of a test for your service, there are a number of factors to consider. The most obvious cost is the initial financial outlay required to purchase the test (this might comprise a manual, forms, test materials etc.). The cost of standardised tests varies considerably; some brief tests are published in professional journals and are freely available; others can be purchased cheaply, but some are very expensive. You will need to justify to the budget holder that the financial outlay will bring sufficient benefit to your service. In addition, you may need to purchase some of the equipment required for test administration if this is not provided with the test. This is more common with tests described in journal articles where the equipment required is described. The expertise required of the rater is another cost factor. Some tests specify that the rater has to have specific qualifications or levels of experience, which may mean that only qualified staff or more senior staff can use the test, or may require that all test administrators undertake a training course. Training courses can be a major financial outlay. Training courses for specific tests can vary in both length and cost and may involve a one-day training session, a part-time course or a week-long residential course. In addition, some tests require administrators to undertake follow-up training to stay up to date or to be recalibrated as raters. Therapists should also estimate the ongoing costs for any supplies that need to be replaced for each assessment, for example food for a kitchen assessment, paper or scoring forms. Some tests have copyrighted scoring forms and you should estimate the cost of replacement test forms if copyright does not allow these to be photocopied.

TIME

The most obvious time factor to consider is the time required to administer the test. Some standardised assessments comprise lengthy test batteries. These testing procedures can be tiring for people. Poor stamina can affect test performance and the reliability of test results. A good test manual will indicate the range of time taken by subjects undertaking the test and/or recommend the length of time you should make available for testing. In addition, you need to allow for the time required to prepare for test administration each time, such as the time needed for setting up the test environment and materials or for purchasing supplies (for example food for a meal preparation assessment). The time required to score the test, interpret results and write up any reports also needs to be estimated. Another time factor, which can be overlooked when considering clinical utility, is the initial time required to learn to administer the test; this might be through attendance on a training course or be undertaken individually by reading the test manual and practising test administration, for example through role play with colleagues.

Some tests incorporate timings into the scoring of test items, but this does not always add to the clinical usefulness of the measure. For example, McAvoy (1991) states that 'activities that are timed, as in the Northwick Park Index, are of little value when safety or control or quality of movement are the key issues, but these qualities are not included in any of the standardised forms' (p. 385).

ENERGY AND EFFORT

The ease with which the therapist can learn to administer the test and the ease of each test administration will influence how much a test is used in a therapy service. Some tests seem complex initially and administration is hard to get to grips with, but most tests become easier to administer with practice, so that an expert administrator can undertake the test without undue effort. Some physical assessments, where a client may require a lot of assistance with mobility and transfers, can place a high physical demand on the therapists administering the test.

PORTABILITY

Therapists need to decide in advance the settings in which a test is to be used as some tests are heavy and/or bulky. If testing is always to occur in a therapy department, then a test with lots of heavy equipment may be appropriate. However, if therapists will need to use the test in several different environments (for example on the ward, in a day hospital or in the person's home, school or work setting), then portability becomes critical. You need to consider how easy it will be to move the test between potential testing environments. If the test has lots of components and does not come with its own case, you may need to purchase some kind of bag or case for carrying. The health and safety of staff must be ensured; so, if the test is very heavy, it may be worth purchasing a trolley for pulling/pushing it between test environments. For example, the Chessington Occupational Therapy Neurological Assessment Battery (COTNAB; Tyerman *et al.*, 1986) comes in a large wooden box on castors and when packed with all the required test equipment is very heavy. Therapists tend to administer the COTNAB in their therapy depart-ment or outpatient clinic environment, as it is very difficult to transport it between hospital wards or in the community between clients' homes.

ACCEPTABILITY

The concept of acceptability overlaps that of face validity. Therapists should consider whether the assessment fits with the philosophy, theoretical frameworks and practice used within the therapy service or by a particular clinician. Whether the test looks professional is another aspect of acceptability. You also need to identify whether the test will be acceptable to the client: will the person see the relevance of the test and is the test likely to cause stress and test anxiety? When judging a test's acceptability, you should also consider how acceptable it will be to manag-ers, service purchasers and lay observers, such as the person's family.

An example of a clinical utility study is provided by Laver (1994), who demonstrated that the SOTOF (Laver and Powell, 1995) had good clinical utility with a sample of people with a primary diagnosis of stroke. A letter requesting volunteers for the study was placed in the *British Journal of Occupational Therapists* (*BJOT*). Therapists were sent a covering letter, a copy of the SOTOF manual and test forms, a questionnaire for the therapist to complete related to clinical utility and content validity, a structured interview for the therapist to give to clients to look at face validity and a stamped addressed return envelope. Sixty-six therapists responded to the *BJOT* letter and a further 38 were recruited through meetings and lectures where the test developer was presenting work on the development of the SOTOF. Forty-four out of the 104 therapist sample completed the study, giving a response rate of 42.3 per cent; this is in line with expected response rates for postal surveys, which Bennett and Ritchie (1975) give as 40 to 60 per cent.

Therapists used the SOTOF with at least two clients and then completed a postal question-naire that covered a wide range of clinical utility issues, including ease of use, materials, time required and appropriateness for their clients. The therapist samples included staff of all grades, ranging from a basic grade through to a head I therapist, and they were working across a number of different clinical areas, including neurology, gerontology, medical, outpatients, rehabilitation unit, surgery and orthopaedics, and medicine and surgery. Most of the clinical utility question-naire items used a five-point rating scale, for example for the 'ease of use' section therapists were asked to rate four questions:

1. 'Were the SOTOF instructions easy to understand?'
2. 'Were the SOTOF instructions easy to follow?'
3. 'Were the SOTOF protocols easy to follow?'
4. 'Were the SOTOF forms easy to fill in?'

Using the same five-point scale:

- impossible
- difficult
- fair
- easy
- very easy

Laver (1994) reports that:

- 54.5 per cent of therapists rated the SOTOF as fair and 34.1 per cent as easy to under-stand
- 52.3 per cent rated the SOTOF instructions as fair and 38.6 per cent as easy to follow
- 52.3 per cent rated the SOTOF protocols as fair and 34.1 per cent as easy to follow
- 34.1 per cent rated the SOTOF forms as fair, 50 per cent as easy and 2.3 per cent as very easy to fill in.

A dichotomous yes/no scoring system was used to examine the clinical utility of materials re-quired for the SOTOF (Laver, 1994), with questions related to the nature of the materials used (Table 6.1).

Table 6.1 Dichotomous scoring system for the SOTOF

Question	Yes, %	No, %
Easy to obtain?	72.7	22.7
Appropriate for the client?	86.4	6.8
Easy to carry?	86.4	4.5
Easy to clean?	90.9	2.3
Easy to store?	88.6	2.3

Therapists were asked to record the length of time taken to administer the SOTOF. Laver (1994) reports that the majority of therapists took an hour or less to administer the SOTOF, with therapist times ranging from 30 minutes to two hours 15 minutes, and with only four therapists taking over an hour to complete the test.

EXAMINING VALIDITY AND CLINICAL UTILITY ISSUES: TEST EXAMPLES

In this section, a few therapy assessments are evaluated in terms of their validity and/or clinical utility as examples of the factors that therapists should consider when reviewing potential tests for their clinical practice.

THE MAYERS' LIFESTYLE QUESTIONNAIRE (2)

Mayers has undertaken studies to examine aspects of the clinical utility, face validity and content validity of the original Mayers' Lifestyle Questionnaire and contact letter (1998) and an adapted version for use in mental health services (2003). In the first study, a questionnaire format was used to gather feedback. A sample of 92 occupational therapists were sent copies of the tool and asked to give it to three clients each, giving a potential sample of 288 clients. Data were returned by 45 therapists (48.9 per cent) and for 132 (45.8 per cent) clients. Mayers (1998) summarises key issues in three tables divided into: comments from therapists on the usefulness of the contact letter, comments from therapists on the usefulness of the Lifestyle Questionnaire and responses from clients. In terms of face validity, she reports that 68 of the 132 (51.5 per cent) clients made comments indicating that the tool had been 'easy to complete/understand'. In terms of clinical utility, she reports that:

> Twenty-five (55.6%) occupational therapists stated that the Lifestyle Questionnaire was useful and relevant as he or she discussed occupational therapy with clients; 10 (22.2%) said it was not useful. There was no response from the remaining 10 (22.2%). (p. 394)

In the second study, an adapted Delphi technique involving a disability action group, comprising six members, was used. For the first phase, each group member was sent questions to consider (see Box 6.1) and a copy of the contact letter and Lifestyle Questionnaire to read and complete. For the second stage, group members met and each person presented his or her ideas in turn. In the final stage, the group discussed the issues raised and priorities were identified and ranked. Both individual written reflections from the first stage and group discussions were analysed.

Box 6.1 Mayers' Lifestyle Questionnaire and contact letter face validity study: questions used in the Delphi approach with a disability action group sample (Mayers, 1998, p. 397)

- What was your initial reaction when you read the contact letter and Lifestyle Questionnaire?

- Do you think that a client would have a clearer idea of the role of the community occupational therapist after reading the contact letter?

- Do you think you would have any problems with the wording and with completing the Lifestyle Questionnaire (it may help you to answer this question by completing it yourself)?

- Do you think that having the opportunity to prioritise your needs beforehand would prepare you better for the community occupational therapist's first visit?

In the discussion, Mayers (1998) reflects on the results of the two studies and notes changes that were made to the tool as a result of feedback from therapists, clients and the disability action group. She concludes that the 'Lifestyle Questionnaire gives the client the opportunity to state his or her individual need(s) and to prioritise these' (p. 397).

Mayers reports that the original version of the Mayers' Lifestyle Questionnaire (1998) was found to be suitable for people with problems caused by physical disability. Following requests from community occupational therapists working with clients with enduring mental health problems, the tool was modified and the application of the adapted version, Mayers' Lifestyle Questionnaire (2), was examined (Mayers, 2003). As part of this study Mayers examined aspects of clinical utility, content validity and face validity. Out of a volunteer sample of 83 therapists who received copies of the tool, 33 returned clinical utility and content validity data; in addition, these therapists submitted face validity feedback from a total sample of 75 clients who had completed the Lifestyle Questionnaire. Data were collected via therapist and client questionnaires. Questions for therapists are provided in Box 6.2. Questions for clients are provided in Box 6.3.

Box 6.2 Mayers' Lifestyle Questionnaire (2) study: clinical utility and content validity questions for therapists (Mayers, 2003, pp. 390–391)

Clinical utility
The purpose of the Lifestyle Questionnaire is for clients to identify, record and prioritise their needs before you commence intervention.

- Has this been useful to you?
- If yes, please state how and why.
- If no, please give reasons.

Clinical utility
Do you think the Lifestyle Questionnaire will be helpful for the majority of your clients?

- Yes/No.
- If no, please give reasons.

Content validity
Having used the Lifestyle Questionnaire, please state any important area(s) or topics(s) that you think have been omitted.

Box 6.3 Mayers' Lifestyle Questionnaire (2) study: face validity questions for clients' feedback (Mayers, 2003, pp. 390–391)

Each therapist was asked to record feedback on the following three questions from three clients who had completed the Lifestyle Questionnaire.

Did the wording of the Lifestyle Questionnaire include all areas that affect your quality of life and are important to you?

- Yes/No.
- If no, please indicate any area that has been omitted.

Please state any problems that you had in completing the Lifestyle Questionnaire.

Mayers (2003) reports that 28 (84.8 per cent) of therapists reported that the Lifestyle Questionnaire had been useful and 23 (69.7 per cent) had indicated that the tool would be helpful for the majority of their clients. In her paper, she provides summary tables of comments related to these questions. In terms of reasons why the tool might not be useful, only one factor was identified by more than one therapist; this related to the length of the questionnaire being quite long for people with poor concentration. Mayers also summarises the important areas or topics therapists identified as omitted in the content validity question. Of these, only two areas were identified by more than one therapist, eight (24.2 per cent) suggested the inclusion of a 'comment box after the final column' and two suggested an item on 'coping with physical/mental health problems'.

In terms of face validity, Mayers (2003) reports that 67 (89.3 per cent) of the clients who completed the questionnaire said that it included all areas that were important to them and that affected their quality of life. In addition, clients had been asked to use asterisks (*) to mark those items on the questionnaire that indicated their top priorities, and 51 (68 per cent) of the sample did this. Mayers lists the 14 top priorities provided by clients in a table and notes that these are similar to areas identified by a number of authors in her literature review. Following analysis, Mayers made some changes to the wording of a number of items. As each item had been prioritised by at least one client, all the original items were included in the final version. Overall, the study supported the clinical utility, content validity and face validity of the measure. Mayers notes that a larger sample would have been desirable and has continued to send out evaluation forms when copies of the test are requested.

RIVERMEAD PERCEPTUAL ASSESSMENT BATTERY (RPAB)

The RPAB (Whiting *et al.*, 1985) was designed to assess deficits in visual perception following a stroke or head injury. Normative data enable the therapist to evaluate whether a person has difficulty with visual-perception tasks greater than that expected prior to brain damage. The aspects of visual perception addressed by the battery can be summarised under eight headings: form constancy, colour constancy, sequencing, object completion, figure/ground discrimination, body image, inattention and spatial awareness. The test comprises 16 short subtests. Fifteen of these tests are timed activities administered at a table on a layout guide and comprise activities such as picture cards, block designs, jigsaws and drawing. The RPAB has been found to lack ecological validity (Laver, 1994). The test environment is very structured and formal and the activities used lack everyday meaning as they are not drawn from clients' normal repertoire of tasks. Age appropriateness was also considered a weakness. Some of the tasks, such as the object matching subtest that includes toy cars, were perceived as childish by some clients (Laver, 1990). Another issue involves the timing of the written and drawn subtests. Many people with stroke experience hemiparesis to an upper limb; in some cases this affects a previously dominant hand. In these circumstances, the client has to perform the subtests using a non-dominant hand to hold the pen. As assessment usually occurs as soon as possible after diagnosis, and precedes intervention, the client rarely has had an opportunity to practise writing with the non-dominant hand prior to testing. Therefore, many people were found to fail these tests as a consequence of the length of time taken rather than actual ability (Crammond, Clark and Smith, 1989). Further limitations include the difficulty of administering the test to clients with severe cognitive impairment (short-term memory, attention and concentration are required) or aphasia. The formality of the test administration procedures increases test anxiety and can have a detrimental effect on performance. Many older clients have visual and auditory acuity loss as a result of primary ageing. The RPAB protocol does not permit the repetition of instructions or the use of additional verbal and visual cues; some clients fail subtests as they do not comprehend the instructions. The colour matching task has been criticised (Laver, 1990). There is poor differentiation between the colours of some items on the tasks. For example, RPAB involves the differentiation of several pieces in blue and green shades but, as a person's colour vision alters with age owing to yellowing of the lens, older clients may find the perception of the blue/green end of the spectrum difficult. Many older clients failed this subtest but could name and point to colours on command. The task requires more complex functioning than the simple identification of colour.

THE MIDDLESEX ELDERLY ASSESSMENT OF MENTAL STATE (MEAMS)

The MEAMS (Golding, 1989) was developed as a screening test to identify gross impairment of cognitive skills (Golding, 1989). MEAMS includes 12 subtests that assess orientation, comprehension, verbal language skills, short-term memory, arithmetic, visual perception and motor perseveration. This is a useful screening test, which is quick and easy to administer and relatively well accepted by clients (Laver, 1994). However, the line drawings used for the remembering pictures subtest are problematic as they are very small and do not account for decreased visual acuity, which is a common deficit occurring as a result of primary ageing. Some subtests, such as the name learning, are age-appropriate; photographs of older people are used for this test and the ability to remember names is a relevant skill. Other subtests, such as the tapping task used to assess motor perseveration, are contrived and lack relevance to everyday activity.

CLIFTON ASSESSMENT PROCEDURES FOR THE ELDERLY (CAPE)

The CAPE was developed by Pattie and Gilleard (1979). Reviews of the research potential and clinical utility of CAPE have been undertaken by Bender (1990) and Pattie (1988). The CAPE is designed to evaluate cognitive and behavioural functioning. The test consists of two parts: the Cognitive Assessment Scale (CAS) and the Behavioural Rating Scale (BRS). These two scales can be used separately or together. The CAS comprises three sections: (1) an information/orientation subtest, an interview covering 12 questions pertaining to orientation of time, place and person and three questions on current information, (2) a mental ability test involving counting, reading, writing and reciting the alphabet, (3) a psychomotor task requiring the completion of the 'Gibson Spiral Maze' to assess fine-motor performance and hand–eye coordination. The BRS is administered as a survey to the primary carer (for example nurse or relative) of the client. Questions on this scale relate to four main areas: physical disability, apathy, communication difficulties and social disturbance.

The limiting aspect of the CAPE is the psychomotor subtest. Pattie (1988) acknowledges that 'at a practical level some users have questioned the usefulness of the Gibson Spiral Maze' (p. 72), while Bender (1990) refers to the maze as 'the least successful element of the CAS' and reports that 'many clinicians manage without it' (p. 108). The maze is not drawn from the usual repertoire of activities carried out in everyday life by older people, and it lacks ecological validity. The score from the maze indicates level of impairment and does not identify causes for dysfunction. Fine-motor performance and hand–eye coordination are complex skills based on the interaction of motor, sensory, cognitive and perceptual functions. A complex range of deficits, including comprehension, apraxia, loss of visual acuity and restricted range of movement, could affect performance on this test. Clinicians, therefore, need to observe the performance of the test informally to identify cues pertaining to performance-component dysfunction. Further assessment is required to evaluate the specific type of neuropsychological dysfunction.

The CAPE writing task has greater ecological validity than the maze, as clients need to be able to sign their name for financial independence. However, the task indicates the ability/inability to perform the task. The dysfunction could arise from a range of deficits and requires further investigation. The information/orientation questions do not indicate the effects of cognitive impairment on occupational performance, and some people find it demeaning to be asked such questions. The BRS is based on report rather than therapist observation, thus the reliability of the results is dependent on the observational skills and memory of the proxy respondent selected. Pattie (1988) admits that administrators of the CAPE have disputed the factor structure of the BRS and also queried the CAPE grading system.

APPLYING CONCEPTS OF VALIDITY TO YOUR OWN PRACTICE

At the back of this book, you will find templates for a series of worksheets designed to assist you in applying principles of assessment and outcome measurement to your own practice. Please now turn to Worksheet 6 (pp. 401–488).

For this reflection, you will need to select a published assessment. This could be a test that you are already using in your clinical practice. Often, therapists inherit assessments when they start work in a different clinical setting or department; this will be a particularly useful exercise if you are using a test that was already available in your department and which you have not critiqued. You might select a test that you are considering purchasing/using in the future. If you are a student, select a test you have seen used on clinical placement or one available at your university or college. Look to see what information (test manual, journal articles, handouts from training courses etc.) is available on your chosen test. If there is very little, which can be the case when you have inherited an assessment, you might need to conduct a literature search in order to complete the worksheet.

The worksheet takes you through a series of questions about different types of validity and prompts you to record key evidence and to form opinions about whether the published evidence indicates adequate levels of validity for your clinical needs.

STUDY QUESTIONS

6.1 Describe one method to examine the content validity of a test.
6.2 Define *construct validity*.
6.3 List one type of criterion-related validity and describe a method for evaluating this type of criterion-related validity.
6.4 What is predictive validity and why is it important to therapists?
6.5 What is face validity and why should therapists consider it?
6.6 What factors would you examine if you wanted to evaluate a test's clinical utility?

You will find brief answers to these questions at the back of this book (pp. 391–2).

7

Reliability

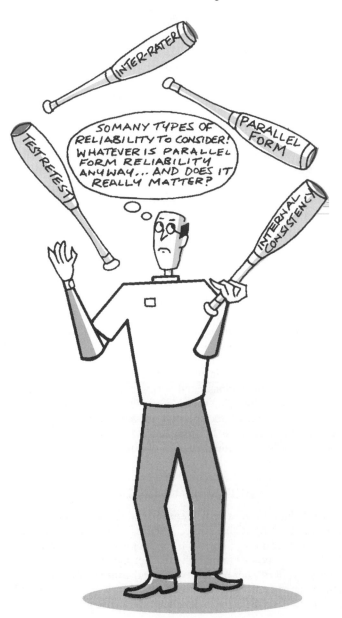

CHAPTER SUMMARY

This chapter will define the main types of reliability of relevance to therapists (test–retest reliability, inter-rater reliability, intra-rater reliability, internal consistency and parallel form reliability) and consider how these are evaluated and what levels of reliability are considered acceptable for clinical practice. The chapter will also explore the concepts of rater severity, sensitivity, specificity and responsiveness. Finally, standard error of measurement and floor and ceiling effects will be described. It will also endeavour to answer the following questions: 'How do I ensure my measurements are reliable?' and 'How can I ensure my outcome measures are responsive to a clinically relevant degree of change?'

INTRODUCING THE CONCEPT OF RELIABILITY

It is critical for occupational therapists and physiotherapists to consider the reliability of an assessment. Frequently, therapists will wish to evaluate the effectiveness of a treatment programme, by retesting a client on an assessment administered prior to treatment to establish whether desired changes in function have occurred. It is, therefore, important that changes in a person's performance on the test are not affected by the time interval or by the rater. The degree of established reliability informs the therapist how accurately the scores obtained from an assessment reflect the true performance of a person on the test (Opacich, 1991). When a therapist uses a test with evidence of high levels of reliability obtained through a robust reliability study design, she can be confident that the scores obtained on the test will reflect her client's true performance.

If an assessment was totally reliable, a therapist could obtain the same result each time she used that assessment under exactly the same conditions. In reality, the results obtained from the vast majority of assessments will differ across administrations owing to error. Pynsent (2004, p. 4) describes measurement as an equation in which:

$$[Measurement = \text{true value} + \text{error}]$$

Reliability data are used to provide an index of the amount of measurement error in a test. The aspects of people evaluated by therapists are open to many variables that may act as so-called sources of error during an assessment. Pynsent (2004) lists four main sources of error: 'error from the rater, from the instrument itself, random error and error from the patient' (p. 4). Errors can occur because of the way the therapist administers, scores and interprets the results of a test. Errors can also occur because of fluctuating or temporary behaviour in the person being tested. For example, the client may guess the answer or may remember the answer from a previous test administration. Errors can occur when the person is distracted during testing. In addition, a person's true ability may not be demonstrated during assessment if his performance is affected by test anxiety. Potentially confounding variables may include the person's motivation, interests, mood and the effects of medication. Because such variables may influence the person's performance to some degree, they can never be completely discounted. Therefore, therapists need to know how likely it is that these potential sources of error will influence the results obtained on a test (de Clive-Lowe, 1996).

DEFINING RELIABILITY

In broad terms, the 'reliability of a test refers to how stable its scores remain over time and across different examiners' (de Clive-Lowe, 1996, p. 359), and reliability studies are undertaken to try to separate measurement errors from the person's true value or score on a measure (Pynsent, 2004). The main types of reliability of relevance to therapists are test–retest reliability, inter-rater reliability, intra-rater reliability, internal consistency and parallel form reliability. Other terms such as agreement, concordance, repeatability and reproducibility are sometimes used in test literature to describe aspects of reliability (Pynsent, 2004).

Dunn (2002) defines *reliability* more specifically as:

> the consistency of scores obtained under the theoretical concept of repeated testing of
> the same individual on the same test under identical conditions (including no changes
> to the individual). This could never be done, and various estimates of reliability are
> obtained in practice. (p. 59)

Reliability should be examined at the test development stage if a measure is being designed
either to be used by more than one therapist and/or to be administered more than once to provide a measure of outcome. Many test developers present reliability data in the test manual and
related publications. This knowledge is produced through studies of reliability. Methodology
required to evaluate reliability varies depending upon the type of reliability to be examined.
The basic method involves a test being administered by different therapists to large numbers of
people at different times and statistical analyses of the similarities and differences in the scores,
obtained from these various test administrations, are calculated. The clinician needs to be able
to understand the differences between various types of reliability, ascertain whether these have
been adequately studied and judge whether the quoted reliability is adequate for the context of
her clinical practice.

RELIABILITY COEFFICIENTS AND STANDARD ERROR
OF MEASUREMENT

COEFFICIENT AND CORRELATION

A reliability coefficient is used to indicate the extent to which a test is a stable instrument that
is capable of producing consistent results. Reliability is usually expressed as a correlation coefficient and varies between zero and one. Correlation is the term used to describe a 'measure
of association that indicates the degree to which two or more sets of observations fit a linear
relationship' (McDowell and Newell, 1987, p. 327). Various statistical formulae can be used for
estimating the strength of correlation and produce correlation coefficients. A correlation coefficient is 'the numerical index expressing the degree of relationship between two sets of data'
(Asher, 1996, p. xxxi). For all methods, a finding of no correlation is indicated by zero (0) and
means that no relationship was evident in the two sets of data being compared. Perfect reliability
is represented by a coefficient of 1.0, but in real life this is hardly ever achieved. The therapist,
therefore, needs to judge the acceptable amount of error when making clinical decisions from
test results. For ordered test variables, as measured on ordinal or interval scales (see Chapter 4),
the correlation statistic is cited with a positive or negative sign and can range from minus one to
plus one (-1.0 to $+1.0$). This indicates whether the correlation is negative or positive. Very few
test administrations will produce perfect correlation, unless they are two different measures of
the same thing. For example, a person's height measured in feet and inches should have perfect
correlation as when measured in metres and centimetres (Saslow, 1982). Negative correlations
are obtained when one test variable has the opposite effect to another, for example 'the correlation between the outside temperature and the size of our heating bill over a year should show
a near perfect negative correlation. A near-zero correlation is likely to be found between our
height and the size of our heating bill' (Saslow, 1982, p. 193). In testing, a negative correlation
indicates 'that the same individual will score high on one test and low on another' (Asher, 1996,
p. xxxi). So the closer the reliability coefficient is to 1.0, the more reliable is the test.

LEVEL OF SIGNIFICANCE

Some authors refer to level of significance when reporting their reliability studies. Asher (1996)
states that level of significance is obtained through a statistical procedure that 'identifies the
amount of objectivity of data by determining the probability that chance influences the results'

(p. xxxi). The lower the level of significance reported, the greater the confidence that you may place in the results. In therapy psychometric literature, the most frequently cited levels of significance are 0.05, which equals a 5 per cent chance, and 0.01, which equals a 1 per cent chance. Figures are often cited with a less than ($<$) sign. Levels of < 0.001 and < 0.0001 are considered highly significant.

ERROR OF MEASUREMENT

A score that would represent entirely all observations of an individual's behaviour on a test is know as the person's universe score or true score (Asher, 1996). No one test administration can represent the person perfectly, and a person's test scores are expected to vary to some degree from one test administration to another. Therapists rarely have time to administer more than once at baseline and once for each follow-up measurement. Therefore, therapists need to be able to generalise from the results of a single test administration. The following formula is often used:

$$X = t + e,$$

where: X = the observed score, t = the true score, e = the error score (Royeen, 1989, p. 55).

The goal then 'is to reduce or identify the controllable error to establish confidence that the observed score approximates the true score' (p. 55). Error of measurement is identified by checking the agreement between an original test score and subsequent scores (Asher, 1996).

STANDARD ERROR OF MEASUREMENT AND CONFIDENCE INTERVAL

Bartram (1990b) reminds us that 'no measurement is perfectly accurate but it is accurate within certain error margins. The lower the error margin, the more confidence we can place in the measure; the higher the error margin, the more we need to think about whether we are addressing the right problem, whether we need to delay a decision and search for further confirmation or refutation of our ideas' (p. 3). Some test manuals provide details of the standard error of measurement (SEM), and this can be very useful to therapists in deciding how accurate the test result is likely to be and how much to rely upon this result in decision making. SEM is the estimate of the 'error' associated with a person's obtained score on a test when compared with his hypothetical 'true' or 'universe' score. A range of scores can be calculated from this figure, and this is known as a confidence interval. The confidence interval represents the range of scores within which you can be highly confident that the person's 'true' score lies. The usual confidence interval used is 95 per cent, which means that you can be 95 per cent confident that the 'true' score lies within the interval (range of scores) calculated. To develop a confidence interval, it is assumed that the distribution of scores obtained by a population on a test will be distributed along a normal curve. In a normal curve, 95 per cent of scores lie within 1.96 standard deviations (s.d.) of the mean. To calculate a 95 per cent confidence interval for a client's score, the therapist will need to look up the reported SEM from the test manual. For example, a manual may state that the therapist can be x (for example 95 per cent) certain that a person's 'true' score lies in the range of the obtained score plus or minus y (for example 3). The therapist takes the SEM value y and multiplies it by the desired confidence interval x (that is for a 95 per cent interval multiply y by 1.96 s.d.).

A good example (see Figure 7.1 below) is provided by Dunn (2002) in the Infant and Toddler Sensory Profile manual, where she calculates a confidence interval for a 10-month-old:

> Justin's section raw score total for Section B. Auditory Processing = 30 SEM for this score =1.93 [*Note:* this is provided in the manual in Table 6.2, p. 62] 1.96 × 1.93 = 3.78

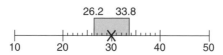

Figure 7.1 Example confidence interval. *Infant/Toddler Sensory Profile. Copyright © 2002 by Harcourt Assessment, Inc. Reproduced with permission. All rights reserved.*

Subtract 3.78 and add 3.78 to Justin's raw score to get the 95% confidence interval.

For Justin these numbers would be:

$30 - 3.78 = 26.2$

$30 + 3.78 = 33.8$

This calculation gives you 95% confidence that Justin's true score lies somewhere between 26 and 34. (p. 63)

A number of therapy assessments have been subjected to Rasch analysis, a statistical procedure that can be used to report the reliabilities of each item in terms of standard error. Fisher (2003a) discusses the advantages of this approach:

> The FACETS Rasch analysis computer program reports the reliabilities of each skill item, task and rater calibration and person measure in terms of standard errors . . . When considered from the perspective of person-centred measurement, the reporting of person by person standard errors of measurement has two advantages. First, rather than applying a single standard error of measurement to an entire sample, we are able to apply a specific standard error of measurement to each person . . . Second, knowledge of each person's error of measurement enables us to determine when that person has made significant gains, beyond chance, as a result of participation in intervention. (p. 39)

INTRODUCTION TO TYPES OF RELIABILITY

There are several types of reliability that the therapist should consider. The main forms of reliability of relevance to therapists described in psychometric and therapy literature (for example Anastasi, 1988; Benson and Clark, 1982; Crocker and Algina, 1986; Ottenbacher and Tomchek, 1993) include:

- test–retest reliability
- inter-rater reliability
- intra-rater reliability
- parallel form reliability (equivalent/alternate form)
- internal consistency.

TEST–RETEST RELIABILITY

Stability is concerned with the consistency with which behaviour occurs (Cromack, 1989). Stability is an important concept for therapists as we need to know whether a behaviour or level of function is stable or has changed over time. In psychometric terms, stability is linked to reliability and relates to whether an assessment can measure the same behaviour or construct repeatedly. One aspect of repeatability, of concern to therapists, is how consistently an assessment can repeat results over time. In order to pick up real changes in function, a therapist needs to know whether the assessment she plans to use at several time points during intervention to monitor her client's function will provide reliability in terms of stability across time. Therefore, tests used as outcome measures should have adequate test–retest reliability.

Test–retest reliability is the correlation of scores obtained by the same person on two administrations of the same test and is the consistency of the assessment or test score over time (Anastasi, 1988). This type of reliability is important because therapists need to examine whether their interventions have been effective, and to do this they administer tests on two or more occasions to monitor changes following treatment. Test–retest reliability is calculated using the correlation between two administrations of the test to the same people with a defined time interval between the two test administrations. When the same clients and therapist are used for a reliability study and the results obtained are consistent over time, then a test is said to have test–retest reliability (McFayden and Pratt, 1997). An acceptable correlation coefficient for test–retest reliability is considered to be 0.70 or above (Benson and Clark, 1982; Opacich, 1991).

A big question that faces researchers, and one which needs to be considered by therapists interpreting reported test–retest data, is: 'How much time should be allowed between test administrations?' There is no perfect answer because the populations assessed on therapy assessments and the purposes of assessments vary considerably. When choosing the most appropriate time interval between test administrations, the purpose of the test should be considered along with the way in which test scores are to be used (Crocker and Algina, 1986). The time period selected needs to be long enough so that any effects from practice or remembering the answers to test items should have faded. But it cannot be so long that a genuine change in function or ability occurs, because then any difference in scores obtained from the test and the retest would result from changes to the person's true scores. The time interval also needs to reflect the likely interval between testing selected by therapists to measure outcomes in clinical practice. For example, a test of infant development will need a short period between test administrations because there is likelihood that maturation will cause frequent changes in an infant's ability and test performance. In addition, it is unlikely that a young infant will remember his previous responses to test items (Crocker and Algina, 1986). Adults, however, are likely to remember their responses over quite long periods and so test developers will need to leave a longer period between test administrations. This may be done when the group of people being tested have a condition that is associated with little or very slow changes in function. However, when a shorter time period is required between test administrations, they will have to develop an alternative form of the test (see section on parallel form reliability, p. 199).

INTER-RATER RELIABILITY

Inter-rater reliability refers to the agreement between or among different therapists (raters) administering the test. Therapists need to be sure that any change in a person's performance on a test represents a genuine change in the person's performance and is not caused by a different test administrator. A reliable measure will need to 'ensure objectivity by using a method of assessment which is not influenced by the emotions or personal opinion of the assessor' (Christiansen and Baum, 1991, p. 854). This is important because clients often move between therapy services, for example from an acute ward to a rehabilitation ward, from in-patient service to a day hospital or outpatient service, or from an intermediate care/rapid-response service to longer-term support by a community team. So a person might be given the same assessment on a number of occasions but each time a different therapist administers the test.

Inter-rater reliability is calculated using the correlation between the scores recorded by two or more therapists administering the test to the same person at the same time. An acceptable correlation coefficient for inter-rater reliability is considered to be 0.90 or above (Benson and Clark, 1982; Opacich, 1991). Many test manuals and journal articles reporting psychometrics deal with inter-rater reliability, and therapists should expect to have easy access to such data when a test is likely to be administered by more than one therapist.

INTRA-RATER RELIABILITY

Intra-rater reliability refers to the consistency of the judgements made by the same therapist (test administrator/rater) over time. Therapists often use tests that require some degree of observation and/or clinical judgement. So they need to know that differences in results obtained for different clients, or the results for the same client obtained at different times, represent a genuine change in the person's performance, or real differences between clients, and is not the result of a fluctuation in the therapist's own consistency in giving and scoring the test. In studies of intra-rater reliability, the interval between ratings by the same examiner is usually brief and the assessment requires some observation or judgement on the part of the rater (Ottenbacher and Tomchek, 1993). One factor that may affect inter-rater and intra-rater reliability is the therapist's level of experience. When reviewing reliability studies, look to see whether the therapists were of the same grade/level of experience or whether the sample used therapists of mixed seniority.

RATER SEVERITY

Some test developers have considered the variation in how lenient or stringent therapists are when judging a person's performance on an observational assessment; this is known as rater severity (Fisher, 2003a; Lunz and Stahl, 1993). For example, therapists wishing to use the Assessment of Motor Process Skills (AMPS; Fisher, 2003a) are required to attend a rigorous five-day training course so that they can be calibrated for rater severity. Therapists view a series of videotapes of AMPS tasks being administered. Some therapists are found to be more lenient in their scoring and give clients higher scores than more severe raters. Knowledge of rater severity scoring the AMPS is accounted for in the determination of the person's ability measure, thus reducing the chance of inter-rater variability confounding the 'true' measure of the person's function (Fisher, 2003a).

PARALLEL FORM RELIABILITY (EQUIVALENT OR ALTERNATE FORM)

Parallel form reliability examines the correlation between scores obtained for the same person on two (or more) forms of a test. A parallel form is an alternative test that differs in content from the original test but which measures the same thing to the same level of difficulty. Parallel forms are used for retesting where a practice or learning effect might affect the test results. Parallel forms are particularly useful when the client group will need regular reassessment, has a condition which is associated with rapid improvements/decline in function or where improvement in scores owing to a practice effect will skew the test results. Several terms are used to describe parallel test forms and you may also see these referred to as 'equivalent forms' or 'alternate forms'. Reliability studies and statistics for this type of reliability can, therefore, be referred to as parallel form reliability, equivalent form reliability or alternate form reliability. Parallel form reliability is calculated using the correlation between two forms of the same test. The correlation coefficient obtained from two sets of scores drawn from parallel (equivalent/alternate) test forms can be called the coefficient of equivalence (Crocker and Algina, 1986). An acceptable correlation coefficient for parallel form reliability is considered to be 0.80 or above (Benson and Clark, 1982; Opacich, 1991).

INTERNAL CONSISTENCY

Internal consistency can be simply defined as the degree to which test items all measure the same behaviour or construct. Cromack (1989) states that internal consistency 'examines how consistently sampled behaviour is assessed over a limited period of time, and how consistently the instrument assesses that behaviour across the elements being measured' (p. 59).

A basic principle of measurement is that 'several related observations will produce a more reliable estimate than one' (Fitzpatrick, 2004, p. 55). If this is to be the case, then the related observations will need to measure aspects of a single construct, attribute or behaviour. When two or more items are included in a test, to measure the same construct or element of behaviour, a comparison can be made between these items to see if they produce consistent results. The more observations of a particular behaviour are made within a test, the more likely it will be that the observed behaviour is not a random incident (Cromack, 1989). However, therapists do not want overly long tests that will tire or bore their clients. So test developers need to select the optimum number and type of test items to adequately evaluate the construct or behaviour of concern. Internal consistency studies enable a test developer to ascertain whether all the items in a test are measuring the same construct or trait. This is known as the *homogeneity* of test items. Items must measure the same construct if they are to be a homogeneous item group and a test is said to have item homogeneity when people perform consistently across the test items. Items may test the same performance domains and constructs but vary in difficulty. Studies of internal consistency examine both item homogeneity and item difficulty and study the effect of errors caused by content sampling. Such studies are undertaken to help the test developer ascertain how far each test item or question contributes to the overall construct or behaviour being measured (McDowell and Newell, 1987).

You may see the term *item-total correlation* used in literature related to internal consistency. This is where the correlation of each test item with the total test score has been used as an indication of the internal consistency/homogeneity of the scales (McDowell and Newell, 1987). Internal consistency coefficients are reported by some test developers and help therapists to consider how homogeneous the item responses are within a scale or assessment (Dunn, 2002). Cronbach's alpha is one of the most frequently used statistical methods for evaluating the internal consistency of a test (McDowell and Newell, 1987). Fitzpatrick (2004) states that values of between 0.70 and 0.90 are considered optimal. Other authors (Benson and Clark, 1982; Opacich, 1991) indicate that 0.80 or above is acceptable for internal consistency. While McDowell and Newell (1987) suggest a slightly higher level, stating that: 'internal consistency coefficients of 0.85 or above are commonly taken as acceptable' (p. 33). So, when reviewing coefficients for internal consistency, you are looking for values of at least 0.70 and preferably 0.85 and above.

Another method of evaluating internal consistency is the split-half method. The test is administered once and items are divided into two halves, which are then correlated with each other. A correction for the shortened length of the tests can be applied. The extent to which the two halves are comparable and the degree to which each represents the whole test is considered to be an estimate of the internal consistency. Some test developers calculate a coefficient alpha; this provides an average of all possible split-halves (Dunn, 2002). A variant of the split-half method is the even–odd system, which involves the test developer comparing the even-numbered test items with the odd-numbered test items (Asher, 1996).

METHODOLOGICAL ISSUES

There is no gold standard for conducting reliability studies, and methodology and sample sizes vary widely across reported studies. Therefore, in addition to examining the reliability coefficient stated for a test, it is important that a therapist, who is deciding whether the test has acceptable levels of reliability, reviews the methodology and sample sizes used. This information is usually published in test manuals or journal articles.

Methodology varies considerably across inter-rater reliability studies. Some test developers only evaluate the reliability of the scoring of the assessment through a method that involves different therapists scoring videotaped administrations of a test, while other test developers consider the reliability between therapists for both test administration and scoring. This is especially important for tests where the therapist uses an element of judgement to guide test administration, such as the provision of prompts or cues or deciding where to start or stop the administration of hierarchical test items.

For example, the inter-rater reliability of the Rivermead Perceptual Assessment Battery (RPAB; Whiting *et al.*, 1985) was evaluated using the videotaped assessment of six people scored by three occupational therapists. Matthey, Donnelly and Hextell (1993) suggest that the small 'sample sizes used by the RPAB authors to calculate the reliability coefficients [make] the reliability data questionable' (p. 366). The methodology used by Russell *et al.* (1993) to evaluate the inter-rater reliability of the Gross Motor Function Measure (GMFM) was more robust as they examined the reliability of testers administering and scoring the test. However, their sample size was still small as they had three pairs of therapists administer and score the GMFM with a sample of 12 children. Laver (1994) undertook two studies to examine the inter-rater reliability of the Structured Observational Test of Function (SOTOF; Laver and Powell, 1995). In the first study, 14 pairs of therapists (n = 28) administered the SOTOF to 14 people with a primary diagnosis of stroke. In the second study, four therapists formed different pairings to administer the SOTOF to a mixed sample of 23 subjects (seven people with a primary diagnosis stroke, 15 with dementia and one with head injury). This gave combined inter-rater reliability data for 32 therapists and 37 clients. In both studies, one therapist administered the test while the second therapist observed the administration and then both therapists scored the person independently.

The experience of the therapists involved in the studies should also be considered in order to identify whether a newly qualified therapist will obtain the same consistent results as an experienced senior therapist. In the RPAB manual (Whiting *et al.*, 1985), the level of experience of the three therapists used for the study is not stated. However, data are provided for the GMFM and the SOTOF inter-rater reliability studies. Both studies report that their samples comprised therapists with a broad range of experience. In the GMFM study (Russell *et al.*, 1993), the six therapists had paediatric experience ranging from 2.5 to 18 years. In the sample for the first SOTOF inter-rater reliability study (Laver, 1994), therapists' experience with elderly clients ranged from one to 15 years and the sample comprised eight basic grade therapists, 11 senior II therapists, three senior I therapists, three head IV, one head III, one deputy head and one therapist who did not specify her grade (n = 28). In the second study, the sample (n = 4) comprised one basic grade, one senior II, one head occupational therapist and the test developer, who was working as a senior lecturer (and had previously been a senior I occupational therapist).

TEST SPECIFICITY

Therapists also need to consider the specificity and sensitivity of tests. Specificity is 'the ability of a measurement to correctly identify those who do not have the condition in question' (McDowell and Newell, 1987, p. 330). Test specificity is important because therapists only want those people who exhibit a specific behaviour or functional deficit to be identified on a test. A false positive result occurs when someone who does not have a deficit is identified on a test as having the deficit. A false negative result occurs when a person who has a deficit is not shown to have that deficit through his performance on the test. *Specificity*, therefore, has been defined as 'the proportion of non-cases according to the agreed diagnostic criteria who are negative' on a test (Green *et al.*, 2005, p. 10). Therapists need to be aware of the risk of a false negative result because this can lead to a person not receiving a correct diagnosis or assessment of the problem, which in turn can result in required treatment being withheld and the person's condition deteriorating unnecessarily. A specific test minimises the number of false positive results that occur when the test is used and will not identify people who do not exhibit the behaviour or deficit being examined (Opacich, 1991). Both types of errors can lead to negative consequences for an individual. A false positive test might result in a person being incorrectly diagnosed and given an inappropriate treatment or suffering discrimination because of the label assigned as a result of the false positive test. In some cases, this could have a serious consequence: a person might be given unnecessary medication and suffer from side effects needlessly or be refused employment or insurance because of his diagnosis.

A good test manual will provide details of potential levels of error, enabling therapists to consider the risk of a false positive or false negative result occurring when they administer the test. For example, the Infant and Toddler Symptom Checklist (DeGangi *et al.*, 1995) provides a table illustrating the classification accuracy for cut-off scores (p. 41) and provides false positive (labelled as false delayed) and false negative (labelled as false normal) percentages for all five age bands covered by the test. These percentages varied considerably across the age bands, for example for children aged 19–24 months, the false positive risk was only 3 per cent and a zero per cent false negative rate indicated that the test should identify accurately all infants with a problem. However, for children in the 25–30 months age band, a false positive rate of 13 per cent and a false negative rate of 14 per cent are given. Therapists would, therefore, be wise to use this test in conjunction with other measures in this age group.

Test developers of therapy assessments often decide that a false negative result will have a greater potential risk to the individual than a false positive result and will select test items in order to minimise false negative scores. For example, DeGangi *et al.* (1995), authors of the Infant and Toddler Symptom Checklist, report that 'the cut-off scores for each subtest were chosen to minimise the false-normal error rate, judged to be the more serious of the two types of error from the perspective of screening and diagnostic decision making' (p. 42).

Abidin (1995) identified three different types of false negative data in parent populations when he analysed his research and clinical experience using the Parenting Stress Index (PSI). He describes these as: type I false negative, defensive individuals; type II false negative, dishonest respondents; and type III false negative, disengaged parents. In the PSI manual, descriptions of the three false negative types are provided to assist therapists in interpreting extremely low PSI total stress scores (scores falling below the fifteenth percentile) in order to decide whether the test results reflect a true picture of a parent under a low level of stress or whether further investigation is required to examine a hypothesis that the parent falls under one of the three false negative types. In order to assist test administrators to identify false negative scores related to defensive responding, Abidin developed a PSI defensive responding scoring system using 15 of the PSI items that are highlighted by shading on the scoring part of the answer sheet. A cut-off score is given, and parents with this score or below are considered to be responding in a defensive manner and so the test administrator then knows to interpret results with caution.

TEST SENSITIVITY

Test sensitivity is important because a sensitive test will identify all those people who show the behaviour or deficit in question. Sensitivity is 'the ability of a measurement or screening test to identify those who have a condition, calculated as a percentage of all cases with the condition who were judged by the test to have the condition: the "true positive" rate' (McDowell and Newell, 1987, p. 330). *Sensitivity* has been defined as 'the proportion of cases according to the agreed diagnostic criteria who are positive' on the test (Green *et al.*, 2005, p. 10). A sensitive test will minimise the chance of false negative results occurring and can identify what it was designed to test. Stokes and O'Neill (1999) state that 'if scales are not sensitive enough to measure change due to physiotherapy, then intervention may be misjudged and undervalued' (p. 562). If a test is not sensitive enough to the target of therapy, then changes that have occurred may be missed, and this can be problematic if intervention appears to be ineffective when significant change has actually occurred. This is sometimes referred to as the degree of *responsiveness* of a test. Responsiveness to change refers to the measure of efficiency with which a test detects clinical change and is distinct from reliability and validity

(Wright, Cross and Lamb, 1998). The responsiveness of a test is critically important to both occupational therapists and physiotherapists because they often need to measure changes in aspects of people's functioning, for example when evaluating the impact of intervention or monitoring the effects of medication. When using evaluative measures, the therapist should ensure that the test used is responsive to picking up both the type and amount of change in behaviour or function that is anticipated, or desired, as the result of intervention. It is important that measures can identify clinically important change, even if this is quite small (Pynsent, 2004). A number of therapists have discussed this issue. Fairgrieve (1992), a head occupational therapist from Dundee working with children with motor-learning difficulties, notes problems with using the Movement Assessment Battery for Children (Movement ABC; Henderson and Sugden, 1992) for monitoring progress, because she had found that 'small differences of performance [were] not reflected in a shift in the pass/borderline/fail scoring criteria [yet] such changes may nevertheless be very significant to parents, to the therapist and to the child concerned' (p. 224). Neale (2004) reports that, in her work setting comprising a rehabilitation ward and stroke unit, her team 'use the Barthel ADL Index (Mahoney and Barthel, 1965) which is completed at the weekly multi-disciplinary meeting . . . but it is not sensitive to the changes we see in patients during rehabilitation . . . the person can have the same score but still be showing marked improvement. We bemoan the Barthel, but the same difficulty arises with the other ADL assessments. If the "score" stays the same week after week, do others recognise the progress? If so, why have a score? If not, aren't there other ways to show progress?' (pp. 25–26).

While an increasing number of therapy measures are now backed by studies of their reliability and validity, 'sensitivity to clinically relevant change over time is often an outstanding property not studied in clinical tools' (Stokes and O'Neill, 1999, p. 562). Yet, when therapists wish to establish the effects of their interventions, it is one of the most important psychometric properties to consider.

Various methods are used to examine responsiveness to change. The simplest method is the calculation of percentage change. Effect sizes and relative efficiency are also accepted methods for comparing the responsiveness to change of different tests (Liang, 1995). Effect size can be applied to evaluate continuous data. Pynsent (2004) states that 'the effect size is usually quoted as a measure of sensitivity to change for instruments whose sample means are reasonably normally distributed' (p. 5), and he provides the following equation:

$$\text{Effect size index} = \frac{\text{Mean at time 1} - \text{mean at time 2}}{\text{Standard deviation (s.d.) at time 1}}$$

McDowell and Newell (1987) describe how the likelihood ratio is used by some test developers in relation to specificity and sensitivity analyses when they state that 'likelihood ratio':

> is an approach to summarizing the results of sensitivity and specificity analyses for various cutting points on diagnostic and screening tests. Each cutting point produces a value for the true positive rate (i.e. sensitivity) and the false positive rate (i.e. specificity). The ratio of true to false positives is the likelihood ratio for each cutting point. (p. 328)

When reviewing research into the responsiveness of tests, therapists should be aware that the larger the effect size, the more responsive the test is to clinical change. An effect size of 0.2 or below is considered small, 0.5 is considered a moderate effect size, while 0.8 or more is considered a large effect size (Wright, Cross and Lamb, 1998). Relative efficiency is particularly useful when you have two potential outcome measures for your service and wish to select the one that will provide the greatest responsiveness. There are both parametric (using a t statistic) and non-parametric (using the z statistic derived from the Wilcoxon sign rank test; Wilcoxon, 1945) methods for calculating relative efficiency between tests. Regardless of the method used, a score of 1 would specify that the responsiveness of the two tests being compared was the same. Scores greater than or less than one indicate that one test is more responsive than the other. To allow comparison of the responsiveness of different tests, raw scores may need to be transformed. For example, to provide comparable scores out of 100, we would divide the person's actual score by the total possible score and then multiply this figure by 100 (Wright, Cross and Lamb, 1998).

Wright, Cross and Lamb (1998) compared the responsiveness to change of the Rivermead Mobility Index (RMI) and the Barthel Index (BI) in a sample of 50 people receiving physiotherapy. They report that both 'the RMI and the BI are responsive to changes in older people having physiotherapy (effect sizes 1 and 0.87 respectively)' (p. 216). They also used both parametric and non-parametric methods to calculate the relative efficiency of the two tests and reported that 'parametric calculation of relative efficiency of the RMI versus the BI was 1.42; non-parametric methods gave a result of 1.25 for the same comparison' (p. 219). 'In both cases, a result greater than 1 would indicate the RMI to be more responsive than the BI' (p. 218). Therefore, they conclude that the 'RMI was more efficient at measuring outcome than the BI' (p. 216).

FLOOR AND CEILING EFFECTS

Floor and ceiling effects can affect the accuracy of an assessment. Measurement of outcome can be confounded when clients either improve or deteriorate beyond the range of functioning tested by the outcome measure. Therefore, therapists need to consider the range of ability expected from their client population and select a suitable measure so as to ensure that their clients will be unlikely to perform above or below the measurement range of the tests used in their service. A ceiling effect occurs when the person scores the maximum possible score on a test and the test does not reflect the full extent of his ability. A floor effect occurs when a person obtains the minimum score on a test and the test does not reflect the full extent of the person's deficits. The size of ceiling and floor effects is established by examining the percentage of a clinical sample obtaining either maximum or minimum scores. When deciding whether any reported ceiling or floor effects could affect the use of a measure for your clients, it is important to look at both the sample used in the study (diagnosis, age range etc.) and the setting in which a test is being used (community, in-patient, outpatient etc.). For example, Wright, Cross and Lamb (1998) examined floor and ceiling effects of the RMI and the BI at three time periods: pre-admission, on admission and at discharge. They used a sample of 50 people receiving physiotherapy for a range of orthopaedic, neurological and cardiorespiratory conditions. They report that when patients were scored before admission 44 per cent achieved the maximum possible score on the BI and 31 per cent scored the maximum possible score on the RMI, indicating that both tests had a ceiling effect when used with patients in the community. However, when the samples were measured on admission to a rehabilitation ward, the 'scores on the BI were evenly distributed around the mid-point of the scale [and] there was no evidence of a floor or ceiling effect' (p. 218). However, on admission 'the average score of the RMI was below the mid-point of the scale and . . . 6 per cent scored the minimum value [and] a floor effect was demonstrated' (p. 218). At discharge, the BI was found to have a 'mild ceiling effect' (p. 219) with 4 per cent of their sample scoring the maximum value and the RMI was found to have a minor floor effect with 6 per cent of subjects obtaining the minimum score. Wright, Cross and Lamb conclude that 'floor and ceiling effects are evident in both the RMI and BI respectively, and . . . this could limit their usefulness for in-patients'. They also state that the BI is limited in its usefulness as an outcome measure in a community-based population because of the marked ceiling effect.

Floor and ceiling effects can be particularly relevant for certain client populations. For example, Saxton *et al.* (1993) report that people who are severely demented 'bottom out' on most neuropsychological tests and are labelled 'untestable'. They state that 'despite pervasive deficits severely-demented patients do show a range of abilities in multiple low-level tasks [and] assessment of these very impaired patients is possible, and indeed necessary' (p. 4). These authors have developed the Severe Impairment Battery (SIB) to 'assess cognitive functioning in patients who are unable to complete standard neurological tests' (p. 4). During test development, they paid particular attention to floor effects and examined test items where subjects scored zero. The authors report 'some questions were dropped from the previous versions of the SIB because of floor effects' (p. 7).

RELIABILITY STATISTICS

The following section provides a brief discussion about reliability statistics to help therapists look at cited correlations critically and make informed judgements about the level of reliability of an assessment and whether this is adequate for their clinical practice. This section is by no means meant as an exhaustive presentation of reliability statistics, and any therapist conducting a reliability study should only use this as a starting point and refer to statistics textbooks and manuals for more detailed guidance. I found the following texts useful when conducting reliability studies as part of my doctoral studies: Royeen (1989), Saslow (1982), Anastasi (1988) and Crocker and Algina (1986). Although these texts are now quite old, they have definitions and descriptions that are still of relevance today. With an increasing emphasis on evidence-based practice, therapists will also find a wide variety of more recently published research, statistics and psychometric texts available.

Statistics is the application of mathematical formulae to order, interpret and analyse a set of empirical data. Statistics enable us to describe the characteristics of our data and to draw inferences from them. Statistical analyses allow the test developer, and the therapist who will be the test administrator, to determine whether the results are due to significant effects or to chance factors (Asher, 1996). Maths was one of my weakest subjects at school and when I embarked on my doctoral studies, and set out to develop the SOTOF, it was undertaking the statistical analyses for the psychometric studies that worried me the most. I found that I was not alone: during my time working with therapy students and clinicians, I've met many who have said that they are no good at maths and feel daunted by statistics. If you fall into this group, *please keep reading on.* As a clinician you need to know enough about reliability statistics to make an informed decision about the value of a test for your clients. Just because a test is published does not mean it has adequate reliability. There are several statistical procedures used in reliability studies, and although many produce correlation coefficients the numbers they produce are not necessarily equivalent and of identical merit. The following section will briefly present some of these statistical procedures and will discuss how the statistics they produce compare. I will try to make it as straightforward as possible.

As stated earlier, reliability is usually expressed as a correlation coefficient ranging from -1.0 to $+1.0$. When you are examining reliability figures quoted in test manuals and psychometric literature, the closer the number is to $+1.0$, the stronger is the reliability of the measure. It is rare to obtain reliability statistics of $+1$ or very close to $+1$. Fox (1969, cited in Asher, 1996) categorises correlations into four levels:

- correlations from 0 to $+$ or -0.50 are low
- correlations from $+$ or -0.50 to 0.70 are moderate
- correlations from $+$ or -0.70 to 0.80 are high
- correlations greater than $+$ or -0.86 are very high

Stein (1976, cited in McFayden and Pratt, 1997) states that, in practice, figures over 0.8 are considered to have acceptable levels of reliability. However, the acceptable level of reliability does vary depending on the type of reliability being examined and must be examined in the context of the variables being correlated (Asher, 1996).

- Test–retest reliability: an acceptable correlation coefficient for test–retest reliability is considered to be 0.70 or above (Benson and Clark, 1982; Opacich, 1991).
- Internal consistency: an acceptable correlation coefficient for internal consistency is 0.85 and above (McDowell and Newell, 1987).
- Inter-rater reliability: 0.90 or above is considered an acceptable level (Benson and Clark, 1982; Opacich, 1991).
- Parallel form reliability: coefficients ranging in the 0.80s and 0.90s are acceptable for equivalent (alternate/parallel) form reliability (Crocker and Algina, 1986).

So when reviewing the reliability literature you are looking for values of at least 0.70 and preferably 0.80 and above.

THE STATISTIC CAN AFFECT THE RESULT

This section explores the different statistical methods used to produce reliability statistics and explains some of the disadvantages and advantages of these methods, which therapists should take into account when evaluating whether the reliability of a measure is adequate for their clinical practice.

There is debate in the therapy literature concerning the 'correct' statistic to use to estimate reliability. The statistic chosen should relate to the level of measurement of the scale used in the test. For example, different statistics should be applied to dichotomous nominal data compared to continuous interval data. Ottenbacher and Tomchek (1993) reviewed 20 articles, which report reliability studies (pulled from the *American Journal of Occupational Therapy* and *Physical Therapy*) in order to examine the 'frequency and type of reliability procedures reported in the therapeutic research literature and to examine issues related to the interpretation of reliability coefficients' (p. 11). They found that the intra-class correlation coefficient (ICC) was the most popular statistical procedure used and this accounted for 57 per cent of all reliability coefficients reported across the 20 studies. Pearson's product-moment correlation (r) was the next most frequently cited statistic and accounted for 15 per cent of the reliability values reported. Kappa's coefficient alpha and percentage agreement were used in a few articles. Ottenbacher and Tomchek report that 'the intraclass correlation approach is most frequently used with continuous data', while 'both Kappa and percentage agreement . . . are used to compute reliability for categorical data or data involving dichotomous decisions' (p. 14). The average values for the five identified reliability coefficients were compared and showed that 'the average value for Kappa is considerably below the average for the other four reliability procedures' (p. 13). All these statistics have a ceiling value of 1.0, or 100 per cent, and so depending on the type of reliability being evaluated and the statistic used you should be looking for values of 0.70 to 1.0 (75–100 per cent).

PERCENTAGE AGREEMENT (P)

P is an expression of the probability of a consistent decision. Percentage agreement is the simplest measure of consistency. It is often applied to criterion-referenced tests that use two-point ordinal scales involving mastery decisions (for example unable versus able, or independent versus dependent). P can be defined as the proportion of subjects consistently classified as either master-master (able-able) or nonmaster-nonmaster (unable-unable) using two criterion-referenced measurements.

INTRA-CLASS CORRELATION COEFFICIENTS (ICC)

ICCs are used to produce measures of consistency or agreement of values within cases. It is useful when more than two raters have been involved in collecting data, for example in an inter-rater reliability study (whereas Pearson's r is used to compare the ratings of a number of assessments undertaken on a sample by only two raters). Pynsent (2004) states: 'ICC should be used for continuous data to measure agreement between or within methods or raters. There are other measures available but the ICC is appropriate and the most commonly used' (p. 4).

PEARSON'S PRODUCT-MOMENT CORRELATION COEFFICIENT

Pearson's product-moment correlation coefficient is used to measure the degree of linear relationship between two sets of observations. Values obtained range from -1.0 to $+1.0$ (Crocker and Algina, 1986). As r indicates the strength of the linear relationship, the highest value of $+1.0$ occurs when all data points fall exactly on the line (Norusïs, 1992). Pearson's r is used for ratio or interval level data (McDowell and Newell, 1987). Ottenbacher and Tomchek (1993) discuss the limitations of this statistic applied to reliability studies: 'because the Pearson product-moment correlation measures linear association or covariation between values, not agreement . . . as long as the raters co-vary consistently, a large actual disagreement in rater scores does not lower the reliability' (p. 13). Pynsent (2004) provides a good example of this problem:

> If a mercury thermometer was compared with a digital thermometer and the mercury device measured exactly the same as the digital equipment but 2° lower, then Pearson's coefficient would be 1, suggesting 100 per cent agreement. It is always worth plotting the results to find systematic biases when comparing data. (p. 4)

For ordinal level data Kendall's tau and Spearman's rho can be used and you may see these referred to as *rank order correlations* (McDowell and Newell, 1987).

COHEN'S KAPPA (K)

Kappa provides a statistical method for producing a 'coefficient of agreement between two raters, kappa expresses the level of agreement that is observed beyond the level that would be expected by chance alone' (McDowell and Newell, 1987, p. 328). The kappa value is easy to interpret; it uses the proportion of agreement and gives the advantage of accounting for chance agreement. Kappa is a measure of agreement that has 'been proposed for categorical variables [and] can be applied to an arbitrary number of raters' (Siegel and Castellan, 1988, p. 284). Kappa provides a transformation of P to a new scale in which the points 0 and 1 are interpretable. A value of 1 indicates that decisions are as consistent as those based on perfectly statistically dependent scores (Crocker and Algina, 1986; Siegel and Castellan, 1988; Norusïs, 1991). A value of 0 does not mean that decisions are so inconsistent as to render the item worthless, but that the decisions are no more consistent than decisions based on statistically independent scores. 'The coefficient K can assume negative values . . . which correspond to the situation in which there is an inverse relationship between the scores on the two forms' (Crocker and Algina, 1986, p. 201). Pynsent (2004) recommends the use of kappa when binary results are to be compared (that is paired/ dichotomous data usually labelled as 1 and 0) and when analysing ordinal data a weighted kappa can be applied where the amount of disagreement is weighted.

Ottenbacher and Tomchek (1993) conclude that kappa was one of 'the preferred methods of computing reliability in applied environments' (p. 14); kappa was preferred to percentage agreement as it corrects for chance agreement. Discrepancies were found between the average kappa values and the average percentage agreement indexes evaluated in their study; all the reliability coefficients in their study had a ceiling value of 1.0, or 100 per cent; kappa had an approximate average value of 0.5 compared to percentage agreement, which had an approximate average of 0.75 (75 per cent).

COMPARING STATISTICAL METHODS FOR EVALUATING RELIABILITY

As part of my doctoral study, I examined the discrepancy of reliability values obtained through several statistical methods when conducting inter-rater reliability and test–retest reliability studies during the development of the SOTOF (Laver, 1994; Laver and Powell, 1995). A comparison of percentage agreement and kappa values obtained in my doctoral research supported the findings of Ottenbacher and Tomchek (1993) that percentage agreement produces values that are consistently higher than kappa values. Average percentage agreement for test–retest reliability of the SOTOF was 0.94, compared with an average kappa value of 0.56. Average percentage agreement for inter-rater reliability of the SOTOF was also 0.94 compared with an average kappa value of 0.63. Comparison of Kappa values with the significance level of values obtained by chi-square, Fisher's and phi showed that items with kappa values of 0.5 and above were usually significant (at the < 0.05 level) for these other analyses. Items with kappa values between 0.34 and 0.65 were significant for chi-square and phi but did not always produce significant values for Fisher's exact test, which can be used to adjust chi-square to account for small expected frequencies. This test was used because it 'evaluates the same hypothesis as the chi-square test, and is suitable for tables having two rows and two columns for small expected frequencies' (Norusïs, 1991, pp. 270–271). Chi-square indicates if an association between variables is significant; the phi coefficient is used to express the degree of association between two nominal variables in a two-by-two table. The value of the phi coefficient ranges from -1.0 to $+1.0$ and can be interpreted as a correlation coefficient (Portney and Watkins, 1993). 'A significance level of 5% (< 0.05) was used to evaluate the significance of chi-square, Fisher's and phi values' (Laver, 1994, p. 305). Items with kappa values less than 0.34 usually had non-significant values for the three other statistical analyses. I concluded that the use of Cohen's kappa, chi-square (adjusted for small sample sizes where necessary) and phi coefficients produce more conservative estimates of reliability than percentage agreement and are, therefore, preferred methods of analysis. The results of this study supported Ottenbacher and Tomchek's (1993) recommendation of kappa as a preferred method of computing reliability in applied therapeutic research (Laver, 1994). Lack of variance in some reliability data may mean that kappa cannot be calculated and it may be necessary for therapists to rely on percentage agreement values; however, they should be treated with some caution as they may give an overly positive image of the test's reliability.

EXAMINING RELIABILITY DATA: TEST EXAMPLES

When making a decision whether to use a test or not based on reliability data, it is important to obtain as much of the evidence as possible. Most test developers will report initial reliability studies in the test manual or journal articles. For some tests, additional reliability data are available, either from later studies undertaken by the test developers or by independent researchers. Studies may not be directly comparable if they evaluate reliability with different diagnostic groups or age groups. But a range of studies will help to build up a picture of the reliability of a measure. The therapist should look for consistency across studies and take particular note of significant differences in reported levels of reliability.

THE RELIABILITY OF THE CANADIAN OCCUPATIONAL PERFORMANCE MEASURE

The Canadian Occupational Performance Measure (COPM; Law *et al.*, 1994) has been developed to measure changes in clients' perceptions of their performance and their level of satisfaction with their performance of self-care, work and leisure tasks. The test–retest reliability of the COPM was originally examined by the test developers and reported in the test manual

(Law *et al.*, 1994). For the original study, test–retest reliability was evaluated in a study of 27 older clients attending a day hospital for rehabilitation for a variety of impairments, including stroke, Parkinson's disease, hip fracture and arthritis. The COPM produces scores for both performance and for the client's satisfaction with his level of performance. The test–retest reliability for the performance and satisfaction scores of the COPM was calculated using inter-class correlation coefficients. Test–retest reliability was reported at 0.63 for performance and 0.84 for satisfaction. The COPM would be considered to have good test–rest reliability for its satisfaction scores, but the reliability of performance scores falls below the recommended 0.70 level. Further studies of reliability for this test, therefore, need to be reviewed. In a more recent study, two British researchers, Sewell and Singh (2001), examined the test–retest reliability of the COPM with a sample of 15 clinically stable patients with chronic obstructive pulmonary disease (COPD). The study was undertaken as the COPM was being considered as an outcome measure for a planned randomised control trial into pulmonary rehabilitation. The retest was conducted after an interval of seven days. Data analysis was conducted to produce mean difference, 95 per cent confidence intervals and correlation coefficients. They used Spearman's rho correlation coefficients (for non-parametric data) and reported 0.81 ($p < 0.0001$) for performance and 0.76 ($p < 0.001$) for satisfaction. They also calculated intra-class correlation coefficients and reported $r = 0.92$ for performance and $r = 0.90$ for satisfaction. Both these figures fall above the accepted level of 0.70, and the authors conclude: 'these are considered to be excellent correlation coefficients and are highly statistically significant, with $p < 0.001$ for both scores' (p. 308). Therapists reviewing this second study would have more confidence using the COPM as a repeated measure. However, they should take the differences in samples into consideration; they could, therefore, have more confidence using the COPM with clients with COPD compared to older clients represented by the original sample. As both studies used relatively small samples of patients, the issue of generalisability needs to be considered. In the case of the Sewell and Singh study (2001), they report that their sample was comparable with other samples from research studies related to pulmonary rehabilitation in terms of their age, male-to-female ratio and level of airflow obstruction. Further reliability values were reported in 2003 by researchers examining the test–retest reliability of the Dutch version of the COPM with stroke patients (Cup *et al.*, 2003). They also used a time period of seven days and report correlation coefficients of 0.89 ($p < 0.001$) for performance and 0.88 ($p < 0.001$) for satisfaction. Sewell and Singh (2001) give a note of caution regarding the use of the one-week time period for their study:

> It was felt that 7 days was enough time between the two COPM interviews and that clients would be unable to recall their previous responses. There is, however, no hard evidence for this and so this issue should be considered as a possible confounding variable. (p. 309)

The test developers reported that four studies had been undertaken to examine the responsiveness of the COPM (Law *et al.*, 1994b). For example, pilot studies conducted by the COPM research group have:

> collected reassessment data for 139 clients for performance scores and 138 for satisfaction scores . . . Differences in the means between initial and reassessment scores for both performance and satisfaction were statistically significant ($p < 0.0001$). The mean change scores in performance and satisfaction indicate that COPM is responsive to changes in perception of occupational performance by clients. (pp. 25–26)

In a recent paper by the test developers (Carswell *et al.*, 2004), which reviews the COPM research literature, they report a further five studies which have evaluated responsiveness (or sensitivity to change) of the COPM. They conclude that:

All five reported that the COPM was very responsive to changes in client outcomes over time and when compared to other measures such as the Short Form-36, the Health Assessment Questionnaire and the FIM, demonstrating improvement in perceived performance and satisfaction. (p. 212)

THE RELIABILITY OF THE GROSS MOTOR FUNCTION MEASURE

The Gross Motor Function Measure (GMFM; Russell *et al*., 1990, 1993) was developed for use by physiotherapists/physical therapists as a measure of change in the gross-motor functioning of children with cerebral palsy, both for use in clinical practice and for research. In a critique of the GMFM, Cole *et al*. (1995) state that it may 'be used to describe a child's current level of function, to determine treatment goals, and to evaluate the effectiveness of therapies aimed at improving motor function' (p. 150). The test comprises 88 items divided into five dimensions, grouped by testing position and arranged in developmental sequence: lying and rolling, crawling and kneeling, sitting, standing, walking, running and jumping. Each item is scored on a four-point ordinal scale. Each dimension provides a raw score, a percentage score and a total percentage score. A goal percentage score may be calculated to reflect the percentage score for those areas that are treatment goals.

Studies have been undertaken to examine the intra-rater, inter-rater and test–retest reliability of the GMFM (Russell *et al*., 1993; Russell, 1987). Six physiotherapists (three from each of two centres) and 12 children were involved in the reliability studies. In addition, 28 videotapes of children's GMFM performance were viewed by therapists who were familiar with the test but unfamiliar with the sample of children. The therapists were blinded to the order in which the tapes were presented. A standardised questionnaire was used for judging change on pairs of videotapes. Reliability was examined using ICC obtained from an analysis of variance (ANOVA) model. The authors selected a correlation of greater than or equal to 0.75 to represent an acceptable level of reliability.

GMFM's inter-rater reliability

Six pairs of therapists evaluated 11 children representative of the ages and severities of cerebral palsy included in a larger study. For inter-rater reliability, 0.90 or above is considered an acceptable level (Benson and Clark, 1982; Opacich, 1991). The ICC for the total score was high at 0.99 indicating excellent inter-rater reliability for the total score. However, individual dimensions ranged from 0.87 to 0.99. As an ICC of 0.87 at the lowest end of the range is only 0.03 below the acceptable level and many ICCs were higher than this, with the highest figure reaching 0.99, the GMFM would be considered to have acceptable levels of reliability across all five domains.

GMFM's test–retest reliability

Test–retest reliability was examined by testing the children on the GMFM on two separate occasions within a two-week period. Six therapists evaluated a sample of 10 children representative of the ages and severities of cerebral palsy included in a study of 111 children. An acceptable correlation coefficient for test–retest reliability is considered to be 0.70 or above (Benson and Clark, 1982; Opacich, 1991). On the GMFM study, ICCs ranged from 0.92 to 0.99 across the five dimensions and the ICC for the total score was very high at 0.99. This indicates that the GMFM has excellent test–retest reliability in a population of children with cerebral palsy. However, as the study involved both a small sample of therapists (n = 6) and children (n = 10) further reliability studies would be very useful.

GMFM's responsiveness

Responsiveness to change was examined by evaluating the child on two occasions six months apart. Judgements of change were made by both therapists and parents. Repeated judgements made by a sample of 23 therapists produced correlations of 0.85 to 0.98 across the five dimensions.

These figures fall above the accepted level of 0.80. Repeated judgements made by a sample of 23 parents produced correlations of 0.67 to 0.92 across the five dimensions. These figures indicate moderate to high levels of responsiveness. The authors conclude that 'the reliability values on repeated testing indicate that the measure can be used very consistently. With the exception of parent judgements of change in sitting and crawling and kneeling, all reliabilities of judgements of change reached acceptable levels' (Russell *et al.*, 1993, p. 18). In a critique of the GMFM, Cole *et al.* (1995) state that:

> the GMFM is responsive to both negative and positive change. In a non-disabled population, those children younger than 3 years showed more change than those older than 3 years (t-test $p < 0.0001$). Those children with acute head injury improved significantly more than the non-disabled children, who improved more than those with cerebral palsy (ANOVA $p < 0.05$). (p. 151)

CONCLUSION

In conclusion, a good measure must have demonstrated validity and reliability. A target analogy can be used to see how a measure may have none, both or only one of these psychometric properties.

In this figure, the bull's eye (which is the shaded circle in the middle of each target) represents the true outcome to be measured and each arrow represents a single application of the outcome instrument. In Figure 7.2(a), none of the arrows has fallen within the bull's eye and the arrows are spread quite widely. This figure represents a measure that is neither valid nor reliable. In Figure 7.2(b), the arrows are clustered very closely together, indicating a reliable measurement, but they are not hitting the bull's eye; so, while reliable, the measure is not measuring what it sets out to measure and is not valid. In Figure 7.2(c), all the arrows fall within the bull's eye, indicating good validity, but the spread of the arrows is still quite wide and so reliability could be improved. Finally, Figure 7.2(d) represents a valid and reliable measure; all the arrows have fallen within the shaded bull's eye and they are clustered close together.

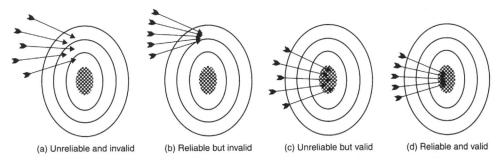

| (a) Unreliable and invalid | (b) Reliable but invalid | (c) Unreliable but valid | (d) Reliable and valid |

Figure 7.2 A target analogy for reliability and validity. *Pynsent P (2004) Choosing an outcome measure. In P Pynsent, J Fairbank, A Carr (eds). Outcome Measures in Orthopaedics and Orthopaedic Trauma (2nd edn.). London, Arnold. © Arnold. Reproduced with permission of Edward Arnold (Publishers) Ltd.*

Note: A target analogy for reliability and validity. The bull's eye represents the true outcome to be measured and each arrow represents a single application of the outcome instrument.

APPLYING CONCEPTS OF RELIABILITY TO YOUR OWN PRACTICE

At the back of this book, you will find templates for a series of worksheets designed to assist you in applying principles of assessment and outcome measurement to your own practice. Please now turn to Worksheet 7 (pp. 405–8).

For this reflection, you will need to select a published assessment. This could be a test that you are already using in your clinical practice. Often, therapists inherit assessments when they start work in a different clinical setting or department; this will be a particularly useful exercise if you are using a test that was already available in your department and which you have not critiqued. You might select a test that you are considering purchasing/using in the future. If you are a student, select a test you have seen used on clinical placement or one available at your university or college. Look to see what information (test manual, journal articles, handouts from training courses etc.) is available on your chosen test. If there is very little, which can be the case when you have inherited an assessment, you might need to conduct a literature search in order to complete the worksheet.

The worksheet takes you through a series of questions about different types of reliability and prompts you to record key evidence and to form opinions about whether the published evidence indicates adequate levels of reliability, specificity, sensitivity and responsiveness for your clinical needs.

STUDY QUESTIONS

7.1 What is reliability?
7.2 What is the difference between inter-rater reliability and intra-rater reliability?
7.3 Define *test–retest reliability*.
7.4 What would be an acceptable correlation coefficient for test–retest reliability?
7.5 What is responsiveness and why is it important if you want to measure outcomes?

You will find brief answers to these questions at the back of this book (p. 392).

8

Test Administration, Reporting and Recording

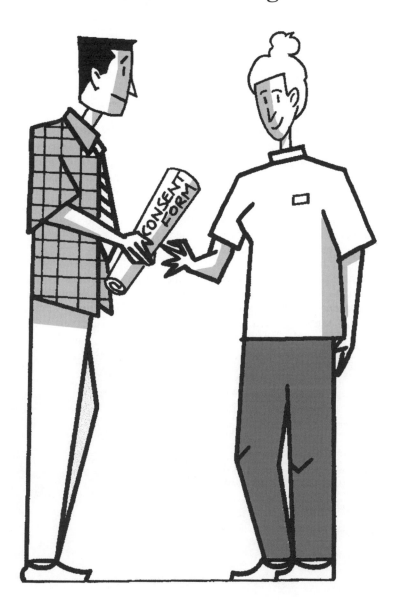

CHAPTER SUMMARY

This chapter will discuss the importance of obtaining informed consent from clients prior to undertaking an assessment. It will consider factors to ensure the most efficient and effective assessment process is followed, such as building rapport, constructing your test environment and communicating the results of the assessment. It will discuss the importance of following standardised procedures and of recording and reporting test results. Suggested content for a report format for standardised test administration is described. The chapter concludes with an example report for a standardised test administration. It will also endeavour to answer the following questions: 'How do I prepare for an efficient and effective test administration?', 'How do I build rapport with my client?', 'How do I ensure that my test administration remains standardised?' and 'How do I communicate the results of my assessment?'

There are eight steps in a rigorous test administration process. These steps are shown in Figure 8.1 below. This chapter provides information on some of these steps or directs the reader to other chapters in this book that deal with the other relevant steps of the process.

STEP 1: PREPARATION FOR TESTING

GAINING CONSENT TO ASSESS

Therapy is rarely as invasive or risky as many other medical procedures, such as general anaesthesia or drug treatments, but it can still be intrusive, stressful and tiring. Before undertaking an assessment or treatment intervention, occupational therapists and physiotherapists have to obtain consent and need to ensure that this consent is valid. Just because the person has signed a consent form does not guarantee that the consent was valid. To be valid, consent must be given voluntarily and with the full understanding and agreement of the proposed assessment or intervention. Clients must be given sufficient information to enable them to make an informed decision. The person must be able to understand and weigh up the information provided. The person must be given the space to act under his own free will. The therapist needs to be aware when consent is being given reluctantly, especially if this is under the influence of another person (and it is unimportant if this other person is a professional or relative). If the therapist suspects that the person's consent has been influenced, she should explain the procedure to the person again, offer him the opportunity to ask more questions and prompt him to raise any concerns. If in doubt, try to allow the person more space to decide and, where possible, raise your concerns about informed consent with colleagues, such as members of the multidisciplinary team. Consent can be given either verbally, non-verbally or in writing. Consent forms are used by some services (although

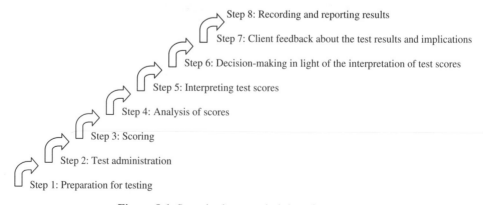

Step 8: Recording and reporting results

Step 7: Client feedback about the test results and implications

Step 6: Decision-making in light of the interpretation of test scores

Step 5: Interpreting test scores

Step 4: Analysis of scores

Step 3: Scoring

Step 2: Test administration

Step 1: Preparation for testing

Figure 8.1 Steps in the test administration process.

generally written consent forms are used for more invasive procedures, such as general an-aesthesia). Therapists should be aware that the person is able to withdraw consent at any time, even after signing a consent form. Before embarking on an assessment process and/or a specific test administration, you should take time to give the person details of the proposed assessment/measurement and to answer any questions the client may have. To gain informed consent, this discussion should include:

- the purpose of the proposed assessment/standardised test/measurement
- a description of how the assessment results will be used – especially talk about how any decisions or treatment plans will be guided by the results. Some assessments lead to de-cisions that have a very profound effect on the person's future life (e.g. results may lead to a decision that the person requires long-term care or a decision that he is no longer competent to drive)
- details of who will be given access to the results of the assessment/test/measurement and what form the results will take (e.g. 'a copy of the test form will be placed in your medical notes and will be seen by the doctors, nurses and therapists involved in your care' or 'a letter summarising the results will be sent to your GP')
- a description of what will be involved (e.g. an interview, observations or tasks to un-dertake). Particularly mention if the person will be required to remove clothing. If the person should be required to undress, a chaperone should be offered, especially if the person is the opposite sex to the therapist
- an explanation of who will be involved in the assessment: will it just be the therapist and client or is the therapist planning to interview/survey the person's spouse, children, other health professionals or social care providers, or a child's teacher?
- information about where the assessment/test/measure will be undertaken (e.g. 'we will need to go down to the therapy department' or 'I will come to assess you at home' or 'we will observe your son at school in his classroom')
- an estimate of how long the assessment/test/measure should take (e.g. 'it usually takes about 30 minutes to complete the tasks involved'). If it is going to be a lengthy assessment, let the person know that he can ask for a break if he starts to feel fatigued
- an explanation of why photographs or video might be taken; sometimes photographs and videos are taken as part of the assessment. This can be useful to monitor change over time and to demonstrate progress to the client. The purpose and proposed use of these must be explained to the person and their consent to use this media as part of the assessment must be gained.

Your clients should be given the opportunity to ask more questions about any proposed assess-ment and also be given more time to make the decision if they appear uncertain. The client may choose to agree to part but not all of the proposed assessment. For example, he may agree to be interviewed but not want to undertake standardised tests, he may be happy to be assessed on the ward or in the therapy department but not want a home assessment or he may not want you to interview a particular family member. Under these circumstances, you undertake the best assessment you can within the parameters agreed to by the client. If you use an assessment pathway in your service, you should document that the pathway was not completely followed in respect of the client's wishes and detail the parts of the pathway for which consent was not granted.

You may decide to develop a consent form for your therapy service. This may be to gain consent to administer a specific outcome measure or to seek consent to undertake a more ge-neric assessment process. For example, a consent form for a joint therapy service for children with physical disability might state:

Physiotherapy and occupational therapy assessments provide information that is evaluated by the physiotherapist and/or occupational therapist and assist in the determination of the need for therapy services, the planning of intervention and the monitoring of progress. The assessment of your child may include any or all of the following elements: use of standardised assessment tools (these are published and validated tests), a structured physical examination (including measurements of joint, range of movement, balance, gait and mobility and other manual activities) requiring that the therapist touch the child and in some cases requiring the child to remove some items of clothing, observation of the child doing everyday activities at home or at school (such as getting dressed, playing, preparing a snack, eating lunch, doing school work), interviews with the child, parents, family members and/or school staff and an examination of the child's equipment or equipment needs (such as wheelchairs, walkers, adapted desks etc.). Photographs and videotape may be taken as part of the assessment (for example to set a baseline and then monitor improvements in gait and mobility or to monitor a contracture during a course of splinting). Results of the assessments will be recorded in the child's therapy notes and a summary report will be sent to the referring doctor.

Once consent has been given, you should document this. If written consent has been obtained, include a copy of the consent form in the medical or therapy notes. If verbal or non-verbal consent is granted, then document that you have explained the reason for the assessment and described the procedure to be followed and that you have obtained consent. Also note that the person was given the opportunity to ask questions about the proposed assessment. Remember to sign and date your entry.

There are a few situations when informed consent cannot be sought or is not sought from the person. The therapist might be part of a multidisciplinary team assessment of an in-patient detained under the Mental Health Act (1983) or the person may not possess the cognitive capacity to understand what is proposed and make an informed decision as to whether or not to agree to the assessment. See the section on capacity assessment in Chapter 3 (pp. 107–9). The therapist will need to judge whether the client has the capacity to consent to the proposed physiotherapy and/or occupational therapy assessment and intervention. Adults are assumed to be competent unless it is demonstrated otherwise. For example, cognitive capacity might be reduced following a stroke, head injury or with the onset of dementia. If you have doubts about a person's competence to give consent, then ask yourself: 'Can this person understand and weigh up all the information required to make this decision?' If cognitive capacity might be an issue, the therapist should consult with medical colleagues and a formal evaluation of capacity may need to be made before the proposed assessment can proceed. Cognitive capacity is not a clear-cut issue: a person may be competent to make some decisions, such as whether to talk to a therapist or allow the therapist to observe him prepare a meal, but not others, such as whether to have an internal investigation involving general anaesthesia with the full knowledge of the potential risk of a negative outcome. The more complex the decision and the greater potential for negative outcomes, the greater the degree of cognitive competency required for informed decision-making. Where a person no longer has the cognitive capacity to provide informed consent, the therapist should check whether the person has made a statement of advanced wishes, a so-called living will or an advanced refusal for a particular intervention. Where this is available, it should be used to judge whether the person would have wanted the proposed assessment/intervention. No one can give consent on behalf of an individual who has been assessed as incompetent to consent, but family members may have useful information about the person's advanced wishes that can assist in making a decision in the person's best interest. Best interests refer to the person's wishes and beliefs when he was still cognitively competent related to his well-being, his medical state and his spiritual and religious beliefs.

If a person feels unable to make a decision about consent, or feels unhappy about an assessment being undertaken without him fully understanding what is involved, then the

Patient Advocacy and Liaison Service (PALS) may be of some help. The person might also be put in touch with an advocate, for example some voluntary agencies provide advocacy for people with specific conditions and some parts of the country have local advocacy services. There are also some national advocacy groups that can be helpful for clients and their families, such as the National Youth Advocacy Service (NYAS), which is a UK charity that advocates children's rights and provides social and legal services, and Rethink Advocacy Services, which works alongside people with mental illness to provide them with impartial, independent information regarding choices available and encourages people to express their own views, needs and choices (http://www.rethink.org/services/advocacy.html, accessed 1.04.06). The Department of Health (DoH) has produced guidelines for clients on consent, for an example see *Consent: what you have a right to expect: a guide for adults* (Department of Health, 2001b).

It is very important to remember that obtaining consent is rarely a one-off process, particularly if you will be working with the client over a period of time. Each time you undertake a new assessment or intervention, you should fully explain what you propose to do and gain consent for that specific assessment/intervention. When undertaking a reassessment, it is good practice to remind the person of the rationale for the original and follow-up assessment and to double-check that the person still consents to this assessment.

TEST SELECTION

Advice on how to select the best test(s) for your client and service is provided in Chapter 11.

ORGANISING THE ENVIRONMENT

The environment and conditions required for an optimum assessment will depend on the purpose of the assessment, the person and the nature of any presenting problems. In the section on the influence of environment on performance in Chapter 1 (pp. 39–42), I discussed how familiarity with an environment may influence assessment results. People will usually behave differently in a familiar environment, such as their home, workplace or school, than in an unfamiliar therapy department, ward or day hospital setting. But assessment in a familiar environment is not always possible or necessary.

Wherever the assessment is to be undertaken, the therapist should ensure the basics are addressed. These include that:

- the room is accessible to the client and any carer who may also be attending the assessment (e.g. lift if not on the ground floor, doorways wide enough for wheelchair or walking aids, clearly signposted – especially if it is in a large district hospital)
- the room is free from hazards, such as a slippery floor, loose mats, toxic substances or potentially dangerous equipment
- there is sufficient room for the person to move around in to the degree required for the assessment
- any furniture or large equipment to be used is appropriate (e.g. the correct height or adjustable-height chair, table, bed, commode, frame)
- there is good lighting; this is particularly important if the person has any visual impairment and/or the task has a visual component, such as reading, writing, drawing or construction
- the room is a comfortable temperature for the nature of the assessment; it will need to be warmer if the person has to undress for a physical assessment
- you have taken steps to limit interruptions (e.g. you put an 'Assessment in progress – please do not interrupt' notice on the door, have turned your mobile phone off or to silent/vibrate or turned the phone onto answerphone and the ringer volume down)

- you have ensured the required level of privacy (e.g. curtains pulled round a cubicle or bed provide visual privacy but the person can still be heard by others outside the curtain)
- if a parent or carer is to be present there is sufficient space and a suitable chair for them to sit on.

If the person has any hearing loss or the assessment requires a significant degree of concentration, then background noise levels should be considered and limited. Remember to check whether the person usually wears a hearing aid, and if so ensure that it is with them and in good working order and switched on. If the person has any visual impairment, the therapist will need to check whether visual aids (contact lenses, glasses, magnifying glass) are used, and ensure that these are clean and being worn. The assessment setting should be well lit and the therapist should check there is no glare. For example, a shiny, white table top might reflect a long strip light and the glare could impede the person's ability to read instructions, fill out a survey or see test materials. Also be aware of the impact of colour uniformity versus colour contrast, for example a white paper on a white table top may be difficult for the person to see. In a home setting, check what lighting the person would normally have on during the task to be observed and assess first with this level of lighting and then if necessary increase the lighting and see if this has an impact on function.

PREPARING TOOLS, MATERIALS AND EQUIPMENT

It is really important to be well organised ahead of any assessment. Allow time for setting up, not just for organising the environment but for ensuring you have the required tools, materials and equipment for the assessment. This means you will be organised and professional, and it will save unnecessary time wasting during the assessment. Ask yourself the following questions.

- Do you need a checklist, test form, blank/lined paper?
- If it is a standardised test, do you have the instructions and/or questions?
- Have you got pens/pencils etc. for you and if relevant for the client – are these working/sharp?
- Do you need a stopwatch or calculator; if so, is the battery working?
- If you are administering a battery of tests, are all the component parts present and in their correct bags/places?
- Do you need ingredients for a cooking assessment?
- If you are assessing the suitability of an aid, do you have the right one or a range of models to try out?

TIMING YOUR ASSESSMENT

Think about the optimum time for conducting your assessment and try to schedule the assessment accordingly. The optimum time will mostly be when the person is able to perform at his best. However, sometimes you may need to evaluate what the person can manage when his performance is at its most compromised, for example when he is fatigued at the end of the day or when the effects of medication are wearing off just before the next dose is taken. You may need this information to judge level of risk or the maximum level of care the person will need. If you are not able to conduct the assessment at the optimum time for the purpose of the assessment, be aware of how a different timing could change the results and remember to take this into account and document any changes. When thinking about optimum timing, consider the following factors.

- Does the person's function fluctuate because of medication?
- Is the person more agitated at a particular time of day?
- Does the person tire easily; if so, what will he be doing before the planned assessment?
- When is the environment you plan to use for the assessment available and when is it most free from interruptions and background noise?

- If a carer, parent, teacher or other care provider is required for the assessment, when are they available?

Lewis and Bottomley (1994) discuss the timing of assessment in relation to mealtimes and recommend that undertaking assessment immediately following a large meal is contraindicated because there is a 'decrease in blood flow to the brain for one hour after a large meal' (p. 290), and they say this is a particular issue for older patients.

CLARIFYING EXPECTATIONS

It is important to be aware of your own expectations. To ensure the client's expectations of the assessment are realistic, you must be very clear about the purpose, nature and format of any planned assessment with the client and, if appropriate, the carer. If you have ensured that the person has sufficient information to provide informed consent for the proposed assessment or measurement, then you are likely to have ensured that the person's expectations about the purpose and nature of the assessment are realistic. Your expectations as to how long you will be able to conduct the assessment for and what you will be able to undertake also need to be realistic, and these will depend on the person (age, diagnosis, anticipated impairments and stamina) and the environment. If you are changing work from one client group to another or from one service to another, your expectations about the timing, nature or pacing of an assessment will almost certainly need to adjust accordingly. This can take time and lead to some initial frustrations. When you are a visitor in a person's home, or at a child's school or client's workplace, you need to allow time for some informal conversation and never forget the fact that you are the visitor. The person may want to give you a guided tour or it may be their culture to serve you a drink or food before you can proceed with a more formal interview or assessment. You may arrive at the environment to discover that you do not have the furniture, equipment or space to conduct the assessment as planned. Therapists have to be flexible.

STEP 2: TEST ADMINISTRATION

DEVELOPING RAPPORT

Rapport is a critical ingredient to ensuring your assessment process or test administration is effective and efficient. But what exactly do we mean by rapport? Rapport should be understood, within the context of a therapy assessment process, to be the ability of the therapist to put the person at his ease by building a relationship based on mutual understanding and empathy. Thus rapport can also be understood as a means of facilitating a person's cooperation with the assessment process by encouraging a conscious feeling of trust in the therapist.

Rapport is very important to ensure a successful assessment. If the person is going to be required to share personal information and feelings, then he is going to need to trust and respect his therapist. Test anxiety can have a big impact on test results and can be alleviated by a good therapeutic relationship. Therefore, it is important to think about the need for developing rapport and to plan strategies for how you will build rapport with the person and, if relevant, the carer, both before and during an assessment. Mosey (1981) identifies the *conscious use of self* as a key therapeutic tool: 'conscious use of self involves a planned interaction with another person in order to alleviate fear or anxiety; provide reassurance; obtain necessary information; give advice; and assist the other individual to gain more appreciation, expression, and functional use of his or her latent inner resources' (p. 95). Developing a therapeutic relationship involves the conscious use of self to build and maintain rapport with the client. There are a number of techniques that a therapist can apply to facilitate building rapport; these include pacing and leading attention by matching, mirroring or cross pacing verbal and non-verbal behaviours (see bullet list below). Many of these techniques are described in literature on neurolinguistic programming (NLP).

For example, see Clabby and O'Connor's (2004) article on teaching medical students to use physical and verbal mirroring techniques from NLP for building rapport with patients.

- Physical mirroring: Physical mirroring requires the conscious and subtle use of body language to place a client at his ease. It is important to differentiate between imitating and mirroring. Overt imitation might make a person feel mocked and can decrease rapport. Mirroring is much more subtle. It might involve using the same gesture or tilting your head to a similar angle of the client's. If sitting opposite the client, you should echo the person's movements so that your position will look similar to the person's if he were looking in a mirror. For example, if the client crosses his right leg over his left, the therapist sitting opposite would cross her left leg over her right. The therapist should leave a little time (seconds to minutes) before mirroring the client's movements and should try to make her position and movements seem as natural as possible (Clabby and O'Connor, 2004).
- Eye contact: the use of eye contact is very important to building rapport. The amount of eye contact the therapist should use will vary depending on what is culturally acceptable for the client. In general, maintaining eye contact is helpful for conveying that the therapist is actively listening to the client.
- Verbal mirroring: Verbal mirroring requires the conscious use of word selection, pace of communication and tone of voice. With verbal mirroring, the therapist tries to echo the person's tone of voice and exactly repeats the person's last phrase or word. It can also be helpful to repeat the phrase or word with a questioning inflection (Clabby and O'Connor, 2004), thus inviting the person to clarify that that was what he meant or to elaborate on what was said. For example, an interview between a therapist and client might go:

> THERAPIST: Do you have any problems with getting dressed?
> CLIENT: No! I can get dressed just fine on my own.
> THERAPIST: OK, you can get dressed fine on your own. Can you bathe or shower on your own too?
> CLIENT: I can manage, but I'm a bit scared.
> THERAPIST: You can manage, but you're a bit scared?
> CLIENT: Yes, I'm scared I'm going to slip and fall again.
> THERAPIST: You're scared you are going to slip and fall again? What happened when you slipped and fell?

- Pace: In addition to mirroring the client's choice of words, mirroring the pace of a client's speech can also aid communication. If the client is speaking fast, with energy and animation, then the therapist should mirror this communication pace and style with quick, animated responses. However, if a client speaks slowly and quietly and leaves gaps between sentences, then the therapist should likewise speak slowly and softly and allow gaps between questions, phrases or sentences.
- Breathing rhythm: Some expert therapists will also adjust their breathing rhythm to match the client's.

USE OF METAPHORS IN BUILDING RAPPORT

People often speak in metaphors to describe their feelings and experiences. Therapists are becoming more aware of how the conscious exploration of metaphors can help build rapport and facilitate an understanding of the person's perspective on his condition or problem (Lawley and Thompkins, 2000). A metaphor is a direct comparison between two or more seemingly unrelated subjects. The metaphor is used because the person associates implicit and/or explicit attributes from the concept to the subject he is discussing. Examples of metaphors include 'I've got butterflies in my stomach' and 'There's a black cloud hanging over me.'

Clients particularly use metaphors to explain feelings (such as pain, anxiety, depression, grief) and experiences (such as discrimination, dependence and loss). Therapists need to be attuned to the use of metaphors because they are not throw-away comments. People often use leading phrases, such as 'You know it's like . . .?' The therapist should pay particular attention to the description the person puts in the '. . .', because this is the metaphor, and the choice of metaphor will have significant meaning for the client. Expert therapists learn to 'converse within the frame of the metaphor' (Lawley and Thompkins, 2000). One technique used by therapists to unpackage metaphors are Clean Language questions. Clean Language questions are simple questions that follow a particular syntax and delivery. The questions are used to prompt and encourage clients to use and explore metaphor to describe their symptoms and problems. Clean Language has been described by James Lawley and Penny Thompkins (1997), who developed the Metaphor Model and related Clean Language questions after studying the work of David Grove, a therapist from New Zealand. Clean Language is applied to both validate the client's experience and facilitate the description and exploration of the person's symbolic ideas, which are normally out of the person's explicit everyday awareness. The aim of using Clean Language early in a therapeutic relationship is to allow an understanding of the client's problems and symptoms to emerge into the client's awareness by exploring *his* coding of *his* metaphor.

Lawley and Thompkins (1997) describe nine basic Clean Language questions, each of which has a specific purpose for facilitating the client to unpackage and understand his use of metaphor further. Two questions are used to request information about the metaphoric symbol's attributes:

1. And is there anything else about . . . ? (For example: 'Is there anything else about that sharp knife?')
2. And what kind of . . . is that . . . ? (For example: 'And what kind of black cloud is that black cloud?' from which the therapist may obtain more information about how big, dark or constant that 'black cloud' feels to the client.)

Two questions are used to ask for locational information:

3. And where is . . . ? (For example: 'And where is that black cloud hanging above you?' which could help the client identify whether this 'black cloud' feels very oppressively just above his head or much further away up in the sky.)
4. And whereabouts? (For example: 'And whereabouts are the butterflies in your stomach?' which may help the therapist understand whether the person feels this 'butterflies' sensation in a very specific spot or more generalised over the centre of his body.)

Two questions which reference the future (from the client's perceptual present) are:

5. And what happens next? (For example: 'And what happens next when you feel butterflies in your stomach?' might prompt the person to describe his feelings of mounting anxiety further: 'And then I start to feel the butterflies are fluttering up my throat and I think I'm going to be sick.')
6. And then what happens? (For example: 'And then what happens after the sharp knife repeatedly stabs you?' can help the therapist to understand whether the pain sensation continues or how the person feels when it stops: 'It feels like I'm stabbed again and again for an eternity and I wait in agony for it to stop.')

Two questions which reference the past are:

7. And what happens just before . . . ? (For example: 'And what happens just before you get but-terflies in your stomach?' can help the therapist understand what triggers the sensation.)
8. And where does/could . . . come from? (For example: 'And where does that black cloud come from?' could prompt a wide variety of responses: 'It comes down from the sky', 'It comes out of my head', 'It just appears out of nowhere.')

The last question offers the client the opportunity to make a lateral, and therefore metaphorical, shift in perception:

9. And that's . . . like what? (For example: 'And that butterflies in the stomach is like what?' could lead to further descriptions of sensations: 'It's like a gentle fluttering feeling' or 'It's like lots of wings beating fast to get out' to the use of an alternative metaphor: 'It's like lots of worms wriggling inside me.')

Some of the techniques described above take considerable practice in order for them to become a refined and habitual part of the therapist's conscious use of self. However, some very simple actions can also help to build rapport. For example, it can be useful to make a phone call to book an assessment yourself, as opposed to delegating this to a team secretary. Ten minutes spent popping up to see a person on the ward the day before you bring him down to the therapy department for an hour's worth of standardised testing can also be ten minutes well spent. You can use this time to explain the proposed purpose, nature and format of the assessment and ob-tain informed consent, and this more informal time can help to build rapport and trust between therapist and client. It can also be helpful to collect a person yourself, for example from the ward or waiting area, and use the time walking down the corridor or waiting for a lift to chat informally and put the person at his ease.

USING STANDARDISED TESTS

Prior to using any new standardised test, therapists should take enough time to 'be fully conversant with the test content, use, reliability and validity before administering the test in order that this is done correctly and that any interpretation of test findings be accurate' (Jones, 1991, p. 179). In addition to reading the test manual and examining the test materials and forms, it can be very helpful to role play test administration with a colleague to familiarise oneself with the test materials and instructions before undertaking the test with a client.

FOLLOWING STANDARDISED PROCEDURES

Chapter 5 defined what is meant by a standardised test and discussed the advantages of using standardised tools. In particular, the use of standardised tests can facilitate objectivity, and this is very important because it is virtually impossible to obtain complete accuracy and objectivity when assessing human functioning. Any standardised assessment should have detailed instruc-tions detailing how and when it should be administered and scored, and how to interpret scores. You should not consider modifying a test in any way unless you are prepared to go through vali-dation and reliability studies again. This is very time-consuming and should not be undertaken lightly (Pynsent, 2004). Following standardised procedures means that you should:

- follow instructions exactly
- repeat instructions to be given to the client word for word
- use the standardised materials and forms provided
- follow precisely the instructions for the test environment, conditions and equipment that should be used.

USE OF PROMPTING AND CUES

The majority of standardised tests have verbal and/or visual instructions. Some standardised tests permit the repetition of instructions and allow the use of prompts and/or cues, but many do not. Most test protocols define, and therefore impose, limitations on the phrasing and repetition of instructions. Sometimes a person may not understand your standardised instruction. You need to have established in advance whether the repetition of instructions or the use of prompts and cues is permissible with that particular test. Many standardised instruction formats do not account for people with multisensory deficits. If instructions are not heard or seen correctly, then the purpose of the task can be misunderstood; the client could fail the test item as a result of limited comprehension. In such cases, the individual could be considered to have a deficit in the area evaluated by the test item and this could lead to unreliable test results. For example, the Rivermead Perceptual Assessment Battery (RPAB; Whiting *et al.*, 1985) involves the timing of the written and drawn subtests. Many people with stroke (who are a primary population for this test) experience hemiparesis to an upper limb; in some cases, this affects a previously dominant hand. In these circumstances, the client has to perform the subtests using a non-dominant hand to hold the pen. As assessment usually occurs as soon as possible after diagnosis, and precedes intervention, the person rarely has had an opportunity to practise writing with the non-dominant hand prior to testing. Therefore, many people were found to fail these tests as a consequence of the length of time taken rather than actual ability (Crammond, Clark and Smith, 1989). Further limitations to the RPAB include the difficulty of administering the test to clients with severe cognitive impairment (short-term memory, attention and concentration are required) or aphasia. The formality of the test administration procedures increases test anxiety and can have a detrimental effect on performance. Many older clients have visual and auditory acuity loss as a result of ageing. The RPAB protocol does not permit the repetition of instructions or the use of additional verbal and visual cues; some clients fail subtests as they do not comprehend the instructions. Furthermore, the colour-matching task has been criticised (Laver, 1990). There is poor differentiation between the colours of some items on the tasks. Colour vision alters with ageing owing to yellowing of the lens; this affects the perception of the blue/green end of the spectrum. RPAB involves the differentiation of several pieces in blue and green shades. Many older clients failed this subtest but could name and point to colours on command. The task requires more complex functioning than the simple identification of colour.

The use of prompts and non-verbal cues is particularly important for some client groups, for example people with communication difficulties associated with problems with visual and auditory acuity, learning disability or cognitive impairment. The use of prompts, cues and repeated instructions may even be part of what is scored on the test, particularly in tests of comprehension and cognitive functioning, for example see the Severe Impairment Battery (SIB; Saxton *et al.*, 1993). Therapists working with people with dementia often need to identify which type(s) of prompts and cues are most successful in supporting the person to achieve maximum functioning.

Hilko Culler (1993) provides an overview of the types of prompts and cues that might be provided. These include:

- printed materials (e.g. prompt cards, written instructions, diagrams and photographs)
- tactile cueing by touching the person to modify or guide their performance (e.g. the therapist could touch the client's lower back to encourage a more upright posture or touch the client's arm to remind him to use a hemiplegic limb following a stroke)
- verbal prompts to repeat the original instruction or guide the person further in the performance of the test item or task
- visual prompts, such as pointing.

Hilko Culler (1993) also breaks verbal cues into two categories: direct cues and indirect cues. She provides an example of the observation of a shopping assessment: 'a direct cue provides the patient with a specific instruction, such as "the spaghetti is here" [while] an indirect cue provides assistance to the patient in a less directive manner, such as "can you find the foods listed on your [shopping] list?" ' (p. 218). In any assessment, whether it is standardised or informal, therapists should record the number and nature of any repeated instructions or supervision, prompts or cues provided. Some tests allow for physical assistance and include a score to represent that physical assistance was provided. The nature and amount of physical assistance should be described in sufficient detail so that another therapist repeating the assessment could ascertain whether more or less physical assistance was given during retesting. Therapists should also record any equipment or environmental modifications made to the prescribed testing method that may affect the test results.

STEP 3: SCORING

When a scoring system has been specified, then a therapist must use it. Pynsent (2004) notes that 'inventing a new system will make the results incomparable, and also greatly detract from the value and efforts made to collect the data' (p. 6). Therapists should also ensure that the instructions for dealing with and recording missing data are followed (Pynsent, 2004). Examples of different types of scoring systems are provided for each of the four levels of measurement (nominal, ordinal, interval and ratio) in Chapter 4, along with a discussion about scoring issues.

STEP 4: ANALYSIS OF SCORES

Where the therapist needs to convert a raw score, for example by referring to normative data, she needs to ensure that she selects the correct table for reference. Where individual test item scores need to be totalled to provide a summary score, the therapist needs to ensure that this addition it accurate. Some standardised tests provide recommendations based on test results, and the scoring method may involve cross-checking the score with a cut-off point that indicates the requirement for further testing or referral to another service.

STEP 5: INTERPRETING TEST SCORES

Test scores are rarely sufficient on their own and must be interpreted within the wider context of the specific testing situation, the influences of the test environment and the client's current situation and personal idiosyncrasies (de Clive-Lowe, 1996). Therapists should not just report results; rather, to add value, a therapist should offer an interpretation of what these results mean in context. The therapist needs to pose a series of questions when examining test scores, such as:

- 'Do I think these scores are a true reflection of the person's function?'
- 'If not, did test anxiety, fatigue, lack of motivation, distractions etc. influence the test results?'
- 'How do these scores compare with other data I have collected about this person (e.g. through interview, proxy report, non-standardised observations)?'
- 'Is there consistency in the data or discrepancies in the picture I am building about this person's ability and needs?'

STEP 6: DECISION-MAKING IN LIGHT OF THE INTERPRETATION OF TEST SCORES

Information on decision-making and diagnostic reasoning is provided in Chapter 10.

STEP 7: CLIENT FEEDBACK ABOUT THE TEST RESULTS AND IMPLICATIONS

It is very important that you share the results and your interpretations of assessment data with the client and, where appropriate, also with the carer. This should be done in a way that the client and carer can easily comprehend; so therapists must be aware of the need to avoid professional jargon and explain any abbreviations or technical or theoretical terms. This feedback enables the client and carer to understand the relevance of the assessment process, the nature of the problems that have been identified and to make informed choices and become actively involved in decision-making about any further assessment, intervention or care package.

STEP 8: RECORDING AND REPORTING RESULTS

It should be remembered that a good test administration is just a beginning and it is critical to document and interpret the results and to share the conclusions drawn from the assessment with the client and other relevant personnel. When reporting on standardised test results, the therapist should state the rationale for administering this particular standardised test. In the report, the therapist should also include a description of the person's responses to and behaviour during testing (for example whether the person was anxious, if he complied with requests or was restricted by pain or fatigue). These additional qualitative observations will provide a context for the therapist's hypotheses about the meaning of the test scores (de Clive-Lowe, 1996). Suggested headings for reporting on a standardised test administration is provided below and an example test report is provided on pp. 228–32.

SUGGESTED HEADINGS FOR A STANDARDISED TEST ADMINISTRATION REPORT

Personal Details Client's name, date of birth, age, diagnoses, address.

Date(s) of Assessment It is important to give the date of an initial assessment and any re-assessment. If appropriate, also state the time of day. For example, if one test was given first thing in the morning and the re-assessment was conducted in the afternoon, fluctuating levels of fatigue or stiffness might influence the test results.

Referral Information The name of the person who made the referral. The reason for referral should influence the selection of assessment focus and methods and have implications for how the test results are interpreted. For example, the referral might be a request to assess the person's safety to be discharged home.

Relevant Background Information Brief information relevant to the selection and interpretation of the assessment, for example the person's occupational history, hobbies and interests, medication (especially if this leads to varying function) and how the person came to be in the present situation. In the example of a home safety assessment, details such as whether the person lives alone would be useful to include here.

Previous Assessment Results (if any) Previous assessment might influence the choice of current assessment and also will be useful for comparison to interpret whether the person's function has improved or deteriorated. If no previous assessment data are available, state 'none known'.

Reason for this Assessment State your rationale for assessing this client with this test at this time. How does this assessment fit into the overall therapeutic process or service pathway? Do you need descriptive, discriminative, predictive and/or evaluative assessment data?

Test(s) Administered State the title of the test(s) given and provide a brief description of the test and its purpose. This is particularly important if the person reading the report is not familiar with the test(s) used.

Behaviour During Testing Describe any behaviour that might have influenced the test results. This information is needed so that anyone reading the report can decide whether the results represent a reliable estimate of the person's ability. Keep descriptions as concise and objective as possible. Include information about apparent fatigue, anxiety, level of cooperation with testing, ability to follow instructions, any distractions or interruptions to the test etc.

Results Give a concise summary of the results. If appropriate, attach a copy of the assessment form and/or summary table or graph to the report. If any parts of the test were not assessed, make a note of this and state the reasons for the omission. If using percentile or standard scores, state which norms have been used so that anyone reassessing the person can use the same norms for future comparison (for example give date of test manual and the page reference for the table). This is very important where there are several editions of an assessment with updated normative data.

Discussion Consider what the results of the assessment mean, whether the results represent a reliable picture of the person's function and hypothesise about what might account for the results. Relate the discussion back to the reason for referral. Give brief examples of observable behaviour and/or specific test results to justify your reasoning. Also refer back to the 'Behaviour during testing' section if this has a bearing on how the results should be interpreted.

Recommendations These should derive directly from the assessment results and should relate back to the reason for the referral and the person's current situation. This may include the need for further assessment to confirm provisional hypotheses. If you recommend further intervention, give timelines and state an appropriate time for re-assessment in order to monitor progress. This may also involve referral to other professionals or services for further assessment, intervention or care packages. Consider whether this same test could be used as an outcome measure to monitor the effectiveness of the proposed intervention. If not, then note that another assessment will be required for monitoring progress during intervention and for measuring final outcomes and recommend an appropriate measure (if possible).

GROUP ANALYSES

It can be useful to aggregate data for groups of clients who have been tested on a particular measure. This can be of particular value when reviewing the appropriateness of referrals or examining outcomes from a specific intervention (see the section on service evaluation in Chapter 3, pp. 116–32). Pynsent (2004) also notes that feedback and the sharing of group results can encourage staff compliance with the administration of a measure, as they can see the benefit to the client group as a whole and to the service.

RECORD KEEPING

Therapists are required to maintain detailed and accurate records of any assessment, plan, intervention, care package and of the person's condition over time. The Chartered Society of Physiotherapy (CSP; 2000) states that a record is anything which contains information (in any media) that has been created or gathered as a result of any aspect of the therapist's work. A 'record may contain information about the current episode of care only, or may be a compilation of every episode of care for that individual' (Chartered Society of Physiotherapy, 2000, p. 2). The College of Occupational Therapists (COT; 2003b) requires all occupational therapy personnel, whatever their clinical setting, to maintain records of 'all occupational therapy activity and intervention made with, or on behalf of, the service user' (p. 35). While the CSP (2000) states: 'record keeping is a professional requirement of all physiotherapy practice and requires specific skills. Failure to maintain a physiotherapy record would cause considerable difficulties in respect of any legal proceedings, e.g. allegations of negligence' (p. 2).

The COT draws therapists' attention to DoH regulations on record keeping (Department of Health, 1999b). Accurate records are an essential part of the provision of evidence-based therapy and support effective clinical decision-making, improve client care through a clear communication of the intervention rationale and progress and facilitate a consistent approach to team working and continuity of care. Records are also required to meet legal requirements, including requests from clients to access their own records and in cases of complaint or litigation. When therapists are working with increasing demands, such as heavy caseloads and waiting-list pressures, record keeping can be delayed or compromised. A record is only useful if it is correctly recorded in the first place, regularly updated and easily accessible when it is needed (Chartered Society for Physiotherapy, 2000). Therapists should remember that record keeping is a useful and critical part of an assessment process and not just a tedious requirement. Sitting down to write a report or note in the person's records provides time to reflect upon and summarise the assessment or standardised test process and results. Accurate records serve a number of important functions (College of Occupational Therapists, 2006); they:

- provide an objective basis to determine the appropriateness of, need for and effectiveness of intervention
- demonstrate the practitioner's professional reasoning and the rationale behind any care provided (see Chapter 10 for more information on clinical reasoning)
- highlight problems and changes in the person's condition at an early stage
- facilitate better communication and dissemination of information between members of health and social care teams
- protect the welfare of clients by promoting high standards of care (p. 2).

Some services require therapists to follow a set format for record keeping. One example is SOAP notes. SOAP stands for:

- S = subjective
- O = objective
- A = assessment (the analysis of data to formulate an understanding of the client's problems)
- P = plan (for intervention/management/treatment).

Pynsent (2004) defines *subjective* as 'pertaining to a perceived condition within the patient's own consciousness' (p. 3) and *objective* as 'a condition of the mind or body as perceived by another' (p. 3). Standardised test scores would be reported as objective entries. Comments that the client has made about the standardised testing experience, for example 'I'm feeling very tired today', would be recorded as subjective entries, while the therapist's interpretation of the test scores within the wider context of her knowledge of the client, the testing environment and circumstances would be recorded as an assessment entry. SOAP notes were described briefly in Chapter 2 (p. 67). Box 2.1 (p. 68) provides an example of a SOAP note entry.

ELECTRONIC CARE RECORDS

Nowadays, records are not necessarily paper-based; rather, many services operate an electronic care records system (Garner and Rugg, 2005). The DoH (1998c) states that paper records resulted in demanding storage requirements and were difficult to retrieve efficiently when needed. In contrast, electronic records were seen as a way to reduce bureaucracy and support more effective and efficient health care. The CSP and COT jointly commissioned an information management project between October 1998 and April 1999 that resulted in the the Garner Report (named after the project's principal investigator Ruth Garner). 'The report identified information management as central to the professions for their clinical practice and for legal, management and academic purposes. It brought together policy context, details about national programmes and an overview of information management needs of both physiotherapists and occupational therapists. The report contained seven key recommendations:

1. Formalise links with the NHS Information Authority.
2. Invest in a centre of excellence for the professions allied to medicine.
3. Make information management more meaningful.
4. Undertake further work on record structures.
5. Provide support, information and advice to members about the development of the Electronic Patient Record (EPR).
6. Develop an information literate, competent and confident workforce.
7. Support the National Electronic library for Health (NeLH)' (Chartered Society of Physiotherapy, 2006a).

CONFIDENTIALITY

'The principles of good management of records apply equally to records created electronically. Any part of any record held on computer must comply with the Data Protection Act (1998) and a procedure must be in place for patients to access their records' (Chartered Society of Physiotherapy, 2000, p. 4). The DoH states:

> One of the main issues in relation to patient records, which applies whether or not [they are] electronically recorded, is patient confidentiality. Issues of confidentiality [are] particularly important in the context of electronic records because of the increased scope for reproduction and dissemination. The recommendations of the . . . Caldicott review reinforce the requirement for adequate safeguards to exist and be maintained. Guidance on this has been issued by the Department in March 1996 (The Protection and Use of Patient Information HSG(96)18). Whilst the guidance does not specifically deal with electronically recorded information, the same principles apply. (Department of Health, 1998c, p. 4)

CASE STUDY: JAMES'S ASSESSMENT OF MOTOR AND PROCESS SKILLS (AMPS) REPORT

By Rachel Hargreaves

ABOUT THE THERAPIST

The therapist completing the assessment and report has worked as an occupational therapist for eight years, practising in a variety of clinical settings including neurology and mental health services for working-age adults and older adults. She had been an Assessment of Motor and Process Skills (AMPS; Fisher 2003a) calibrated therapist for 18 months before performing the assessment. The AMPS is an assessment that is used in the multidisciplinary specialist memory clinic service and also in the community mental health team (CMHT) for older adults in which she is based.

TEST REPORT

ASSESSMENT OF MOTOR AND PROCESS SKILLS (AMPS)

NAME: James

AGE: ••

DIAGNOSES: Parkinson's disease
Bowel cancer, treated surgically three years ago
Under investigation for cognitive impairment

REFERRED BY: Memory Clinic Consultant Psychiatrist

ASSESSED BY: Memory Clinic Occupational Therapist

DATE OF ASSESSMENT: •• •• ••

REASON FOR REFERRAL

- Assessment of performance in activities of daily living (ADL).
- Identification of areas of ability and deficit in ADL.
- Recognition of areas that would benefit from restorative interventions using occupation and adaptation.

REFERRAL INFORMATION

James has an 11-year history of Parkinson's disease, with a one-year history of visual hallucinations and gradually deteriorating memory. All physical causes for memory problems have been ruled out by his GP prior to the referral to the memory clinic. Referred for multidisciplinary team assessment as per memory clinic protocol, with a view to introduction of cholinesterase inhibiters in line with NICE guidance. The occupational therapy assessment is identified as being required because of James's physical health difficulties, along with problems with his memory, which are increasing his dependency on his carer. The referral requests that other appropriate interventions to assist James and his wife with community living are explored.

RELEVANT BACKGROUND INFORMATION

James has lived with his supportive wife in their isolated owner-occupied, three-bedroom, detached property for the last four years. After their retirement, both James and his wife were active members in the local community, being volunteers for several community services. They have found it difficult adjusting to being 'on the other side', and they have resisted asking for help themselves until this time.

Up until the memory clinic appointment, the only service they had accessed was a respite stay for James in a local residential home. James's wife is considering a similar arrangement to allow her to take a holiday with friends later this year, owing to increasing levels of carer stress.

James spends the majority of his time in his bedroom, sitting on the bed watching television. His room is en suite, with a raised toilet seat/free-standing toilet frame *in situ*. He prefers to use the shower in the house bathroom.

PREVIOUS ASSESSMENT RESULTS

Mini Mental State Examination (MMSE) score 24/30. No previous multidisciplinary team assessments completed; no specific occupational therapy assessments, including AMPS, administered.

REASONS FOR USE OF THE AMPS

The AMPS was selected by the specialist occupational therapy team within the memory clinic as the best researched and most robust available tool to measure ADL qualities/deficits in older people reporting cognitive impairment. The occupational therapist who picked up James's referral identified that the AMPS would provide data regarding James's possible process deficits owing to his memory problems and would also illustrate the impact of his Parkinson's disease on his motor skills.

TEST ADMINISTERED

The AMPS (Fisher 2003a, 2003b) is an observational assessment enabling simultaneous evaluation of motor and process skill areas. Motor skills are those observable actions enabling a person to move himself or to manipulate and move objects that are required to complete an activity or task. Process skills are the observable actions that are used to logically organise and adapt behaviour in order to complete a task. The person chooses two or three daily-living tasks to perform, is observed carrying them out and then rated by the occupational therapist. The results are computer-analysed to provide profiles of performance and measures for motor and process skill ability.

The cut-off points on the AMPS motor skill scale (2.0 logits $+/-0.3$ logits) and AMPS process skill scale (1.0 logits $+/-0.3$ logits) are the levels at which the skill deficit begins to affect the performance of daily-living tasks. The majority of people at this level begin to experience difficulties with independent community living. Logits are equal-interval units of measurement that are based on the logarithm of the odds – also called log-odds probability units (Fisher, 2003a). In the case of the AMPS, a logit describes 'the logarithm of the odds of obtaining a given skill item score when a person of a given ability is observed performing a given task' (p. 34).

The tasks negotiated with James for completion within the AMPS contract were:

1. P-4: putting on socks and shoes
2. P-2: brushing teeth.

Both the tasks chosen for the AMPS test administration were within the 'very easy' and 'much easier than average' categories. They were selected as the tasks that were performed regularly. Owing to his Parkinsonian symptoms, James had identified that he limited his performance of ADL.

BEHAVIOUR DURING TESTING

Throughout the assessment, there was no evidence of psychotic symptoms. James cooperated with the occupational therapist throughout the assessment, including negotiating the tasks and then the completion of both tasks. He reflected on feelings of self-worth and purposefulness in being encouraged to undertake tasks to his own standards as opposed to relying on others, which had caused subsequent feelings of powerlessness.

RESULTS

James scored -1.16 logits on the AMPS motor skills scale, which demonstrates a severe level of impairment, with the cut-off being 2.0 logits. He scored 0.07 logits on the process skills scale, which is well below the cut-off point of 1.0 logits. In motor skills areas, a moderate level of disruption was noted throughout all skills, except the items of 'flows' and 'calibrates', where there was a marked disruption.

In process skill areas, James demonstrated no deficit in chooses, heeds, inquires, continues, sequences, searches, gathers and restores. In the remaining 12 areas, there was evidence of moderate disruption, specifically 'energy' and 'adaptation' (the ability to appropriately respond to and modify actions in an environment, to overcome problems and/or prevent them occurring).

DISCUSSION

The results show that James experiences difficulties with both motor and process skills, which affect his ability to perform independent community living. The motor skills score indicate that James needs physical support when completing ADL. James's wife is currently providing this physical assistance, but finding this increasingly difficult. The process skills score means that James needs less support in this area, but that when confronted with a problem he finds it difficult to overcome. Support is, therefore, required to assist James with problem-solving; again, this is being provided by his wife.

James's wife states she was considering the option of respite/day care, during which time her husband would require the support of carers for both his motor and process skills deficits. James highlighted that mealtimes were 'particularly trying' due to dribbling, dropping food and difficulty applying sufficient pressure to facilitate food onto a fork (when brushing teeth, James also experienced difficulty applying the correct pressure effectively). James's wife explained that she was reviewing the option of employing a private cleaner and gardener, as she completes all domestic tasks.

James identified that he perceived himself as a failure in domestic ADL, following a number of incidents and accidents (for example dropping crockery), stating he is 'banned from the kitchen'. This has compounded to reduce his confidence in himself and his abilities. During the latter part of the assessment, James became tearful, when acknowledging all the things he had lost (hobbies, interests, roles). He also reported several falls over the last four weeks. The AMPS showed impairment with mobility owing to a marked short shuffling gait, with difficulty initiating forward movement. At times during the visit, James had problems transferring in and out of the chair, having a poorly controlled descent into the chair.

James became easily frustrated when he was initiating a task but was unable to complete it as he forgets the sequence. He recalled statements made by the occupational therapist during the assessment, including equipment recommendations.

RECOMMENDATIONS

Motor Skills

- Poor grip (manipulates, calibrates, grips, flows and lifts skill areas):
  - Adaptive cutlery assessed for and provided.
  - Advice given regarding alternative methods for brushing teeth; other equipment highlighted to assist (e.g. electric toothbrush).
- Poor mobility (stabilises, aligns, positions and walks skill areas):
  - Referral made for physiotherapy assessment.
  - Referral sent for the fitting of a second banister rail.
- General motor deficits (reaches, bends, calibrates and lifts skill areas):
  - Respite services to be informed of difficulties, ensuring provision of appropriate equipment.
  - Previously provided equipment to be checked.

Process Skills

- Problem-solving (uses, initiates, organises and adaptation skill areas):
  - Education for James's wife regarding management skills/techniques.
  - Identification of the areas that produce the greatest difficulties also grading of activities, to be pursued during further occupational therapist visits.

Support/Other

- Carer stress: referrals to Crossroads, Carers Resource and Social Services.
- James's negative outlook: identification and participation in meaningful tasks with appropriate support as required.
- Medication: liaison with consultant psychiatrist to feedback findings, for consideration in prescribing cholinesterase inhibiters.

WORKSHEET

At the back of this book, you will find templates for a series of worksheets designed to assist you in applying principles of assessment and outcome measurement to your own practice. Please now turn to Worksheet 8 (p. 409). The worksheet takes you through a 'to do' list and can be used by students on placement or therapists to ensure that they have prepared thoroughly for an assessment or test administration.

STUDY QUESTIONS

8.1 What factors should you discuss with the client prior to assessment to ensure you have gained informed consent?

8.2 What factors should you consider in order to ensure that you achieve an effective and efficient assessment?

8.3 What techniques could you apply to help build rapport with your client?

You will find brief answers to these questions at the back of this book (pp. 392–3).

9

Applying Models of Function to Therapy Assessment and Measurement

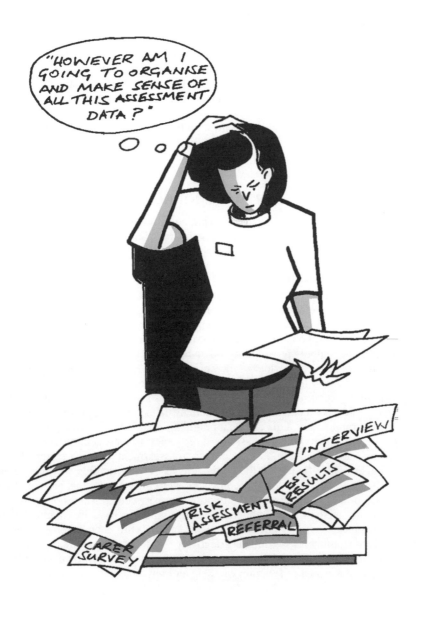

CHAPTER SUMMARY

This chapter will describe and discuss the application of different models used in rehabilitation for categorising dimensions of functioning and disablement. It begins with an overview of systems theory, including open systems theory. The two internationally recognised models produced by the World Health Organization (WHO) will be outlined; these are the *International Classification of Impairments, Disabilities and Handicaps* (ICIDH) published in 1980 and the *International Classification of Functioning, Disability and Health* (ICF) published in 2002. The less-well-known, but useful, National Center for Medical Rehabilitation Research (NCMRR) five-level model of function and dysfunction (which categorises dysfunction in terms of pathophysiology, impairment, functional limitation, disability and societal limitation) will also be presented. This chapter will consider why such models are useful tools for examining an assessment approach in both uni-disciplinary and multidisciplinary settings. The ICF and NCMRR models will be explored in greater depth, and examples of assessment domains and measures that provide information at the different levels of function identified within these models will be provided. When applying these sorts of models, a therapist often needs to decide at what level to begin assessment; so the chapter will offer an exploration of the merits of a top-down versus a bottom-up approach to therapy assessment. The chapter will conclude with a case study showing how the NCMRR five-level model of function can be applied to the case of an elderly woman receiving both physiotherapy and occupational therapy as part of a fast-response service. It will also endeavour to answer the following questions: 'What is the best way to collate and analyse the different types of data obtained through the assessment process to produce a coherent, meaningful picture of the person?' and 'How do I fit my assessment practice into the wider context of a multidisciplinary team and/or interagency approach?'

WHY USE MODELS?

A model is a term used to describe a pattern, plan, chart or simplified description of a system. Models can be used to aid the gathering and organising of information and can act as checklists. Therapists frequently collect multiple pieces of data about a person, his occupations, his environment, his illness and his problems throughout an assessment process. Therapists also obtain assessment data from different sources (the person, his carer, other health and social care professionals) as well as from therapist-administered standardised tests and from informal observational assessment methods. All this information needs to be documented, organised and reflected upon in a meaningful way to result in a thorough and useful assessment. It is important for therapists to understand how their assessment practice fits into the wider context of assessment, intervention and support provided by other health and social care colleagues and independent and voluntary service providers. Therapists need to define their areas of expertise and be able to articulate these to their clients, carers (for example parents, spouse or other relative), multidisciplinary team, referral sources and other agencies involved in the client's treatment and care. Dividing up aspects of a person for assessment by different members of a multidisciplinary team is quite common practice. This can be a pragmatic solution for reducing repetition for the person being assessed and making the best use of resources. However, some therapists view this as a reductionistic, rather than a holistic, approach to assessment. When a therapist directs her focus of attention on a specific part of the body, or aspect of functioning, she may be blinkered and fail to see the person as a whole. This can lead to working on goals that are not of relevance to the person or a failure to understand the relationship between an illness or dysfunction and other aspects of the person's life. Reductionistic thinking can lead to fragmented practice, especially when professionals do not communicate clearly with each other and fail to share information derived from their assessments effectively. Models can be applied to help therapists gain an overview of the whole and understand how discrete parts can or may interrelate. An explicit application of a model of function can help an individual therapist, a therapy service or a multidisciplinary team review their assessment practice and facilitate communication about assessment, outcome measurement and intervention.

The World Confederation for Physical Therapy (WCPT; 2006b) includes the following in its list of important principles and states that physiotherapists should:

- use terminology that is widely understood and adequately defined
- recognise internationally accepted models and definitions (e.g. the WHO's definition of health).

Appling a model of function can assist your assessment process in a number of ways, such as:

- At the stage of problem setting, it can be particularly helpful to categorise the client's problems (identified by the referral or initial interview) in terms of levels of function/ dysfunction and to use the boundaries of a defined level to help focus further data collection, such as the use of standardised observational tests or to help decide if information needs to be collected from proxy sources.
- When critiquing standardised assessments for use within your service or for a particular client, models and hierarchies describing levels of function/dysfunction can be useful for identifying and comparing the levels, domains and scope of different or apparently similar tests.
- Many therapists work as part of a multidisciplinary team and models can be useful to help each team member identify their primary level or domain of concern and for the team to identify areas where there is overlap in the assessment data collected and any gaps or omissions where a level of functioning has not been adequately assessed by team members.

THE COMPLEXITY OF HUMAN FUNCTION

In Chapter 1, I began to explore the challenges of undertaking a rigorous assessment and how some of these challenges were linked to the complexity of human functioning and the intricacy of the relationship between a person and his environment. To begin this chapter on the application of models of function, it is worth thinking about what human functioning entails, because a useful model of functioning will need to encompass both the breadth and intricacy of human function.

Every day, individuals perform basic activities, such as eating, drinking, washing, dressing, cooking, cleaning and travelling. These basic activities of daily living (ADL) support their ability to perform other personally selected activities related to work, play and leisure. The balance or configuration of self-care, work and leisure activities changes as the individual matures from infancy through adulthood to old age. Many basic activities become overlearned routines and become part of that person's habitual repertoire of behaviour. *Occupation* is the term used in therapy literature to describe a person's 'engagement in activities, tasks and roles for the purpose of meeting the requirements of living' (Levine and Brayley, 1991, p. 622). This process of engagement is called *occupational performance* (Christiansen and Baum, 1991). The ability to perform activities is dependent on the interrelation of several levels of function. Each activity requires a combination of skills developed as a result of the normal functioning of the motor, sensory, cognitive and perceptual systems. The functioning of these systems is in turn dependent on the functioning of individual body components, such as nerves, organs, muscles and joints. Participation in occupation affects a person's psychological and biological health. For example, it is through occupation that the musculoskeletal system is exercised and maintained; unused muscles quickly waste. Research investigating the effects of sensory deprivation has shown that when sensory stimulus, usually provided through interaction with the physical and social environment, is withdrawn neurological disorganisation occurs (Rogers, 1983).

Millions of individuals find themselves unable to perform activities independently, owing to illnesses, chronic disease or deficits caused by accidents. Habitual occupational performance is usually taken for granted until an illness, accident or disabling condition makes perform- ance difficult or impossible. The devastation to independent living caused by these deficits is not just experienced by the individual; the effect of disease on an individual also affects their family, friends and colleagues. The impact of an illness, disease or accident on a person's life- style and quality of life can be reduced by the level of support he receives from family, friends and colleagues and by the type of health, social and voluntary services available. The nature of his physical environment also influences the amount of disability experienced, for example if his home has been adapted to be wheelchair-accessible.

The relationship between these many variables is usually very complex and needs to be as- sessed rigorously. Without accurate assessment, it is impossible to plan effective intervention and management. It is important to establish the limitations of performance and the underlying causes of this limited performance. Limited performance can be caused by impaired skills, dys- functional systems and specific motor, sensory, cognitive and/or perceptual deficits. It is, there- fore, essential for clinicians to understand the relationship between an individual's brain and body functioning and their behaviour. To help therapists approach this task in a logical manner, it can be helpful to organise the assessment process in terms of levels of functioning or impact. Several classification systems that define the range of problems and levels of function/dysfunc- tion addressed by professionals working in the field of rehabilitation have been proposed. Many models are based on some sort of hierarchy, and we will begin our consideration of models by looking at the broad hierarchy of living systems.

GENERAL SYSTEMS THEORY AND THE HIERARCHY OF LIVING SYSTEMS

General systems theory forms the foundation of many therapy theoretical frameworks and so is a useful place to begin when considering models of function. For example, the Model of Human Occupation (MOHO; Kielhofner, 1992, 1985; Kielhofner and Burke, 1980) is an occupational therapy model that draws on general systems theory and views humans as open systems. Another example is the Person-Environment-Performance Framework (Christiansen and Baum, 1991). In this framework, occupational performance is viewed as a transaction between the individual as an open system and the environment.

General systems theory emanates from an interdisciplinary base and involves the integration of natural, social, medical and scientific disciplines. The systems approach is concerned with the description of systems, which are integrated wholes that derive their essential properties from the interrelations between their parts. Therefore, the systems approach does not focus on the parts but on their interrelations and interdependencies (Capra, 1982).

From a structural viewpoint, a system, like a person, is a divisible whole. We can divide the person, conceptually, in terms of separate bones, muscles, organs and subsystems, such as the motor, cardiovascular and respiratory systems. However, from a functional perspective, a system

---

Definition of a system

A system is defined as an organised whole comprised of interrelated and interdependent parts. It can be defined as a set of objects together with relationships between the objects and their attributes:

- objects are the components of a system
- attributes are properties of objects
- relationships tie the system together.

is an indivisible whole. A system is indivisible functionally in the sense that some of the essential properties of the system are lost when it is taken apart. When a person experiences some sort of pathology or injury to one part of his body, it can affect the overall functioning and roles of that person. As therapists, we need to understand how a deficit or problem in one part of the person's body or life affects other parts and how some of the disability associated with a deficit can or cannot be remediated through the physical or sociocultural environment. For example, a man in his mid-70s develops chronic obstructive airways disease (COAD), which leads to a symptom of shortness of breath. This makes it very difficult for him to climb stairs. As a result, he and his wife decide to move to a bungalow. He also has to stop his role babysitting his young grandchildren as his son and daughter-in-law live in a three-storey house and his grandchildren's bedrooms are located up two flights of stairs.

Systems involving creative, evolutionary and developmental processes can experience growth. With growth, the system changes in the direction of increasing subdivision into subsystems and sub-subsystems, or differentiation of functions. This is the case for humans, as embryonic development involves the germinated egg progressing from a state of wholeness (a single fertilised egg) to a state of regions that develop independently into specialised organs (Hall and Fagen, 1956), such as heart, lungs and kidneys, that can be viewed as systems in themselves. This process continues after birth, and so paediatric therapists are very concerned with the assessment of an infant's or child's developmental processes. Paediatric therapists will need to consider what would be an expected level of development in different systems, such as the respiratory or motor system, and whether the child has progressed to this expected level of development. In order to do this, therapists apply discriminative tests that are founded on normative data and enable the therapist to compare a child's performance with the norm (expected performance) for children of that age and socio-economic background.

Many systems deteriorate or decay over time, and this is seen in the human ageing process. For example, deterioration occurring in the human visual and auditory systems is associated with age-related changes to vision and hearing. Therapists working with older people will need to assess changes in function related to visual and auditory acuity and be able to differentiate these expected ageing processes from changes due to pathology.

Subsystems can be recognised at various levels of the organisation of a system; these subsystems constitute Gestalt wholes in themselves and are also organised into a larger Gestalt whole according to the laws of the hierarchy. Sykes (1983) defines *Gestalt* as a 'perceived organised whole that is more than the sum of its parts' (p. 414). The organising laws incorporated by each level are used to describe the levels of a system.

- Each level is perceived as comprising of at least one more complex law than the level below.
- Higher levels direct or organise the lower levels.
- Higher levels are dependent upon, or constrained by, lower levels.
- At any level, phenomena belonging primarily to that level incorporate characteristics or mechanisms of lower, less complex levels.
- The purpose of a level is found by examining the level above.

For example, in a hierarchy of human performance (as described by Kielhofner, 2002), which comprises three levels (volition, habituation and performance capacity), the lower level of motor coordination at the performance level is controlled by the higher habituation and volitional levels (Kielhofner, 1985). Volition, at the highest level, is the person's 'pattern of thoughts and feelings... which occur as [he] anticipates, chooses, experiences and interprets what [he] does' (p. 19). Habituation is his 'semi-autonomous patterning of behaviour', which manifests as 'routine, automatic behaviour' that 'is organised in concert with [his] familiar temporal, physical, and social' environments (p. 19). A disturbance or change at one level resonates through the whole system (Kielhofner, 1978); for example, injury to a muscle at the motor performance level will affect the ability to perform controlled movement. Movements that had become embedded as habitual patterns of action, such as driving or brushing teeth, now require focused attention because they cannot be performed with the previous ease. The decision to exercise at a volitional level, for example following a physiotherapist's prescribed set of exercises, will lead to changes in muscle tone and strength and will help to remediate the injured muscle.

Systems may be open or closed. Most natural, or organic, systems are described as open. This means that they exchange materials, energies or information with their environments. According to von Bertalanffy (1968), the theory of open systems is part of a general systems theory. The basis of the open system model is the dynamic interaction of its components. Survival of all living things is dependent on some form of action. Even without external stimuli, or input, humans are not passive but intrinsically active systems. An external stimulus, such as a change in the temperature of the external environment, does not effect a reaction in an otherwise inert system (a rock will become hotter or colder in direct response to the external temperature); however, an external stimulus, such as changing temperature, stimulates modification in a highly active system. People, for example, either sweat or shiver in order to maintain their body temperature.

The human system is involved with continuous, irreversible cycles involving the import and export and construction and destruction of materials. For example, in terms of import and export, we take in oxygen from the air and expel carbon dioxide and we take in food and drink, extract what our body needs and expel waste as urine and faeces (see Figure 9.1). Central concepts in the theory of open systems are the concepts of dynamic interaction and feedback. Feedback allows the system to modify its internal components in response to the demands of the external environment. To do this, the system includes a receptor, such as a sense organ, which receives information by nerve conduction. This information is then processed in the system's controlling centre, such as the brain. The processing of information involves the evaluation of the incoming message and the transmission of an outgoing response message to an effector,

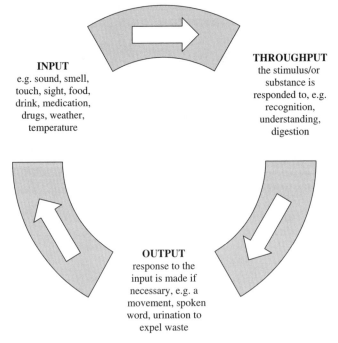

INPUT
e.g. sound, smell,
touch, sight, food,
drink, medication,
drugs, weather,
temperature

THROUGHPUT
the stimulus/or
substance is
responded to, e.g.
recognition,
understanding,
digestion

OUTPUT
response to the
input is made if
necessary, e.g. a
movement, spoken
word, urination to
expel waste

Figure 9.1 A person as an open system.

such as a muscle. The functioning of the effector is monitored back to the receptor. This makes the system self-regulating, for example it guarantees stabilisation or direction of action.

Stephenson (2002) considers the central nervous system (CNS) as a complex adapting system (CAS) and proposes a model of behaviour based on self-organisation. In the article, 'neuroplasticity is explored as the means by which agents in the system interact, with population coding and models of processing being the mechanisms through which behaviour is achieved. Complexity theory is used to construct a holistic model of human behaviour; the total integration model (TIM). Physiotherapy is placed as a "weighted" stressor within a homeodynamic system, with emergent client behaviour reflecting the aggregate influence of all stressors' (Stephenson, 2002, p. 417). Stephenson proposes TIM as a new paradigm for physiotherapy.

The assessment of any complex phenomenon necessitates knowledge of its function as both a part and a whole. Therapists need to encompass a vast field of phenomena from neurons and cells to organs, such as the brain and eyes, to the person as a whole, and to the interaction between people and their social and physical environments. These phenomena can be viewed as an interrelated continuum and can be classified into an ordered hierarchy.

Several taxonomies of phenomena that differentiate levels of complexity have been proposed (Boulding, 1968; von Bertalanffy, 1968). Christiansen (1991) describes a hierarchy of living systems that could be used by therapists (see Figure 9.2). Each of the ten levels in

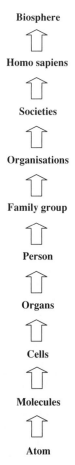

Figure 9.2 Hierarchy of living systems (Christiansen, 1991).

this hierarchy is viewed as a subsystem or component of the next higher level, and there is considered to be increasing complexity as one ascends the hierarchy. The lowest level of the hierarchy of living systems is the level of the atom (1); this is followed by (2) molecules, (3) cells and (4) organs. The level of the person (5) falls in the middle of the hierarchy and is followed by the levels of (6) family group, (7) organisations and (8) societies. The highest levels are (9) *Homo sapiens*, defined as 'biological species which includes existing and extinct humans', and (10) biosphere, which refers to 'habitable parts of the world for living organisms' (Christiansen, 1991, p. 16).

For the majority of therapists, the prime levels of concern, in this hierarchy of living systems, are the organ level, through the assessment and treatment of functioning of organ systems (such as the musculoskeletal system), and the person level, through the assessment and treatment of the person's occupational performance. The impact of the person's social supports is explored at the family-group level; this level is of particular concern to those therapists who educate and support carers, such as the parents of a child with cerebral palsy or the spouse of a person who has experienced a stroke. Therapists work at the organisations level when they signpost or refer people to other organisations (such as voluntary organisations offering appropriate support or activities) or when liaising with a person's employing organisation to negotiate adaptations to the person's work space or adjustments to their work activities. Some therapists work at an organisations level when providing assessment or training for a group of people, for example in the areas of lifting and handling or person–job–environment fit. A few therapists contribute at a societal level, for example by contributing expertise to the development of government policy on topics such as health promotion and social inclusion. In terms of the biosphere, a few therapists are challenging us to consider environmental issues, such as the development of equipment and the furnishing of therapy departments using recycled materials. Another concern for occupational therapists and physiotherapists is the issue of the cleaning and reallocation versus the disposal of equipment and aids to ensure the minimal amount of waste and the use of non-polluting cleaning chemicals.

Law and Baum (2001) suggest that therapists need to understand a number of key concepts to be able to appreciate fully how therapy fits into the larger context of health care and rehabilitation. They cite the conceptual frameworks provided by the WHO, the NCMRR and the work of Nagi (1991) as examples worthy of consideration. These models will now be described and examples from other therapy literature used to illustrate how they have been applied by therapists.

INTERNATIONAL CLASSIFICATION OF IMPAIRMENTS, DISABILITIES AND HANDICAPS

One of the most widely recognised and accepted systems for defining function was developed by the WHO and was called the *International Classification of Impairments, Disabilities and Handicaps* (ICIDH; World Health Organization, 1980). The purpose of the ICIDH was to provide a framework for classifying the consequences of injuries and disease (Hammell, 2004). The WHO originally developed a three-level hierarchy of dysfunction (1980). The ICIDH described function in terms of a three-level hierarchy (1980) comprising impairment, disability and handicap.

Townsend, Ryan and Law (1990) state that 'the ICIDH provides an internationally accepted language, conceptual framework and system of classification, coding and rating to differentiate categories of disablement. The ICIDH is an epidemiological tool for measuring health status in terms of performance rather than traditional measures of prevalence and incidence of disease' (p. 17). Cole *et al.* (1995) report that 'along with the whole field of medical rehabilitation, physical therapists have widely accepted the *International Classification of Impairments, Disabilities and Handicaps* . . . it helped stimulate physical therapy to increase its earnest efforts to develop valid standards of practice based on the present state of the art and science, and it provided

Handicap

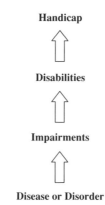

Disabilities

Impairments

Disease or Disorder

Figure 9.3 The consequences of disease and disorders as conceptualised by the WHO in their ICIDH (World Health Organization, 1980).

a conceptual model which made sense in rehabilitation' (p. 2). A number of therapists have considered how this model can be used to define areas of assessment (for example Christiansen, 1991; Coster and Hayley, 1992):

Impairment the lowest level of this hierarchy is impairment; this level involves the function of organs and organ systems. Dysfunction at this level is defined as limitation or abnormality in anatomic, physiologic or psychological process (for example, paralysis of muscle groups, impairment of visual or hearing acuity). A deficit at this level may or may not affect a person's ability to accomplish tasks.

Disability the middle level of function is disability; this involves the performance of ADL, (for example washing, dressing and feeding). Dysfunction at this level results in a deficit in which task accomplishment is affected.

Handicap the highest level of the hierarchy is handicap. Dysfunction at this level involves interference of social roles leading to a decrease in quality of life (for example an inability to maintain a work role, access leisure facilities or participate in social events). An inability to satisfactorily perform tasks often hinders successful role performance and can result in social disadvantage.

Functional Assessment This, as perceived within the WHO's ICIDH framework, evaluates 'any restriction or lack of ability to perform an everyday activity in a manner or within the range considered normal for a person of the same age, culture, and education' (World Health Organization, 1980, p. 143).
Clifford (2002) provides a good clinical example.

> ICIDH makes a distinction between impairment, handicap and disability. The concept of 'impairment' referred to the underlying physical problem or condition e.g. a cataract; the concept of 'handicap' referred to the restriction in function caused by the impairment e.g. blurred vision, and the concept of 'disability' referred to the limitation in activity resulting from the handicap e.g. being unable to read the newspaper. (p. 33)

These three components of function are hierarchic in the way that they represent increasingly complex integrated activities. The presence of difficulties at one level, however, does not automatically result in difficulties at the other levels. For example, a person can have impairment but not have a disability or handicap. A simple, everyday example is that the prescription of a hearing aid can overcome hearing deficits and enable people to carry out their daily activities. One of the most frequently used aids in the Western world are glasses, or contact lenses, which enable people to function with a visual impairment and continue with daily activities, such as driving, and maintain their social roles (such as driving to collect his child from football practice). Clifford (2002) provides examples of how a problem can be addressed at each of the three levels of function.

> The 'problem' [cataracts] may be addressed in several ways: by addressing the underlying physical cause (e.g. removing the cataract); by compensating for the resulting handicap e.g. providing glasses; or by compensating for the disability e.g. reading the newspaper to the patient. (pp. 33–34)

There are multiple influences in addition to impairment that affect a person's functional capability. A handicap can be caused by the social and physical environment with which the person needs to interact. For example, a person's ability to maintain a work role is a function of his functional capacities, the acceptance and encouragement of his management and peers and the accessibility of his physical work environment.

In the past, measures applied in health care mostly focused upon negative outcomes, such as death and impairment. The ICIDH placed increased focus on the concepts of disability and handicap and led to greater measurement at these levels. Jette (1994) reports that measures started to examine disability regardless of the underlying impairment or the need to use assistive devices to achieve independence in ADL. Stokes and O'Neill (1999) recommend that therapy outcomes can be 'measured at the level of impairment, disability and handicap' (p. 562), although they note: 'measurement of outcome at the level of impairment in older people may not be optimal' and suggest: 'it may be best measured at the level of disability and/or handicap since it is at this level that patients experience difficulties associated with daily life' (p. 562).

Jeffrey (1993) applied the ICIDH 'as an objective base for [reviewing] the content of ten measures as part of a project to select appropriate measures for the West Lothian NHS Trust occupational therapy service'. Jeffrey notes that many outcome measures evaluate at the impairment level and some provide information related to disability. Jeffrey was particularly interested in assessments that addressed the handicap level as she felt this was the level where comprehensive rehabilitation needed to focus. The ICIDH description of six survival roles (orientation, physical independence, mobility, occupation, social integration and economic self-sufficiency) were felt to be important and should be represented in the content of the outcome measure used by their service. Jeffrey, therefore, analysed the content of potential measures against this six-item WHO handicap scale. During her review, she identified the Craig handicap assessment and reporting technique (CHART; Whiteneck *et al.*, 1992) as a rehabilitation outcome measure that used the ICIDH definition of handicap and five of the six survival roles (orientation is omitted).

An example of a therapy outcome measure based on the ICIDH is the Therapy Outcomes Measure (TOM; Enderby, John and Petherham, 1998). The conceptual foundation from the TOM was based on the WHO model; the therapist records baseline and post-test scores for four test domains: impairment, disability, handicap and distress/well-being. TOM provides a global measure of health outcomes and can be used with clients across the age range and with a wide variety of diagnoses. Scoring is undertaken using an 11-point ordinal scale.

The ICIDH model, although widely recognised, was not generally embraced by therapists. Several inadequacies have been identified in the distinctions among different components of the model (Pope and Tarlow, 1991; Coster and Hayley, 1992). Clifford (2002) considers that 'whilst the underlying conceptualisation is plausible in the case of a clearly-identifiable physical problem there are problems in generalising this approach to mental health and, more broadly, social problems' (p. 34). He gives a number of reasons to support this assertion. First, Clifford maintains that the underlying impairment of mental disorders cannot be as readily identified as with the majority of physical conditions. He notes that frequently there is debate about the underlying causes of some mental health problems. Because of this, Clifford suggests that 'impairment cannot be assessed independently of the handicap' (p. 34). Secondly, he asserts that the uni-directionality of causation that is implied in the ICIDH model (that is from impairment to handicap to disability) fits less well when working with people with mental health problems because 'interactions between the individual and the environment can lead to causality going in both directions e.g. depressed mood might lead to irritability with others, resulting in lowered levels of interaction with others, resulting in turn in more severely depressed mood' (p. 34). Jette (1995) also suggests that a linear relationship does not exist between impairment and disability. Thirdly, Clifford (2002) feels that the model did not appeal to clinicians because:

> from a practical point of view, the subtlety of the underlying conceptual distinctions, even if logically correct, make the framework awkward to use in routine practice: ground level staff are interested in identifying the 'problem' which can be addressed as directly as possible and tend to be relatively disinterested in either causality (except insofar as this points towards a possible mode of intervention) or the finer points of conceptualisation. (p. 34).

A model proposed by Nagi (1991) was considered to be conceptually clearer than the ICIDH model, because Nagi interposed a level that bridges the WHO model's levels of impairment and disability. This intermediate level was termed *functional limitations* and relates to limitation experienced at the level of the whole organism. Disability, within this model, relates to social functioning and is defined as 'an inability or limitation in performing socially defined roles and tasks' (Nagi, 1991, p. 315). However, the Nagi model was still considered to leave some conceptual difficulties at the higher end of the hierarchy.

Jette (1995) applied concepts in the disablement model developed by Nagi (1991) and also used the ICIDH. He reports that these models 'provide an excellent lens through which we can view the traditional research paradigm guiding physical therapy research' (p. 967). He concludes that 'viewed from the terminology used within these conceptual frameworks, the dominant research paradigm guiding physical therapy research and practice can be characterized as one that focuses on *impairment outcomes*' (p. 967). He goes on to offer a number of impairment level outcomes of interest to physiotherapists, including restriction in range of motion, muscle weakness and pulmonary function. He suggests that physiotherapists are becoming increasingly interested and involved with *disability outcomes*. At a disability level, therapists focus 'outcome attention at the level of the individual's behaviour or his or her functioning in social roles within society' (p. 967).

WADE'S FOUR-LEVEL MODEL FOR PEOPLE WITH STROKE

Wade (1988) presents a four-level hierarchical model of dysfunction to identify the levels of function that should be addressed following stroke. Wade's approach uses three levels related to the original WHO (1980) ICIDH with the addition of a first level of pathology (similar to the NCMRR model level of pathophysiology that is described later in this chapter, pp. 245–51). Wade describes his model as follows.

> The first level is that of *pathology*. Not only does this arise first in time, but a pathological diagnosis is vital before undertaking any further actions . . . The second level is that of direct neurophysiological losses arising from the area damaged pathologically. These are the symptoms and signs, but they are also referred to as *impairment*. Usually these are used to deduce pathology. The third, vital level of stroke management is that of *disability*. This refers to *functions that are lost* as a consequence of the impairments: inability to walk or dress, difficulty using the toilet, etc. The *behavioural and emotional* sequelae form an important part of this level.

The fourth level is that of handicap; this refers to the wider social consequences of stroke such as loss of job, need to change house, loss of friends, inability to pursue leisure interests etc. (pp. 1–2)

The level of pathology has usually been addressed before the person is referred to occupational therapy and physiotherapy and, prior to interaction with the person, the diagnosis of stroke is the therapist's starting point from which to frame the case (Rogers and Masagatani, 1982). Using Wade's model, therapists working with someone who has had a stroke will focus on people's motor, sensory, cognitive and perceptual losses at the level of impairment and consider how any impairments affect occupational performance, which is addressed at Wade's level of disability. Therapists then evaluate how loss of independence in ADL affects occupational roles at the handicap level. Therapists will, therefore, require an assessment, or group of assessments, that addresses the impact of brain dysfunction on performance across these levels (impairment, disability and handicap).

FIVE-LEVEL MODEL OF FUNCTION AND DYSFUNCTION

Drawing upon the work of both the WHO (1980) and Nagi (1991), the NCMRR (1992) broadened the functional and dysfunctional hierarchy to a five-level model. Differentiation was made between pathophysiology, impairment and functional limitation. Disability remained and handicap was re-conceptualised as a 'societal limitation'. The NCMRR drew upon the expertise of a multidisciplinary group (which included therapists) to develop its five-level model of function/dysfunction. The NCMRR model's five levels are presented in a hierarchy (Figure 9.4).

The NCMRR model recognised that the progression of dysfunction was not 'always sequential or unidirectional' but should be viewed as a 'complex feedback loop that integrates the whole person as an entity who must adjust to problems in many of these areas simultaneously' (National Center for Medical Rehabilitation Research, 1992, p. 31). The NCMRR has identified the need to apply 'findings from studies of pathophysiology and impairment to the functional limitations they engender' (p. 33). The specification of these five levels of function was an important advance within the field of rehabilitation as it assisted clinicians and researchers to define their domains of concern and clearly identify which level or levels of function they were addressing in their assessment and intervention.

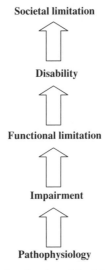

Societal limitation

Disability

Functional limitation

Impairment

Pathophysiology

Figure 9.4 NCMRR's five-level model of function and dysfunction.

DESCRIPTION OF THE FIVE LEVELS OF FUNCTION AND DYSFUNCTION

At the societal limitation level, dysfunction is caused by restriction, attributable to social policy or barriers (structural or attitudinal), which limits the fulfilment of roles or denies access to services and opportunities that are associated with full participation in society (National Center for Medical Rehabilitation Research, 1992). The level of impact is societal. Areas assessed at this level include roles, cultural background, physical and social environment and carer issues. Roles may be related to personal relationships (such as being a parent or spouse) and also related to work/volunteer occupations (such as being a therapist/helping out at her child's school) and leisure activities (such as being a member of a sports team or drama group). In terms of physical environment, therapists might be considering how different flooring affects mobility or establishing the distances within which a person needs to mobilise in order for the fulfilment of roles. Therapists might consider the height of furniture, fixtures and fittings in the person's home environment or the width of doorways or location of hand rails. Assessment of a social environment can involve exploring the person's social networks and likely levels of support available from family, friends, neighbours, colleagues, voluntary and statutory services. The ability and willingness of a close relative or friend to adopt the role of carer is important in some cases, and the therapist may need to consider the carer's physical, emotional and financial resources and assess any emotional or physical burden.

The level of occupational dysfunction experienced by an individual depends, to a large extent, on the roles he wishes to fulfil and the nature of the physical and social environment he has to master. For example take two people, who we will call Jack and Jill, whose work involves operating computers. Jack develops severe rheumatoid arthritis in his upper extremities and Jill has a spinal cord injury, which results in paraplegia. Jack's rheumatoid arthritis will prevent him from managing the computer keyboard, although computer adaptations might be used to facilitate performance initially. His condition is progressive, and it is likely that he will be unable to maintain his original work role. Jill, however, has upper extremity function and should still be able to operate the computer. She would be able to maintain her previous worker role, provided she had a work environment that was accessible to a person in a wheelchair (Laver, 1994). As the therapist who was assessing these two people, you would need to seek information about their previous worker roles and undertake an assessment of their physical work environment. In addition, the attitude of their employers and colleagues would play an important part in how their job specification and physical and social work environments could be adapted to enable them to remain in employment.

At the disability level, dysfunction is defined in terms of an inability or limitation in performing socially defined tasks and activities within a physical and social environmental context resulting from internal or external factors and their interplay (National Center for Medical Rehabilitation Research, 1992). Impact is felt at an individual level. Areas assessed include the identification of the activities and tasks the person undertakes related to each of his roles followed by an assessment of the person's level of independence in these identified areas. This includes the domains of personal and domestic ADL and activities and tasks related to work, leisure and play. The disability level relates to limitation in performing tasks and activities. The therapist needs to understand the underlying causes of occupational dysfunction in order to plan effective treatment. To understand the reasons for impaired occupational performance at the disability level, it is imperative to assess functioning at the levels of functional limitation, impairment and pathophysiology. If assessment at these levels is not the therapist's domain of concern, then information about functioning at these levels is sought from other members of the multidisciplinary team.

At the functional limitation level, dysfunction is exhibited by a restriction or lack of ability, resulting from impairment, to perform an action or skill in the manner or range considered normal for stage of development and cultural background (National Center for Medical Rehabilitation Research, 1992). The impact is seen at a functional level. Areas assessed are skill components of tasks. Activity analysis is conducted to break down tasks into their skill components at this level, for example the ability to reach, grip, manipulate, scan, initiate, recall, sequence and name. Balance and gait are assessed at this level.

At the impairment level, dysfunction is exhibited as loss and/or abnormality of cognitive, emotional or anatomical structure or function, including all losses or abnormalities, not just those attributable to the initial pathophysiology (National Center for Medical Rehabilitation Research, 1992). The impact is felt at the level of organs or organ systems. Areas assessed at the impairment level include the neuromusculoskeletal, sensory, cognitive, perceptual and psychosocial performance components. Weakness of a muscle group or reduced joint range of motion would be addressed at this level. For example, Adams (2002) cites the Joint Alignment and Motion Scale (Spiegel, Spiegel and Paulus, 1987), which measures joint deformity in people with rheumatoid arthritis, as an example of an impairment measure.

At the pathophysiological level, dysfunction is exhibited by interruption of, or interference with, normal physiological and developmental processes or structures (National Center for Medical Rehabilitation Research, 1992). The level of impact is cells and tissues. The pathophysiological level is usually assessed by the doctor. The therapist needs to understand the underlying pathology to know how the medical diagnosis will translate into functional deficits. For example, the identification of a fracture or a bleed in a specified location of the brain would be diagnosed at this level.

Therapy assessment processes rarely address all five levels of dysfunction (societal limitation, disability, functional limitation, impairment and pathophysiology), and so therapists are dependent upon other team members for information in order to understand the inter-relationships between function and dysfunction across all levels. Using a model, such as that developed by the NCMRR, can assist multidisciplinary teams to look at their assessment processes more critically and identify which team members are obtaining assessment data at which levels. This can help to highlight both areas of unnecessary overlap and gaps in the assessment. As an example, a person admitted to hospital with a possible stroke will be assessed by a number of health professionals; these could include a neurologist, physiotherapist, occupational therapist, nurse, social worker, psychologist, speech and language therapist and radiologist. This team might examine their assessment practice in light of the NCMRR model and identify at which level(s) their assessment is undertaken and provide examples of areas of assessment at these levels (see Table 9.1 below). This could be the starting point for better communication within the team about areas of overlap and clarification of exactly what is being assessed and the purpose of this assessment. For example, the occupational therapist and social worker would see that they are both undertaking assessment with the carer. However, on further exploration the social worker is using a county council carers' assessment that leads to the identification of services, such as respite, and benefit entitlements, while the occupational therapist is assessing the carer's resources (for example physical and cognitive ability) to learn new techniques and strategies to manage their loved one at home, such as the use of a wheelchair or cueing the person to use a one-handed dressing method. The occupational therapist is also examining physical and emotional burden in case an aid, such as a hoist to assist transfers, is required. The speech and language therapist, nurse and occupational therapist all identify eating as an assessment area; however, on closer exploration it transpires that the speech and language therapist is focused on the impact of problems with swallowing and dribbling because of paralysis on one side of the face, the nurse is focused on the person getting adequate nutrition while an in-patient and the occupational therapist has been examining how the person attempts eating and is providing a plate guard, non-slip mat, spork and is teaching one-handed feeding techniques.

The application of a model, such as the NCMRR hierarchy of function and dysfunction, helps therapists to understand the inter-relationships between function and dysfunction across

Table 9.1 A stroke rehabilitation team apply the NCMRR model to examine their assessment practice

Societal limitation	Disability	Functional limitation	Impairment	Pathophysiology
Social Worker *e.g. social supports, carer assessment, benefits eligibility* Occupational Therapist *e.g. roles, physical and social environment to assess person-environment-occupation fit, carer's resources and emotional and physical carer burden*	Occupational Therapist *e.g. tasks, activities and occupations, such as personal care, domestic chores, work and leisure activities* Physiotherapist *e.g. mobility and transfers* Social Worker *e.g. level of independence in activities to assess for long-term care needs* Speech and language therapist (SLT) *e.g. eating and drinking* Nurse *e.g. sleep, feeding, washing and dressing*	Physiotherapist *e.g. balance and gait, gross movement patterns such as bridging and rolling – focus on lower limb* Occupational Therapist *e.g. reaching, manipulating, bilateral integration, sequencing task – focusing on upper limb* SLT *e.g. mastication, swallowing, coordination of movements of mouth and tongue* Psychologist *e.g. recall, attention, recognition*	Doctor *e.g. neurological tests for vision, coordination, sensation and assessment of pain* Physiotherapist *motor system (e.g. range of movement) and sensory system (e.g. pain)* SLT *e.g. cognitive and motor functioning* Psychologist *e.g. cognitive and perceptual functioning* Nurse *e.g. blood pressure, temperature, pain*	Doctor *e.g. diagnosis of the type, location and possible cause of stroke, neurological tests for muscle strength and reflexes* Radiologist *e.g. Magnetic Resonance Imaging (MRI).* Physiotherapist *e.g. at a tissue level examines specific muscle weakness and tone (spasticity and flacidity)* SLT *e.g. choking and swallowing reflexes, diagnosis of neurological deficits (dysphasia and dysarthria)*

all levels. For example, a dressing assessment (undertaken at a disability level) could highlight a client's inability to don his shirt independently. There could be several different reasons for such dysfunction. The client may be unable to manage the skills of reaching the shirt and manipulating fastenings (functional limitation) because of a motor deficit (impairment) caused by spasticity in the flexor group of his upper-extremity muscles. Alternatively, he may have perceptual deficits (impairment) that result in his being unable to perceive the shirt against the background of the bed and being unable to discriminate the arm holes and collar from the shirt as a whole (functional limitation). Many other deficits, such as reduced visual acuity or apraxia (impairment), could result in an inability to don the shirt independently. With a person who has cognitive deficits associated with dementia, difficulty with dressing could be related to the person forgetting to get dressed or having difficulty selecting appropriate clothes to wear or putting the garments on in the wrong order. Treatment plans to improve independence in dressing will be different if the cause of dysfunction is a motor deficit as opposed to a perceptual or cognitive deficit.

The NCMRR's hierarchy of dysfunction was used by Laver (1994) during her doctoral research to develop the Structured Observational Test of Function (SOTOF; Laver, 1994; Laver and Powell, 1995). See Tables 9.2 and 9.3 to see how four of the NCMRR levels were used to assist the categorisation and definition of the test domains and items assessed by the SOTOF.

Table 9.2 The assessment domains and items covered by the SOTOF

Level of function/ dysfunction	Disability	Functional limitation	Impairment	Pathophysiology
Definition of level	Inability or limitation in performing socially defined activities and roles within a social and physical environment resulting from internal or external factors and their interplay	Restriction or lack of ability to perform an action or activity in the manner or range considered normal that results from impairment	Loss and/or abnormality or mental, emotional, physiological or anatomical structure or function, including secondary losses and pain	Interruption or interference of normal physiological and developmental processes or structures
SOTOF assessment question	*HOW?*	*WHAT?*	*WHICH?*	*WHY?*
SOTOF assessment domain	Occupational performance	Specific skill or ability, task subcomponents	Performance components	Neurological deficit
SOTOF specific assessment areas	Personal ADL – four basic tasks: • feeding • washing • drinking • dressing	Examples of skill subcomponent include: • reaching • scanning • sequencing • naming	Performance components assessed include: • perceptual • cognitive • motor • sensory	Example deficits assessed include: • apraxia • dysphasia • agnosia • spasticity

Note: Table 9.2 is adapted from Laver (1994) PhD thesis 'The development of the Structured Observational Test of Function (SOTOF)' p. 191 and was based on an assessment model by Laver and Baum (1992). The definitions of the four functional levels are modified from the work of NCMRR (1992).

Note: in Table 9.3 below levels shown in bold are assessed through direct observation of task and skill performance and levels shown in italics are postulated through a diagnostic reasoning process and structured hypothesis testing process provided in the SOTOF Instruction Cards (Laver and Powell, 1995). For more information on diagnostic reasoning see Chapter 10.

Table 9.3 SOTOF: overview of direct and indirect assessment of levels

Level of dysfunction	Level of living systems	Levels of occupation	Levels of functional assessment
Disability	**Person**	**Occupational performance (activities and tasks)**	**Task performance**
Functional limitation	**Person**	**Skills**	**Skill performance**
Impairment	*Organs*	*Performance components*	*Components of task performance*
Pathophysiology	*(Not addressed)*	*Neuropsychological functions*	*(Not addressed)*

As can be seen in Tables 9.2 and 9.3, the SOTOF identifies information related to four different levels of functioning, which are:

- disability: the person's residual occupational performance in the domain of ADL through structured observation to assess his ability to perform simple ADL tasks (e.g. feeding and dressing)
- function limitation: the person's residual and deficit skills and abilities within ADL performance; activity analysis was used to break down each ADL task into its component parts and these are assessed through structured observation (e.g. reaching, scanning, grasping and sequencing)
- impairment: SOTOF provides a method for identifying the performance components (perceptual, cognitive, motor and sensory) that have been affected
- pathophysiological: at this level a diagnostic reasoning process leads to the identification of the specific neuropsychological deficits that are affecting ADL self-care function (e.g. apraxia, agnosia, aphasia and spasticity).

Assessment at each of these four levels is used to address different assessment objectives through different assessment questions (see Table 9.2 above).

- Disability level: *how* does the person perform ADL tasks – independently or dependently?
- Functional limitation level: *what* skills and abilities does the person have intact, and what skills and abilities have been reduced or altered by the neurological damage?
- Impairment level: *which* of the perceptual, cognitive, motor and sensory performance components have been affected by the neurological damage?
- Pathophysiology level: *why* is function impaired? At this level the cause is identified through the naming of the specific neurological deficits and underlying pathology.

Laver (1994) also used the NCMRR model as a basis from which to compare and contrast three other observational assessments with the SOTOF (Laver and Powell, 1995). The three standardised tests critiqued were the Arnadottir OT-ADL Neurobehavioural Evaluation (A-ONE; Arnadottir, 1990), the Assessment of Motor Process Skills (AMPS; Fisher, 2003a) and the Kitchen Task Assessment (KTA; Baum and Edwards, 1993). A summary critique of these measures (at the point of their development in 1994) can be found in Table 9.4.

Using the NCMRR model as a basis for comparison of the test domains addressed by the four measures, the A-ONE was found to address similar domains to the SOTOF across the levels of disability (occupational performance), functional limitation (skills), impairment (performance components) and pathophysiology (neuropsychological deficits) and, at the level of impairment, both addressed the function of the perceptual, cognitive, motor and sensory systems. The AMPS focused on levels that could be directly observed and addressed the levels of disability (occupational performance – instrumental ADL) and functional limitation (motor and process skills). The KTA provided assessment at the levels of disability, functional limitation and impairment, but at the level of impairment the KTA focused only on cognitive function.

Laver's work was used as a starting point by McFayden and Pratt (1997) in a review of measures of work performance. Table 9.5 shows how McFayden and Pratt applied the NCMRR model to provide a conceptual framework for planning assessment and interventions related to work performance.

However, despite its obvious uses, the NCMRR model does not offer an adequate working model for practice and research on its own as it only provides broad descriptions of the levels. A conceptual model of functional performance and performance dysfunction also needs to encompass those personal factors (such as age, gender and cultural, social and educational backgrounds) that can affect performance. The model needs to account for the social and physical environment available to support (and in some cases hinder) functional performance. Life span and cultural and environmental issues are considered important within the therapist's domain of concern.

Table 9.4 Critique of A-ONE, AMPS and KTA. *Taken from Laver (1994) PhD thesis 'The development of the Structured Observational Test of Function (SOTOF)' Figure 2v, p. 132*

Test critique criteria	A-ONE	AMPS	KTA
NCMRR (1992) Levels of function addressed *(Focus level in italics)*	*Disability* Functional limitation Impairment Pathophysiology	*Disability* Functional limitation	*Disability* Functional limitation
Occupational performance domain	4 PADL tasks: dressing, grooming and hygiene, transfers and mobility, and feeding.	3 IADL tasks selected from a list by client and OT, e.g. making a bed, vacuuming and fixing a salad	1 IADL task: making cooked pudding. Test focuses on the identification of cognitive components (e.g. initiation, safety, organisation and sequencing)
Ecological validity related to test environment	Can be performed in client's own setting at home or in hospital	Can be performed in client's own setting at home or in hospital	Performed in OT kitchen or client's own kitchen
Ecological validity related to test task and materials	Tasks are basic, universal PADL tasks, which are relevant to all ages, both sexes and clients from different cultural backgrounds	Clients have some choice in the tasks used, but choice is restricted to a list and method for performing task is prescribed	No choice in task. Method prescribed by instructions. May lack relevance and familiarity for some clients
Clinical utility related to availability and cost	Test described in a published book, forms have to be purchased, therapists have to pay to attend a training course. Need to purchase test materials, e.g. food items.	Test outlined in an unpublished manual, which is provided by the author on completion of a 1-week training course. Need to purchase test materials.	Test published in *AJOT* and is freely available. No training required. Need to purchase test items.
Subject group for whom test designed	Adult and older adult clients with suspected CNS damage.	Adults and older adults.	Adults with suspected dementia.
Normative standards	79 volunteers of both sexes age range 19–89. Normative standards for older adults 60+ years based on a sample of 35.	Studies on various adult populations are still in progress.	No normative data.
Suitability of test for early intervention	Low-level PADL, but client needs to mobilise to a sink/bathroom.	Higher-level IADL, client has to mobilise to gather test items.	Can be used to identify how cognitive deficits affect performance on an IADL task and what cues are required for independent function.

PADL = personal activities of daily living
IADL = instrumental activities of daily living
CNS = central nervous system
AJOT = American Journal of Occupational Therapy

Table 9.5 Application of the NCMRR model to measures and interventions for work performance. *Adapted and reproduced with permission from McFayden and Pratt (1997) Understanding the Statistical Concepts of Measures of Work Performance. British Journal of Occupational Therapy 60(6), p. 280, Table 1: 'A conceptual framework for planning assessment and interventions', which was adapted with permission from Laver (1994) 'The Development of the Structured Observational Test of Function (SOTOF)'. Unpublished doctoral thesis, Guildford: University of Surrey. Definitions of the five levels are based on NCMRR (1992) definitions.*

Societal limitation	Disability	Functional limitation	Impairment	Pathophysiology
Restriction attributable to social policy or barriers (structural or attitudinal), which limits fulfilment of roles or denies access to services or opportunities.	Inability or limitation in performing socially defined activities and tasks within a social and physical environment as a result of internal or external factors and their interplay.	Restriction or lack of ability to perform an action or activity in the manner or range considered normal that results from impairment.	Loss and/or abnormality of mental, emotional, physiological or anatomical structure or function, including secondary losses and pain.	Interference of normal physiological and developmental processes or structures.
Performance of roles and occupations by the person in societal context.	Performance of activity or task by the person in physical and social context.	Performance of subcomponents of tasks or activities.	Organs or organ systems.	Cells and tissues.
Example roles: worker, friend, parent, spouse.	Performance areas: productivity, including work-related activities and educational activities, personal and instrumental ADL leisure activities.	Process components: initiate, organise, sequence, judge, attend, select. Gross-motor components: sit, roll, lift, scoop, squat, stand, reach. Fine-motor: pinch, grip, grasp, hold, release. Interpersonal components: relate, interact, cope, manage.	Physiological and psychological functioning related to the cognitive and perceptual systems, sensory system and motor system.	Physiological deficits, neurological deficits, immunological deficits.
Barriers/issues: recreation, attitudes, accommodation, quality of life	Context: physical environment, social environment, cognitive environment.			
Examples of work performance measures: Role and interest inventories, Occupational Stress Inventory, Community Profile.	Examples of work performance measures: Functional Capacity Assessment (FCAs), e.g. ERGOS, EPIC, WEST, Valpar work samples.	Examples of work performance measures: General Clerical Test (GCT-R), vocational aptitude tests.	Examples of work performance measures: McGill Pain Questionnaire, Perceived Stress scale.	Examples of work performance measures: Goniometry, strength capacities.

INTERNATIONAL CLASSIFICATION OF FUNCTIONING, DISABILITY AND HEALTH

The (WHO) worked to revise the original ICIDH, and documents published for review and field trials initially referred to this revision as ICIDH-2. The finalised version of the revised model was entitled the *International Classification of Functioning, Disability and Health* (World Health Organization, 2002), and this revision is known as the ICF (although some papers still refer to the ICIDH-2). ICF has been developed to provide 'a standard language and framework for the description of health and health-related states' (WHO, 2002, p. 2). The WHO spent seven years and involved people from 61 countries in the development and trials of the ICF (Chard, 2004). The original ICIDH (World Health Organization, 1980) was revised for a number of reasons, which were:

- health and social care systems needed a uniform terminology
- there was a need for a tool that supported communication between people with disabilities and health and social care professionals
- there was a need to produce 'a tool that documents outcomes using a classification system that is appropriate for and acceptable to all who use it' (Chard, 2004, p. 1).

The ICF is a classification system that aims to provide a common language for understanding and researching health and health-related states. Chard (2004) states that 'the intended application of the ICF is to provide a tool for clinical use, research, statistics and education towards raised awareness of social inclusion' (p. 1). The ICF is considered to be a particularly valuable tool for therapists because it provides an integration of the medical and social models. The WHO (2002) provides the following introduction to the ICF.

> It is a classification of health and health-related domains – domains that help us to describe changes in body function and structure, what a person with a health condition can do in a standard environment (their level of capacity), as well as what they actually do in their usual environment (their level of performance). These domains are classified from body, individual and societal perspectives by means of two lists: a list of body functions and structure, and a list of domains of activity and participation. In ICF, the term *functioning* refers to all body functions, activities and participation, while *disability* is similarly an umbrella term for impairments, activity limitations and participation restrictions. ICF also lists environmental factors that interact with all these components. (p. 2)

Table 9.6 provides an overview of the key components of the ICF showing the components, domains and constructs covered and delineating the related contextual factors that require consideration. It also contrasts the positive and negative aspects.

In Figure 9.3 (p. 241) we saw the hierarchical relationship between the components of the ICIDH (World Health Organization, 1980), that is disease/disorder ⇒ impairment ⇒ disability ⇒ handicap. Figure 9.5 shows a representation of the model of disability that is the basis for the ICF. This model has been referred to as a biopsychosocial model that draws upon both a social model of disability and a medical model of disability. The WHO has moved away from a hierarchical model to a model that shows the interconnections between all the key components.

Many therapists have welcomed the WHO's revised classification; for example, McDonald, Surtees and Wirz (2004) state: 'the ICF is an important and exciting development because of its holistic framework and concentration on function and health, rather than disease-based models of disability, and places the individual . . . at the core of the health care process' (p. 299). Clifford (2002) concurs that the new model is an improvement on the original ICIDH because it 'has the benefit of a more neutral conceptual framework and a conceptualisation that does not appear to pre-judge the issue of causality' (p. 34).

The WHO defines the key concepts within the ICF as follows.

Definitions of key terms used within the ICF

- Body functions: are physiological functions of body systems (including psychological functions).
- Body structures: are anatomical parts of the body, such as organs, limbs and their components.
- Impairments: are problems in body function or structure, such as a significant deviation or loss.
- Activity: is the execution of a task or action by an individual.
- Participation: is involvement in a life situation.
- Activity limitations: are difficulties an individual may have in executing activities.
- Participation restrictions: are problems an individual may experience in involvement in life situations.
- Environmental factors: make up the physical, social and attitudinal environment in which people live and conduct their lives.

Definitions reproduced with permission from World Health Organisation (WHO; 2002, p. 10) Towards a Common Language for Functioning, Disability and Health (ICF). Geneva, WHO. All rights are reserved by WHO.

Table 9.6 An overview of the ICF (World Health Organization, 2002). *Table from World Health Organization (WHO) 'International Classification of Functioning, Disability and Health: Introduction'. Table 1: Overview of the ICF (p. 11). Geneva, WHO. All rights reserved by WHO.(Available as a PDF file, http://www3.who.int/icf/intros/ICF-Eng-Intro.pdf)*

	Part 1: Functioning and Disability		**Part 2: Contextual Factors**	
Components	Body Functions and Structures	Activities and Participation	Environmental Factors	Personal Factors
Domains	Body function Body structures	Life areas (tasks, actions)	External influences on functioning and disability	Internal influences on functioning and disability
Constructs	Change in body functions (physiological) Change in body structures (anatomical)	Capacity executing tasks in a standard environment Performance executing tasks in the current enviornment	Facilitating or hindering impact of features of the physical, social and attitudinal world	Impact of attributes of the person
Positive aspect	Functional and structural integrity	Activities Participation	Facilitators	not applicable
	Functioning			
Negative aspect	Impairment	Activity limitation Participation restriction	Barriers/ hindrances	not applicable
	Disability			

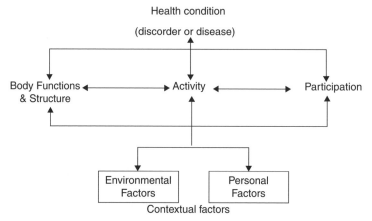

Figure 9.5 Representation of the model of disability used as the basis of the ICF. *Model of disability reproduced with permission from World Health Organization (WHO; 2002, p. 9) Towards a Common Language for Functioning, Disability and Health (ICF). Geneva, WHO. All rights are reserved by WHO.*

The ICF has been adopted by therapists in many countries; for example, in the UK the College of Occupational Therapists (COT) has published guidance on the use of the ICF along with the Ottawa Charter for Health Promotion in occupational therapy services (College of Occupational Therapists, 2004). As client-centred practitioners, there is a good fit between occupational therapy practice and the ICF model's mandate to place attention in health evaluation and research to insider perspectives of people with a disability (McGruder, 2004). Figure 9.6 provides a diagram that demonstrates how the concepts of the ICF are embedded in the structure and process of occupational therapy practice.

Roberts (2004) reports: 'embracing the International Classification of Functioning, Disability and Health . . . has allowed the [occupational therapy] profession to be proactively descriptive of all people and not just those with illness or disability. Inherent in this, and when set within a wider context of the Ottawa Charter for health promotion, it offers a broader way at looking at how the profession might better address the needs of local populations not only in the UK but worldwide' (p. 13). McDonald, Surtees and Wirz (2004) perceive the ICF as a basis for therapists to use to evaluate their practice and that use of the ICF 'encourages a powerful dialogue with funders and managers and provides a means of communication with [clients] and their families' (p. 299).

The ICF has not been without some critics. Chard (2004) reports that the ICF definition of disability is based on a concept of function, whereas some people in the disability movement do not accept this definition of disability and consider that the attitudes of individuals and society have a greater link with disability than impairments. Hammell (2004) offers: 'a sceptical inter-rogation of the classificatory practices of the ICF' (p. 408). She reminds therapists that the ICF only offers a classification system and a scientific coding system that are 'systems for classify-ing and documenting deviations from assumed norms' and 'are not needs assessments' (p. 410). Hammell reviews literature from disability theorists and warns:

> Although the intent of classifying, measuring and statistically analysing the divergence from assumed norms may, at times, be benign, the consequence for those classified as abnormal can be devastating . . . On the basis of classification, disabled people are denied medical interventions . . . physically segregated within their communities . . . and confined within institutions . . . The ICF is not a client-oriented tool, but one to enable professionals to code, to categorise and to compile statistics. (pp. 409–410)

With this in mind, care needs to be taken to maintain an overall holistic focus throughout the assessment process that values the views of the client and carer as paramount throughout and in which the therapist thinks explicitly about her clinical judgements and has a clear rationale for the frameworks she selects to help gather data and form these judgements.

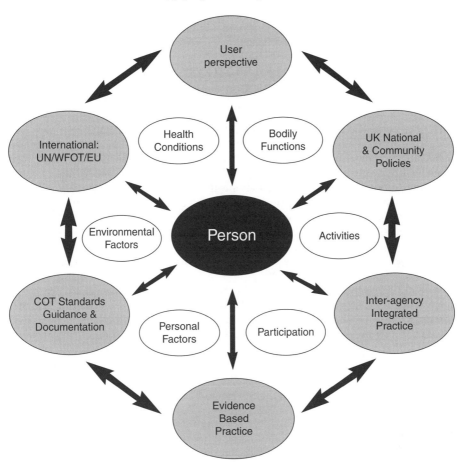

Figure 9.6 ICF concepts embedded in the structure and process of occupational therapy practice. *Reprinted with permission from the College of Occupational Therapists (COT; 2004) Guidance on the Use of the International Classification of Functioning, Disability and Health (ICF) and the Ottawa Charter for Health Promotion in Occupational Therapy Services, Diagram 1, p. 12.*

Clifford (2002) also offers some cautions to clinicians applying the ICF. He notes that content has been organised on 'general classificatory grounds rather than on psychometric or measurement grounds' (p. 34) and asserts that this 'results in a subtlety of distinction that one suspects will prove awkward to carry over into clinical practice' (p. 34). As an example, he notes that the 'control of voluntary movement functions' has been classified under 'Movement functions', and this has been placed in the 'Musculoskeletal' section of the 'Body functions' chapter. However, he notes that the area of 'mobility' has been assigned a section on its own in the 'Activities and Participation' chapter. Clifford feels that 'whilst it may make sense from a classificatory perspective to separate the impairment of bodily function from the impact of that impairment upon mobility, it would seem probable that the average practitioner would assess the two together' (p. 35).

Clifford (2002) expresses particular concerns regarding the application of the ICF to mental health problems. He describes how functions relating to both 'caring for others' and 'caring for personal objects' (for example possessions) have been grouped together in a section called 'Caring for household objects and assisting others', and this has been classified under 'Domestic life'. Clifford notes that 'from a mental health perspective, two quite separate domains, one relating to performance of basic activities of daily living in the home and the other concerning the person's relationships with others have been grouped together for convenience because they both take place in the home' (p. 35).

APPLYING THE INTERNATIONAL CLASSIFICATION OF FUNCTIONING, DISABILITY AND HEALTH TO THERAPY ASSESSMENT

The WHO has published a number of classifications internationally. One of the best known is ICD-10 (World Health Organization, 2004). In health care, the ICD-10 is used predominately by doctors as an aetiological framework for the classification, by diagnosis, of diseases, disorders and other health conditions. By contrast, ICF classifies functioning and disability associated with health conditions. The ICD-10 and ICF are therefore complementary. The WHO (2002) encourages professionals 'to use them together to create a broader and more meaningful picture of the experience of health of individuals and populations' (p. 3). The WHO states that the 'ICF is useful to understand and measure health outcomes. It can be used in clinical settings, health services or surveys at the individual or population level. Thus ICF complements ICD-10 . . . and therefore is looking beyond mortality and disease'. Figure 9.7 provides a diagram showing the relationship between the ICF and ICD-10.

The WHO (2002) reported that studies showed that diagnosis alone did not predict service needs, length of hospitalisation, level of care or functional outcomes. In addition, the presence of a disease or disorder is not 'an accurate predictor of receipt of disability benefits, work performance, return to work potential, or likelihood of social integration' (p. 4). A medical classification of diagnoses on its own is not sufficient for making an individual prognosis and treatment plan or for wider service planning and management purposes. What are also required are data about levels of functioning and disability. Therapists with an understanding of the ICF can supplement the information provided by the diagnosis (which may be classified using the ICD-10) and help to demonstrate how this diagnosis affects the person or diagnostic group in daily life. The model can also provide a framework for exploring how access to physical and social supports has an enabling or disabling effect on an individual or group.

The WHO (2002) provides a section on how the ICF can be applied for service provision at the level of individual clients, at a service or institutional level and can be applied more widely for a population, community or at a social policy level. The applications identified by the WHO at each level are provided in the following three boxes along with the focus question for each application.

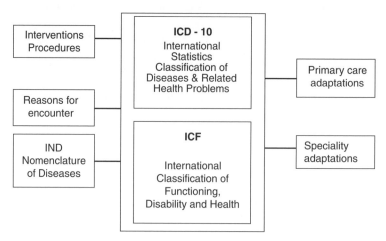

Figure 9.7 WHO family of international classifications: ICF and ICD-10. *Figure reproduced with permission from World Health Organization (WHO; 2002, p. 4) Towards a Common Language for Functioning, Disability and Health (ICF). Geneva, WHO. All rights are reserved by WHO.*

Applying the ICF at the individual level

- For the assessment of individuals:
  - ◦ *What is the person's level of functioning?*
- For individual treatment planning:
  - ◦ *What treatments or interventions can maximise functioning?*
- For the evaluation of treatment and other interventions:
  - ◦ *What are the outcomes of the treatment?*
  - ◦ *How useful were the interventions?*
- For communication among physicians, nurses, physiotherapists, occupational therapists and other health workers, social service workers and community agencies.
- For self-evaluation by consumers:
  - ◦ *How would I rate my capacity in mobility or communication?*

Applying the ICF at the service/institutional level

- For educational and training purposes
- For resource planning and development:
  - ◦ *What health care and other services will be needed?*
- For quality improvement:
  - ◦ *How well do we serve our clients?*
  - ◦ *What basic indicators for quality assurance are valid and reliable?*
- For management and outcome evaluation:
  - ◦ *How useful are the services we are providing?*
- For managed care models of health care delivery:
  - ◦ *How cost-effective are the services we provide?*
  - ◦ *How can the service be improved for better outcomes at a lower cost?*

Applying the ICF at the population/community/social policy level

- For eligibility criteria for state entitlements such as social security benefits, disability pensions, workers' compensation and insurance:
  - ◦ *Are the criteria for eligibility for disability benefits evidence-based, appropriate to social goals and justifiable?*
- For social policy development, including legislative reviews, model legislation, regulations and guidelines, and definitions for anti-discrimination legislation:
  - ◦ *Will guaranteeing rights improve functioning at the societal level?*
  - ◦ *Can we measure this improvement and adjust our policy and law accordingly?*
- For needs assessments:
  - ◦ *What are the needs of persons with various levels of disability-impairments, activity limitations and participation restrictions?*
- For environmental assessment for universal design, implementation of mandated accessibility, identification of environmental facilitators and barriers, and changes to social policy:
  - ◦ *How can we make the social and built environment more accessible for all people, those with and those without disabilities?*
  - ◦ *Can we assess and measure improvement?*

Table 9.7 Using the ICF Framework for Occupational Therapy Measurement. *Reprinted with permission from Law M, Baum C (2001) Measurement in Occupational Therapy. In M Law, C Baum, W Dunn (eds) Measuring Occupational Performance: Supporting Best Practice in Occupational Therapy. Thorofare, NJ, Slack, p. 11*

ICF Dimension	Body Function and Structure	Activity	Participation	Enviornmental Factors
Occupational Therapy Classification	Performance components	Occupational performance	Occupational performance; role competence	Environmental/ contexual factors
Examples of Attributes	Attention Cognition Endurance Memory	Dressing Eating Making meals Manipulation tasks	Community mobility Education Housing Personal care	Architecture Attitudes Cultural norms
	Movement patterns	Money management Socialization	Play Recreation	Economic Geography Light Resources
	Mood Pain Range of motion Reflexes Strength Tone	Shopping Walking Washing Writing	Social relationship Volunteer work Work	Health services Institutions Social rules Sound Weather

Law and Baum (2001) draw upon the ICF recommendations for application and apply this specifically for therapists. They provide three tables that show how the ICF framework can be used to organise the focus of measurement in occupational therapy. The first table considers the application of the ICF for occupational therapy measurement, the second applies this to assessing individuals and the third considers how therapists can apply the ICF to wider measurement contexts at a societal level when working with organisations, such as schools, day care facilities, industry (see Tables 9.7, 9.8 and 9.9).

Table 9.8 Using the ICIDH Framework for Occupational Therapy Measurement – for the individual. *Reprinted with permission from Law M, Baum C (2001) Measurement in Occupational Therapy. In M Law, C Baum, W Dunn (eds) Measuring Occupational Performance: Supporting Best Practice in Occupational Therapy. Thorofare, NJ, Slack, p. 11*

Population	Occupational Need	Required Measurement Approach
Persons with chronic disease	Productive living and quality of life	Person, environment, and occupational influences including family and community participation
Children with chronic or neurological conditions	Opportunity to develop into a productive adult	Person, environment, and occupational influences including family and community participation
Individuals with acute injuries	Return to productive living	Person, environment, and occupational influences including family and community participation

Table 9.9 Using the ICIDH Framework for Occupational Therapy Measurement – for society. *Reprinted with permission from Law M, Baum C (2001) Measurement in Occupational Therapy. In M Law, C Baum, W Dunn (eds) Measuring Occupational Performance: Supporting Best Practice in Occupational Therapy. Thorofare, NJ, Slack, p. 12*

Population	Occupational Need	Required Measurement Approach
Industry	Productive workers	Capacity for work, person/ environment fit
Social Security Administration	Eligible recipients	Functional capacities evaluation
Hospital/community health system	Healthy communities	Community participation, absence of secondary conditions
School	Children with the capacity to learn	School participation
City and county government	Housing and resources for older adults	Capacity for community living
Architecture or engineering firm	Consumers, universal design	Person/environment fit
Retirement communities	Satisfied residents, least support	Person, environment, and occupational influences including family and community participation
Day care facilities (child and adult)	Enhance performance	Person, environment, and occupational influences including family and comunity participation
Universities/colleges	Support learning	ADA – disability access officers

Law (2001) recommends that therapists identify the focus of a measurement and 'use the ICF framework to indicate the focus of the measurement instrument that is being reviewed' (p. 287). She provides brief definitions for *organic systems, abilities, participation* and *environmental factors* to help therapists rate the measure according to the ICIDH framework.

A number of therapists and therapy organisations have used the ICF model to assist with the classification of various assessments and measures in terms of the domains and levels of functioning addressed. The COT (2004) provides a table of common outcome measures categorised within an ICF framework. This is provided in Table 9.10 below.

Table 9.10 Common therapy outcome measures categorised within an ICF framework. *Reprinted with permission from the College of Occupational Therapists (COT; 2004) Guidance on the Use of the International Classification of Functioning, Disability and Health (ICF) and the Ottawa Charter for Health Promotion in Occupational Therapy Service, Table 5, p. 30*

	Body function/ structure	Activity	Participation	Contextual factors
Barthel Index (Mahoney and Barthel 1965)	•	•		
Canadian occupational performance measure (Law *et al.* 1998)		•	•	
Community dependency index (Eakin 1993, cited by Eakin and Baird 1995)			•	•
Mini mental state examination (Folstein *et al.* 1975)	•			
Bayer ADL (Hindmarch *et al.* 1998)		•	•	
Structured observational test of function Laver and Powell 1995)	•			
Falls efficacy scale (Tinetti *et al.* 1990)		•	•	

The Chartered Society of Physiotherapy (CSP; 2002a), in its guidance document on outcome measures for people with depression, states that the measures critiqued in its 'report cover the range of levels as identified by the International Classification of Functioning, Disability and Health, that is, impairment, activity and participation' (p. 4).

McDonald, Surtees and Wirz (2004) offer a detailed case for using the ICF model as a theoretical basis for adaptive seating system assessment and provision. The authors state that the ICF allows them to address the possible conflicts that arise 'between the medical model of reducing or delaying impairment of body functions and structures and the social model of children and families accessing life and environmental situations through mobility and seating equipment' (p. 293). Their paper uses the domains of the ICF to structure their literature review. They conclude that applying the ICF model in clinical practice when providing adaptive seating gives therapists 'both a powerful tool for communicating with children and families as well as managers and a basis for evaluating practice' (p. 293).

Fisher (2003a) describes the relationship of her Assessment of Motor and Process Skills (AMPS) to the ICF. At the activities level, therapists use the AMPS to 'evaluate activity and activity limitations when they implement performance analyses and evaluate the quality of the goal-directed actions performed as part of a complex activity (e.g. daily life task)' (p. 27). At the level of participation, Fisher notes that the 'interpretation of the performance analysis . . . yields information at the level of participation' when the therapist addresses the question 'is the quality and the level of the person's performance at an expected level of achievement given the personal, environmental, and societal factors that may be facilitating or hindering the person's performance?' (p. 27). As an example she states: 'Once we progress to the idea that a person experiences increased effort and decreased efficiency when buttoning because the size of the buttons on the shirt are hindering his ability to manipulate buttons, we have progressed to analysis at the level of participation' (p. 27).

Research is being conducted in Australia to develop outcome measures based on the ICF. Commonwealth Government funding has enabled researchers to adapt the TOM (Enderby, John and Petherham, 1998) to be compatible with the ICF and to produce separate scales for occupational therapy and physiotherapy (Unsworth, 2005). The occupational therapy version, Australian Therapy Outcome Measures for Occupational Therapy (AusTOMs-OT), comprises four domains, with the first three drawn from the ICF model.

- impairment
- activity limitation
- participation restriction
- distress well-being

The fourth domain 'distress/well-being' was added to the original version of TOM (Enderby and John, 1997) because therapists involved with the test development felt that they supported clients to reduce their levels of distress and worked to increase clients' well-being, and that these were also important therapy outcomes that should be measured. The TOM comprises 12 scales. Of these the therapist selects only those that relate to agreed therapy outcomes. In practice, this tends to range from between one to five outcome scales being used per client.

1. learning and applying knowledge
2. functional walking and mobility
3. upper-limb use
4. carrying out daily life tasks and routines
5. transfers
6. using transport
7. self-care
8. domestic life: home

9. domestic life: managing resources
10. interpersonal interactions and relationships
11. work, employment and education
12. community life, recreation, leisure and play

Freeman (2002), in describing the physiotherapy management in a case history of a patient with multiple sclerosis, describes how she uses the ICIDH-2 (World Health Organization, 1997) framework of impairments, activities and participations to identify appropriate outcomes for measurement. She states that 'in measuring impairments I would undertake goniometry measurements of lower limb joint range (Norkin and White, 1975); a spasm frequency score (Penn *et al.*, 1989); a self-rating visual analogue scale to quantify low back pain (Wade, 1992)' (p. 215). Freeman (2002) goes on to identify a number of functional ability measures that are useful when working in a multidisciplinary setting and also recommends a couple of physiotherapy measures that would be relevant in an outpatient setting where the physiotherapist was the main health care provider.

Unsworth (2000) provides an overview of what outcomes research is and lists examples of outcomes assessments in a variety of practice areas. This article adopts ICDH-2 as an organising framework and promotes the use of this framework when undertaking outcomes research.

TOP-DOWN VERSUS BOTTOM-UP ASSESSMENT APPROACH

Rogers and Holm (1989) propose a functional assessment hierarchy. This hierarchy consists of four levels (see Figure 9.8 below).

When the therapist is framing the problem, selecting a theoretical framework and choosing related assessment strategies and tools, an important decision to be made is whether to take a top-down or bottom-up approach to the assessment process. Some assessments simultaneously collect data from several levels of function, but usually an assessment tool or strategy just focuses on data at one or two levels of function. The therapist, therefore, has to decide at which level to begin the assessment process.

A top-down assessment begins at the Role Performance level of the Rogers and Holm (1989) hierarchy and 'determines which particular tasks define each of the roles for that person, whether he or she can now do those tasks, and the probable reason for an inability to do so' (Trombly, 1993, p. 253). If you were using an NCMRR (1992) model as a framework for assessment, then a top-down approach would start assessment at the levels of societal limitation and disability. If you were using the ICF (World Health Organization, 2002) model as a framework for assessment, then a top-down approach would start assessment at the levels of participation, contextual and environment factors.

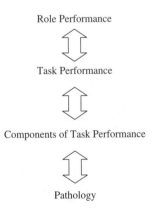

Figure 9.8 Hierarchy of functional assessment (Rogers and Holm, 1989).

A bottom-up assessment begins at the levels of pathology and components of task perform-ance on the Rogers and Holm (1989) functional assessment hierarchy. Note this is called bottom-up and *not* bottoms up; the latter being what a bartender says to customers when he has called last orders and needs to close up! A bottom-up approach 'focuses on the deficits of com-ponents of function, such as strength, range of motion, balance, and so on, which are believed to be prerequisites to successful occupational performance' (Trombly, 1993, p. 253). If you were using an NCMRR (1992) model as a framework for assessment, then a bottom-up approach would start assessment at the levels of pathophysiology and impairment. If you were using the ICF (World Health Organization, 2002) model as a framework for assessment, then a bottom-up approach would start assessment at the levels of body structures and functions and impair-ments. The bottom-up approach can be associated with a medical model and has been popular in the past. Its advantage is that it provides the therapist with important information about the underlying performance component functioning of the individual. However, a disadvantage to the bottom-up approach is that the purpose of the assessment, and ensuing treatment plan, may not be obvious to the person and may, therefore, lack meaning and relevance.

> An example of the bottom-up approach is when the occupational therapist detects that a client who is referred to occupational therapy for remediation of occupational dysfunction (e.g. lack of independence in self-care) lacks sitting balance. Because sitting balance is considered to be an ability required to dress independently, the therapist may begin treatment by engaging the client in activities to improve balance. The occupational therapist may not make clear to the client the connection between the component deficit and occupational functioning. The outcome desired by the occupational therapist may or may not be congruent with important goals of the client or even with the client's perceived reason for receiving occupational therapy services. Confusion and dissatisfaction may result. (Trombly, 1993, p. 253)

Rogers (2004) also expresses some reservations about a reliance on a bottom-up approach.

> For example, knowing that a client has rheumatoid arthritis, the evaluation may begin with measures of pinch strength. Having ascertained that the client exerts 1.5 pounds of pinch on the right (dominant) and 5 pounds on the left, the practitioner might infer that the client is unable to prepare meals due to inadequate pinch strength. This is a weak diagnostic statement because it is based on prediction or inference about performance supported by impairment testing but not activity testing. (p. 27)

In contrast, the top-down approach begins at the level of the person as a whole and starts by investigating past and present role competency and by evaluating the person's current ability to perform meaningful tasks from his previous daily activities. Fisher (2003a) recommends thera-pists take a top-down approach.

> [We] must stress a top-down approach to assessment that begins with the ability of the individual to perform the daily life tasks that he or she wants and needs to perform to be able to fulfil his or her roles competently and with satisfaction. These are the daily life tasks that commonly are meaningful and purposeful to the person who performs them. In contrast to a bottom-up approach that focuses on impairments and capacity limitations, a top-down approach focuses on quality of occupational performance as the person interacts with the physical and social environment in the context of his or her roles. (p. 2)

A top-down approach helps the therapist to gain an early understanding of the person's val-ues and needs. When the person experiences a discrepancy between previous role and task performance during the assessment process, then he can see the need for treatment and will find greater meaning and relevancy in the resultant treatment plan (Trombly, 1993). A top-down approach facilitates the development of a partnership between the therapist and client, in which the person feels valued and understood as a unique individual. Explaining clearly to the person the rationale for both assessment and treatment is essential for joint decision-making and the negotiation of goals and is a critical part of client-centred practice (Sumsion, 2000). The therapist needs to ensure that the person can make a truly informed choice as to whether to engage with the therapist's proposed assessment and treatment. If the person understands and accepts the therapist's rationale, this helps to build trust and rapport and to enhance his motivation to engage with rehabilitation. The top-down approach, thereby, helps to clarify the purpose of therapy for the person. The approach also assists the therapist in the formation of an accurate picture of the person and his problem(s), which is critical for the identification of relevant and meaningful treatment goals. In a review of research and clinical literature pertaining to the Canadian Occupational Performance Measure (COPM), Carswell *et al.* (2004) found that the COPM was 'ideally suited to what . . . Trombly . . . called the top-down approach to assessment, where occupational performance problems are identified first, and then the underlying causes are further assessed using measures of performance components' (p. 219).

CONCLUSION

The models presented are not assessments in themselves but rather frameworks for assisting health care professionals to classify domains and constructs of concern. Models can aid communication between different professionals and can support the identification and documentation of unmet needs. Frameworks, such as the ICIDH, NCMRR and ICF, enable health care professionals to identify when people vary in some aspect of function from culturally specific norms. It is important to remember that some of these models are criticised by people within the disability movement (Chard, 2004; Hammell, 2004). When using such models for pragmatic reasons to assist in your assessment processes, it is important to maintain a wider systems perspective that keeps considering the whole as well as the parts and stays focused on a client-centred approach.

CASE STUDY: 'MARY'

By David Jelly and Alison Laver Fawcett

INTRODUCTION TO THE THERAPIST AND HIS SERVICE

David is a superintendent physiotherapist and team leader of the Fast Response Service. He qualified in Leeds in 1993 and since then has spent much of his career working with the elderly client group.

INTRODUCTION TO THE FAST RESPONSE SERVICE

The Fast Response Service is an intermediate care service that was set up in December 2003. The mission statement of the team encapsulates its primary objectives: 'the goal of the Fast Response Service is to try to prevent avoidable hospital admissions and to facilitate early discharge using a patient-centred approach . . . providing a tailored package of care and rehabilitation for a period of up to six weeks' (for a copy of the full operational policy, contact David Jelley at david.jelley@hdft.nhs.uk).

The main client group is made up of older people in crisis in the community owing to an acute illness, an exacerbation of a previous medical condition or who have had an accident.

The Fast Response Service is based in a rural market town with a population of 17,000 and a rural hinterland of 100 square miles and a scattered population of 8,000. The area is covered by eight GP practices, two social services offices and community nursing staff based in each GP practice. Fast Response is staffed by a part-time team leader who is also the superintendent for the physiotherapy service at the community hospital, a full-time social worker, a part-time senior I occupational therapist, a part-time occupational therapist technical instructor, a full-time senior I physiotherapist, a full-time G grade nurse and four full-time support workers. The service accepts referrals from 8 a.m. to 6 p.m. Monday to Fridays and from 9 a.m. to 1 p.m. on a Saturday. Referrals made outside these times can be supported by 72-hour Fast Response beds in the community hospital. Support workers work on a rota system seven days a week from 7.30 a.m. to 6 p.m. There is an evening and night service staffed by one E grade nurse and one support worker. All services share one base and there is a brief handover period for work and patient information to be passed between staff.

The aims of the Fast Response Team are:

- to prevent unnecessary admission to hospital of patients who with support could be safely looked after at home
- to facilitate the discharge of patients who have been in hospital less than 72 hours and are no longer in need of hospital-based medical intervention and who could be discharged with a package of care and rehabilitation
- to provide a time-limited service that will normally be from two days to no longer than six weeks
- to reduce the likelihood of admission or re-admission to hospital or care home by the use of a problem-solving and multidisciplinary assessment leading to individual care and treatment plans that prioritise rehabilitation goals
- to liaise fully with all other existing community services and work flexibly to avoid duplication and unnecessary hand-offs of the patient from service to service
- to fully assess the needs of the patient (and carers where appropriate) before formulating goal-orientated and time-limited care and treatment plans
- to regularly review the caseload and provide timely and appropriate referral where either rehabilitation has not been effective and long-term care is necessary or where rehabilitation will need to continue substantially longer than six weeks
- to offer training and support for carers to continue rehabilitation work.

Referrals can be made by any health care professional, social services or voluntary sector agency. However, if the client has not been referred by a GP and there has not been a very recent medical assessment, the GP will be contacted and will usually be asked to check the client medically at the earliest opportunity. Following acceptance of a referral, the Fast Response Service undertakes an initial assessment to assess the patient's presenting needs and evaluates whether the referral is appropriate. If a need is identified that can be addressed, then a care plan is drawn up and agreed with the client. The overall aim of intervention, and any package of care provided, is to facilitate and improve independence. The client and carer are made aware from the outset that the Fast Response Service provides a short-term, intermediate care service that will usually last no more than six weeks.

THE ASSESSMENT PROCESS

The *National Service Framework for Older People* published by the Department of Health (DoH; 2001a) 'proposes the development of a single assessment process (SAP), in Standard Two 'Person-centred care'. The Fast Response Service has recently become one of the demonstration sites for SAP. The SAP documentation that has been agreed upon is EASY-Care (Philp, 2000; Richardson, 2001), one of the DoH-approved providers for SAP. 'EASY-Care was originally developed on behalf of the European Regional Office, World Health Organisation, for use in Europe as a first-stage assessment of older people in primary or community care settings (including day care) by nursing staff, social work staff, therapists and care assistants' (EASY-Care, 2006a).

> EASY-Care is a tool for integrating the assessment of a service user's physical, mental and social well-being. It has been designed to give a broad picture of a service user's needs from the viewpoint of the service user. It incorporates the assessor's and the carer's view where appropriate. EASY-Care helps assessors to identify needs and supports person-centred care. It includes sections for contact and overview assessment, planning care, risk assessment and providing consent . . . The University of Sheffield has been working with a software development company, Liquidlogic Limited, to develop an electronic version of EASY-Care, addressing Department of Health criteria for information systems, particularly linkage to the national electronic health record, currently under development. (EASY-Care, 2006b)

EASY-Care can be administered by any health or social care assessor. When a client is re-ferred, their details are logged as an EASY-Care contact assessment via the software program provided by Liquidlogic. This information is not stored on the computers in the Fast Response offices, but is transmitted via a secure server to the Liquidlogic Internet site. The second level of assessment is the EASY-Care overview assessment. Overview assessment is divided into sections.

1. Seeing, hearing and communicating
2. Looking after yourself
3. Safety and relationships
4. Your accommodation and finance
5. Looking after your health
6. Your well-being
7. Your memory
8. Additional personal information

The overview assessment addresses a number of different levels of function, for example Sections 1 and 7 look at an impairment level (National Center for Medical Rehabilitation Research, 1992), Sections 3 and 4 address the societal limitation level and Section 2 assesses function at the disability level.

The overview assessment provides a database that can then be shared by all profession-als involved with a client. It is hoped that this will end the frequent repetition of questions which normally occur when different agencies and professionals are working with one indi-vidual. The overview assessment can be completed by any of the qualified staff working in Fast Response, regardless of professional background. If further assessments are needed by specific professionals, these can be requested using the Internet links between all the local services in the SAP demonstration site (social services, community nurses, voluntary sector providers). Because the Fast Response Service includes four different professional groups, each of these has their own specialist toolkit of standardised and informal assessment procedures. For example, the physiotherapist may wish to undertake a Berg Balance assess-ment (Berg *et al.*, 1992) or the nurse a Waterlow pressure ulcer risk assessment (Waterlow, 2005). All of these can be added to the SAP database and shared with other professionals.

INTRODUCTION TO THE CASE OF 'MARY'

Mary was an 83-year-old lady living alone who fell in the night when she got up to go to the toilet. She was unable to get herself up and had lain on the floor for four and a half hours. She was found when one of her daughters, Anne, popped in to check on her the next morning. Mary was cold and shaken and complained of severe pain in her left forearm. Anne telephoned her sister Liz for help; she felt her mother needed to go to hospital but also had the responsibility of taking her young children to school. Liz lived in a village 15 minutes' drive away. When she arrived, she agreed with her sister that their mother needed to see a doctor and discussed the possibility that she could have broken a bone in her arm. They persuaded Mary that she should go to the Community Hospital's Minor Injury Unit (MIU) and be checked over. When Liz and Mary arrived at the MIU, she was assessed promptly and sent to have her arm X-rayed. The X-ray showed that Mary had sustained a Colles' fracture.

So at the pathophysiology level of the NCMRR (1992) model of function, the doctor identified damage to bone; a Colles' fracture occurs at the lower end of the radius and occurs with posterior displacement of the distal fragment. Colles' fractures are most often sustained when a person is moving forwards with their wrist in supination, for example reaching out a hand to help break a fall. Colles' fractures are particularly common in older people, and an increased risk of sustaining a Colles' fracture is associated with osteoporosis and falls (Hughes, 1983).

Mary's wrist was put in a plaster, which she was told would need to stay on for about six weeks while her fracture healed. Mary wished to return home, but Liz told the doctor in the MIU that her mother would find it very difficult to cope at home alone, particularly as she doubted that her mother would be able to manage her walking frame with a plaster on her arm. Liz was very anxious about her mother being discharged home and keen to see her admitted to hospital, at least for a few days. The daughter reported that she and her sister already needed to visit their mother two or three times a day prior to the fall and that she had been barely copying at home on her own for the last year.

REFERRAL

Staff in the MIU explained to Mary and Liz that there was a new Fast Response Service that might be able to help their mother return home safely. They both agreed, and the MIU nurse rang the Fast Response office, which is on the same site. The social worker was on duty and after taking contact details on the telephone came straight to the MIU to discuss the situation with Mary and her daughter. The social worker began the EASY-Care contact assessment in the MIU by completing the personal background information section. She also sought some basic details from Mary and her daughter about the home situation prior to the fall and the problems that they both anticipated if Mary did return home with her arm in plaster. She established that Mary definitely did want to return home and had good insight into the constraints that she would be under with the plaster on her arm. The social worker decided that this was an appropriate referral. She explained to Mary that the team could put in visits to help her with aspects of her personal care that she could not manage and that they would try and help her to regain her confidence and independence so that she could continue to live independently in her own home. The social worker also reassured Liz that she would not be expected to do more than she was already doing, and that the team would visit as many times as necessary to keep her mother safe. When both Liz and her mother agreed to the involvement of the Fast Response Service, the social worker helped Liz to get her mother to the car and informed them that members of the team would meet them at Mary's house within an hour. The social worker returned to the office to discuss with the occupational therapist and physiotherapist what would be the best approach to maintaining Mary's safety and independence at home.

INITIAL VISIT AND FIRST ASSESSMENT

When a new referral occurs, the Fast Response Service will endeavour to allocate the most appropriate workers to undertake the initial assessment. However, because the team is small and staff are spread to provide a service over six days, there are some occasions where the professional who would be the obvious first choice to assess is not available. However, because there has been a great deal of joint working between professionals and shared training sessions, all professionals have increased their generic skills. On this occasion, the occupational therapist was not available on the day that Mary suffered her fracture and, therefore, David, the physiotherapist, elected to do the initial visit with Claire, one of the support workers. David continued to complete the EASY-Care contact assessment begun by the social worker; this involved interviewing Mary and her daughter to obtain a medical history, medication history and a history of services currently or previously received.

Mary lived in a three-bedroom cottage in a village in the Yorkshire Dales. On presentation, she appeared upset about her fall and her time at the MIU and was extremely anxious about being forced to give up her home and move into a residential or nursing home. She was seated in an armchair by the coal fire. She was still in considerable pain from her arm and she had not yet had any lunch. Her daughter Liz was obviously anxious about the situation.

INTERVIEWING A PROXY TO IDENTIFY SOCIAL SUPPORTS AND NEEDS

David and Claire began the assessment process by introducing themselves to Mary and her daughter and explaining the role of the Fast Response Service. Liz offered a cup of tea and the support worker went into the kitchen with her to obtain an informal proxy report of Mary's needs and the current level of care provided by Liz and her sister. At a societal limitation level (National Center for Medical Rehabilitation Research, 1992), they needed to assess the support available to Mary to enable her to live safely on her own at home. Liz reported that she and her sister shared the care of their mother and that her need for support had increased significantly over the past year. Mary had not received any regular visits from any health or social services staff prior to her fall. Carer burden needed to be assessed as both Mary's daughters had young children to support and, as their husbands were farmers, they both also had responsibilities with farm work. It appeared that her daughters would not be able to offer all the support that Mary would require at home while her arm was in plaster.

COLLECTING SELF-REPORT DATA TO OBTAIN HISTORY
OF THE PRESENT CONDITION

David began by interviewing Mary in the living room. He observed that Mary had an electric armchair that moved her into a semi-standing position to assist transfers. On enquiry, Mary stated that she had purchased the chair three years ago and found it very comfortable and useful. David began seeking information at a pathophysiological level by asking Mary and her daughter to outline any past medical problems. They reported that Mary had widespread osteoarthritis. She reported that her left hip had been replaced eight years ago and her right knee had been replaced three years ago. Mary had some degree of heart failure, which was monitored by her GP. David observed that she had signs of oedema, particularly in her feet and calves, and he enquired whether Mary had any problems with swelling. Mary reported that her 'legs felt heavy all the time' and she said that she often had difficulty getting her shoes on because of the swelling. Mary explained that she had been told to keep her legs up and this was another reason that she had bought the electrically operated chair as it enabled her to get her legs into a raised position. Her daughter informed David that Mary had developed cellulitis last year and the district nurse had visited regularly until this had cleared up. Cellulitis is an acute inflammation of the connective tissue of the skin, caused by infection with staphylococcus, streptococcus or other bacteria. Cellulitis is most common on the face or, as in Mary's case, the lower legs. David undertook an informal observational assessment of Mary's physical function; this included assessment of:

- strength
- range of movement (ROM)
- pain
- posture
- abnormal tone.

When David undertook a physical examination of Mary's lower limbs, he found that her left knee was now very stiff with reduced ROM, but her replaced knee had good ROM. Decreased ROM can affect balance when the restricted ROM leads to postural compensations that affect the ability of the person to react quickly to losses of balance.

INITIAL INFORMAL OBSERVATIONAL ASSESSMENT

At a societal limitation level, David needed to assess the physical home environment, particularly looking for factors which would increase the risk of falls or hamper Mary's independence. Mary had very steep stairs with a banister on only one side (banister to the left side when going up stairs). David felt that an immediate referral was required to the Stay Put service (a local organisation that undertakes minor works for elderly and disabled clients for the cost of the supplies) to have a stair rail put up on the wall on the other side so that Mary could have a banister to hold onto with her right hand both going up and down the stairs. Mary's house had a bathroom and toilet upstairs and her bedroom was next door to the bathroom. The bathroom had a small shower cubicle in it and a bath. The bedroom contained a single bed and was reasonably spacious.

At a disability level, David needed to assess Mary's ability to perform transfers on and off her chair, bed and toilet as well as risk assess the safety of ascending and descending the stairs. He was also concerned about how Mary would be able to use the toilet in the night when she would be alone. David explained to Mary that it was important to see how well she could move about her home and to assess her ability to get on and off her chair, bed and toilet. Mary could use her electric armchair well to get on and off the chair and managed to stand safely with the walking frame. However, she had great difficulty walking unaccompanied as she found it hard to lift the frame with her arm in plaster. With the help of one person, she walked to the base of the stairs, but she was not able to safely ascend the stairs as the banister was on the side of her fractured wrist. There was no possibility of bringing a bed downstairs as both downstairs rooms were very small. Therefore, David suggested Mary tried to ascend sideways up the stairs, using her good hand on the banister. This took a long time, but David was reassured that at all times Mary was safe. David then asked Mary to attempt to get on and off the toilet. This presented her with more difficulties as she was used to pulling herself up using her now fractured arm and the basin. David hypothesised that the purchase of an electrically operated armchair had led to a decrease in quadriceps strength because she no longer had to use muscles actively to go from sitting to standing. Finally, David assessed Mary's transfer on and off the bed. This was not easy while Mary had her wrist in plaster and, because her abdominal muscles were weak, she had difficulty getting from lying to sitting. Mary reported that she usually liked to go to bed quite early (by 9 p.m.). She also reported that she had fallen twice in the night.

David had also taken a commode in the back of his car in case this was needed. He assessed Mary's ability to transfer on and off the commode independently; however, when he assessed Mary's transfer between her bed and the commode, he felt this was not safe while Mary had her wrist in a pot. Therefore, in order to remain at home while her arm was in plaster, Mary was going to require a night-time visit. David asked Mary how often she usually got up in the night to go to the toilet and whether the time varied or was at a similar time each night. Mary reported that she usually got up once and this tended to be between 3 and 4 a.m. David made a note to refer Mary to the night nursing service for a 3 a.m. visit to assist with toileting and decided to leave the commode at the bedside as a transfer from bed to commode would be less demanding for Mary in the night than moving across the landing to the toilet.

The journey downstairs was safer as the banister was on the side of the unaffected arm. But by the time Mary had returned to her seat she was exhausted and rather tearful.

Mary did have a downstairs toilet, but this was outside in the yard and necessitated a step down at the backdoor and a step up into the toilet. David, therefore, decided to recommend Mary had a second a commode in her living room for daytime use. Mary would also need assistance to transfer on and off this commode and regular visits throughout the day would be required to prevent problems with incontinence or risk of falls if Mary attempted the transfer alone.

At the end of the assessment, David and Claire analysed the information collected and considered potential solutions for identified problems. Mary's presenting problems are summarised in Table 9.11.

One model for prioritising areas of need for intervention is Maslow's hierarchy of need model (Maslow, 1943). The lowest level of need is the physiological level; at this level, basic needs, such as food, drink, warmth and sleep, must be addressed. The next level is the safety level (the need for security from danger and providing a roof over your head are considered at this level). Once these basic needs are addressed, the next level is social needs (these include experiencing love, belonging, friendship and being able to engage in social activities). The fourth level in the hierarchy is the esteem level; at this level, people need to achieve self-respect, respect from others and a sense of achievement. Finally, the highest level of needs is self-actualisation, and this relates to the need for personal growth and development, the opportunity for creativity and for using our talents to their full potential. See Figure 9.9 for the assessment of Mary's hierarchy of need.

At the most basic physiological level of need, Mary needs to be warm, to eat, to drink, to pass urine, to open her bowels, to wash and dress and to sleep. The assessment had identified specific areas of difficulty at this level. At the safety level, the assessment highlighted some significant areas of risk related to difficulties with mobility and transfers. Mary showed that she had insight, cognitive capacity to make an informed choice about areas of risk and determination to remain in her own home. The problem areas needed both an immediate problem-solving approach and also a more long-term analysis of how the environment might be altered to create a safer living situation. Taking each area of essential need and considering it over a 24-hour period is a useful method of assessing a problem and searching for solutions.

1. Nutrition: Breakfast – her daughter will come and organise after taking her children to school. Lunch will be made by a support worker. Evening meal – her other daughter will come at about 6 p.m. to prepare Mary's tea.
2. Elimination: Mary will need to use the toilet when she wakes, after breakfast, lunchtime, late afternoon, early evening, before going to bed and during the night. A support worker will assist Mary to get out of bed in the morning and use a commode (to be supplied by Fast Response Service). After breakfast and in the evening, her daughters can supervise use of downstairs commode/toilet. Lunchtime and late afternoon: the support worker can supervise use of downstairs commode or outside toilet. The evening service will visit at between 8 and 9 p.m. and supervise going upstairs and use of the toilet and help Mary out of her clothes and into bed. The night service will visit at 3 a.m. and help Mary out of bed and onto the commode. (Key will need to be signed for and handed over to night service.)

Table 9.11 Using the NCMRR model to provide a conceptual framework for describing Mary's presenting problems

Societal limitation	Disability	Functional limitation	Impairment	Pathophysiology
Restriction attributable to social policy or barriers (structural or attitudinal), which limits fulfilment of roles or denies access to service or opportunities. Social support: supported by two carers, daughters Anne and Liz. Socially isolated does not go out and mix with peers. Environmental issues: very steep stairs – banister on only one side. Only indoor toilet upstairs. Needs grab rails by toilet, shower, front and back door. Safety issue: unable to summon help following her fall in the night; Mary had lain on the floor for 4 ½ hours waiting for her daughter to come at breakfast time.	Inability or limitation in performing socially defined activities and tasks within a social and physical environment as a result of internal or external factors and their interplay. Mobility: difficulty walking unaccompanied, unable to manage walking frame with her arm in plaster. Not able to safely ascend the stairs as the hand rail was on the side of her fractured wrist. Transfers: difficulty with toilet and bed transfers. Personal care: will have difficulty with washing and dressing while her left arm is in plaster. Needs perching stool for strip washing. Meal preparation: difficulty making snacks and drinks one-handed while wrist in plaster.	Restriction or lack of ability to perform an action or activity in the manner or range considered normal that results from impairment. Mary had limitations with motor components of tasks such as: • pushing up to stand • turning around • reaching.	Loss and/or abnormality of mental, emotional, physiological or anatomical structure or function, including secondary losses and pain. Motor system: • decrease in quadriceps' strength • abdominal muscles weak • left knee very stiff with reduced ROM (but replaced knee has good ROM) • reduced static and dynamic balance	Interference of normal physiological and developmental processes or structures. Presenting problems: • oedema • Colles' fracture (left arm) Past medical history: • widespread osteoarthritis • left hip replaced 8 years ago • right knee replaced 3 years ago • cellulitis

3. Locomotion/exercise: Support worker will supervise Mary descending the stairs. Mary was told that the support worker will not be standing below her as this would present a risk for the support worker if Mary were to fall on top of her. At the lunch-time and late-afternoon visits, the support worker will be instructed to encourage Mary to do some walking around the ground floor of the house and to do some chair-based exercises.

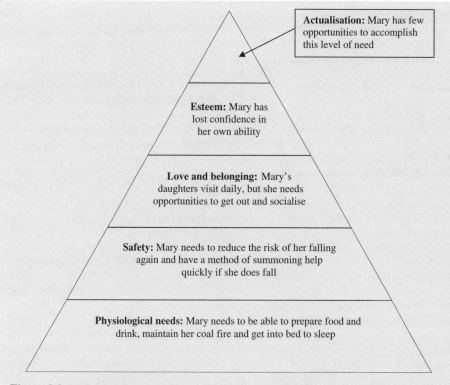

Figure 9.9 Mary's needs categorised using Maslow's Hierarchy of Needs (Maslow, 1943).

4. Warmth: The support worker will light the coal fire in the morning and Mary's daughters will feed it on their visits, as will the support workers.
5. Cleanliness: Support worker will supervise washing in the morning, and the evening service will do the same when getting Mary ready for bed.

All these issues were thoroughly discussed with Mary and her daughters. Mary agreed to this proposal as she was still determined that she wanted to stay at home rather than be placed in a recuperation bed in a local residential home.

IDENTIFYING CARE NEEDS

At a societal limitation level, it was clear that Mary was going to need social care and support from her daughters for a considerable length of time, and David reflected that this might also be an opportunity to broach the subject of more long-term help to reduce the strain on Mary's daughters. David, therefore, felt that it would be very useful to involve the social worker in this case. There may be possibilities of day-care attendance, voluntary sitters, respite care and ongoing carer support. David also felt that the whole living environment could be made safer by a range of adaptations and aids to daily living. He therefore wanted the occupational therapist to visit as soon as possible. However, the immediate need was to write a care plan for the support workers and the evening staff and to get the essential items of equipment. While David wrote the initial care plan, the support worker returned to the joint equipment store at the hospital to get a second commode and a form for Mary to sign to hand over a key to the house. This key was to be kept in a key safe in the hospital base. David informed Mary and her daughter that he would be asking the social worker and the occupational therapist to contact them on the following day.

THE SUPPORT WORKER'S ROLE

When an assessment identifies the need for involvement of the Fast Response team's support workers, a care plan is drawn up that is aimed at encouraging independence, and the plan is discussed and agreed with the client. Support workers provide a variety of social care, occupational therapy, physiotherapy and nursing tasks. They are not asked to perform any tasks without documented training for the specific task and are supervised by the qualified team members. All the support workers can take a monitoring as well as a rehabilitation role as they are trained to re-assess a client's progress prior to continuing their care plan. If the support worker is concerned that the client has deteriorated since a previous visit, she informs the most relevant person (for example her supervisor at Fast Response, the community nursing team, the client's GP or will call for emergency services where necessary). Support worker involvement is time-limited to usually no more than six weeks, and Mary and her daughters were made aware of this.

When the support worker returned with the second commode, David educated her daughter on how to supervise Mary transferring on and off it, and he placed it in the living room. Final arrangements were made for the times of the visits and consent was obtained for the key and the sharing of notes on the SAP database. David booked a follow-up visit to undertake some more specialist balance tests and to complete a Falls Risk Identification assessment.

When David got back to the team office, he gave the social worker a verbal description of Mary's first assessment and then began inputting the information that he had gathered so far onto the SAP system. He asked the social worker to continue with gaining details for the SAP overview assessment when she visited Mary the next day.

PHYSIOTHERAPY ASSESSMENT OF BALANCE AND RISK OF FALLS

Balance problems can result from a wide range of causes (Browne and O'Hare, 2001), and it is very important for the physiotherapist to assess balance to identify the root cause of any balance disorder. Browne and O'Hare (2001) give three important reasons for assessing balance.

1. 'First, it is an aid to understanding how the postural control system works' (p. 489); this addresses an assessment question at the level of impairment.
2. Second, it is an aid to clinical diagnosis and the assessment of treatment efficacy' (p. 489), and so may help with providing the diagnosis at the pathophysiological or impairment levels and provides a baseline for outcome measurement across the level(s) where intervention will be targeted.
3. 'Thirdly, it can be used to identify elderly people with a history of falls and areas where they are at risk of falling' (p. 489); this risk assessment provides predictive data that can inform the intervention and help identify those people who might most benefit from a falls programme to reduce their future risk of falls.

Methods for assessing balance can be broadly divided into two groups (Browne and O'Hare, 2001): the first group comprises functional assessments of standing balance, such as the Functional Reach Test (Duncan *et al.*, 1990), the Berg Balance Test (Berg *et al.*, 1992), The Fugl-Meyer test (Fugl-Meyer *et al.*, 1975) and the Fall Risk Index (Tinetti, Williams and Mayewski, 1986), which focus at the functional limitation and disability levels of the NCMRR (1992) model of function and dysfunction; the second group comprises physiological assessments of balance (such as sway magnetometry, mechanical ataxia meters and potentiometric displacement tranducer to record sway patterns, multi-sensor polymer insoles, three-dimensional video analysis, muscle electrodes, static force platforms and dynamic force platforms); these assessments focus at an impairment level. The Fast Response team have selected two of the functional assessments as balance measures that can be used in the person's home: the Functional Reach Test (Duncan *et al.*, 1990) and the Tinetti Fall Risk Index (Tinetti, Williams and Mayewski, 1986).

Functional Reach Test

David used the Functional Reach Test (Duncan *et al.*, 1990) to measure how far Mary could reach without taking a step forward or falling. The physiotherapist uses this assessment to provide quantitative dynamic data about the person's ability to maintain standing balance by asking them to move their centre of gravity towards the edge of their base of support. Browne and O'Hare (2001) report that the Functional Reach Test is 'mostly used for elderly people with balance problems resulting from the ageing process or associated with conditions such as Parkinson's disease. It is quick to administer and is therefore useful as a screening tool which is demonstrated by its routine use in physiotherapy departments' (p. 490). Duncan *et al.* (1992) report strong predictive validity for the Functional Reach Test for subjects at risk of falls, while Duncan *et al.* (1990) report good levels of reliability with an inter-rater reliability ICC of 0.98 and an intra-rater ICC of 0.92.

David followed these instructions for administering the functional reach test.

1. Stand with right shoulder just touching the wall – do not lean on the wall.
2. Bring the arm up to 90 degrees (parallel to floor).
3. Make a fist.
4. Mark where the furthest point of the hand reaches.
5. Say to the patient: 'Reach as far forward as you can without moving your feet but do not lose your balance.'
6. Again measure the furthest point that the hand reaches.
7. The difference between the two points is the distance of the reach.
8. Measure this distance in millimetres.

OCCUPATIONAL THERAPY ASSESSMENT

Sarah, the occupational therapist, visited Mary the following morning with the support worker to undertake a more thorough assessment of Mary's abilities in all personal and domestic activities of daily living (ADL); this was an observational assessment undertaken at a disability level (National Center for Medical Rehabilitation Research, 1992). The occupational therapist planned to assess Mary's ability to:

- get dressed/undressed
- wash
- transfer on/off the bed, upstairs toilet, chair in living room, chair in kitchen, outside toilet
- get up and down stairs
- get in and out the front and back doors
- prepare a drink and snack
- access help in the event of another fall.

During this assessment, the therapist had two considerations: first, a short-term analysis as to what Mary would be able to manage during the six weeks her arm was to be in plaster and an assessment of what aids, equipment and support would be required to maintain Mary safely at home during the period and, second, a longer-term focus in terms of what changes might be useful to maintain Mary's independence and safety once she was out of plaster. In the short-term, Sarah identified a need for a toilet frame for both upstairs and downstairs toilets. These frames would both raise the seat by three inches, which would decrease the power needed by the quadriceps to get Mary up into a standing position and also the frames provided arms that Mary could use to push up on rather than pulling herself using the basin. Sarah also tried a bed rail inserted under the mattress and on the side of Mary's non-fractured arm. This enabled Mary to pull herself up into a sitting position over the side of the bed with less difficulty and also gave her something to hold onto as she transferred to the commode. Sarah amended the care plan to ask the night staff to supervise this transfer and, if it were done safely for three nights in a row, they could cease their visits. Sarah also provided a perching stool for the bathroom for Mary to perch on at the basin when strip washing.

The occupational therapist identified a longer-term need for grab rails in the toilet, shower, outside the front and back doors and a stair rail to complement the original banister. Mary was asked if she was in agreement to having these fitted as she owned the property. She was keen to have this done, and Sarah marked all the positions of the rails and put the order in to Stay Put.

When Mary had fallen, she had been unable to get herself up and had lain on the floor for four and a half hours. Sarah described the local Community Alarm Scheme to Mary and explained how it provides a way for people like her to summon help in an emergency at home. The scheme would supply Mary with:

- a small pendant that she could wear around her neck or carry with her; this has a red button, which, when pressed, sends a signal to the telephone
- a new telephone to replace Mary's old one; it can receive the signal sent from the pendant from anywhere in Mary's house or garden.

Sarah explained that 'when you press your pendant's red button the telephone automatically calls the control centre where an operator is always waiting to alert the nominated people to provide help as soon as your call comes in. Depending on the problem, they can also alert the doctor or ambulance service. The operator will see on his computer screen some brief medical notes, which you supply when you join the scheme, and the names and addresses of three friends or relatives you have named. So you could put both your daughters down, for example. He will contact the nearest available person on your list to come to your house with a key to deal with your problem and to let professional help in when it arrives.'

Sarah also explained that these 'new telephones also include a clever device to make conversation much clearer for people who wear a hearing aid and, if it rings, you can answer it by pressing your pendant button, so there is no need to rush to the phone'. Mary was told that she could choose to either rent or buy the equipment. Mary thought the Community Alarm Scheme sounded like a very good idea and agreed to having it set up.

Also Sarah instructed the support worker about how to facilitate Mary to maximise the activities that she was still able to do herself. It is an important element of the service that clients are continually encouraged to maintain their independence even though it would often be quicker for the support workers to do the task for the person.

SOCIAL WORK ASSESSMENT

In the afternoon, the social worker met with Mary's daughter Liz to undertake a carer's assessment. For EASY-Care a carer is defined as a friend or relative of the person who provides support and who is unpaid (EASY-Care, 2006b). EASY-Care is derived from a collection of published instruments. The Carers' assessment in EASY-Care is the Carers of Older People in Europe (COPE) Index (McKee *et al.*, 2003), and it is usually administered as part of an overview assessment and can be used to evaluate whether a carer would need a more in-depth specialist assessment and benefit from emotional and/or practical support with their caring role. The social worker also added to the assessments undertaken by the physiotherapist and occupational therapist to complete the EASY-Care overview assessment.

Mary was adamant she wanted to live at home but did admit that she felt a bit isolated and would enjoy getting out. Therefore, the social worker said she would try and arrange a weekly day-centre place and transport to get there. This would also give Liz a day when she was free to be out all day. A revised care plan was draw up jointly by the physiotherapist, occupational therapist and social worker and a review date set for the following week.

INTERVENTION

During the next six weeks, Mary was supported by an intensive package of care involving her daughters, the Fast Response Service and the evening nursing service. She only needed visits during the night for four nights. She gained in confidence over the six-week intervention period, and the support workers undertook a programme of falls prevention exercises with her, which improved her strength and balance (Campbell *et al.*, 1997). The support workers advised David and Sarah about Mary's progress, and the care plan was amended three times to reflect her improving abilities.

After Mary's plaster was removed, David assessed her wrist and printed out a programme of home exercises to improve ROM and muscle strength. These exercises were complemented by the work that the support workers were then doing with Mary to increase her independence in all aspects of her personal and domestic ADL. It was evident that if some of the caring pressure was to be reduced for Liz and Anne then Mary was going to continue to need regular daily visits even when her wrist was no longer immobilised. The social worker organised direct payments to be made for Mary to use the local personal assistance scheme to employ a carer who lived in the village to visit twice a day for an early-morning and late-evening call.

While the Fast Response team usually provides an intermediate care service of about six weeks' duration, the team stayed involved for a total of eight weeks because of the need to maximise Mary's independence after the plaster had been removed. Finally, because Mary had a history of falls, she was invited for a falls assessment at the local hospital. This led to Mary being offered a place on an eight-week Falls Group Service to improve her balance and mobility. The Falls Group Service was initially set up as a pilot in response to the *National Service Framework for Older People* (DoH, 2001a), which stipulates in Standard Six that Trusts should have an integrated falls service in place by April 2005. In addition to this national policy driver, the Fast Response team had found that over 30 per cent of people referred to the Fast Response Service had suffered a fall.

FALLS GROUP SERVICE

The Falls Group Service programme was based on evidence obtained from a thorough review of literature on falls rehabilitation. The team reviewed information on implementing the *NSF for Older People Falls Standard* (Department of Health, 2003). A number of studies influenced the components of the programme. First, two meta-analyses of falls studies provided a starting point for reviewing the evidence: Chang *et al.* (2004) undertook a systematic review and meta-analysis of randomised clinical trials exploring the evidence on interventions for the prevention of falls in older people, and Gillespie *et al.* (2003) led a Cochrane review on interventions for preventing falls in elderly people. The issue of combating the fear of falls was identified in a paper by Bruce *et al.* (2002). Several studies were found that provided evidence that group exercise was a means of reducing falls, for example a study by Rubenstein *et al.* (2000) to examine the effects of a group exercise programme on strength, mobility and falls among fall-prone elderly men. Some studies also examined the use of home exercise programmes to reduce falls, for example the Falls Service drew upon the work of Campbell *et al.* (1997), who describe a randomised controlled trial of a general practice programme of home-based exercise to prevent falls in elderly women, and Day *et al.* (2002), who describe a randomised factorial trial of falls prevention among older people living in their own homes. Muscle strengthening was also included as an outcome for the falls programme; the team also drew on the work of Chandler *et al.* (1998), who describe a study to explore whether lower-extremity strength gain is associated with improvement in physical performance and disability in frail, community-dwelling older people, and Hurley and Roth's (2000) work on strength training in older people.

Mary attended the day hospital at her local community hospital, where the Falls Service was based. Initially, she undertook a screening assessment to establish her suitability for the falls programme and to identify any needs requiring referral to other services, such as a podiatrist or optician (for intervention at an impairment level). The initial assessment also included three standardised measures that the Falls Service staff had selected as outcome measures for the group programme; these were the Timed Up and Go test, the Tinetti Balance Scale and a 12-metre walk test.

The Timed Up and Go Test

The Timed Up and Go (Podsiadlo and Richardson, 1991) is an observational test that is used by both clinicians and researchers. It covers aspects of assessment across the impairment, functional limitation and disability levels of the NCMRR model of function/dysfunction (National Center for Medical Rehabilitation Research, 1992): and is used to:

- assess aspects of one impairment level system (motor performance)
- examine specific motor skills (such as the ability to rise, turn, sit down, balance and mobilise a short distance) at a functional limitation level
- observe at the disability level the tasks of walking and transferring on/off.

Cole *et al.* (1995) provide a brief overview of the test and state that the Timed Up and Go 'is a quick and practical method of testing basic mobility manoeuvres' (p. 38). The Timed Up and Go can be used with older people with a wide range of conditions, including osteoarthritis, stroke, Parkinson's disease, rheumatoid arthritis, multiple sclerosis, hip fracture, cerebellar degeneration and general de-conditioning. It is an inexpensive test as only a stopwatch is required. It is quick to administer as the test comprises only one short multi-phase task. The test has established test–rest reliability. Podsiadlo and Richardson (1991) conducted a study in which 20 geriatric clients were evaluated on the Timed Up and Go by the same observer on consecutive visits and the test–retest agreement was calculated to be high (ICC 0.99). The test also has established inter-rater reliability. Mathias, Nayak and Isaacs (1986) conducted a study in which 22 geriatric clients were evaluated separately by three raters on the same day and found a high level of agreement between raters (ICC 0.99). In addition, Podsiadlo and Richardson (1991) report a study in which 40 clients aged 52–94 years were videotaped undertaking the Timed Up and Go and were rated by physiotherapists and doctors. The inter-rater reliability for physiotherapists was acceptable (Kendall's coefficient W, 0.85) but lower levels of agreement were reported for the doctors (0.69) (Cole *et al.*, 1995). A concurrent validity study reported by Podsiadlo and Richardson (1991) showed correlations between the Timed Up and Go and other measures; 'the longer the time for the Up and Go test, the lower was the score on the Berg Balance Scale, the Barthel Index and gait speed' (Cole *et al.*, 1995, p. 39).

Mary was asked to start the test seated in an armchair. She was then told to stand up from the chair, stand still momentarily, walk to a line (which had been taped on the floor three metres away from the chair), turn, return to the chair and turn around and sit down again. Mary was scored according to the time in seconds that it took her to successfully complete the task. The therapist scoring the test makes a qualitative judgement about the person's risk of falls using a five-point ordinal scale:

1. normal
2. very slightly abnormal
3. mildly abnormal
4. moderately abnormal
5. severely abnormal.

Tinetti Balance Scale

The Tinetti Balance Scale is part of the Performance Orientated Mobility Assessment developed by Mary Tinetti (1986). It comprises nine test items, each scored on either a two-point or three-point ordinal scale with a maximum possible score of 16. Balance is assessed with the person sitting, moving from sitting to standing, standing and turning around. The person's ability to maintain balance against attempts at disruption (a nudge and without a horizontal reference when the eyes are closed) are also tested. The nine test areas are (Tinetti *et al.*, 1995):

1. sitting balance
2. arises
3. attempts to arise
4. immediate standing balance (first five seconds)
5. standing balance
6. nudged (subject at maximum position with feet as close together as possible; examiner pushes lightly on the subject's sternum with palm of hand three times)
7. eyes closed
8. turning 360 degrees
9. sitting down.

Numbers are assigned to behavioural descriptors for scoring, for example the scoring method for the standing balance items is:

- 0 = unsteady
- 1 = steady but with wide stance (medial heels more then four inches apart) and uses cane or other support
- 2 = steady without walker or other support.

Mary scored six out of a possible 16 on the Tinetti Balance Scale.

Twelve-metre walk test

Worsfold and Simpson (2001) provide an overview of distance-limited timed walking tests and state that 'there is evidence that [they] are useful indicators of functional mobility in elderly people' (p. 125). They report that 'slower walking times are associated with increases in disability, postural instability and risk of falling' (p. 125). As physiotherapists use this test to assess usual performance, the person is allowed to use their own walking aid. Although some studies have found the use of a walking aid to be associated with slower speeds (for example Friedman, Richmond and Baskett, 1988), it was felt by the Falls Service that this should be the person's choice, with the main issue being that the physiotherapist records what walking aid (if any) is used for the baseline assessment and ensures the same walking aid is used for follow-up assessments to provide consistency. If the person has improved so much that a walking aid is no longer needed at re-test, then this should be recorded clearly on the assessment.

When discussing distance-limited timed walking tests, Worsfold and Simpson (2001) state that 'standardisation is especially necessary when very old people are the test subjects as variability in almost all abilities is greater among them than among younger people. Therefore, if results are to have any meaning beyond the individual person, the possible sources of variation in test administration within and between subjects should be reduced to a minimum' (p. 125). David has typed out test administration instructions for the 12-metre walking test to be used by staff at the Falls Service.

1. Six metres' distance is marked out along the day hospital corridor.
2. The person is told: 'The purpose of this test is to find out how long it takes you to walk 12 metres. You will start from this point,' indicates the start of the measured six metres 'walk down the corridor to this point,' (indicate the end of the six-metre distance) 'turn round and walk back to the starting point. Walk at the fastest pace you can go *safely*.' The patient is also told: 'Do not hurry so much that you are unsafe, and use the walking aid that you would usually use for walking.'
3. The therapist starts the person standing at the line with both feet together and finishes timing when the lead foot goes over the line.

It took Mary 102 seconds to complete this 12-metre walk.

Mary was considered to be a suitable candidate for the Falls Service and after the assessment was given a start date for her falls group programme. The group sessions were run by an occupational therapy technical instructor, who also had an exercise instructor qualification, and Claire the support worker from the Fast Response team.

Mary received eight weekly sessions, at the local community hospital. At a societal limitation level, transport was provided via Red Cross Ambulance to enable Mary to access the Falls Service. The group sessions delivered interventions across several levels of function, which included:

• at the disability level, Mary engaged in walking practice
• at a functional limitation level, she was given training and advice in how to cope if she did fall at home, including movements to use to attempt to get up off the floor and strategies to stay warm
• at an impairment level, she engaged in group sessions to improve balance and strengthening exercises to increase her muscle strength and stamina
• at a societal limitation level, Mary was given a booklet about safety in the home and advice on nutrition (feeding and nutrition is addressed at a disability level); in addition, group participants watched a video about falls and received advice and information regarding falls prevention.

During the eight-week period, two home visits are usually undertaken. The first visit is conducted by the occupational therapist to undertake a home hazard assessment. Mary had already received this assessment from the Fast Response team occupational therapist following her fall. The second visit is undertaken by one of the physiotherapists to prescribe a home exercise programme. The team felt that the exercise programme should be individually prescribed to take into account the person's home circumstances and abilities. The team have found that, by visiting the person at home and personalising the exercise programme, participants become more motivated to continue to exercise at home after the group sessions have ended. Mary had already been prescribed an exercise programme by David when she was referred to the Fast Response Service. David felt that it was relevant to review Mary's progress during her eight-week programme and modify her exercise programme to increase Mary's strength and stamina further. The progression of falls prevention exercises is based on strength training following the principle of overload, and this is best achieved by an ankle-weight system that allows extra weights to be added. These systems are relatively inexpensive, and a variety of hip, knee and ankle exercises have been devised by the New Zealand Falls Prevention Research Group (Gardner *et al.*, 2001), which have been reproduced by AGILE (2004.) This programme of exercises can be purchased and copies of the exercises given to clients so that carers/relatives and friends can help and encourage the person to continue to practise them. Mary was given a printed sheet of exercises, and her daughters were instructed to encourage her to follow her exercise programme regularly. Four controlled trials of the home exercise programme have been undertaken and analysed by the falls prevention research group (Robertson *et al.*, 2002), and a meta-analysis showed that 'the overall effect of the programme was to reduce number of falls and number of fall-related injuries by 35%' (p. 905). The home exercise programme was found to be 'equally effective in reducing fall rates in those with or without a previous fall' and 'was most effective in reducing fall-related injuries in those aged 80 and older' (p. 905).

At the end of the eight sessions, Mary was re-assessed again on the three outcome measures (see scores in Table 9.12). Mary had improved on all three measures.

Mary was discharged back to her GP. Copies of her falls group baseline and follow-up scores were included in the discharge letter and the GP was asked to re-refer if he felt Mary had deteriorated at a future date. Mary was followed up three months after discharge from the Falls Service for re-assessment on the outcome measures, and to discover if Mary had any falls since she completed the programme. Sarah also uses this opportunity to re-check for home hazards and to promote the continuation of her exercise routine.

Table 9.12 Mary's baseline and follow-up scores

Assessment Conducted by	Date	Timed Up and Go	12-metre walk	Tinetti Balance
J	2/8	45 secs	102 secs	6/16
J	29/9	27 secs	40 secs	15/16

WORKSHEETS

Please now turn to Worksheet 9. There are two versions of this worksheet: 9.1 (p. 410) allows you to apply the NCMRR model (National Center for Medical Rehabilitation Research, 1992) and 9.2 (p. 411) allows you to apply the ICF model (World Health Organization, 2002). For this reflection, you will need to review the range of unstandardised and standardised assessments and outcome measures used within your occupational therapy or physiotherapy service or by your multidisciplinary team. If you are a student, reflect on the range of assessments and outcome measures that you have seen used on one of your clinical placements. Worksheet 9.1 lists the five levels of the NCMRR model of function and dysfunction in the left-hand column, while

Worksheet 9.2 lists four of the key dimensions from the ICF model. Both worksheets pose a number of questions or instructions to be completed for each level/dimension.

STUDY QUESTIONS

9.1 Why can it be useful to apply a model of function as a framework for your assessment process?

9.2 What are the 10 levels in the hierarchy of living systems, described by Christiansen (1991)?

9.3 In the ICF model (World Health Organization, 1992), how are the terms *body functions*, *body structures* and *impairments* defined?

9.4 In the ICF model (World Health Organization, 1992), how are the terms *activity*, *participation*, *activity limitations* and *participation restrictions* defined?

9.5 What are the five levels proposed by the NCMRR (1992) model of function and dysfunction?

You will find brief answers to these questions at the back of this book (pp. 393–4).

10

The Importance of Clinical Reasoning and Reflective Practice in Effective Assessment

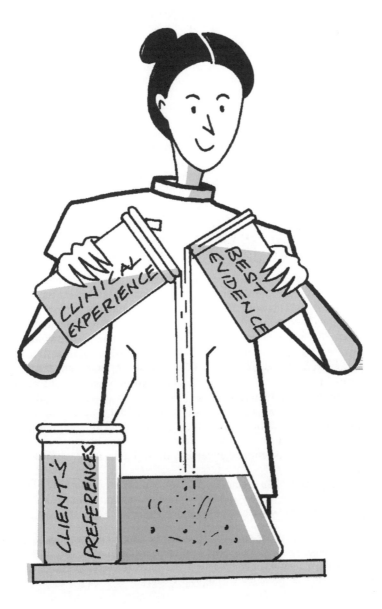

CHAPTER SUMMARY

The aim of this chapter is to highlight to therapists the importance of reflecting upon how they and others think about and make clinical decisions related to assessment and measurement. This chapter will define clinical reasoning and show how it is an essential component of assessment and required for interpreting measurement data. It will also define and describe different types of reasoning, for example diagnostic reasoning, procedural reasoning interactive reasoning, conditional reasoning, ethical reasoning and narrative reasoning and discuss the importance of reflective practice. The chapter concludes with a case example as an illustration of how a therapist thinks in practice when assessing a client. Finally, it will endeavour to answer the following question: 'How do I combine the best available evidence with my clinical experience and my knowledge of my client's preferences?'

> To practise well requires a strong sense of vision to guide us. We need expert clinical judgement – the ability to grasp and interpret what is unfolding, and skilful action to respond appropriately and effectively. We then need to evaluate and reflect in order to learn from the situation and apply such learning and new experiences within a reflexive spiral of being and becoming. This is professional practice. Within that spiral, we draw on relevant theory to inform us, theory that we then assimilate into our personal knowing. (Johns, 2004, p. 3)

So how do occupational therapists and physiotherapists develop expert clinical judgement? How do we learn to reflect upon and improve our clinical practice? How do we form this 'strong sense of vision' to guide our practice wisely? The following text provides some basic answers to these questions, but as professional judgement, clinical reasoning and reflective practice are complex areas of study this chapter can only serve as a basic introduction to a fascinating and important subject – suggestions for further reading are provided in case this chapter whets your appetite for greater understanding!

CLINICAL REASONING AS AN ESSENTIAL COMPONENT OF PRACTICE

Problem-solving in therapy can be directed, as in medicine, to problem identification and diagnosis, but it also often refers to 'the invention of the unique solutions for the complex problems and issues the client faces' (Unsworth, 1999, p. 53). So problem-solving by therapists involves reasoning directed towards solving a goal, the goal usually being to understand the nature of the problem and to organise a response that will be therapeutic. The problems identified by therapists during assessment usually are framed as problems of understanding, for example identifying the cause of observed behaviour. Information from several assessment sources is gathered to research the presenting problem(s) and then integrated into a single clinical image through clinical reasoning processes. Fleming (1994a) identifies and describes a variety of reasoning strategies used by therapists to determine clients' problems and to select appropriate treatments. Both the explicit and tacit reasoning that guides therapy problem-solving processes has been called 'clinical reasoning' (Mattingly, 1991). Other synonymous phrases seen in therapy, health and social care literature include clinical expertise, clinical judgement, clinical decision-making and reflective thinking.

Clinical reasoning is seen as an essential and important component of effective practice, and not just occupational therapy and physiotherapy practice but across the spectrum of health and social care. The World Confederation for Physical Therapy (WCPT) states that it:

> champions the principle that every individual is entitled to the highest possible standard of culturally-appropriate health care provided in an atmosphere of trust and respect for human dignity and underpinned by sound clinical reasoning and scientific evidence. (World Confederation for Physical Therapy, 2003)

While the College of Occupational Therapists (COT; 2003a) refers to clinical reasoning in its definition of evaluation as:

> the process of using clinical reasoning, problem-analysis, self-appraisal and review to interpret the results of assessment in order to make judgements about the situation or needs of an individual, the success of occupational therapy or the therapist's own performance. (p. 53)

Donaghy and Morss (2000), in their paper on reflective practice within the discipline of physiotherapy, recommend that the physiotherapy profession should encourage therapists to engage in systematic critical inquiry and to focus their attention on problem-solving and clinical reasoning. They stress the importance of linking reflection to higher-order cognitive processes, such as memory schema, illness scripts and clinical knowledge. White (2004) notes that 'clinical decision making is inextricably linked to therapist/patient interaction and the reflective/analytic phase of clinical reasoning which takes place during and after contact' (p. 28). White goes on to state that 'reflection is an area that was once undervalued by physiotherapists but has now been given recognition for its contribution to clinical reasoning and decision making. This has been achieved by the amalgamation of empirical and phenomenological philosophies and the development of critical reflection' (p. 29).

In Chapter 1, we examined the demand for therapists to deliver an evidence-based practice (EBP). Clinical reasoning plays a critical role in enabling a therapist to marry practice based on best evidence with practice that is client-centred and based upon a person's unique presentation of problems and needs. Sackett *et al.* (1996), in their discussion about the nature of evidence-based medicine (EBM), emphasise that practitioners undertaking EBP cannot take a 'cookbook' approach. EBP requires an 'approach that integrates the best external evidence with individual clinical expertise and patients' choice; it cannot result in slavish, cookbook approaches to individual patient care' (p. 71). External clinical evidence is used to inform clinical decisions, but should not replace individual clinical expertise. Clinical reasoning is the process by which clinical expertise is applied to individual client problems; the therapist engages in clinical reasoning to decide whether available external evidence applies to the individual client's presentation. When the clinician decides external evidence does apply, clinical reasoning is required to establish how this evidence should be applied in this particular case and underlies clinical decision-making around how the evidence should be integrated into this client's assessment, management and/or intervention.

The underlying knowledge base and experience that a therapist brings to an assessment is critical, but it is not sufficient to address the complexity of assessment. Kielhofner (1992) notes that 'the use of theory is not a simple mapping of theory onto reality; it is a much more complex, indeterminate, and artful process' (p. 260). Each assessment requires the therapist to engage in original thinking.

> Therapists must recognize the unique conditions presented by each patient and make careful observations and interpretations to find the best strategies for resolving each patient's particular set of problems. Clinical reasoning takes place as therapists attempt to understand the nature of patients' problems and develop individualized therapy directed towards the future life for each patient. (Cohn and Czycholl, 1991, p. 161)

Clinical judgement should be informed by the use of objective, preferably standardised, assessment processes. The therapist needs to address a number of assessment questions. These will vary depending upon the nature of the referral, service and diagnosis but may include:

- What are the person's strengths or abilities? (Rogers, 2004)
- What are the client's deficits or needs? (Rogers, 2004)
- What is the person's occupational profile? (Rogers, 2004)

- What degree of independence does the person have?
- Why is performance affected?
- How does the person perform the task?
- When is the person functioning at his best?

The specific questions to be addressed will vary from person to person and will depend upon the diagnosis, presenting problems and whether the therapist is a physiotherapist or occupational therapist. It is important to recognise the unique conditions that are presented by each person, and the assessment should involve careful observations and interpretations in order to identify the optimum strategies for resolving each person's particular problems.

CLINICAL JUDGEMENT AND CLINICAL REASONING

Clinical judgement has been defined as 'the ability of professionals to make decisions within their own field of expertise using the working knowledge that they have acquired over time. It is based on both clinical experience and the theoretical principles embedded in their professional knowledge base but it may remain highly subjective' (Stewart, 1999, p. 417). Clinical judgement is exercised through both theoretical and clinical reasoning, which are defined as:

- theoretical reasoning is learned from sources such as text books and lectures and relates to generalities, to what the therapist can predict (Unsworth, 1999)
- clinical reasoning occurs as the therapist works to understand the nature of the person's problems and to construct individualised client-centred interventions (Cohn and Czycholl, 1991).

Clinical reasoning has been described as 'the thinking or cognitive processes and decision making that therapists use to guide their work' and is 'a practical know-how that puts theoretical knowledge into practice' and is concerned 'with deliberating over appropriate action and then putting this in place' (Unsworth, 1999, pp. 45–46). The Chartered Society of Physiotherapy (CSP, 2001b) draws upon the work of Higgs (1990) to define clinical reasoning as 'the thinking and decision making processes associated with a physiotherapist's assessment and management of a patient' (p. 4). Simply put, clinical reasoning is 'the process used by practitioners to plan, direct, perform and reflect on client care' (Schell, 1998, p. 90). So when a therapist is involved in planning, doing or thinking about therapy she is engaged in clinical reasoning.

The American Occupational Therapy Association (AOTA; 1984, cited in Hopkins and Smith, 1993a, p. 914) defines clinical reasoning as 'the process of systematic decision making based on an identifiable professional frame of reference and utilizing both subjective and objective data accrued through appropriate assessment/evaluation processes'. The COT (2003a) draws upon the work of a number of authors to define clinical reasoning as:

> the mental strategies and high-level cognitive patterns and processes that underlie the process of naming, framing and solving problems and that enable the therapist to reach decisions about the best course of action. Clinical reasoning translates the knowledge, skills and values of the therapist into action and ensures that occupational therapists practise occupational therapy and not some other form of intervention. (p. 51)

This definition will be the one used in this text as a starting point for understanding clinical reasoning. In terms of physiotherapy, clinical reasoning involves exactly the same process, only one that is exercised within a physiotherapy context.

SCIENTIFIC REASONING

The basic process of reasoning is considered to be universal: 'all human beings reason' (Roberts, 1996, p. 233). Problem-solving is a fundamental process that is undertaken by people faced by some sort of problem. However, the precise nature of the problem-solving process can vary depending on the nature of the problem, the context in which problem-solving is undertaken and the expertise of the problem solver. The two most commonly discussed forms of reasoning in scientific literature are deductive and inductive reasoning. Both types of reasoning are used by therapy clinicians and researchers.

DEDUCTIVE REASONING

Discussion about deductive reasoning dates back to Aristotle. Deductive reasoning involves reasoning from the general to the particular (or from cause to effect). The deductive reasoning process begins with statements that are accepted as true and then applies these held 'truths' to a new situation to reach a conclusion. Deduction, therefore, is seen as reasoning based on facts. Deductive reasoning is the process of reaching a conclusion that is guaranteed to follow, if the evidence provided is true and the reasoning used to reach the conclusion is correct. The conclusion must be based only on the evidence previously provided; it cannot contain new information about the subject matter. Deductive reasoning is seen as a top-down approach to reasoning (see Figure 10.1).

Therapists use deductive reasoning in assessment. For example, a clinician may start from theories of perception and knowledge that perception can be affected by a stroke. One type of perceptual deficit she has seen in previous clients with stroke is figure/ground discrimination deficit. The therapist forms a hypothesis that the client has figure/ground discrimination perceptual deficit. She forms a further more specific hypothesis which states that this figure/ground discrimination deficit will negatively affect the person's ability to retrieve the previously recognised object of a spoon from a drawer full of cutlery. The therapist then sets about to test

Theory

Hypothesis based upon the theory

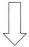

Observation: the collection of data based on what is expected to be true or false based on the hypothesis

Testing: the hypothesis is tested using the collected data

Decision: confirmation or refutation of the hypothesis either supports or negates the theory

Figure 10.1 Deductive reasoning.

her hypothesis by presenting the client with a drawer of knives, forks and spoons and asks him to take out a spoon. The client fumbles about in the drawer, complains that it is such a muddle and finally takes out a fork. He recognises it is a fork once it is the only object of his attention and puts it back. He looks at the drawer again but struggles to see each individual item of cutlery from the other pieces of cutlery and the background of the base of the drawer. The therapist concludes from these observations that her hypothesis is confirmed and makes a diagnosis of figure/ground discrimination deficit.

With deductive reasoning, we can make deductive conclusions based on known facts (that if x is present and x and y are know to occur together, then if x is present then y will also be present). For example, it is known that if it rains then the ground below becomes wet; so if we observe from a window that it is raining we can reliably deduce that the ground below will be wet. However, we cannot necessarily deduce the opposite (that if the ground is wet it must be raining), because there are a number of other causes of wet ground. If we begin with the observation that the ground is wet, then we would need to use an inductive reasoning process to problem-solve the cause.

INDUCTIVE REASONING

Inductive reasoning is a system of reasoning based on observation and measurement. Inductive reasoning works in the opposite way to deductive reasoning: the reasoning process works from specific observations to broader generalisations and theories. Inductive reasoning involves observing patterns and using those observations to make generalisations. Therapists use inductive reasoning to draw a general conclusion based on a limited set of observations. With inductive reasoning, therapists begin with specific observations and measurements; from these they detect patterns and regularities and then formulate some tentative hypotheses that can be explored and tested, and finally they produce some general conclusions or theories. Inductive reasoning is seen as a bottom-up approach to reasoning (see Figure 10.2).

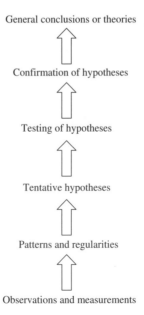

General conclusions or theories

Confirmation of hypotheses

Testing of hypotheses

Tentative hypotheses

Patterns and regularities

Observations and measurements

Figure 10.2 Inductive reasoning.

In inductive reasoning, the person may start with the observation that the ground is wet. There may be several causes for this: a sprinkler may have been on, a river may have flooded, a drain may have overflowed, a container of liquid may have spilt or it may have been raining. A measurement of how much ground has become wet and observation of the nature of the dampness (for example whether it is clear or muddy or smelly) will aid the narrowing of these possible hypotheses. The person may observe over time that whenever it rains the ground is wet; this becomes a pattern. Rain may also be noted as the most frequent reason the ground becomes wet. Other observations may also be associated with this pattern, for example that other objects higher up, such as trees and buildings, also become wet. This additional information can be used as an observation to be made when narrowing and testing out hypotheses for the causes of wet ground in the future. So the inductive process would go: observation that the ground is wet, hypothesis that it has been raining, hypothesis tested by further observation that the ground is wet as far as the eye can see and that the trees and plants are also wet with a clear, clean liquid, which all lead to a general conclusion that it has been raining.

GENERALISATION

Generalisation is a type of inductive reasoning of relevance to therapists. It is known as inductive generalisation. This type of reasoning proceeds from a premise about a sample of people to a conclusion about the whole population. So if a proportion of the sample has a particular attribute, then we generalise that the same proportion of the total population has that same attribute. How accuate these generalisations are depends on two main factors, first the number of people in the sample group compared to the number in the population and, second, the randomness of the sample. This is of relevance when using normative data obtained from a sample of the population for comparison of a client's score on a norm-referenced test (for more information on norm-referenced tests, see the section on norm-referenced tests in Chapter 5). It is also of relevance when applying prevalence data for a diagnosis or a problem, drawn from research on a sample, to a wider population, for example in order to estimate the level of demand on a therapy service.

If a therapist is starting from the position of individual client-based observations, then she starts with an inductive reasoning process, but if she receives a referral and reads the name of a diagnosis or problem that leads her thinking straight to a theory or frame of reference, then she starts her assessment process with deductive reasoning. Both forms of reasoning are useful in clinical practice. How these types of reasoning have been implemented and adapted by therapists has become the focus of some studies on therapist's clinical reasoning.

In therapy, scientific reasoning is undertaken by clinicians to understand the client's presenting condition and to decide which interventions would produce the best desired effect for removing or reducing the impact of the presenting condition for the client. Scientific reasoning in therapy 'is a logical process, which parallels scientific inquiry' (Schell, 1998, p. 93). In the therapy clinical reasoning literature, two types of scientific reasoning are discussed; these are diagnostic reasoning (Rogers and Holm, 1991; Rogers, 2004) and procedural reasoning (Fleming, 1994b).

PROCEDURAL REASONING

Procedural reasoning is an 'umbrella term that describes a therapist's thinking when working out what a client's problems are and what procedures may be used to reduce the effect of those problems' (Unsworth, 1999, p. 54). Therapists use procedural reasoning to understand the person's problems and to consider ways to alleviate, or reduce the impact of, these problems. Fleming (1994a), in her research into procedural reasoning, found that:

> In situations where problem identification and treatment selection were seen as the central task, the therapists' thinking strategies demonstrated many parallels to the patterns identified by other researchers interested in problem solving in general, and

clinical problem solving in particular. The typical medical problem-solving sequence – diagnosis, prognosis, prescription – was commonly used. However, the words the therapists used to describe this sequence were problem identification, goal setting and treatment planning. (p. 121)

Fleming also found that the therapists she studied utilised the three problem-solving methods that had been previously described by Newel and Simon (1972, cited by Fleming, 1994a): the methods of recognition, generate and test and heuristic search. These methods have also been identified in Rogers and Holms' (1991) study of therapists' diagnostic reasoning and their formulation of a therapy diagnosis.

DIAGNOSTIC REASONING AND THE THERAPY DIAGNOSIS

Many professions use the process of diagnosis (Schön, 1983) and apply the scientific model that involves hypothetical reasoning (Fleming, 1991). For example, Benner (1984) describes the diagnostic reasoning and treatment decision-making processes in nursing. Diagnostic reasoning becomes a unique occupational therapy process or physiotherapy process when it is applied to profession-specific concepts. For example, in occupational therapy, diagnostic reasoning 'is applied to profession-specific concepts . . . such as occupational performance' and 'as diagnosticians, therapists seek to learn about a patient's functional performance and to describe it so that intervention can be initiated' (Rogers and Holm, 1989, pp. 8–9). In a problem-solving process, the problem is some sort of malfunction that you are trying to track down. In therapy, the client comes to you with suboptimal functioning in some area of his life. So, for therapists, diagnostic reasoning 'is concerned with clinical problem sensing and problem definition' (Schell, 1998, p. 93). It is similar to, although not exactly the same as, medical problem-solving (Mattingly, 1994b). The product of an initial therapy assessment is the formulation of a problem statement. Therapists use various clinical reasoning processes to develop problem statements. The case method, for example, 'is a problem-solving process that fosters the application of knowledge for defining and resolving problems. Data are collected, classified, analysed and interpreted in accordance with a clinical frame of reference and transformed into a definition of the problem and subsequently an action plan' (Line, 1969, cited by Rogers, 2004, p. 17).

In occupational therapy literature, the problem statement has been called the 'occupational therapy diagnosis' (Rogers and Holm, 1991). This is defined as a 'concise summary of a client's disruptions in occupational role that are amenable to occupational therapy' (Rogers, 2004, p. 18). Physiotherapy literature also talks about a physiotherapy diagnosis. In the 'Description of physical therapy: what characterises physical therapy?' section of its website, the WCPT (2006c) states: 'diagnosis arises from the examination and evaluation and represents the outcome of the process of clinical reasoning. This may be expressed in terms of movement dysfunction or may encompass categories of impairments, functional limitations, abilities/disabilities or syndromes.' The WCPT goes on to state:

> Diagnosis within physical therapy is the result of a process of clinical reasoning which results in the identification of existing or potential impairments, functional limitations and abilities/disabilities. The purpose of the diagnosis is to guide physical therapists in determining the prognosis and identifying the most appropriate intervention strategies for patients/clients and in sharing information with them. In carrying out the diagnostic process, physical therapists may need to obtain additional information from other professionals. If the diagnostic process reveals findings that are not within the scope of the physical therapist's knowledge, experience or expertise, the physical therapist will refer the patient/client to another appropriate practitioner.

The thinking that leads to a therapy diagnosis is referred to as *diagnostic reasoning*. Diagnostic reasoning involves the therapist creating a clinical image of the person through cue acquisition, hypothesis generation, cue interpretation and hypothesis evaluation (Rogers and Holm, 1991). It has developed from scientific reasoning, following the process of hypothesis generation and testing (Unsworth, 1999). The diagnostic reasoning process can be explicated in two ways, in terms of steps taken and in terms of strategies used (Rogers and Holm, 1989). First, in terms of the steps involved in functional assessment, such as data collection and the analysis and synthesis of that data, such as the steps in a problem-orientated reasoning process (see description later on in this chapter, p. 291). Second, in terms of the principles and strategies that therapists use to collect, analyse and synthesise data, this includes the use of hypothesis generation, testing and validation and the application of heuristics (the use of hypotheses and heuristics will be explored below).

If a person is unable to perform activities independently, the therapist will note a lack of mastery or independence and will also need to explore the underlying causes for the dysfunctional interaction. The function of performance components will, therefore, need to be evaluated. In order to do this, the therapist has to understand what the requirements of the interaction were. When a therapist analyses an activity, both the individual and non-human components of the activity are unpackaged. Many therapists draw upon models that are founded upon general systems theory and view the person as an open system. Open systems theory is an interdisciplinary approach used by both occupational therapists and physiotherapists. In my own work (Laver, 1994) on assessment and diagnostic reasoning, I drew upon early work on systems theory from von Bertalanffy (1968), Mackay (1968) and Allport (1968) to form an understanding of open systems theory and explored the later work of Kielhofner (1978 and 1992), who applied these ideas to occupational therapy concepts. To summarise, the person (as an open system) takes in information and stimuli (referred to as input) from both his internal systems and external environment and converts or acts upon this information (a process referred to as throughput) to produce some sort of response, which may include observable behaviour (known as the person's output). The outcome of this behaviour in turn produces more information and stimuli and provides feedback as a cyclical process (for more information on open systems please see the section on general systems theory and the hierarchy of living systems and Figure 9.1 in Chapter 9). The person repeats this cyclical process of input $\Rightarrow$ throughput $\Rightarrow$ output $\Rightarrow$ feedback throughout life to meet the demands of a constantly changing external environment. In this way, the repertoire of a person's actions develops throughout his life. People learn to associate stimuli (input) with action responses (for example presentation of food with eating). Based upon this developed repertoire, the person has a limited number of responses (output) to a specific stimulus (input). The repertoire of an individual's acts develops throughout the life span as the result of interaction with his environment. The limitations of such a repertoire means that there are a limited number of responses (output) an individual can make to a given stimulus (input). Humans learn to associate stimuli and action responses, for example presentation of food with eating. These associations form a conceptual framework of normal stimulus–response interactions. The observation of the demands of an individual's environment provides information about the nature of the information (input) received by that individual. The observation of the output produced in response to this environmental input provides the therapist with an indication of the nature of the person's internal organisation (throughput). As therapists, we have a conceptual framework of normal stimulus–response behaviours for the culture in which we live and work. When a therapist engages in observational assessment, she needs to note the demands of the individual's environment to gain information about the nature of the information/stimuli (input) presented to the person. The observation of the person's behavioural responses (output), related to the observed input, provides the therapist with an indication of the nature of the person's internal organisation (throughput). As we have a repertoire of normal stimulus–response behaviours, we can predict what an acceptable behaviour response will be for a person of a particular age and background. Unusual output provides observational cues that prompt hypothesis generation. When a therapist observes an unpredicted output, this alerts her to the possibility of dysfunction. Unexpected output (which could take the form of an abnormal action, facial expression or spoken word) prompts the diagnostic reasoning process, and the therapist begins a journey of questioning and hypothesising, which starts with a simple question such as: 'Why did he do that?', 'Why did he say that?' or 'Why did he react in that way?'

As an example, I will describe the diagnostic reasoning process used in the Structured Observational Test of Function (SOTOF; Laver and Powell, 1995), a test I developed as part of my doctoral research (Laver, 1994). The SOTOF is based on an error analysis assessment approach in which the therapist acts as a data processor who collects, sorts, selects and then interprets assessment data obtained through both observation and interview. Cue acquisition is selective, based on the observer's expectations of the client's performance. The therapist observes the client's behavioural responses to defined stimuli and then selects any unexpected behavioural cues, or observed error, as the focus of the diagnostic reasoning process. Reasons for the observed errors are generated in the form of hypotheses, which are then tested against further observational cues, and theoretical and tacit knowledge.

For example, if a person is presented with a cup and asked, 'What is the name of this object?' the expected response would be 'A cup.' There are many reasons why the person may not have responded correctly, and the therapist is faced with a differential diagnosis. A differential diagnosis (sometimes abbreviated DDx or ΔΔ in therapy and medical notes) is the systematic method used by health care professionals to identify the causes of a person's problems and symptoms. If the client fails to respond correctly to a question or test item, the therapist would list the most likely causes and start to formulate a range of hypotheses that could explain the person's behaviour. The therapist then asks questions and performs tests to eliminate possibilities until she is satisfied that the single most likely cause has been identified. For example, when the person failed to identify the cup, the therapist might consider the most likely reason to be that he has reduced hearing acuity and did not hear the instruction. Otherwise, he might have heard but have a language deficit, such as receptive aphasia, and did not understand the instruction. A less common but possible cause, if receptive language and hearing are intact, is that the problem might still lie in the language domain, but be one of expressive aphasia. Alternatively, the therapist could hypothesise that if hearing and language are intact the problem might have a visual origin, for example visual acuity, visual attention or visual field loss. Further cues that would provide information about hearing, vision and language would be sought and then used to evaluate each of these hypotheses. If hearing, vision and language were all found to be intact, the therapist would need to generate further hypotheses to explain the original observed behavioural error (failure to name the cup). A further hypothesis could be visual object agnosia, which is the failure to recognise familiar objects although vision is intact. All these hypotheses are related to performance component dysfunction (sensory, cognitive, perceptual components). A further explanation could lie with the volitional subsystem.

Dysfunction in a performance subsystem is only one explanation for unexpected responses. Motivational factors, arising from the volitional subsystem, can have a profound effect on behaviour. For example, if the therapist is hypothesising about why the client did not name the cup when he was shown a cup and asked what it was, she would also need to consider that perhaps he felt too depressed to answer or that he just could not be bothered to respond. Another explanation could be that he considered it was a trite question and was offended, or it was such an easy question he thought it was a trick question and a much more complicated response was required and he was too anxious to reply in case he made himself look stupid. The volitional subsystem should be considered to place observed behavioural cues into the context of the individual's internal, as well as external, environment. It is essential to engage the individual's motivation. If judgements made from observational assessment are to be reliable and valid, then optimum performance needs to be elicited. The selection of an assessment domain must be made with reference to the interests, roles and habits of the population on which the test is to be used. Motivation may be enhanced by allowing the individual some choice in the assessment activity to be performed. However, the benefits of individual choice have to be balanced against the requirements of standardisation.

PROBLEM-ORIENTATED CLINICAL REASONING PROCESS

Roberts (1996) states that 'in the process of clinical reasoning, there is usually a problem' and that 'the goal of the reasoning . . . is to solve the problem' (p. 233). It should be remembered that in many instances in therapy the product of a clinical reasoning process is not the definitive answer but a 'best guess'. Roberts acknowledges that therapists cannot solve problems in the complete way that a mathematician solves a mathematical problem and acknowledges that 'there is not necessarily a right answer to problems posed by humans who are ill' (p. 233). The problem-orientated clinical reasoning process is applied by therapists to establish the most likely cause of the complex problems posed by their clients and to assist with the identification of the most appropriate intervention plan to attempt to address identified problems. Opacich (1991) describes six key steps in a therapy problem-orientated clinical reasoning process; these are:

1. problem-setting (context)
2. framing the problem(s)
3. delineating the problem(s)
4. forming hypotheses
5. developing intervention plans
6. implementing treatment.

Diagnostic reasoning, as a component of clinical reasoning, primarily occurs during the first four steps of this process. These first four steps will now be described.

PROBLEM-SETTING

Problem-setting involves naming the phenomena/constructs that are to become the target of assessment. Defined problems are constructed from observed and reported problematic situations that are experienced by clients. Rarely in clinical practice do problems present themselves to the therapist as clear, obvious cause-and-effect relationships. These problematic situations can be puzzling, messy and uncertain. The therapist needs to unravel the person's experience of a problematic situation in order to name the problem to be investigated. This involves selecting what will be perceived as the 'things' of the situation. The therapist then sets boundaries to focus the remit of the assessment and imposes upon it a coherence that enables the statement of what is 'wrong' and how the problematic situation needs to be changed (Schön, 1983).

FRAMING THE PROBLEM

This stage of framing the problem is where theory and conceptual frameworks play a key role. Framing the problem involves illuminating the problem(s) within a context (Opacich, 1991). The process of framing involves the selection of an initial frame of reference to guide the therapist's reasoning. This is followed by the critique (see section on test critique in Chapter 11) and selection of assessment tools designed to address the named constructs. The assessment tools selected should be consistent with the chosen theoretical framework (Rogers and Holm, 1991). Assessment should be carefully structured in order to identify specific deficits/constructs. Constructs often are complicated, and it can be hard to discern whether dysfunction can be attributed to one or more constructs. This is why the therapist needs to select a frame of reference to structure the assessment and use sensitive, valid and reliable measures in order to develop and test out hypotheses about the relationships between dysfunction and underlying deficits/constructs. This process of beginning with a theory, or conceptual framework or a frame of reference, then proceeding to the formation of hypotheses, then selecting methods of assessment to collect data required to test the hypothesis is a deductive reasoning process (see Figure 10.1 above).

DELINEATING THE PROBLEM

The stage of delineating a problem involves the implementation of the therapist's chosen assessment methods and strategies. Therapists often use multiple measures of performance and a range of data-collection tools (see Chapter 2). Once data are collected, they are organised and categorised for interpretation. Standardised assessment should provide clear guidelines for the scoring and interpretation of data. With non-standardised assessments, the therapist should provide clear details and rationale for how data have been analysed.

PATTERN RECOGNITION, HYPOTHESES AND HEURISTICS

Earlier in this chapter, I drew your attention to the work of Fleming (1994a), who found that the therapists she studied utilised the three problem-solving methods previously described by Newel and Simon (1972, cited by Fleming, 1994a). These three methods were described as 'recognition, generate and test and heuristic search' (p. 121). Recognition occurs to some degree when the therapist frames the problem. It occurs further when the therapist observes and selects cues related to the problem to help generate and test hypotheses. Payton (1985), who undertook research on clinical reasoning processes in a sample of ten peer-designated expert physiotherapists, found they used a hypothetico-deductive model. Rivett and Higgs (1997), who undertook a comparative study with a small sample of 11 expert therapists and eight non-experts therapists, report that all therapists in their sample generated hypotheses consistent with the use of the hypothetico-deductive reasoning process.

Social perception is the process by which someone infers other people's motives and intentions from observing their behaviour and deciding whether the causes of the behaviour are internal or situational. Social perception helps people make sense of the world, organise their thoughts quickly and maintain a sense of control over the environment. It helps people feel competent, masterful and balanced because it helps them predict similar events in the future (Lefton, Boyles and Ogden, 2000, p. 457). Therapists will already have acquired skills in social perception before they even train to become physiotherapists or occupational therapists. During their training and subsequent clinical practice, therapists draw upon and refine social perception processes to aid their assessment. Therapists need to develop a more refined process for identifying the likely causes of a client's observed behaviour or reported problems. This process involves hypothesis generation and testing and the application of heuristics.

Therapists use hypotheses and heuristics to reduce the complex task of identifying the underlying causes of a client's problems into a simpler one. Therapists need to simplify the task because of the limits of working memory: 'working memory is the memory system component where active processing of information occurs . . . several cognitive activities take place in working memory. These include encoding, rehearsal, recording/chunking and transfer of information to and from long-term memory' (Carnevali and Thomas, 1993, p. 18).

ENCODING

Carnevali and Thomas (1993) state that 'accuracy and precision in encoding stimuli associated with one's professional practice is one dimension of clinical expertise and a necessary element of diagnostic reasoning and decision making' (p. 20). They describe how 'encoded bits of mental information coming in from sensory memory are further processes by assigning more precise meaning or interpretation to them' (p. 18). The therapist will be receiving multiple data into her working memory from all her sensory systems: vision, touch, smell and hearing.

For example, a therapist moves a client's arms through a passive range of movement (ROM) and senses resistance in the client's muscle as she reaches the outer range. Therapists use language to encode and they also link newly acquired data into systematic relations with previous knowledge. In this example, the therapist might label the sensory data from the passive movements in terms of 'normal tone', 'stiffness', 'spasticity' or 'flaccidity'. Therapists can undertake encoding consciously when the sensory data received are unfamiliar and complex, but as they become more experienced more and more encoding will become more automatic. So 'encoding expertise in [working memory] involves recognition of information from sensory memory and adequate professional language or imagery to further encode them' (p. 20).

REHEARSAL

Rehearsal has been described as 'a mental recycling activity serving to retain stimuli in' working memory (Carnevali and Thomas, 1993, p. 20). *Maintenance rehearsal* requires repeating information a number of times in order to help keep the information in working memory for a bit longer. For example, the therapist might rehearse a client's response to a test question, or goniometric measurements taken to assess ROM. A second type of rehearsal is *elaborative rehearsal*; this 'is a process reorganising new information using the information's meaning to help store and remember it' (p. 20). This is achieved by drawing on knowledge the therapist already has in her long-term memory and forming relationships with this previous knowledge and the current information in the working memory.

RECODING AND CHUNKING

The working memory only has a limited capacity. Most people can only remember between five to nine pieces of information at a time. These pieces of information are referred to as *chunks*. A chunk can comprise one item of information/data or it can be formed of many related items of information. Therapists recode separate pieces of data by grouping them together and then remember this group of information as one chunk. Often therapists do this by grouping cues together linked to a recognised pattern. Pattern recognition is the therapist's ability to:

- 'observe a phenomenon
- identify significant characteristics (cues)
- perceive a relationship among cues (a configuration)
- compare a present configuration to a previously learned category or type (template)' (Fleming, 1994b, p. 145).

The recognition of patterns assists therapists with the generation of hypotheses. There are two types of hypotheses generated by therapists: familiar hypotheses retrieved from the long-term memory that have been used before and proved successful in identifying a client's problem which was linked to the same pattern of cues and new hypotheses generated when the therapist perceives this to be a novel situation. Fleming (1994b) states that therapists particularly use heuristic search when new hypotheses are required or when they need to invent a particular solution for a client. She found that therapists 'often use heuristic search methods in the problem resolution phase of problem solving' (p. 147).

A hypothesis has been defined as a tentative explanation of the cause(s) of observed dysfunction (Rogers and Holm, 1991). The delineation of the problem as a hypothesis involves the acquisition and interpretation of cues drawn from the assessment data.

Heuristics is a problem-solving technique in which the most appropriate solution is selected using rules. Usually, these are simplified rules used for processing information on a rule-of-thumb, trial-and-error basis. Heuristics help us to access information and make decisions more quickly because they reduce the amount of data to be processed, reduce processing time, move us beyond the presenting cue and enrich the information accessed in the therapist's memory by inference. Therapists use heuristics as a problem-solving method by drawing upon what they have heard and seen in their past clinical practice to develop their own rules of thumb from how people with a particular diagnosis or problem have presented in the past and from what the underlying causes and solutions proved to be. Reoccurring patterns become embedded as rules of thumb that are then accessed to help formulate hypotheses about the current client. The therapist reflects on the cues acquired and searches previous theoretical and experiential knowledge for rules of thumb, recognisable patterns and metaphors to direct the formation of hypotheses.

While heuristics can be very helpful, therapists need to be aware that they can lead to suboptimal decision-making, faulty beliefs and systematic errors. First, the formation of oversimplified categories can lead to stereotypes. Secondly, if a faulty belief underlies a rule of thumb used by a therapist, then significant and persistent biases will occur in the hypotheses she is likely to generate for particular client scenarios. One faulty belief relates to how common or frequent we perceive a particular client presentation, which we have formed as a category, to be.

People tend to judge the likelihood of an outcome based on how easily they can imagine that likelihood; this is called the *availability heuristic*. The danger with this approach is that outcomes which are easier for us to imagine, because they are vivid in our memories or associated with strong feeling, will be perceived as more likely than those outcomes we find harder to picture, remember or comprehend. This leads to a cognitive bias in our estimations of the probability of different outcomes.

In clinical practice, a group of clients whose presenting features are readily available to the therapist's memory might appear to be more numerous than they really are, and events that easily come to mind might be judged more likely than they are, for example a client falling at home and having to be readmitted after being assessed as fit for discharge by a therapist might lead to this therapist being overly cautious about the readiness of future clients for discharge because her perceived risk of falling in this client group is higher owing to this clearly remembered negative outcome. The availability of certain information may be biased because the therapist has had limited exposure to clients/interventions of a certain kind, or because the clients/outcomes are more remarkable and attract more attention, or because the therapist has stored the information in her memory in a particular fashion. The availability heuristic is of significance for therapists and something of which we should be mindful. When we are presented with a new client, we are more likely to match him to clients we have worked with recently because these cases are in our recent memory and easier to recall than clients treated a long time ago. So we will suppose his problems and related outcome will be similar to these easily recalled clients. In addition, if a particular past client made a significant impression on us, for example because the case was perplexing or the outcome achieved was very positive or characteristics about the client resonated with us (they had the same hobby, liked the same television programme, looked like our father etc.), this client will be more vivid in our long-term memory and becomes easier to recall than less memorable clients. We all have particular clients who stick in our minds, some because we really enjoyed working with them and others because they really challenged us and we struggled with their therapy. Because these clients are memorable and easier to recall, the danger is that we will perceive the features of their presentation as being more common/frequent (Toft and Reynolds, in press). When we perceive the presentation of these cases to be more frequent, we are more likely to use them to generate rules of thumb that then drive the development and analysis of clinical hypotheses. So if a new client has a couple of features that fit the heuristic generated by more recent and/or memorable clients, we will match the client to this category, and might ignore another set of features that would lead us to a category group which have a much rarer presentation. This is where standardised tests can help us, because a useful measure should address the full range of behaviours or presenting features under the domain concerned in equal measure, and such tests will prompt us to consider deficits that we might have never or only rarely seen, such as ideational apraxia or colour agnosia.

Following the formation of a hypothesis, the therapist should conduct further assessment to test out her hypothesis. This is the process of validating the hypothesis. Testing hypotheses helps to reduce the impact of bias. Care must be taken to be very objective during the hypothesis testing process because a person is more likely to see what they expect to see (because they perceive it as more common and, therefore, more likely) and ignore data that refute their beliefs. Cue interpretation and acquisition is often focused on the identification of confirmatory cues. As well as considering what behaviour would be observed if the hypothesis were true, therapists also need to consider what behaviour would be observed if the hypothesis were false and then plan their further assessment to collect evidence to help confirm or refute the hypothesis. So, when validating a hypothesis, you need to see if there are symptoms and signs that cannot be explained by your hypothesis and also think about whether your hypothesis would lead to the presence of any symptoms or signs that are not present in this case. The more discrete and targeted the tools and strategies used in the assessment, the easier it is for the therapist to test out her hypotheses and to make valid and reliable clinical decisions.

Standardised test results can be used to help confirm or refute a hypothesis. For example, a standardised test might be selected to assist the evaluation of a hypothesis generated during an initial interview and/or from a review of presenting information, such as a referral letter and medical notes. Standardised test results can also provide the cues that lead to further hypothesis generation. It is critical that standardised test results are used within the context of the whole assessment process and are not used for decision-making in isolation. The therapist's clinical reasoning skills help her to examine the test results in terms of the context in which they were obtained and apply them to the wider context of the client's presentation and situation. The test results need to be examined in the context of this particular client, tested in a particular test environment and at a particular time. A number of variables (fatigue, medication, test anxiety, motivation, time of day, distractions etc.) could have influenced the obtained results. The results should also be examined alongside other client information, such as the client's self-report, informal observations and proxy report. Consistencies or discrepancies that show up once data from different sources are triangulated are given particular attention during the diagnostic reasoning process. Some standardised assessments offer guidance to therapists on how the test results should be interpreted and applied. For example, Abidin (1995), author of the Parenting Stress Index (PSI), provides interpretative guidelines in the PSI manual that are based on a combination of qualitative data drawn from clinical judgements and clinical literature (what he refers to as interpretations drawing upon the art of therapy) and quantitative data drawn from research conducted on the PSI and upon the relationship of individual PSI items to research outcomes reported in child development literature (drawing upon science-based therapy). Abidin states that 'the interpretations suggested [for PSI scores] should be viewed as working hypotheses, the validity of which will need to be established by further inquiry with a particular parent' (p. 5).

Diagnostic reasoning produces a therapy diagnosis that reflects not just the pathology but also the observed performance deficit and the postulated causes of that deficit. A diagnosis (such as ideomotor apraxia resulting from stroke) formulated from formal neuropsychological testing tells us neither the client's exact pattern of functional deficit nor his motivation and potential for independence. The flexibility provided by observational assessment allows the therapist to use judgement and improvisation in moving from theory to the requirements of a client's unique experience. This produces a unique therapy diagnosis for each person.

THERAPY DIAGNOSIS

A diagnosis can be viewed in terms of both a process and a product (Rogers and Holm, 1989); 'it is simultaneously the complex sequence of reasoned thought that moves forward from problem sensing to problem definition, and the product of that reasoning' (p. 8). In occupational therapy, some authors refer to the diagnosis as the occupational diagnosis. An 'occupational diagnosis refers to both the cognitive processes used by the occupational therapy practitioner to formulate a statement summarizing the client's occupational status, and the outcome of that process, the diagnostic statement' (Rogers, 2004, p. 17).

DIAGNOSTIC STATEMENT

The therapy diagnosis can be presented as a diagnostic statement. This statement consists of four components: 'descriptive (functional problem) + explanatory (aetiology of the problem) + cue (signs and symptoms) + pathological (medical or psychiatric)' (Rogers, 2004, p. 19).

DESCRIPTIVE COMPONENT

The descriptive component should describe the specific deficits identified at each level of function that are affecting the person's ability to engage successfully in their chosen roles and activities. It articulates the identified problems that are addressed by either occupational therapy and/or physiotherapy. Rogers (2004) states that this component should name 'task disabilities, such as difficulty dressing, or social role dysfunctions, such as difficulty working as a seamstress'. She clarifies that 'a task disability occurs at the level of individual tasks, while a social role dysfunction occurs at the level of social role, which is comprised of many tasks' (p. 18). (*Note:* for more information on assessment at different levels please refer to Chapter 9.)

EXPLANATORY COMPONENT

The diagnosis should contain an explanatory component that indicates the therapist's hypothesis or hypotheses about the possible and most likely cause(s) of the defined problem described in the descriptive component. This is a very important aspect of the diagnostic statement because the cause of the problem may require a specific solution and different therapy interventions will be selected for different causes of the same problem. A person's problem can be the result of an interaction between a number of impairments or hindrances, and so the therapist may need to list several causes in the explanatory component. Rogers (2004, p. 18) provides, as a useful example, how a dressing disability might be caused by:

- sensory impairment (e.g. low vision, paraesthesia)
- physical impairment (e.g. limited movement or strength)
- cognitive impairment (e.g. apraxia, amnesia)
- affective impairment (e.g. lack of motivation, fear of injury)
- physical contextual hindrance (e.g. architectural barrier)
- social contextual hindrance (e.g. restrictive attitude of carer).

CUE COMPONENT

This identifies the observed and reported signs and symptoms that lead the therapist to conclude that there is a problem requiring therapy intervention and to hypothesise the nature and cause of the identified problem. A symptom is a condition that results from the problem. Data on symptoms are usually obtained through self-report and proxy data-collection methods. For example, the client may inform the therapist that 'I can't reach to put on my socks and shoes', or a carer may explain: 'He gets in a muddle in the garden. He gets out the wrong tools for the job, and I caught him pulling out well-established plants the other day instead of the weeds.' Some clients or carers may be able to provide the therapist with a further explanation of why they have this problem: 'I can't put on my shoes as I'm too stiff and because it's too painful to stretch down' or 'He had such a good knowledge of plants and was such an avid gardener but now he's pulling up plants instead of weeds because he doesn't remember and can't tell the flowers from the weeds now he has dementia.' In some cases, the therapist will wish to verify this explanation with an observational assessment method, and where the cause is unclear she will definitely need to undertake further assessment to elicit the underlying causes. This may include the use of standardised measures or setting up a task the client/carer has described as problematic and undertaking an informal observation to analyse the difficulty with performance. Data collected by the therapist using observational methods are referred to as *signs* (Rogers, 2004). (*Note:* for more information on different methods of data collection please refer to Chapter 2.)

PATHOLOGIC COMPONENT

This provides the pathological cause, if any, of the functional deficit (this part of the diagnosis often relates to, or is drawn from, the medical diagnosis). This is useful for therapists because 'the nature of the pathology, the prognosis and pathology related contraindications establish parameters for . . . therapy interventions' (Rogers, 2004, p. 19). Interventions will be tailored not just to the underlying cause of the problem (as identified in the explanatory component of the diagnostic statement) but also by factors such as whether the person is terminally ill (diagnosis of cancer), has a long-term irreversible condition (diagnosis of dementia) or has a curable illness (diagnosis of anxiety).

COMPONENTS OF THE DIAGNOSTIC STATEMENT

To illustrate the components of the diagnostic statement, two examples are provided (Boxes 10.1 and 10.2). These two examples show how the same deficit and pathology can arise from different causes; both examples have the same descriptive and pathologic components (the client has had a stroke leading to dependence in dressing), but the cues leading to the explanatory component of the diagnosis are quite different and will lead on to different therapeutic interventions.

Box 10.1 First example of a diagnostic statement

Mr A

Descriptive component
Unable to get dressed independently.

Explanatory component
Related to:

- reduced sensation in left upper limb
- reduced active ROM in left upper limb
- spasticity in left upper limb.

Cue component
As evidenced by the following symptoms described by Mr A.

- 'My arm feels numb and heavy. If I concentrate really hard, I can move it a little bit, but I can't feel things properly and I can't pick up fiddly things.'

As evidenced by the following signs identified through observational assessment.
- inability to identify objects through touch in left hand with eyes closed
- inability to report temperature or pin prick on left hand and arm on testing
- inability to move left elbow, wrist and fingers through full ROM on command
- inability to pick up and manipulate objects with left hand
- when left arm is moved through a passive ROM, full range is present but resistance and increased tone is felt

Pathologic component
Owing to a right cerebral vascular accident (CVA).

Box 10.2 Second example of a diagnostic statement.

Mrs B

Descriptive component
Unable to get dressed independently.

Explanatory component
Related to:

- left unilateral neglect.

Cue component
As evidenced by the following symptoms described by Mrs B.

- 'The nurse came along and said "*Eat up, Doris, you need a good meal*", and I was annoyed because I had finished it all up and I said: "*What do you mean eat up? I've eaten it all up today*", and she laughed and said: "*We're having a joke today, are we? Have you finished then?*" and then I felt really cross because I wasn't joking around and I said again: "*I've eaten it all up!*" So then the nurse looked thoughtful and she said very seriously: "*I'm not joking, Doris; so bear with me. Before I take your plate away, can you take another look and tell me whether you see any food left on your plate?*" I felt confused and annoyed because it seemed such a stupid question, but she's a nice girl, you know, and she was so serious, so I thought I'd humour her. I took another look and when I replied: "*Of course not!*" she said: "*Oh*" and then moved my plate a bit and told me to look again, and do you know what? I'd left some food after all – I think I'm going mad!'

As evidenced by the following signs identified through observational assessment.
- ignores objects to the left of the midline
- does not attempt to dress left side of the body
- puts both sleeves on right arm

Pathologic component
Owing to a right cerebral vascular accident (CVA).

Rogers (2004) also provides an example of a diagnostic statement.

> Mrs Bright is unable to prepare meals for herself (description) related to a memory deficit (explanatory) as evidenced by: her repeated requests for instructions; inability to remember salting the soup; failure to remove the soup when boiled; and burning the corner of the potholder (cues); caused by dementia of the Alzheimer's type (pathological). (p. 19)

In formulating the diagnosis, the therapist also considers the person's strengths, interests and resources, and notes those physical and verbal prompts and cues that appear to facilitate function. So a therapy diagnosis is elaborate and is broader than the medical diagnosis as it also encompasses the person's physical and social environment, motives and values. In addition to a diagnosis, the therapist formulates a prognosis in terms of projecting both the person's likely response to treatment and future functional ability.

The formation of a working diagnosis is just the beginning of the therapeutic journey with a client. As the therapist implements her chosen interventions and management strategies, she reviews her original therapy diagnosis in light of the client's response to the intervention. If her chosen interventions do not remedy the problem, she may decide to revisit her hypothesis and double-check that she had discovered all the relevant signs and symptoms during her initial diagnostic reasoning process. She may generate and test alternative hypotheses to explain the client's problem and try interventions linked to these alternative hypotheses to see if these deliver the desired outcome. In complex cases, the therapist may need to revisit the diagnostic reasoning process several times before she is convinced that she has identified the correct cause(s) of the client's problem and has selected the best intervention to address this underlying cause.

INTRODUCTION TO OTHER FORMS OF REASONING

As part of the assessment process, therapists need to learn about people's individual experiences of their illness or disability. In the underlying philosophies of both occupational therapy and physiotherapy, every individual is perceived as a unique person. This philosophy needs to be carried out in practice. Therefore, therapists need to take a person-centred approach to understand the unique way in which diagnoses affect the lives of the people who receive therapy. Two people may be of the same age, sex, socio-economic background and have the same diagnosis, but their experiences of, and responses to, that diagnosis may be completely different. Therefore, therapists need to engage in assessment and intervention in a phenomenological way. With a phenomenological approach, a person's experience of his body is inseparable from his experience of the whole world and disability is viewed as an interruption or injury to a whole life (Mattingly, 1994a). So the therapist needs to assess a person in the context of how he did, does and hopes to live his life. Assessment is used to provide an understanding of a person in terms of his daily practices, life history, social relationships and long-term goals and plans that give him meaning in his life and his self-identity (Mattingly, 1994a). In order to obtain this complex image of a person, and understand the impact of the diagnosis on his functioning, therapists need to engage in several types of clinical reasoning during the assessment process. Mattingly and Fleming (1994a) found that 'therapists shift rapidly from one type of reasoning to another' (p. 18).

> The reasoning style employed changes as the therapist's attention is drawn from one aspect of the problem to another. Therapists process or analyze different aspects of the problem, almost simultaneously, using different thinking styles but do not lose track of their thoughts about other aspects of a problem as those components are temporarily shifted to the background and another aspect is dealt with immediately in the foreground. (p. 18)

Fleming (1994a) describes this ability to utilise multiple modes of reasoning as 'the therapist with the three-track mind' (p. 119). Through her research, she identified three distinct forms of reasoning, which she labelled as procedural reasoning (this has been described briefly earlier on in this chapter), interactive reasoning and conditional reasoning. Other types of reasoning of particular relevance to assessment processes described by other authors include narrative reasoning (Mattingly, 1994b), pragmatic reasoning (for example Schell, 1998; Schell and Cervero, 1993) and ethical reasoning. While the forms of reasoning identified in the literature have some distinct strategies or components, there is some overlap between different types of reasoning as described by these different authors, and the following types of clinical reasoning are not completely discrete.

INTERACTIVE REASONING

Both occupational therapy and physiotherapy require very interactive and collaborative relationships between the therapist and the client. Interactive reasoning occurs during the therapist's face-to-face interactions with clients and is used to create the collaborative therapeutic relationship. Other types of reasoning, such as procedural reasoning, are usually factually based; in contrast interactive reasoning is often intuitive (Unsworth, 1999). Creating an effective collaborative relationship is a very skilled process that requires a therapist to evaluate a wide range of cues to understand the client's motives, meanings and what he wants from therapy (Mattingly and Fleming, 1994b). Therapy involves an active doing *with* process, as opposed to a passive doing *to* process. This doing *with* clients means that therapists encourage and allow the person to do as much as he can for himself. The therapist creates a relationship that empowers the client to stretch himself; this is achieved by staying near to the client, coaching, encouraging, prompting and cueing and only offering physical assistance when required. During assessment, the therapist needs to assess both what the client is capable of doing and what the client is willing to do. At certain times, the therapist may appear to be sitting back and doing nothing during an observational assessment, but much negotiation may have led to this point, and active observation and clinical reasoning will be ongoing as the therapist 'sits back' while the client attempts the agreed activity or task. Mattingly and Fleming (1994b) explain:

> They often do not seem to be actually doing something themselves but are 'doing with' the client to help them in the transition from dependent patient to (as they say) 'independent living'. Doing with the patient also means having patients practice exercises in the hospital during times when they are not being seen by the therapist. Clients are asked to take an active role in their treatment. (p. 179)

CONDITIONAL REASONING

Mattingly and Fleming (1994a) perceive conditional reasoning as 'a complex form of social reasoning' that is used by therapists 'to help the patient in the difficult process of reconstructing a life that is now permanently changed by injury or disease' (p. 17). In their studies of therapists' reasoning, they saw how this 'reasoning style moves beyond specific concerns about the person and the physical problems and places them in broader social and temporal contexts' (p. 18). They selected the term *conditional* because they perceived therapists were thinking about 'the whole condition, including the person, the illness, the meanings the illness has for the person, the family, and the social and physical contexts in which the person lives' (p. 18). Unsworth (1999) noticed that Mattingly and Fleming (1994a) utilise the term conditional in three different ways when discussing therapist's reasoning.

1. Conditional reasoning involves the therapist reflecting on the whole condition; this includes the client's illness or problem, the meaning the client and his family attach to this illness and the client's whole context.
2. The therapist imagines how the condition could change, both positively and negatively, and thinks about what this might mean for the client. These imagined outcomes are conditional on other factors and may or may not be achieved.
3. The therapist considers whether or not the imagined outcomes can be achieved and understands 'that this is conditional on both the client's participation in the therapy program and the shared construction of the future image' (Unsworth, 1999, p. 61).

Conditional reasoning has some overlap with both narrative reasoning (Mattingly, 1994b) and pragmatic reasoning (for example Schell, 1998; Schell and Cervero, 1993), both of which will be briefly discussed below.

NARRATIVE REASONING

Narrative reasoning is used by therapists to help them make sense of the illness experience of their clients. 'Narrative reasoning is so named because it involves thinking in story form' (Schell, 1998, p. 94). Through narrative reasoning, the therapist 'uses story making and story telling to assist . . . in understanding the meaning of disability or disease to the client' (Unsworth, 1999, p. 48). Kielhofner (1992) suggests that 'narrative thinking is orientated to making sense of human experience in terms of understanding motives' (p. 260). He sees the therapist as being 'drawn into the personal drama of the unique individual' with a particular condition. He uses the example of arthritis. If the therapeutic process is to be successful, the therapist must 'figure out' how this individual 'is going to live with arthritis in the context of everyday occupations' (p. 261). So the therapist is very interested in the person's struggle to engage in his everyday activities and roles as an arthritic person. In order to help solve the problems faced by this person with arthritis in his unique physical and social environment, the therapist must not only understand the condition of arthritis but also seek understanding of the 'particular situation of the individual' (p. 261). People's personal narratives are a key part of their identity (Smith, 2006) and are of critical importance to a therapist trying to undertake a comprehensive, client-centred assessment. Therapists are encouraged to seek narratives from their clients because the person's construction of his situation enriches the therapist's understanding of:

- how the client experiences the condition
- how the lived experience of the condition is shaping and constraining the client's day-to-day experiences
- how other key people, such as family members, have reacted to the person since he developed this condition
- how experiencing the condition has changed the person's priorities
- what solutions are desired by the client.

CLIENT–THERAPIST STORIES

Through narrative reasoning, the therapist is empowering the person as the expert in his own story. Smith (2006) recommends that 'if we listen from the not-knowing position, people's stories will emerge as they begin to trust us. This is a transformative process through which their stories lead us to what is important to the individual. It is a process in opposition to the process of labelling, which leads to us seeing people in terms of only one or two categories' (p. 307). He goes on to suggest that when the client's 'story has emerged, we have to let the person pick it up and make the process of doing and becoming his or her own. We do not create our clients' future lives, but we make space within which they can create their lives for themselves . . . good therapy is not about observation but about negotiation, leading to interaction, shared memories and co-creation' (Smith, 2006, p. 307). This is how therapists use narrative reasoning beyond the assessment process to help clients engage in the therapeutic process. Schell (1998) notes that therapists often 'work with individuals whose life stories are so severely disrupted that they cannot imagine what their lives will look like' (p. 94). For many clients who experience disability as the result of an accident or the sudden onset of an illness, such as a heart attack or stroke, this unexpected onset/accident can make them feel like their life has to all intents and purposes ended. The therapist works to help the person see that this is not the end to his life but rather the marking of the end of a chapter in his life story. The process of rehabilitation can be like turning to a fresh page to start a new chapter. The plot has taken a dramatic and often unexpected turn, but the story still goes on and the unexpected can lead to positive as well as negative changes if the person can be helped to face the future with optimism and creativity. Therapists interweave treatment goals and interventions based on activities that have meaning for their clients to assist their clients to start to imagine what their lives could be in the future. Mattingly (1994b) describes how therapists 'reason about how to guide their therapy with particular patients by using images of where the patient is now, and where this patient might be at some future time when the patient will be discharged' (p. 240). To move the person through a therapeutic process from his current ability to a position of greater ability, the therapist needs more than the know-how to perform a set of tasks, rather she needs to be able to conceptualise a temporal whole that captures the continuum from seeing the person as he functions at the beginning of the therapeutic story to the desired outcome, by imaginatively anticipating what the person could be in the future. Mattingly refers to this as a 'prospective treatment story' (p. 241). This prospective treatment story helps the therapist to organise the tasks and activities that will form the intervention and to sell these tasks and activities to the client as worthy of engagement. In her research examining the clinical reasoning of therapists, Mattingly (1994b) found that these prospective stories 'were useful not because they were completely accurate predictions of what would happen, but because they were plausible enough to give therapists a starting point' (p. 242). Mattingly continues:

> The clinical stories therapists projected onto new situations often ran into trouble because the new situation was often resistant to the mold. Clinical practice is idiosyncratic enough and illness experiences are contextually specific enough that stories created from other times and for other patients often fall short in providing ideal guides to new situations. While clinical stories are rarely ever applied wholesale – the therapist is always tinkering, always improvising to make the fit appropriate. (pp. 242–243)

As the therapist engages with the client through interventions, she engages in informal assessments of the client's responses to her treatment approach. She may also undertake a formal evaluation of his progress. During this re-assessment, the therapist may find that her prospective treatment story does not fully fit the actual unfolding therapeutic story with this particular client. When therapists experience a misfit between their original prospective story and the unfolding story, Mattingly found that 'they would revise the story accordingly, redirecting therapeutic interventions so that they were more in line with what was actually unfolding' (p. 242). However, this readjustment of the story is not always sufficient to achieve the desired outcome. In these cases, Mattingly found that 'therapists experience the anxiety and frustration of falling out of the story, of losing their way' (p. 242). When this happens, therapists find that their prospective story for this client no longer makes sense and they start to 'lose faith in their strategies and plans for the patient because the outcomes are too far afield from the ones they consider desirable' (p. 243).

Not all therapeutic stories have happy endings; as therapists we have success stories we like to share with our colleagues and students, but we also have our failures – the clients with whom we failed to build rapport or for whom the problem remained elusive or the chosen interventions did not deliver the desired outcomes. These are the cases where our attempts to revise the prospective story, to mould it to this client, did not work out. In such cases, Mattingly (1994b) discovered:

> If therapists were . . . never able to locate and enact a story they considered clinically meaningful, the stories they told retrospectively were often explorations or justifications for who was to blame. When things go wrong in therapy . . . therapists are no longer narrators with their images of the ending well in tow. Through difficult and unexpected turns in the therapeutic process, therapists become readers of the story . . . they struggle to understand what has gone wrong and, sometimes, what another story might be that could substitute for the one they have had to abandon. (p. 243)

These problematic clinical stories are the ones from which we have much to learn. These are the stories we should pay particular attention to and reflect upon and puzzle over. The clinical stories where we felt muddled and frustrated are useful to share with our peers and supervisors, to learn as much from what does not work as from what does and also to learn from the experience of others so that when faced with a similar client we do not construct the same unsuccessful prospective story as our starting point. Later in this chapter we discuss the importance of reflective practice and Box 10.5 provides a clinical story analysis format that may help you to write down and reflect upon a problematic clinical story of your own.

THERAPISTS SHARING STORIES

Another aspect of narrative reasoning relates not to how the therapist and client share stories but to how therapists share stories with each other. In their studies on clinical reasoning, Mattingly and Fleming (1994a) observed that 'therapists often traded stories about patients' (p. 18). Other writers have noticed this sharing of stories amongst therapists, for example Barnett (1999) notes 'today in every therapy department and staff room, communicating through stories can be observed as the favoured method of social discourse' (p. vii). Mattingly and Fleming (1994a) noticed that 'this was not gossip' (p. 18) but had two important functions. First, it was a method used by therapists to puzzle out a problem. The problem might relate to how to engage a person in therapy, or which intervention to select, or figuring out the nature of underlying deficits that are affecting observed functional problems. Therapists will informally discuss cases over coffee or lunch as a way of figuring out things in their own mind, but also to seek help in an informal manner: 'I saw a client this morning and . . .' Their colleagues often respond through storytelling: 'I had a patient like that and what I did was' or 'When I had a person with . . . what worked was . . .' Through these stories, therapists offer each other suggestions, strategies and solutions. The second function for sharing stories identified by Mattingly and Fleming (1994a) was that it was 'a way to enlarge each therapist's fund of practical knowledge through vicariously sharing other therapists' experience . . . these stories form a bond between therapists and also teach them much more than they could learn in a classroom or through their own personal experience' (p. 19).

PRAGMATIC REASONING

Pragmatic reasoning relates to the therapist's clinical practice setting and personal context. Pragmatic reasoning is how the therapist obtains an understanding about how the personal context and the practice setting affect the assessment and treatment processes she implements. It takes into account organisational, political and economic constraints and opportunities that place boundaries around the assessment and treatment that a therapist may undertake in a particular practice environment (Schell and Cervero, 1993; Unsworth, 1999). Therapists 'actively consider and are influenced by the situations that occur in their . . . practice' (Schell, 1998, p. 94). The content of a therapist's pragmatic reasoning related to her practice setting may include:

- the availability of assessment and treatment resources
- time limitations owing to her caseload and the priorities placed by other clients on her current caseload
- the culture of the organisation within which she works
- power relationships with her supervisor, manager, other therapists and across members of the multidisciplinary team
- trends in clinical practice within her profession
- financial issues and constraints, for example to pay for equipment, adaptations, placements or services that may be of benefit to the client.

The personal context that a therapist brings to her practice also plays a part in her pragmatic reasoning; this might include thinking related to her:

- clinical competence and confidence undertaking particular assessment procedures or interventions
- preferences, which can include her preferences for working with particular types of clients or in particular environments (such as the therapy department versus the client's own home) or for working with particular colleagues (e.g. she has a very collaborative and mutually respectful relationship with nursing staff but feels undermined by the physician in charge)
- level of commitment to her job and her profession
- work life versus home life balance and the demands she is facing outside of work (e.g. her child is at home sick and her husband was unhappy about missing his work to take care of their child).

Schell (1998) explains how personal issues can drive clinical decisions on a daily basis:

> For instance, if a practitioner does not feel safe in helping a client stand or transfer to
> a bed, he or she is more likely to use table-top based activities. (p. 94)

So in an assessment process, this therapist might opt for a bottom-up approach using a standardised battery of tests that can be administered at a table to explore performance component functioning, as opposed to a top-down approach that might involve observing the person undertake the activities that were of most importance to him, such as moving from his bed to the bathroom, transferring on and off the toilet and toileting independently. Schell (1998) goes on with her examples to suggest:

> Alternatively, another practitioner may feel uncomfortable in dealing with depressed
> individuals, and avoid treating them, suggesting that such individuals are not
> motivated for therapy. (p. 95)

In this example, we see how the hypothesis selected by the therapist to explain the client's presentation is one related to motivation as opposed to a hypothesis related to low mood as the causal factor. In examining this hypothesis, the therapist's pragmatic reasoning is likely to guide her subconsciously towards cues that support her hypothesis related to the client's lack of volition and ignore cues that would pertain to a problem with depression. Finally, Schell (1998) offers the example of a therapist who:

> has a young family to go home to, he or she may opt not to schedule clients later in the
> day, so that he or she can return home as soon as possible. (p. 95)

In this example, we might find the therapist who phones a community-based client for monitoring and discovers the situation has worsened deciding that a home visit is not necessary that day and can be delayed until tomorrow. Alternatively, if she decides a face-to-face assessment is required today and perceives that she might get involved with complicated factors and a time-consuming visit, she may decide to refer to an out-of-hours crisis intervention team, even though they are not familiar with her client. Another example is a hospital therapist who on undertaking an initial assessment towards the end of the working day decides to administer a brief screening test rather than a lengthier standardised test battery, even though the presenting information and initial interview point towards the more rigorous battery being necessary.

It is challenging to be consciously aware of how pragmatic reasoning shapes our decisions, but if we truly want to act in the best interests of our clients, as opposed to the best interests of ourselves and/or our employing organisations, then we need to practise the art of reflection and look critically at the underlying reasoning behind our clinical decisions. However, although pragmatic reasoning may lead to actions that are not in the best interests of the client, it can be very useful in helping us to answer practical questions that shape our therapy positively; these include (modified and developed from Schell, 1998, p. 96, Figure 9.1: Aspects and examples of clinical reasoning process):

- Who referred this client for therapy and why was this referral made?
- Who is paying for this treatment, and what are their expectations of the outcome of therapy?
- What family/carer support does the client have and what are these people's expectations and abilities: can they provide resources (practical support, physical help, encouragement, finances) to assist with the client's intervention?
- How much time will I have available to work with this client?
- What clinical and client-based environments are available for therapy and what standardised tests, equipment and adaptations can I access to support the therapeutic process?
- What are the expectations of my manager, supervisor and multidisciplinary colleagues?

- What are my clinical competencies and will these be sufficient to provide the client with the therapy he needs?

ETHICAL REASONING AND MORAL REASONING

Barnitt (1993) notes that the terms ethics and morals and ethical reasoning and moral reasoning are used interchangeably in the literature and she offers some helpful definitions:

> *Ethics* refers to identifiable statements about norms and values which can be used to guide professional practice. Codes of conduct, ethical guides and guides to standards in professional practice are examples of this . . . Professional ethics are the rules and recommendations about appropriate behaviour in clinical work. *Moral reasoning* refers to a more philosophical enquiry about norms and values, about ideas of right and wrong, and about how therapists make moral decisions in professional work. Moral issues have to be resolved through reflective thinking and problem solving because guidelines to ethics cannot cope with specific instances. (p. 402)

Schell (1998) uses the term ethical reasoning and describes this as thinking that is concerned with the question of 'what should be done?' (p. 95). Schell perceives that therapists engage in ethical reasoning to help them to select morally defensible courses of action, particularly when faced with competing interests. Rogers (1983) contends that the assessment process is concluded by ethical decision-making. Once the therapist has analysed the person's presenting problems, formulated a therapeutic diagnostic statement and has identified a range of relevant interventions or management strategies, she will have engaged in pragmatic reasoning around the resources available to her and the client and will then move onto ethical reasoning to decide on the most appropriate application of treatment approaches and available resources. Schell (1998) provides examples of the types of value-laden questions that therapists try to address through ethical reasoning.

- 'What are the benefits and risks to the person related to service provision and do the benefits warrant the risks?
- In the face of limited time and resources, what is the fairest way to prioritize care?
- How can I balance the goals of the person receiving services with those of the caregiver, when they don't agree?
- What should I do when other members of the treatment team are operating in a way that I feel conflicts with the goals of the person receiving services?' (Schell, 1998, p. 96).

REFLECTIVE PRACTICE

In this chapter we have explored various types of clinical reasoning. We have seen how different modes of reasoning are undertaken for different purposes or in response to particular features of a problem or interaction with the client (Mattingly, 1994b). These different types of reasoning are not undertaken in a sequential manner, but are rather interwoven during the complex thinking that the therapist undertakes as she engages with a client during assessment and re-assessment. The therapist must draw together the thinking that results from these various modes of reasoning to form 'a coherent understanding of the patient and of what the therapy will be' (Kielhofner, 1992, p. 261). The ability to pull together, synthesise and make sense of the myriad pieces of information (from the referral, the client, the carer, other colleagues) and marry these with standardised test results and informal observations is what therapists learn through carrying out therapy over time; expertise comes with practice. This is why clinical placements form such a critical part of any therapist's education, and why ongoing reflection on practice is so important for any qualified therapist who wants to develop and improve her clinical skills. To reflect upon clinical reasoning involves metacognitive analysis – that is engagement in 'thinking about thinking' (Schell, 1998, p. 90). Finding a language to explain and unpackage your clinical reasoning helps you to become a more cognisant therapist and helps your students and colleagues to learn from your experience and expertise.

All therapists need to engage in reflective practice to ensure that what they are doing, and why they have made decisions to do this, is supported as far as possible by the evidence base and that this leads to safe and effective practice. Schön (1983, 1987) considers reflection to be a critical part of developing expertise in clinical practice and clinical decision-making. His work has been drawn upon by both occupational therapy writers (for example Kielhofner, 1992; Mattingly and Fleming, 1994a; Unsworth, 1999) and physiotherapy writers (for example Larin, Wessel and Al-Shamlan, 2005; White, 2004). Schön (1983) differentiates between reflection *in* action, which occurs while the therapist is engaged in an encounter with a client – this is thinking on one's feet or 'online reflection' (White, 2004) and reflection *on* action, which is a retrospective process that occurs after the therapeutic encounter when the therapist pauses to interpret and analyse what has occurred; this it what White (2004) refers to as 'off-line reflection' (p. 29).

The CSP defines reflective practice as a process by which the therapist, as a practitioner, stops and thinks about her practice, consciously analyses her decision-making processes and draws on theory and relates it to what she does in practice. This process of critical analysis and evaluation refocuses the therapist's thinking on her existing knowledge to generate new knowledge and ideas. This may lead to a change in her actions, behaviour, assessment approach, treatments and/or learning needs (Chartered Society for Physiotherapy, 2006b). I would add to this that the therapist needs to draw from the evidence base as well as from theory and relate both to her practice. Swain (2004) defines reflective practice as 'the capacity of a therapist to think, talk or write about a piece of practice with the intention to review or research a piece of practice with clients for new meanings or perspectives on the situation' (p. 217). Swain's definition shows that reflective practice is not just about thinking individually; it can also be communicated and shared with others through conversation and written documents. Both definitions touch on the outcome of reflection, either in terms of understanding or in terms of action. Tate (2004) provides a simple figure for the reflective learning cycle (Figure 10.3 below).

This figure has been adapted by Tate from work by Boud, Keogh and Walker (1985). They note that experience alone is not sufficient for learning and posed the following questions.

- What is it that turns experience into learning?
- What specifically enables people to gain the maximum benefit from the situations they find themselves in?
- How can people apply their experience in new contexts?

Boud and colleagues suggest that structured reflection is the key to learning from experience. They were particularly interested in the application of reflection during training. They linked the timing of reflective activities to the three stages in experience-based learning – preparation, engagement and processing – and highlighted the importance of including reflective activity at each stage. During the preparatory phase, students are prompted to examine what is required of them and consider the demands of their clinical placement site; during their experiences on placement, students are encouraged to process a variety of inputs arising from their clinical practice; finally, once back in the academic setting, students are given time to consider and consolidate what they have experienced on placement (Boud, Keogh and Walker, 1985).

Reflection, in both students and qualified therapists, is undertaken all the time during interactions with clients as they make adjustments to their assessment approach and treatments based on feedback from the client and the clinical reasoning that draws upon their tacit knowledge and skills. Sometimes, this tacit reflection is made explicit when students/therapists have to discuss decision-making about a client, for example with their supervisor, their student or another member of the multidisciplinary team. But the speed of decision-making required during interactions

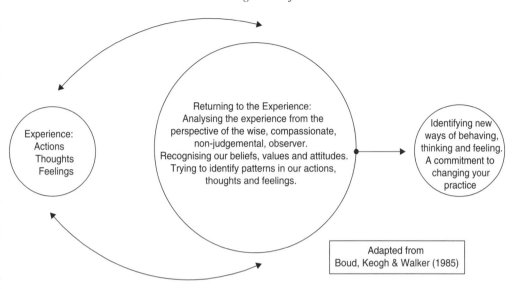

Figure 10.3 The reflective learning cycle. *Reprinted with kind permission from Sylvina Tate taken from Tate S (2004) Using critical reflection as a teaching tool. In Tate S, Sills M (2004) The Development of Critical Reflection in the Health Professions. London, Learning and Teaching Support Network (LTSN) at the Centre for Health Sciences and Practice (HSAP).*

with clients does not provide the time out required for a therapist or student to reflect deeply on what she is doing. This is why students and therapists need time outside of their day-to-day practice to think more deeply about what they are doing and why they are doing it. Reflection on action, therefore, requires a student/clinician to make time to step back from a particular client–therapist interaction, case or experience in order to reflect upon and question her decisions, feelings and actions. Being a reflective practitioner should involve the therapist taking a long, hard look at the why, what and how of a particular aspect of her practice, the way she handled a specific case or a significant incident, because in order to be most beneficial reflection requires 'exploring deep-seated beliefs and taken-for-granted assumptions' (Swain, 2004, p. 216).

Swain (2004), in a chapter on interpersonal communication from a text on psychosocial approaches for physiotherapists, highlights the relationship between reflection, effective communication and social constructivism. 'The effectiveness of physiotherapy practice is not just dependent on the technical skills of a physiotherapist but on the whole complex process of interpersonal communication through which physiotherapy practice is realized' (p. 216). Social constructivism, in very simple terms, is a viewpoint in which knowledge is not purely objective but is at least partly socially constructed. Swain states that social constructivism 'is one way of viewing personal and social worlds that can inform the standpoint of physiotherapists seeking to reflect critically on their practice as socially constructed encounters through and within interpersonal communication' (p. 216). When social constructivism is used by therapists to support reflection, 'at a personal level, it can help therapists to examine the beliefs and values they bring to their practice for signs of stereotyping or prejudice' while 'at a professional level, it can provide a framework for evaluating theories and models of practice in terms of their potential to oppress or marginalize people' (p. 217).

REFLECTIVE PRACTICE AS A COMPONENT OF CONTINUING PROFESSIONAL DEVELOPMENT

Physiotherapists and occupational therapists practising in the UK are required to undertake continuing professional development (CPD) activities and keep a record of them as part of their registration with the Health Professions Council (HPC). The requirement for undertaking and documenting CPD for registration to practise as a physiotherapist or occupational therapist has existed for longer in some other countries. Other health care professionals are also required to evidence their CPD, and this can include an explicit requirement for reflection on action, for example all nurses practising in Ontario are required to complete a Reflective Practice programme and declare their participation in the programme. In the UK, the HPC's (2006) guidelines on standards for CPD list reflective practice as an example of a work-based-learning CPD activity. The CSP recommends that therapists record reflective activities because written evidence of reflective practice can demonstrate to others how the therapist has kept her practice under regular, critical review and how her practice has developed safely and effectively. In addition, the CSP (2006b) states that keeping a record of reflections:

- provides written evidence of what you learned during your reflections
- can clarify your thoughts more succinctly as you put your reflections in writing
- can be shared with others at a later date.

The CSP (2006b) also encourages therapists to share their reflections with others as:

- when 'you share your experiences and learning with others, so they can learn from you
- another's thoughts about your experience can help you to draw out more from the experience
- another's point of view takes away some of the subjectivity of reflective practice.'

There are a number of ways in which reflections can be documented; these include diary entries, reflective journals, significant incident analyses, case analyses, clinical stories and notes from supervision, mentorship or peer reflection sessions. A good place to keep such reflections is in your portfolio of continuing development. Reflective journals are used across a number of health professions. For example, in nursing reflective learning journals are recognised as significant tools in promoting active learning among nursing students (Thorpe, 2004). Nursing, occupational therapy and physiotherapy educators all use reflective journals to encourage their students to think about past experiences, current situations and expected outcomes of their actions in order to assist students to find a language for explaining what they do in the clinical setting and why. Guidelines for structuring a reflective journal entry or for undertaking a significant incident analysis, either alone or in a group setting, are provided below.

Therapists can be extremely busy and not have time to stop and reflect immediately after a significant incident; unless you have an excellent memory, it can be very useful to jot a few key facts and feelings down in your diary as soon as possible and then complete a significant incident analysis later. White (2004) uses the reflective cycle developed by Gibbs (1988) as a format for reflecting on an incident that she uses with physiotherapy students on clinical placement. This comprises the following sections:

1. Description of the incident
2. Explanation – how did it feel?
3. Evaluation – what was good or bad about the experience?
4. Analysis – what can you learn from the event?
5. Conclusion – could you have done anything differently?
6. Action plan – if it happens again, what would you do? (White, 2004, p. 30)

Similar questions are posed by Larin, Wessel and Al-Shamlan (2005) in their guidelines for physiotherapy students writing a weekly reflective journal entry while on clinical placement. These are provided in Box 10.3 (below).

Box 10.3 Guidelines for writing a reflective journal

Reflective journals should include observations, impressions, and reactions to what you have learned in the academic portion of the semester and how you are applying it to clinical practice. How does the clinical experience change what you thought, felt, or did in the past, and how you may respond in the future?

1. Describe the learning event, issue or situation. Describe prior knowledge, feelings or attitudes with new knowledge, feelings or attitudes.
   What happened?
2. Analyse the learning event, issue or situation in relation to prior knowledge, feelings or attitudes.
   What was your reaction to the learning event, issue or situation? Your response may include cognitive and emotional reactions. Why did it happen?
3. Verify the learning event, issue or situation in relation to prior knowledge, feelings or attitudes.
   What is the value of the learning event, issue or situation that has occurred? Is the new knowledge, feeling or attitude about the learning event, issue or situation correct?
4. Gain a new understanding of the learning event, issue or situation.
   What is your new understanding of the learning event, issue or situation?
5. Indicate how the new learning event, issue or situation will affect future behavior. Determine the clarification of an issue, the development of a skill or the resolution of a problem.
   How will you approach the same or similar event, issue or situation in the future?

Reprinted from Larin H, Wessel J, Al-Shamlan A (2005) Reflections of physiotherapy students in the United Arab Emirates during their clinical placements: A qualitative study. BMC Medical Education 5 (3).

As a modernisation manager working in the NHS, I find the following headings useful for focusing my reflections on incidents and interactions that I want to learn from.

- What happened and why?
- How did you behave, think and feel as it was happening?
- What were the main learning points from the experience?
- Could you have anticipated the situation?
- What will you do differently as a result of this reflection?

These reflective journal entry headings were given to me and other NHS managers attending a middle managers development centre run by the National Institute for Mental Health for England (NIMHE) and the NHS Modernisation Agency Leadership Centre (February 2004, Darlington). They also provided a useful process for teams or groups of people who have shared a significant experience or incident to follow to guide reflection and help the team/group identify lessons and any actions or changes that they should make (see Box 10.4 below).

Writing and analysing case studies and clinical stories can be very useful for helping you undertake reflection *on* action. Mattingly and Fleming (1994a) provide a number of case examples and clinical stories throughout their text. They also provide an appendix of clinical stories (pp. 343–359) that have been written by different therapists. Each clinical story is followed by some discussion questions to prompt reflection. Unsworth (1999) also structures much of her text around case studies, through which therapists' reasoning related to the evaluation and intervention of a range of cognitive and perceptual dysfunctions are explored. Box 10.5 provides a clinical story analysis format to help you write and reflect on a clinical story of your own.

Box 10.4 After action review process

Step 1: Fix a time for the review – allow at least 20–30 minutes
Step 2: At the start of the review, propose some ground rules; for example:

- Everyone's experience is valid, irrespective of status in the organisation.
- Don't hold back: share what you saw, heard, experienced.
- No 'thin skins' – don't take anything personally, focus on the impact of the experience on the team/group.
- Propose changes – what could be done differently or better?

Step3: Work through the basic questions of the After Action Review. Ask each person to make brief notes on the following questions.

- What was supposed to happen?
- What actually happened?
- What accounts for the difference?

Step 4: Taking each question in turn, ask each person present to comment, and note down the points on which most people agree on a flip chart.
Step 5: When all the questions have been dealt with ask:

- 'What could we do differently next time?'

Note any ideas and actions that are feasible and you agree could improve practice.
Step Six: Close the meeting, thank everyone for their input and give all participants in the process a copy of the results.

There are advantages and disadvantages to undertaking reflective activities individually or with colleagues in pairs or groups and between unsupervised and supervised reflection (Tate and Sills, 2004). These advantages and disadvantages are presented in Table 10.1 (below).

Reflective practice has traditionally been seen as an individual or small group activity undertaken by professionals. Swain (2004) reports that Anderson (1992) 'has developed an approach in which professionals reflect in the presence of those who consult them and then invite the clients to reflect on their reflections. The advantage of this approach is that it encourages the client to have a voice in what is usually regarded as professional territory. It also provides an opportunity to privilege the issues and concerns of clients in negotiating priorities in physiotherapy practice' (Swain, 2004, p. 218). In a health care environment in which systematic and embedded client and carer involvement is being increasingly highlighted as essential to good practice, the involvement of clients in your reflective activities should be implemented.

COGNITIVE DISSONANCE

Finally, in this discussion about reasoning, reflection and decision-making, it is important to draw your attention to cognitive dissonance. We do not like to have inconsistencies between our attitudes/beliefs and our behaviours. When this happens, we experience an uncomfortable feeling known as cognitive dissonance. Cognitive dissonance is a psychological phenomenon first identified by Leon Festinger in 1956 (see Griffin, 1997). It occurs when there is a discrepancy between what a person believes, knows and values, and persuasive information that calls these into question. The discrepancy causes psychological discomfort, and the mind adjusts to reduce the discrepancy. This leads some people who feel dissonance to seek information that will reduce dissonance and avoid information that will increase dissonance. People who are involuntarily exposed to information that increases dissonance are likely to discount that information,

---

Box 10.5 Clinical story analysis format

1. **Identification of themes**
   a. Develop a descriptive title for the client's point of view.
   b. Develop a descriptive title for the therapist's point of view.
   c. Who is constructing the plot; what are they doing to emplot (make the story 'come true')?
   d. Describe the motives and morals, desires and passions reflected in the story.
   e. Discuss the following:
      i. Does the story explain and/or blame or not explain and blame?
      ii. Does the story take credit or not take credit?
   f. Does revision take place? If so, describe the process.
2. **Action and inquiry**
   • What are the puzzles/questions being worked upon?
   • What actions make a pivotal point – insights/inferences promoted by the therapist or client?
   • Describe action and reaction clusters, together with reciprocity of action on the part of each.
   • Describe the revisions made in the therapeutic process as a result of inquiry.
   • Describe the inquiry that resulted from action, and vice versa.

This story analysis format has been adapted from a handout used with occupational therapy students at the Occupational Therapy Program at Washington University School of Medicine, St Louis, USA. The handout was developed by colleagues Karen Barney and Christine Berg in 1991.

---

either by ignoring it, misinterpreting it or denying it. Cognitive dissonance can affect our judgement and decision-making (Toft and Reynolds, in press).

One way of dealing with dissonance is to change our viewpoint. But changing our views to agree with another person's can be very problematic in clinical situations and can work to the disadvantage of the client. For example, a therapist may find her views, beliefs or assessment result in conflict with those of other members of her department or multidisciplinary team. Cognitive dissonance is likely to occur under these circumstances, particularly if she is less experienced or less qualified than her colleagues. Changing her views, beliefs or conclusions by deferring to the superiority of senior colleagues, such as a consultant or senior therapist, will help to reduce the feeling of dissonance.

To justify such a change, she may rationalise that the senior colleague has more experience, greater qualifications, is wiser and/or further up the organisational hierarchy and responsible for her supervision/management. This type of reasoning is known as *argument from authority* and is a type of inductive reasoning. An argument from authority draws a conclusion about the truth of a statement based on the proportion of true propositions provided by that same source. It has the same form as a prediction. So if the therapist has found 99 per cent of the claims of authority by her senior colleague to have been true, then she inducts that there is a 99 per cent probability that this claim from the same colleague is also true. However, this situation may be the 1 per cent occasion when the senior colleague is wrong.

Toft (2001), in an external inquiry into an adverse incident, found cognitive dissonance to be one of the factors leading to the death of a client. Toft's report provides a stark example of the consequences of junior staff not questioning senior colleagues; in this case, a junior doctor was passed a drug to administer through lumbar puncture by a senior doctor. The drug administered in this way proved fatal. When interviewed, the junior doctor admitted that he had responded to being handed the drug by repeating the drug's name in a questioning manner, he received

Table 10.1 Advantages and disadvantages of different methods of critical reflection. *Reprinted with kind permission from Sylvina Tate. Taken from Tate S (2004) Using critical reflection as a teaching tool. In Tate S, Sills M (2004) The Development of Critical Reflection in the Health Professions. London, Learning and Teaching Support Network (LTSN) at the Centre for Health Sciences and Practice (HSAP).*

Method	Advantages	Disadvantages
Unsupervised		
Individual	• Not threatening • Can be undertaken according to individual needs • May be able to be more honest • Concentrates on personal issues	• More difficult to challenge self • Have only one world perspective • May become negative • May self deceive
Pairs	• More than one world perspective • Can feel supported • Can provide a more objective view of the experience	• May collude rather than challenge • Need to consider another when engaging in the process
Group	• Many world perspectives • Have a support group when initiating action • Can learn from the experiences of others	• Need to adhere to ground rules • May be scape-goated • May develop 'cliques'
Supervised		
Individual	• Can be undertaken according to individual needs • May be able to be more honest • Concentrates on personal issues • Can be undertaken according to individual needs • Have the experience of a facilitator • May be more motivating for supervisee	• May respond to please the facilitator • Need to find a personal facilitator • Need to trust and respect the facilitator • May be costly
Pairs	• More than one world perspective • Can feel supported • Can provide a more objective view of the experience • Have the experience of a facilitator • May be more motivating for supervisee	• Need to consider another when engaging in the process • May respond to please the facilitator • Need to find a personal facilitator • Need to trust and respect the facilitator • May be costly
Group	• Many world perspectives • Have a support group when initiating action • Can learn from the experiences of others • Have the experience of a facilitator • Less costly than individual supervision • May be more motivating for supervisee	• Need to adhere to ground rules • May be scapegoated • May develop 'cliques' • Need to consider another when engaging in the process • May respond to please the facilitator • Need to find a personal facilitator • Need to trust and respect the facilitator • Participants may be at different developmental stages • Personal needs may not be the priority for the group.

an affirmative response and repeated the drug's name with the method of administration in a questioning manner but then proceeded after receiving a further affirmative response from the senior doctor. The junior doctor felt his limited experience of the type of treatment and his junior status meant that he was not in a position to challenge a senior colleague. Had he followed his initial convictions and refused to administer the drug as a spinal administration, the client would not have died.

While it can be uncomfortable to challenge senior colleagues, our responsibility as therapists to act in the best interest of our clients demands that we handle our dissonace and make challenges if needed. I had a positive experience of making such a challenge in a ward round when I was a basic grade occupational therapist who had just joined a well-established multidisciplinary team. I had just started working on an elderly medical ward and had undertaken a brief interview with a client I was taking over. The lady had sustained a fall that had led to a fractured neck of femur. My previous rotation had been in a psychiatric day hopsital and so I was experienced in assessing for mental health problems. In my brief interview with the lady I found her to be very keen to get better and to be well enough to live at home again, but also anxious of returning home because of her fear of falling again. Overall, she presented with signs of a low mood: she was rather tearful, complained of feeling tired and of not sleeping well and of having little appetite. I developed a hypothesis that she was suffering from mild depression and anxiety.

During the ward round, the doctor stated that the X-rays showed she had made a good physical recovery from the fracture and should now be ready for discharge. The nursing staff reported that she was more dependent than anticipated and still required assistance with washing, dressing and transfers. The team felt frustrated at the lack of motivation the client had for her rehabilitation and felt her attitude was hampering her recovery. The team debated the way forward with her rehabilitation but no mention was made of her mental state. In the end, I cautiously asked what was being done about her anxiety and probable depression. The team looked surprised and asked me what I meant. I hesitated and then reported on my brief interview stating that I had found her very anxious about returning home, owing to her fear of falling, and exhibiting symptoms of mild depression. I hypothesised that her mental state was affecting her physical and functional rehabilitation. I also explained that she had told me that her greatest wish was to return home, but she was worried about how she was going to manage now her legs felt so weak following the fracture and that she was very frightened that she would fall and break her leg again. I asked whether we had access to a psychiatrist.

The consultant agreed to seek a second opinion from a psychiatrist, and the lady was then formally diagnosed with depression and anxiety. I also worked closely with my physiotherapy colleague to focus on the psychological aspects of her rehabilitation related to her confidence and fear of falling. Once the team focused on her mental state, the lady began to make significant progress with all areas of rehabilitation and was discharged back home. Prior to discharge, I took the lady on an assessment home visit to evaluate her environment for hazards that might increase her risk of future falls. The physiotherapist gave her strengthening exercises to continue with at home after discharge and we also referred her for a pendant alarm.

This example shows how those cases that are more accessible to our recall are more likely to shape the hypotheses we generate during assessment. As I had been working in a mental health field, it was easy for me to recall cases of people with anxiety and with depression and to match the patterns of symptoms presented by those cases to those signs exhibited by the lady. For the rest of my colleagues who had been practising in a physical rehabilitation setting for some time, the same cues had led to a hypothesis of lack of motivation. Had I not found the confidence to share my conflicting hypothesis, this lady would have been labelled as unmotivated and the team's approach and her path to recovery may have taken a less productive course.

This positive outcome early in my career helped to give me the confidence to contribute my views in other team meetings when I felt I had information or conclusions that ran counter to a senior colleague. Several times in such multidisciplinary team meetings other members of the group would support my stated viewpoint, such as a client was unsafe to be discharged home, and I found they also had questioned the senior colleague's decision to discharge but had not felt confident to challenge openly. When I was working in a geriatric day hospital, I was fortunate to work with a forward-thinking consultant geriatrician who realised that staff in his team were hesitant to challenge his views. One day, he pretended to have lost his voice and asked me to chair the multidisciplinary meeting. He observed that all the team members contributed much more actively and confidently in the discussion when he was not stating his views first and stood back from taking a lead role at the meeting. As a result of this experience, he asked the multidisciplinary team to share the chairing of the group and we took turns to lead the meeting. This meant that we became more aware of allowing each team member to have a voice and also more comfortable with voicing alternative viewpoints.

Undertaking an analysis of your approach to conflict can be useful. The Thomas–Kilmann Conflict Mode Instrument (Thomas and Kilmann, 1974) is an interesting self-report instrument that is designed to assess a person's behaviour in conflict situations. The test taker chooses from a series of paired statements related to her most likely response in a series of conflict situations. The test results provide a profile for how often the person is likely to use each of five responses to conflict. These are labelled as the competing, collaborating, compromising, avoiding and accomodating modes. These modes fall into two behavioural dimensions, assertiveness and cooperativeness. Therapy is a very collaborative process and client-centred therapy involves a great deal of cooperativeness, negotiation and accomodation on the part of the therapist. A competing stance, where the therapist has to be assertive and uncompromising, may not come naturally, and therapists may need to work on developing skills in assertiveness in order to become effective advocates for clients receiving health or social care in a disempowering system.

As the use of self is so important as a therapeutic tool for building a therapeutic relationship (Mosey, 1981) and for how you handle yourself as a member of a multidisciplinary team, a reflective activity – analysis of therapeutic self – can be very valuable. The purpose of this activity is to help you to become more aware of the personal resources you can bring to your therapeutic relationships. Box 10.6 (below) provides a format for describing your personal style as a therapist.

NOVICE TO EXPERT CONTINUUM

'Professional expertise is a goal of health care professionals and an expectation of health care consumers' (Higgs and Bithell, 2001). Expertise is hard to measure. In an exploration of clinical reasoning in physiotherapy development, Roskell (1998) comments that expertise is often measured in terms of a therapist's length of clinical experience, seniority and academic qualifications but that it *should* be measured in terms of knowledge, skills and qualities. King and Bithell (1998) highlight the quality of a therapist's advanced clinical reasoning skills as being a significant factor in separating an expert from a competent practitioner, while Higgs and Jones (2000) recommend that clinical expertise should be considered as a continuum along multiple dimensions. Jensen *et al.* (2000), in their qualitative study to identify the dimensions of clinical expertise in physical therapy practice, drew upon their findings to develop a theoretical model of expert practice in physical therapy. This model comprises four dimensions:

1. 'a dynamic, multidimensional knowledge base that is patient-centered and evolves through therapist reflection
2. a clinical reasoning process that is embedded in a collaborative, problem-solving venture with the patient
3. a central focus on movement assessment linked to patient function
4. consistent virtues seen in caring and commitment to patients' (p. 28).

Box 10.6 Analysis of therapeutic self

1. Describe your personal style in terms of the qualities listed below. In your descriptions, try to include examples of behaviours you have demonstrated in clinical helping relationships. The following qualities are listed in alphabetical order – but you do not have to follow this order. You may wish to undertake this activity over time, reflecting on one or two qualities at a time. Comments, in brackets, are provided after each quality to give you some ideas and/or clarify concepts.
   a. affect, emotional tone (e.g. are you enthusiastic, energetic, serious, low key)
   b. attending and listening (including your ability to reflect back and/or add to what the speaker has said)
   c. cognitive style (detail- or Gestalt-orientated, abstract or concrete, ability to understand diverse points of view)
   d. confidence (not only what you feel, but what you show to others)
   e. confrontation (can you do it and with whom)
   f. empathy (for what emotions, in what situations)
   g. humour (do you use it and, if so, how)
   h. leadership style (directive, facilitative, follower)
   i. non-verbal communication (facial expressiveness, eye contact, voice tone and volume, gestures)
   j. power sharing (need to control or comfortable with chaos)
   k. probing (when you are comfortable doing it, with whom and about what)
   l. touch (do you use it automatically or consciously, when, where and with whom)
   m. verbal communication (vocabulary, use of vernacular, ease of speaking)
2. Write a summary of what you see as your strengths and weaknesses relative to establishing therapeutic relationships.
3. Review your reflections on your personal style and your strengths and weaknesses, which areas or skills would you like to improve upon? Prioritise these and suggest strategies for improving your top two priorities. Draw up an action plan for implementing these strategies for improvement.

This activity has been based on a handout provided to me when I visited colleagues engaged in clinical reasoning research at Tufts University, Boston (April 1992). The handout does not acknowledge an author or date. It was developed as an activity for occupational therapy students.

A number of therapy writers have drawn upon the work of Dreyfus and Dreyfus (1986) to understand the journey taken as clinicians move from being novice to expert practitioners. This novice to expert continuum comprises five stages and is outlined in Figure 10.4 (below).

Schell (1998) drew on the work of a number of authors, including Mattingly and Fleming (1994a) and Benner (1984), to apply the novice to expert continuum proposed by Dreyfus and Dreyfus (1986) to clinical reasoning in occupational therapy practice. She perceives the novice as someone with no experience who has to be dependent on theory to guide her practice. Such a person would use rule-based procedural reasoning to guide her clinical decisions and would not yet be able to recognise contextual cues. At this stage, Schell perceives narrative reasoning to be apparent when forming social relationships but not being used to inform clinical practice. A novice will recognise overt ethical issues. Schell states that at this stage 'pragmatic reasoning [is] stressed in terms of job survival skills' (p. 97).

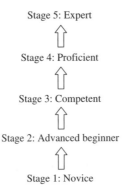

Stage 5: Expert

⇑

Stage 4: Proficient

⇑

Stage 3: Competent

⇑

Stage 2: Advanced beginner

⇑

Stage 1: Novice

Figure 10.4 The novice to expert continuum. *Based on the Dreyfus model of skill acquisition (Dreyfus and Dreyfus, 1986).*

An advanced beginner is likely to have less than one 'year of reflective practice' under her belt (Schell, 1998, p. 97). At this stage, the therapist starts to 'incorporate contextual information into rule-based thinking' and is able to start recognising the differences between expectations from theory and real clinical problems. A lack of experience means that the therapist has yet to form patterns/heuristics to help prioritise her competing hypotheses. An advanced beginner is developing skills in both pragmatic and narrative reasoning. At this stage, Schell believes the therapist 'begins to recognize more subtle ethical issues' (p. 97).

The competent therapist will have been engaged in reflective practice for about three years (Schell, 1998). A therapist at this stage is able to perform more therapeutic skills automatically and so can focus attention on more issues. She is more efficient at sorting data and at setting priorities. Her planning becomes 'deliberate, efficient and responsive to contextual issues' and a competent therapist can use 'conditional reasoning to shift treatment during sessions and to anticipate discharge needs' (p. 97). At this stage, Schell states that the therapist can recognise 'ethical dilemmas posed by [her] practice setting, but may be less sensitive to justifiably different ethical responses' (p. 97).

The proficient therapist is likely to have engaged in reflective practice for around five years (Schell, 1998). This therapist will have developed a wealth of experiences that enables her to be more targeted in her assessment approach, efficient in diagnostic reasoning and flexible in alternating between different treatment options. These therapists are able to 'creatively combine different diagnostic and procedural approaches'; they also have more refined narrative reasoning skills and become 'more attentive to occupational stories and the relevance [of these stories] for treatment' (p. 97). In terms of pragmatic reasoning, a proficient therapist becomes better at accessing and negotiating resources to meet her clients' needs. At this stage, Schell states that the therapist has become sophisticated in her ability to recognise the 'situational nature of ethical reasoning' (p. 97).

Finally, an expert therapist will have undertaken ten or more years of reflective practice (Schell, 1998). Schell states that for an expert 'clinical reasoning becomes a quick and intuitive process which is deeply internalized and imbedded in an extensive store of case experiences'; she says that this 'permits practice with less routine analysis, except when [the therapist is] confronted with situations where [her] approach is not working' (p. 97). An expert therapist will have become highly skilful in her use of stories and will have refined the narrative reasoning skills that she applies to her assessment and intervention.

Where are you on this novice to expert continuum? Are you a first-year occupational therapy or physiotherapy student working at a novice level or a third-year student moving towards the stage of advanced beginner? Have you recently graduated into the profession and while competent can see that you have much to learn still? Have you come to this text as a post-graduate student with a wealth of clinical experience, or as an educator or clinical supervisor and perceive yourself to be proficient or expert in your practice? Try to place yourself on this novice to expert continuum and then reflect on some goals to help you move your skills to the next stage.

FURTHER READING

Clinical reasoning is a vast and complex subject. This chapter has only provided a brief overview; so you may find it helpful to undertake some further reading. A good starting point is *Clinical Reasoning: Forms of Inquiry in a Therapeutic Practice* (Mattingly and Fleming, 1994a).

In order to understand how this clinical reasoning process works in practice, it can be helpful to examine several different therapists' reasoning related to specific client cases. Detailed case examples that outline therapists' thinking during assessment can be found in several chapters in Carolyn Unsworth's (1999) textbook *Cognitive and Perceptual Dysfunction: A Clinical Reasoning Approach to Evaluation and Intervention*. Rogers and Holm (1989) provide a useful case example that demonstrates cue interpretation and hypothesis evaluation. Schell (1998) has written an overview chapter for occupational therapists that includes a case example (Can she go home?) at the start of the chapter, which is then unpackaged in terms of different types of clinical reasoning.

Another interesting chapter is 'Professional identity and clinical reasoning' in Kielhofner (1992). Ryan and McKay (1999) discuss the role of narratives in practice and education. Their book provides an introduction to clinical reasoning. In particular see 'Section 2: Describing Practice', which contains four chapters made up of:

- Lillian and Paula: a treatment narrative in acute mental health by Elizabeth Anne McKay
- Jenny's story: exploring the layers of narrative reasoning by Rachelle Coe
- The team's story of a client's experience of anorexia nervosa by Ruth Erica Living
- A support group for head-injured individuals: stories from the peer leader and facilitator by Alice Lowenstein and Sharan L. Schwartzberg.

The Development of Critical Reflection in the Health Professions is one of a series of occasional papers produced by the Learning and Teaching Support Network (LTSN) at the Centre for Health Sciences and Practice (HSAP). It includes chapters on 'Using reflective practice in the physiotherapy curriculum' by Patricia White (2004) and 'Reflective practice within the occupational therapy curriculum' by Rebecca Khanna (2004). It also contains some useful figures showing the experiential learning cycle (Figure 1.1, p. 9) and reflective learning cycle (Figure 1.2, p. 11) and a very helpful table listing the advantages and disadvantages of different methods of critical reflection (Figure 1.3, p. 12). There are lots of useful appendices, including examples of reflective writing, journal guide, portfolio criteria and reflective questions to consider after an activity. This resource can be accessed online (see White, 2004).

For more information on reflective practice, for physiotherapists in the UK who are members of the CSP, access the members' section of the website (Chartered Society of Physiotherapy, 2006b) where you can read sections on:

- what reflective practice actually means and the theories behind it
- useful ways to reflect on your practice
- proformas for reflective practice
- additional guidance papers.

CASE STUDY: MRS ELLIS' INITIAL ASSESSMENT PROCESS

By Karen Innes and Alison Laver Fawcett

This case study has been provided by Karen Innes and written jointly with Alison Laver Fawcett. It has been written to illustrate the therapist's clinical reasoning related to the initial assessment of a client with whom she is likely to work over many months. The case is provided to illustrate several of the different types of reasoning outlined earlier in this chapter. It is a detailed study in order that students and novice therapists can see an example of how a therapist frames and explains her assessment approach. The therapist's thinking is mostly provided in boxes to separate the reasoning from the description of what happened during the assessment process for this case.

INTRODUCTION TO THE OCCUPATIONAL THERAPIST

The therapist had worked as a qualified occupational therapist for five years. Prior to that she has had 12 years' experience as a technical instructor working with people with learning disabilities, working-age adults with mental health problems and older adults with mental health problems; she worked across in-patient, outpatient and community settings. Presently, the therapist is a community mental health team (CMHT) member, together with a consultant psychiatrist, physiotherapist, community psychiatric nurse, social worker and health care assistants, based in a rural location.

MODELS AND APPROACHES THAT GUIDE THE THERAPIST'S PRACTICE

The two main models used by this therapist are:

- the Model of Human Occupation (MOHO; Kielhofner 1985; Kielhofner and Burke, 1980). 'MOHO seeks to explain how occupation is motivated, patterned, and performed. By offering explanations of such diverse phenomena, MOHO offers a broad and integrative view of human occupation. Within MOHO, humans are conceptualized as being made up of three interrelated components: volition, habituation, and performance capacity. Volition refers to the motivation for occupation, habituation refers to the process by which occupation is organized into patterns or routines, and performance capacity refers to the physical and mental abilities that underlie skilled occupational performance. MOHO also emphasizes that to understand human occupation we must also understand the physical and social environments in which it takes place. Therefore, this model aims to understand occupation and problems of occupation that occur in terms of its primary concepts of volition, habituation, performance capacity and environmental context' (Model of Human Occupation, 2006).
- the Canadian Model of Occupational Performance was developed by a group of therapists associated with the Canadian Association of Occupational Therapists (CAOT; 1991). The Occupational Performance Model promotes working in a client-centred way, respecting client choice and autonomy and advocating for the client's needs and wishes. This model focuses on the dynamic relationship between people, their environment and their occupations (activities related to self-care, productivity and leisure). It provides a framework for enabling occupation in all people and can be applied across age groups, diagnoses and clinical settings. Using this model, client-centred practice is based on a collaborative assessment of occupational needs of the person within his specific physical and social environment (Canadian Association of Occupational Therapists, 2006).

The therapist also draws upon a mixture of approaches such as problem-based (Hagedorn 1997), activities of daily living (ADL; Hill, 1993), compensatory, graded activities, group work (Creek 1996b) and cognitive approaches (perceptual and behavioural) (Hagedorn, 1997).

The process of change that the therapist hopes to elicit from the clients is through the use of rehabilitation (although not applied as frequently with people with a terminal illness such as dementia), education, which is mainly undertaken with the carers, adaptation and facilitation (MacRae, 2005) and risk management (Thom and Blair, 1998), especially risk related to the environment and the activities that the client is engaged with. Often the treatment process is a combination of most of these models, approaches and processes, as the needs of the client are considered and changes occur.

In relation to the models and approaches used by the therapist in this case study, the main standardised tests used by the occupational therapist are:

- Assessment of Motor and Process Skills (AMPS; Fisher 2003a, 2003b): The AMPS is a specialised assessment of function that requires the occupational therapist to attend a one-week intensive training course. The course costs approximately £900 (which in this case was funded by raising money through the local training consortium and sponsor money through a drug company). The test assesses motor and process skills deficits, which affect a person's ability to perform tasks. It can be administered in the person's own environment.
- Safety Assessment of Function and the Environment for Rehabilitation (SAFER Tool; Community Occupational Therapists and Associates, COTA, 1991): The therapist found the SAFER Tool an excellent tool to use, as it provides a comprehensive environmental prompt list, and it gives some good pointers to help the therapist with solutions to environmental risk factors. However, it can be time-consuming and can enable people to stray from the purpose of the assessment; therefore, the therapist has to remain focused upon the purpose of using the assessment and guide the client through it.
- Canadian Occupational Performance Measure (COPM; Law *et al.*, 1991): This is a self-report tool used to evaluate a client's self perception of occupational performance. However, for clients with organic impairment, depending on what stage the client is at with the dementia, this tool may not be appropriate, owing to a client being unable to think through a situation in an abstract manner. This tool is used alongside the Canadian Model of Occupational Performance (Canadian Association of Occupational Therapists, 1991).
- Mini Mental State Examination (MMSE; Folstein, Folstein and McHugh, 1975): This assessment is a short test that is easy to use, and it provides an indication of the level of cognitive function and is good for test/retest purposes.
- Mayer's Quality of Life Scale (Mayers, 2002): This covers the areas of activities of daily living (ADL) and social activities. The scale can be done together with the therapist or as a self-report tool for the client to complete on his own. This scale provides a good prompt for conversation; however, it can be too abstract for people who have lost the ability to think more abstractly.
- The Activity Card Sort (Baum, Perlmutter and Edwards, 2000): This gives visual prompts that help a person with cognitive impairment, and it can be easier for the person to identify levels of activity with this test compared to checklist formats.
- Bradford Well Being Profile (University of Bradford 2002; Bruce, 2000): This is an observational assessment that subtly identifies small changes in a person's well-being in those with moderate to moderately severe cognitive decline level. It is a relevant assessment for therapist as it assesses the person's well-being.

- Zarit Caregiver Burden Survey (Zarit, Todd and Zarit, 1986): This is a proxy measure that the therapist uses as a prompt to encourage conversation with the carer to assess for carer burden and to find out where they are having difficulties in caring for the client.
- Memory and Behaviour Problems Checklist (MBPC; Zarit, Todd and Zarit, 1986): This is a proxy report checklist used to identify memory and behavioural problems observed by carers of people with cognitive impairment. The checklist collects data on the presence and frequency of problems/behaviours.
- Interest Checklist (Matsutsuyu, 1969; Katz, 1988) and Role Checklist (Oakley *et al.*, 1986) were tools the therapist used in a previous clinical setting and are measures that fit with the Model of Human Occupation (Kielhofner, 1985).

These standardised tools, together with the structured and semi-structured interviewing techniques and informal observations, are the assessment tools used by the therapist in this case.

The therapist usually begins her assessment following a top-down approach (see the section on 'Top-down versus bottom-up assessment approach' in Chapter 9, pp. 261–3). The top-down approach helps the therapist to build an understanding about who the client is and involves gathering information in a semi-structured way about the life story of the client and his family. The therapist investigates the person's roles, values, interests, social supports and then explores functioning in associated activities. From this foundation, the therapist moves on to an exploration of the client's perceived difficulties, and identifies any stress or anxiety linked to these difficulties. This is a very client-centred approach. It takes time to build up a comprehensive image of the client, and this initial assessment is usually conducted over a couple of sessions. It is at this stage that the therapist is engaged in problem-setting and then framing and delineating the identified problems. As she takes a client-centred approach, she draws upon narrative reasoning to form a clinical image of the person and to understand his story. Through narrative reasoning, she attempts to understand the person's struggle to engage in his everyday activities and roles as an older person with a mental health problem, such as dementia.

From the information gathered at initial assessment, the therapist then forms some hypotheses around the underlying causes of the stated problems. She then switches to a bottom-up approach and engages in diagnostic reasoning to test her working hypotheses. This may involve searching for further cues, and these are obtained by conducting appropriate standardised assessments and undertaking further interviews with the client and carer to gain a more detailed history of symptoms. At the end of the diagnostic reasoning process, she has developed an idea as to why, how and where the client's problems are occurring. She then engages in conditional reasoning to develop treatment goals linked to her prognosis and then builds a treatment plan to deliver these goals.

CASE HISTORY: MR AND MRS ELLIS

REFERRAL INFORMATION RECEIVED AND FURTHER INFORMATION GATHERING

A very brief written referral was received from the GP by the CMHT requesting support for a gentleman struggling with his wife's care during her three-year history of an Alzheimer's type dementia. During a multidisciplinary team meeting, it was decided that it was important to determine the level of difficulty being experienced. This information could come from two sources: the GP and the husband of the lady with the illness. On receiving the referral, the therapist's reasoning moved towards her prior experience of working with people with Alzheimer's disease. She was able to consider the types of problems that the lady and her husband might be experiencing and hypothesised that given the lady had been diagnosed three years ago she was likely to be at a moderate stage of dementia. The community occupational therapist decided to start the information-gathering process off by investigating the referral further to establish a more in-depth history to get a flavour of where the difficulties lay. This information would start a procedural reasoning process to understand the person's problems and to consider ways to alleviate, or reduce the impact of, these problems. She also wanted to phone the GP to clarify the GP's expectations of what role the CMHT might play in the care of this couple. This approach is linked to pragmatic reasoning and attempts to address the questions of 'Who referred this client for therapy and why was this referral made?'

A telephone call was made to the GP to acknowledge the referral and to request further information about the situation and what had triggered the referral. It transpired that the family had been known to the practice for approximately 30 years. Mrs Ellis' recent illness had been treated by a consultant privately after relations had broken down with the local hospital at the start of the illness. The GP also reported that the family were willing to accept help from the team because they wanted to be in closer proximity to their care providers. The GP said that the family were well respected within the community having been very actively involved with local groups in the past. This involvement had reduced over recent years. It was also established that the main problems reported to the GP were around the patient's disturbed sleep pattern; some sleeping tablets had been prescribed.

> **Pragmatic reasoning:** the therapist's immediate impression was one of caution. It was going to be very important to start off on the correct footing to establish a trusting therapeutic relationship in order to be able to engage effectively with this couple to meet the care needs of the client and her family. The therapist wondered what 'relations had broken down with the hospital' meant. She wondered whether this implied that some sort of formal complaint had been made and decided that she should be very thorough with all her documentation pertaining to this case.

The next step was to contact the client's husband over the telephone to make an introduction and to set up a mutually appropriate appointment to meet him and his wife. This phone call was made. Mr Ellis was polite and appeared to be expecting a call from the team. He seemed pleased she had phoned promptly, and a date was agreed and the therapist followed this up with a letter of confirmation.

> **Pragmatic reasoning:** The therapist was very conscious of the importance of following a correct and thorough procedure to build up an efficient and effective client-centred first impression, and to provide information of the role of the occupational therapist and the CMHT. She was relieved that Mr Ellis had been expecting her contact and appeared pleased to be receiving a home visit. Some of her initial anxieties about building an effective therapeutic relationship were reduced after she had spoken to Mr Ellis and had a positive initial contact.

FIRST HOME VISIT AND INITIAL ASSESSMENT

> **Procedural reasoning:** It is important that each client's circumstances are considered as a unique case; therefore, prior to the home visit the therapist had to determine what the objectives of the initial assessment were and the information to be gathered. In this scenario these included:
>
> - establishing a trusting therapeutic relationship
> - gaining a history about the couple and finding out how the family are coping

- establishing where both Mrs and Mr Ellis see their difficulties
- informally assessing Mrs Ellis' orientation and perception of her difficulties
- determining what the action plan formulation is to be for future care needs.

Problem-orientated clinical reasoning process: The therapist decided an observational assessment approach would be used to gather information about physical and social environmental factors – this assessment would be informal but her observations would be framed in terms of SAFER Tool items (Canadian Association of Occupational Therapists, 1991). She also planned to observe how the couple communicated with each other and to seek cues related to the quality of the couple's relationship. The Interest Checklist (Katz, 1988) and a Role Checklist (Oakley *et al.*, 1986) can be used during the initial interview to help gather client-centred information. This information can help inform narrative reasoning and is useful for both assessment and treatment planning processes. The therapist decided to take these checklists with her and then see once she was there whether their use in the first interaction would be appropriate.

Pragmatic reasoning: As with any home visit, it is important to set a realistic time scale to conduct the visit, allowing enough travelling and interview time. For an initial home visit, the therapist usually allows two hours (it can take a while for the client/therapist to settle down to the assessment). One hour is normally allowed for subsequent visits unless complex assessments are conducted. Care was taken by the therapist to create the right impression of the service offered, particularly because the relationship had broken down with another service in the post.

The couple's home was a large luxury bungalow. They said they had lived there for over 45 years. Access to it was via a long drive and there were five steps up to the entrance. Mr and Mrs Ellis appeared at the door at the same time and greeted the therapist with polite formality inviting her into their home. The therapist waited for the couple to decide where it was convenient for the interview to take place. Mr Ellis allowed Mrs Ellis to determine this and whether she wanted him present throughout the visit also. Both of them were very well dressed and Mrs Ellis was well groomed, her hair looked like it had been professionally set and she wore understated but expensive-looking jewellery (the therapist noted that there were no obvious signs of self-neglect but wondered how much support her husband offered to maintain this standard of presentation and whether a special effort had been made for her visit). The bungalow was immaculately presented in terms of decor, tidiness and cleanliness (the therapist wondered who undertook domestic chores in this household). There were photos of the couple in exotic locations (what appeared to be on safari in Africa, by Ayres Rock, in front of a pyramid and on a tropical island) and items of interest collected from their travels as well as many family photographs around the room. A grand piano stood in one part of the room.

Narrative reasoning: The therapist started to construct a story around this couple's past life experience. The photos of their travels appeared to have been taken since their 50s and they were clearly well travelled. She postulated that the couple had a very active life together. She hypothesised that the onset of dementia had reduced their trips abroad and wondered how they were coping with the changes in their lifestyle. She also wondered if anyone played the piano. The therapist observed that this was a couple that considered each other's needs and made decisions jointly. They took pride in their surroundings and appeared to have a large family and a range of personal interests. She decided to proceed with a semi-structured interview to start building rapport and initiate a working relationship and to seek some insight into the difficulties being experienced.

During the interview, it was revealed that Mrs Ellis was 81 years old, and she and Mr Ellis had been married for 62 years after being childhood sweethearts. Mrs Ellis lost her mother at a very young age. The couple had four children and 15 grandchildren. Mrs and Mr Ellis had been very accomplished in their respective professional careers, as a headmistress and doctor of engineering respectively. Both individuals had continued with interests in music, travel and languages once they had retired. Mrs Ellis was an accomplished pianist and continued to play the piano up to the present time; however, Mr Ellis had to prompt her to play now and he said she was no longer interested in picking up new tunes but preferred to play old favourites from memory.

Procedural reasoning: The therapist wondered how much prompting was required to initiate other activities. She wondered how much Mrs Ellis' range of interests could be maintained through drawing on long-term memory, such as the years of practice that had led to her ability to read music and play a wide variety of tunes from memory.

Diagnostic reasoning: The therapist took cues from this initial conversation and began hypothesis generation. Her experience of working with other people with organic impairment was that when a client with dementia required prompting to initiate one task or activity this impairment was generalised to other areas of functioning; so she hypothesised that Mrs Ellis had impairments in the area of task initiation that would affect ADL as well as leisure activities. She also hypothesised that Mrs Ellis showed little interest in learning new tunes because she experienced difficulties with attending to an unfamiliar piece of music and that her ability to learn a new tune would be affected by cognitive deficits, particularly problems with short-term memory and working memory, related to her Alzheimer's disease.

The therapist continued with her interview asking more specific questions to ascertain which interests had been relinquished or reduced since the diagnosis. The couple reported that up until four years ago they had lived very full lives with lots of time spent with their family and frequent visits from grandchildren as they had liked to babysit and have their grandchildren who lived further away to stay. Mrs Ellis had been heavily involved with the local Girl Guides for many years. She had taught languages and after her retirement had become a member of a local interest group speaking French and Italian and enjoying exchange visits. The couple had enjoyed entertaining, going to the theatre and had frequent holidays abroad, both as a couple and with family. The therapist asked more about the onset of problems that had prompted them to seek medical help. Short-term memory problems (mainly with forgetting names) were reported to have started approximately four years ago. A diagnosis of Alzheimer's type dementia had been made. Cognitive functioning had been maintained for a couple of years with the help of drug therapy, following the couple seeking help through a consultant psychiatrist.

Diagnostic reasoning – cue acquisition: The therapist noted that both Mr and Mrs Ellis were happy to talk and appeared confident in their views and their account of the history of her illness. Mrs Ellis had an extensive vocabulary, was articulate and presented socially very well owing to her high intellectual ability. However, as the interview unfolded, it became evident that, although Mrs Ellis could cover up some of the difficulties she was experiencing in a brief conversation, when a conversation was continued over several minutes repetition and confabulation became evident. Repetition of some information, such as her being a headmistress and having four children, occurred several times over the duration of the hour's interview and occasionally Mrs Ellis would speak in a distressed and tearful manner of her husband still having to go away on dangerous reconnaissance missions in the war. This was something that had happened in the past, and the distress that this had caused her then was still vivid for her in the present time, even though her husband had been out of active service for over 45 years. Mrs Ellis also appeared to tire towards the end of the interview, allowing her husband to answer more of the questions and staring vacantly at times. The therapist hypothesised that Mrs Ellis' role of mother and teacher were very important to her sense of self; she also felt that her initial hypotheses about problems with attention and short-term memory had been supported further.

The therapist asked if Mrs Ellis was feeling tired and would prefer to end the visit for today. Mr Ellis suggested they leave her to rest for a moment while they went to the kitchen and made them all a cup of tea. Once he was alone with the therapist, he explained that his wife had been a very energetic person but that she did tire quickly these days. He reported that he often had to speak for his wife when she was tired or appeared to have difficulty replying. He described how her speech had become very quiet, almost inaudible on occasions, and said that this coupled with her confabulation and repetition was extremely frustrating.

Procedural reasoning: The therapist wondered about the causes of the reduced speech volume and decided to ask Mrs Ellis if she was aware of any communication problems. She did not have expertise in the area of communication and thought a referral to a speech and language therapist might be required.

Mrs Ellis was aware that she had problems but was unable to identify what they were specifically. She appreciated that her husband found it frustrating when he could not hear what she was saying. She agreed to have an assessment on her communication difficulties and said she would see a speech and language therapist if it might help the situation for her husband's sake.

As the interview unfolded further, some emotional distress was expressed by Mrs Ellis. This was in the form of fear and anxiety, relating to the delusional belief that when her husband left her for any length of time she believed that he would not come back. Mrs Ellis became quite tearful.

Pragmatic reasoning: The therapist wondered about potential separation problems should day or respite care be required in the future for the couple. The therapist had to be particularly sensitive to these verbal and non-verbal communication signs. She also had to achieve a balance between acknowledging the client's expressed fears and emotion but without turning the interview into a counselling situation.

Physically, Mrs Ellis' mobility did not initially cause any concerns to the therapist, as she appeared to move quite well. However, Mr Ellis reported that his wife had experienced a couple of minor falls lately, and was on occasion unsteady on her feet. He explained that she also had started to drop things. The therapist was informed that Mrs Ellis had experienced two heart attacks over the last three years and was unable to participate in any strenuous activity.

> **Diagnostic reasoning:** In terms of the reported falls, the therapist hypothesised about neurological changes occurring as a result of the disease and postulated about deficits in movement and balance. She also thought about person–occupation–environment fit and the possibility of environmental risk factors. She decided that a detailed home environment assessment to seek further cues around physical hazards would be useful.
>
> **Pragmatic reasoning:** She did not consider herself a specialist in falls and felt she should suggest to the couple that an assessment around balance, strength, falls risk and prevention with the team's physiotherapist would be helpful.

Mr Ellis was very informative during the interview, reporting that his wife no longer participated in complex levels of decision-making for ADL. He explained that he did try to involve her in making decisions where he could, for example in meal choice, daily clothing and where they should go if they went out for the day.

> **Conditional reasoning:** The therapist was aware of the insight and interest Mr Ellis had and took about his wife's abilities and the importance of retaining her independence as much as he could. However, her intuition questioned his emotional acceptance of the situation, how much he was actually doing around the house and what degree of carer stress he was under.

> **Procedural reasoning:** The therapist thought about the assessments that might be appropriate to use to gain some further insight into the abilities of Mrs Ellis so that some constructive interventions could be used to help Mr and Mrs Ellis perform some tasks together and maintain Mrs Ellis' role about the house in a safe and least-restrictive way – retrieving past theoretical knowledge, she drew on the work of Wheatley (1996) in formulating this plan. She felt this course of action might also allow Mr Ellis to gradually come to terms with his wife's failing abilities. Tests that would help to provide valuable information for the therapist included the MMSE (Folstein, Folstein and McHugh, 1975), which would give an indication of Mrs Ellis' cognitive function. The therapist was keen to observe Mrs Ellis directly in the performance of familiar tasks, so she chose the AMPS (Fisher, 2003a) as a measure that would help her to identify what the impact of her cognitive function was having on functional abilities. The dilemma for the therapist was how not to insult the couple's intellectual integrity while highlighting the deficiencies; she decided to focus the interview upon Mr Ellis and think about that later.

As she talked to Mr Ellis about the couple's daily and weekly routines, it became apparent that all the ADL tasks were left to Mr Ellis to undertake. He reported his wife had difficulty following instructions and would often 'end up in a confused muddle with familiar things if she was left to her own devices'. Mr Ellis had initially presented with strong composure throughout the interview, but at this point his eyes filled up with tears and it became apparent that he was struggling to come to terms with his wife's illness and difficulties. He explained how capable his wife had once been, his distress over the change that he was seeing his wife go through and the helplessness he felt about the situation. Mr Ellis explained that he found it very difficult coping with the disrupted sleep patterns that his wife was experiencing and how the sleep deprivation was affecting him negatively. He said he had gone to his GP because he was suffering from severe headaches, which his GP felt were linked to sleep deprivation and stress. He explained that his GP had told him that it was quite common for partners of people with dementia to begin grieving even while their loved one was alive because you lose the person you knew and the roles between you change. He said his chat with the GP had 'been very supportive and reassuring' as he was distraught by his wife's loss of ability and was feeling increasingly fearful about his ability to care for her adequately and was concerned about their future.

REASON FOR INTERVENTION – NEEDS IDENTIFICATION

> **Narrative reasoning:** The lived experience of dementia was proving distressing for both the client and her husband. It was becoming apparent that it was not only a practical supporting role that may be required but also an emotional one, for both Mrs Ellis and her husband needed support to come to terms with the losses in function associated with her dementia. She started to construct a prospective treatment story, imagining what the intervention might look like and what the outcome could be. The therapist felt confident that, owing to the candour with which the couple had described their situation, a therapeutic relationship based on trust was starting to develop.

The therapist then summarised her initial findings from the information given by the couple and her preliminary observations. She explained that, from what they had told her, it was clear that the memory problems that Mrs Ellis was experiencing were causing some reduction in her independence, which, together with the recent falls, had affected her confidence. The therapist also expressed her concerns over how distressed Mrs Ellis sometimes became over her anxieties and how the change in role for Mr Ellis, coupled with the impact of sleep deprivation, was affecting them both. The therapist stressed the value of continuing their involvement in social activities together and gave positive reinforcement to this. The therapist explained that she would use the information gained at the visit to identify further assessments required to formalise a treatment and intervention plan. She explained that this intervention plan would be developed in accordance with their priorities and agreement. The therapist followed the CMHT referral procedures and protocol for confidentiality and explained that the next step would be to discuss her findings with the consultant psychiatrist and the other members of the CMHT, which included a nurse, social worker and a health care assistant. She gained their permission to make referrals to the physiotherapist and speech and language therapist. She told them that she would then set up another home visit to discuss her ideas for addressing identified problems and needs.

> **Pragmatic reasoning:** On this occasion it was felt by the therapist that it was inappropriate to use either the Role or Interest Checklists as the time was at a premium. However, she felt they would provide useful data and be acceptable to Mr and Mrs Ellis. Therefore, she left the two checklists with the couple to complete as a self-report/proxy assessment and to give them some control and involvement over the assessment. Using Mrs Ellis' roles and interests would help her to tailor the treatment process and ensure any activities selected as the basis for intervention were meaningful to the client.

IDENTIFYING THE PROBLEMS AND FOCUSING THE ASSESSMENT

The therapist now engaged in problem-setting; this involved naming the phenomena/constructs that were to become the targets of an assessment. Defined problems were constructed from the observed and reported problematic situations that were identified from the referral information, discussion with the GP and the initial home visit interview. From the initial contact, a lot of information was gleaned without the use of standardised tests. From this information, the therapist developed a problem list around the difficulties that the couple were experiencing. She then selected appropriate assessments to provide the data required to explore these further and test out related hypotheses.

Problem list

From the information given by Mr and Mrs Ellis, the therapist identified that:

- Mrs Ellis had short-term memory problems and presented some challenging behaviour towards her husband by being easily distracted, confused, disorientated, and presenting with disrupted sleep patterns.
- Mrs Ellis had become increasingly dependent for some personal activities of daily living (PADL) and most domestic activities of daily living (DADL).
- Mrs Ellis had communication difficulties, confabulation and quietness of speech.
- There was some evidence of delusional beliefs and insightfulness exhibited by Mrs Ellis, which made her feel tearful and anxious.
- The therapist hypothesised that there may be perceptual and cognitive changes occurring. Related cues of falls and dropping items could result from such changes.
- Physically, Mrs Ellis was quite frail as a result of a history of cardiac problems; related to this, her lack of regular exercise reduced her stamina and possibly muscle tone.
- Mr Ellis was rational and realistic in the care for his wife; however, he was experiencing emotional difficulties in association with increased responsibility of being a carer, struggling to come to terms with the changes his wife was going through and struggling with the increased lack of sleep he was enduring.
- Mr Ellis was taking increased responsibility in all DADL.
- The couple still enjoyed a social life, mainly focused around their family and long-standing friends; however, both Mr and Mrs Ellis were becoming more isolated from social involvement owing to this situation.

FEEDBACK TO THE TEAM

In the past, drug therapy had been the main focus of intervention; however, as there had been deterioration in the well-being of Mrs Ellis, a joint care approach was taken following discussion with the consultant psychiatrist and CMHT.

DELINEATING THE PROBLEMS

The stage of delineating a problem involves the implementation of the therapist's chosen assessment methods and strategies. The therapist needed to apply multiple measures related to these various problems, these were to look at:

- **Occupation:** The therapist needed to assess Mrs Ellis's remaining abilities in personal care (washing, dressing), domestic involvement and role activity. She wanted to understand the underlying causes of any dysfunction and to see how Mrs Ellis tackled tasks and to assess whether any particular cues or prompts facilitated her function. Therefore, she decided to assess Mrs Ellis' functional ability through use of the AMPS (Fisher, 2003a). From the assessment results, the therapist anticipated she would be able to identify ways of working with Mrs Ellis to maintain her capabilities.

- **Challenging behaviour:** Mrs Ellis was exhibiting a number of challenging behaviours. The therapist wanted to assess the frequency and intensity of these problems further. She thought she would ask Mr Ellis to complete an MBPC (Zarit, Todd and Zarit, 1986). She anticipated that carer education would be invaluable in explaining to Mr Ellis why such behaviours may be occurring and as a means of trying to minimise the displayed behaviours.
- **Communication:** Communication appeared problematic, particularly in social situations; therefore, investigation into extent and support opportunities could be included in the treatment process of speech problems. A referral to a *speech and language therapist* was made.
- **Physical function:** Mrs Ellis was experiencing difficulties that were putting her at risk of falls and accidents and limiting her involvement in activity. The therapist felt physiotherapy intervention would be extremely helpful to the couple to maintain their mobility and physical well-being. A referral to a *physiotherapist* was made.
- **Environment:** An occupational therapy environmental risk assessment could be used to minimise further hazards around the home. The therapist planned to use the SAFER Tool (Canadian Association of Occupational Therapists, 1991).
- **Carer stress:** Mr Ellis seemed to be experiencing carer stress, and the nature of his physical and emotional burdens needed to be investigated to gain some insight to their extent, and appropriate support was to be offered where necessary. The therapist decided to tell Mr Ellis about the *Alzheimer's Society* and *Carer's Resource*. She would encourage engagement with these services but give him the option of self-referral so that he could take control over the extent and timing that he engaged with these agencies. The therapist considered that a referral to a day-care service would offer Mr Ellis some respite and Mrs Ellis socialisation, but she wondered whether this would be an acceptable option for the couple at this time.

Pragmatic reasoning: The therapist was aware that this battery of assessments would be too much for Mr and Mrs Ellis to undertake all at once. She was also aware that the sudden involvement of health care colleagues (physiotherapist and speech and language therapist) and of workers from voluntary agencies (Carer's Resource and Alzheimer's) may be too much straight away, as the couple seemed to like to make considered decisions about things that happened. It would, therefore, take a number of visits to follow the assessment and intervention process through with the full approval and support of Mr and Mrs Ellis.

A second home visit was planned by the occupational therapist with consent from the couple.

The objectives for the visit were to:

- discuss the couple's thoughts about the previous meeting
- discuss the findings of the first contact and agree some prioritised goals with Mrs and Mr Ellis
- collect the Role and Interest Checklists and use these as the basis for looking at some options of intervention

- conduct an environmental risk assessment
- conduct an MMSE (Folstein, Folstein and McHugh, 1975) to gain a baseline figure to monitor any cognitive changes later in treatment.

From the data gathered from the initial meeting with the client and the outcome of the team meeting, the next visit was primarily to discuss the proposed assessment, treatment and management. The therapist felt that it was important to keep the couple informed of ideas and thoughts about CMHT intervention so that the couple did not become increasingly anxious in an already emotional situation.

The next visit was again conducted by the therapist alone. The couple were pleased to see her and happy to discuss their thoughts of the last visit. Mrs Ellis was very pleased at the thought of some help for her husband and she recapped her concerns over how she felt a burden to him because of her memory problems.

Mr Ellis again presented calmly initially when discussing the care of his wife; however, the tears were evident again as the discussion progressed. The therapist wondered about the use of the Cruse bereavement care counselling service to help with the loss/helplessness he was feeling but felt that this was not the time to discuss this. She also wondered whether Mr Ellis might be suffering from a mild reactive depression and wondered whether it would be worth using a brief depression screen. The therapist discussed some of her thoughts about the previous meeting and suggested that this meeting was about prioritising goals for the couple and the therapist to work together on. The therapist's approach was to look both at the couple's joint needs and also at their individual problems.

The therapist discussed the history of falls previously mentioned, and the couple were happy that a referral to a physiotherapist for a falls assessment had been made. In conjunction with this, the couple allowed the therapist to make an assessment of the environmental factors in the couple's home. This would identify any potential risks that could be elevated prior to the physiotherapist's visit.

The tool that the therapist used was the SAFER Tool (Canadian Association of Occupational Therapists, 1991). This is a comprehensive checklist that addresses an individual's occupational performance tasks in their own home. The therapist found that all furniture was of a suitable height for safe transfers. From the assessment, a few problems were highlighted and addressed. For example, the therapist suggested removing the scatter rugs in the home. Mr Ellis reported that his wife used to be a magnificent cook but that now she found it difficult even to make a cup of tea or use the toaster. Mr Ellis reported that he felt that his wife would be unable to identify the need to put together a nutritional meal. Mr Ellis also reported that he usually carried hot food and drinks for her, for fear of Mrs Ellis falling while transferring hot items to the table. The therapist suggested using a compensatory technique in the form of a kitchen trolley; this was gratefully accepted. Mr Ellis informed the therapist that he was considering getting an au pair to help with domestic tasks so that he could devote more time to the more pleasurable side of life with his wife. He felt that this might take the pressure off himself as he did not enjoy domestic tasks. In the area of PADL, Mr Ellis reported that his wife spent a lot of time in the bedroom 'fidgeting' and would often require help with dressing as she would get dressed inappropriately, selecting the wrong items of clothing or mislaying items that she was looking for.

Procedural reasoning: The therapist wondered what level Mrs Ellis was functioning at, where the difficulties were in performing tasks and how her function was affected by Mr Ellis protecting his wife's feelings over her reduced abilities. Again, the therapist had to be subtle in performing any assessments so that some positive outcomes could be developed from the results. She decided that she would like to undertake an AMPS (Fisher, 2003a) as soon as possible.

Narrative reasoning: During this visit, the therapist was aware that Mrs Ellis had said very little. She wanted to keep engaging with her lived experience of dementia and maintain rapport with her client, as well as with her husband; so the conversation was directed more towards her to try to identify what her priorities were. The therapist gave Mr Ellis the MBPC (Zarit, Todd and Zarit, 1986) and suggested he might want to do this at the kitchen table. She said that she would chat to Mrs Ellis in the living room while he was doing the checklist. The therapist used the completed Role Checklist and Interest Checklists as a focus for her conversation with Mrs Ellis, as she did not feel that the COPM (Law *et al.*, 1991) would be a valuable tool in Mrs Ellis' case, owing to the possibility that confabulation would affect the reliability of her self-report. She felt Mrs Ellis might struggle with the ten-point rating scale and this could cause distress. She hoped that the Interest and Role Checklists would help her engage Mrs Ellis in exploring her past life history and current lifestyle and future wishes.

The Role Checklist indicated that Mrs Ellis had enjoyed being a mother and now loved being a grandmother. She was proud of her professional achievements and work with various charities. She also enjoyed participating in regular worship at her church.

From the Interest Checklist, the therapist discovered that Mrs Ellis had enjoyed the arts, theatre, dance and cookery. She continued to be involved with a local language group, which she got a lot of pleasure from as she attended with her husband. Mrs Ellis also reminisced about the camping holidays that the family used to take. Mrs Ellis stated that she would love to remain involved in many of these pleasurable activities for as long as possible as they gave her a sense of usefulness. The therapist explained that another questionnaire would provide an even more detailed picture of Mrs Ellis' quality of life and would help them monitor her participation in these important activities. She then administered the Mayers' Lifestyle Questionnaire (Mayers, 2003) as an interview. Mrs Ellis appeared to enjoy one-to-one conversation with the therapist and did not appear to tire. As they explored her lifestyle and quality of life, she became quite animated and was fully engaged in the conversation. The therapist wondered whether Mrs Ellis would enjoy formally working on recording her life story and might benefit from reminiscence work.

Narrative reasoning: The therapist noted that Mrs Ellis had a strong sense of self and, when speaking about these roles, exhibited a strong sense of self-esteem about her past and current contribution to her family life and past community participation.

The areas of priority for goals identified by Mrs Ellis were to:

- maintain her personal care skills
- assist her husband with some light household tasks
- continue to be involved with her family
- continue to engage in the language group
- enable her to be a companion for her husband.

Conditional reasoning: The therapist felt that this had been a valuable visit as it had opened up some possible areas of occupational therapy intervention. It appeared that although there were difficulties with domestic activities outside help in the form of an au pair would help to support Mr Ellis with these. The couple identified that the most important areas for them to enjoy were around pleasurable pursuits. The therapist felt that, given the degenerative nature of the disease, this was a sensible and philosophical way of moving forward once the safety issues were tackled.

ACTION PLAN

- Arrange a visit to introduce the physiotherapist.
- Conduct a baseline assessment for cognitive function using the MMSE (Folstein, Folstein and McHugh, 1975). This would give an indication of any cognitive changes that may affect drug therapy decisions (the therapist had planned to do this last time but had chosen to undertake the Mayers' Lifestyle Questionnaire and thought it had been too much to do this afterwards).
- Conduct an AMPS (Fisher, 2003a) to investigate quality of occupational performance to identify areas that could be modified and enable the couple to do activities together or to enable Mrs Ellis to perform her own personal care independently.
- Speak with Mr Ellis privately about carer stress and possible support available.

During the next week, the occupational therapist took the physiotherapist to visit the couple. He conducted assessments that took the form of gaining a verbal history from the client and her husband about physical functioning, environment, habit and ADL in conjunction with measuring intact balance through two measures – the Berg Balance Scale (Berg *et al.*, 1992) and the Get Up and Go Test (Mathias, Nayak and Isaacs, 1986), which identify people with poor balance, either sedentary or dynamic, who are at risk of falling. The outcome from these assessments indicated that Mrs Ellis had relatively good dynamic balance, but on rising from a seated position she would occasionally feel unsteady. Advice was given on this and some general t'ai chi based exercises were prescribed for the couple so that Mr Ellis could support his wife in performing exercises routinely. It was also suggested that a six-week attendance at a local day hospital for older people with mental health problems would enable monitoring of progress and allow further physiotherapeutic assessment and treatment to be conducted. Mrs Ellis would also be able to join a group exercise class at the day hospital. Mrs Ellis was happy to consider this option. The therapists also felt this short-term intervention would provide Mr Ellis with some much-needed respite.

Prior to the next occupational therapy home visit, there was a telephone call from Mr Ellis requesting some help with night-time wandering. He sounded quite exasperated by the experience of his wife wandering around the house and even trying to leave the house at night. The therapist suggested that he call into the team's office after dropping his wife at the day hospital for her preliminary visit so that they could talk without Mrs Ellis being present and she could give him the time that he needed to discuss his worries without feeling that he had to protect his wife's feelings. In the meantime, the therapist sent out some information about wandering and sleep problems related to dementia and reinforced the availability of the Carer's Resource team and Alzheimer's worker for advice. This was the start of the educative role that the therapist would play, and it was also an indication of the trust that had been built up between carer and therapist. The therapist noted that the skill would be to keep the relationship a positive therapeutic one that supported Mr Ellis but prevented dependence.

During the visit to the day hospital, Mrs Ellis met the rest of the team and participated in some of the activities that occurred; she was particularly good in quizzes and enjoyed the baking, requiring verbal prompts throughout. Mrs Ellis was slightly anxious when her husband left her to speak with the therapist but became distracted by the rest of the group enough to alleviate her separation anxiety. During her visit, the nurse administered the MMSE and agreed to share the results with the therapist. Mr Ellis took the opportunity to speak frankly about the strain he was under through lack of sleep and how sad and frustrated he was feeling about being helpless in respect of being unable to help his wife.

Procedural reasoning: The therapist had a few thoughts about what was going on and what may help. She decided to encourage setting up a Life-story Book about their life together, as it might help to consolidate some of their feelings and celebrate their life together as well as giving the couple a joint activity to perform. It might also involve other family members to support Mr Ellis. Also, it refocused the therapist's role in this person's treatment; as the occupational therapist was aware that while being a generic CMHT member her professional expertise was with occupational performance, role engagement and activity analysis. The need to assess the quality of functional performance by using the AMPS could determine the level of involvement that Mrs Ellis could function at and provide one way of allowing Mrs and Mr Ellis to achieve some level of satisfaction in occupation, as this has been a major theme throughout the couple's life. Mr Ellis was partly grieving at the diminished functional performance that his wife was now subject to after a life of high achievement.

The therapist requested that she conduct the Zarit Caregiver Burden Survey (Zarit, Todd and Zarit, 1986) and undertake this as an interview. She found that, while he wanted to do the best he could to help his wife, Mr Ellis was finding it increasingly tiring. He understood that it was important to maintain her independence and sense of individuality but had concerns over her safety; this was a huge worry to him. The therapist acknowledged his concerns and discussed her thoughts about the Life-story Book and undertaking an AMPS assessment with a view to providing advice on cues and prompts to maximise functional ability. Both suggestions were accepted by Mr Ellis, but the therapist felt that there was a lack of confidence in the suggestions. It was also explained that, once a treatment plan was set up, support could be initially offered to the couple from the therapist but ongoing support from the CMHT would be provided by the health care assistant. The assistant would follow through with some of the treatment plan, for example supporting Mrs Ellis to prepare a drink and snack, so that Mr Ellis did not feel that it was another thing to overwhelm him in caring for his wife.

FOCUSING THE TREATMENT

The next home visit was conducted early in the morning so that options for selecting AMPS tasks for assessment could be broadened. One of the priorities identified by Mrs Ellis had been about personal care activities, and the therapist agreed she would arrive before Mrs Ellis had got dressed. On arriving, the therapist was greeted at the door by an unfamiliar lady, who introduced herself as the new au pair who had been employed by the family to help with domestic tasks and meals. The impact upon Mr Ellis was obvious; he looked much more relaxed as he now felt he could devote himself to spending productive and quality time with his wife. Mrs Ellis was pleased that as a result of her husband having more free time they had initiated a Life-story Book, which had brought back some lovely memories, and the therapist observed lots of photographs scattered on the coffee table.

The therapist explained the process of the AMPS and sought consent from Mrs Ellis to conduct the assessment. Mrs Ellis grasped most of what was being asked of her and agreed to participate; however, the therapist sensed that Mr Ellis still had reservations over assessing his wife undertaking tasks and the possibility of highlighting her inabilities. The therapist explained that she only assessed activities that the person wanted to do and that the assessment looked at the quality of the performance so that the process could be modified to maintain success and indicate possible risk. The therapist was aware of the tentative beginnings and how these had developed into a positive relationship. It was important that a full explanation was given to this couple at every stage of assessment and intervention to ensure fully informed consent and to maintain trust and rapport.

Based upon the priorities identified by Mrs Ellis on the Mayers' Lifestyle Questionnaire, the tasks offered for assessment were limited to those of an average complexity to provide a reasonable challenge to Mrs Ellis. The AMPS tasks identified were upper and lower body dressing and preparing a cold cereal and drink.

INTERPRETING THE RESULTS

The results of the AMPS assessment indicated that in the dressing task Mrs Ellis found difficulty locating appropriate clothing and required some prompts to help her choose her clothing and struggled on occasion with fine-finger dexterity and grip. She was slow in conducting the process of the task and had difficulties with starting the various parts of the task, for example she would stop in between putting on her blouse and then her cardigan, requiring assistance to select the garment. Mrs Ellis asked questions frequently. The preparation of cold cereal and drink indicated difficulties finding items and returning them to their original positions, and she had problems gauging the distance and speed of pouring the liquid. Again, prompts were required to assist Mrs Ellis through the process, but she completed the tasks successfully.

Procedural reasoning: The therapist determined from the results that Mrs Ellis was inefficient in performing tasks graded by the assessment as being of average difficulty; however, when given verbal prompts and only items that she required to complete the tasks, she could succeed. The physical difficulties with her motor control meant that activities required grading so that she could achieve desired levels of performance; for example, the therapist decided she should educate Mr and Mrs Ellis not to fill jugs too full so that she could pour without spilling fluid. The repeated deficits seen across both tasks of being unable to find items and with sequencing problems meant that only items required should be in view so that Mrs Ellis could respond to verbal cues in an uncluttered environment. Mrs Ellis did not compensate for her actions, and there was potential to create a risk situation.

NEGOTIATED GOAL-SETTING

The therapist discussed her findings with the couple and they agreed to the following treatment goals.

- Education for Mr Ellis regarding setting up the environment so Mrs Ellis could perform personal care tasks and simple domestic tasks safely and with minimal verbal prompting. Mr Ellis was to assist by choosing items and tools to be used in a task and setting them up in view for Mrs Ellis to use.
- Mr Ellis would use simple verbal cues to help Mrs Ellis complete the tasks.
- The therapist undertook some environmental modifications required to help Mrs Ellis to perform ADL.

After the assessment, the therapist explored the environmental changes required to assist in Mrs Ellis' independence. These included de-cluttering surfaces and cupboards to cut down inappropriate stimuli, setting out tools required for the task and the modelling of an activity with Mrs Ellis to show Mr Ellis how to reinforce task processes and cut down on the need for prompts.

The therapist also discussed the use of orientation prompts to help address the sleep problems, for example using notices to prompt Mrs Ellis to return to bed, going to bed later in the evening, bladder management to minimise the need to go to the toilet etc.

SUMMARY OF THE ASSESSMENT PROCESS

The therapist had gathered her information to explore the referral from various sources, discussed the proposed visit formally over the telephone with the carer, started initial assessment procedures during the first home visit and worked on developing the therapeutic relationship from initial telephone contact and during home visits. The therapist was aware of the limits of her own expertise and attempted to provide treatment boundaries with the couple by involving appropriate other professionals and focusing her support upon both the client's and the carer's needs.

Although the therapist had a list of assessments she wanted to use and a preferred order of administration, in a complex condition like dementia where contact with the client and family is likely to be long term the assessment process rarely follows a linear route. Instead what often happens is that the assessment pathway can be one of exploring and revisiting options time after time in a client-centred way, even though the therapist's experience may already contain a certain predicted path of treatment options (the prospective story). The client's unique treatment process comes from the priorities set from the initial assessments, and these will change over time as an illness develops or circumstances alter. Sometimes a therapist can feel as if the treatment is on a designated route but then things happen to make the treatment route change; there is a constant reviewing of the situation and a flexible approach needs to be adopted.

In this case, the therapist administered her chosen assessments over a number of visits with Mr and Mrs Ellis, trying to work in a client-centred way to engage in problem-solving and risk assessments. Her assessment process included professional expertise from other team members to gain a holistic view of the individual's perceived and observed difficulties. The selection of assessments provided a combination of observational, self- and proxy reported data. Initially, the focus was upon gaining verbal information through a semi-structured interview with both client and carer. Standardised measures, such as the Mayers' Lifestyle Questionnaire, the Memory and Behaviour Checklist and the Zarit Caregiver Burden Survey, helped to gain specific proxy and self-report data. These helped to identify the client's and carer's perceived priorities and negotiate what they wanted to work upon. The next step was to conduct some observational standardised assessments in the form of the AMPS and the physiotherapy balance scales. This enabled baseline measurements of function and movement to be taken so that treatment could be discussed with the couple together and a joint working approach could be adopted in the planning stage.

This case provides an example of the complexity of assessment and of the various reasoning forms that the therapist undertakes to make sense of the presenting condition and move towards negotiated goals and treatment plans.

WORKSHEET

At the back of this book, you will find templates for a series of worksheets designed to assist you in applying principles of assessment and outcome measurement to your own practice. Please now turn to Worksheet 10 (p. 412). The worksheet takes you through a series of headings to guide you to write a therapy diagnostic statement. Use the worksheet to develop a therapy diagnostic statement for one of your clients. If you are a student, write a therapy diagnostic statement for a client you have worked with on placement. Refer to diagnostic statement examples for Mrs A and Mr B earlier in this chapter (pp. 297–8).

STUDY QUESTIONS

10.1 What is clinical reasoning?
10.2 What type of questions do therapists attempt to answer through pragmatic reasoning?
10.3 What are the four components of diagnostic reasoning?
10.4 How could you document your reflections on your practice?

You will find brief answers to these questions at the back of this book (p. 394).

11

Implementing the Optimum Assessment and Measurement Approach

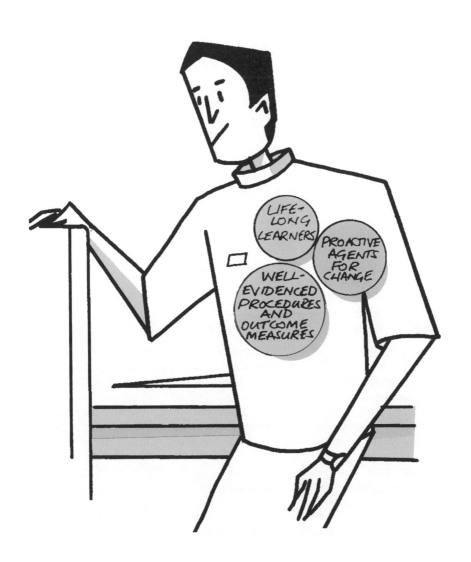

CHAPTER SUMMARY

In this chapter, we shall look at the factors that therapists should consider when choosing an assessment and measurement approach for an individual client, client group or service. The chapter will describe the process for identifying the strengths and limitations of potential published assessments through test critique and provide an example of a detailed test critique. Guidance on how to find details of potential tests for your client population and/or practice setting is included. The chapter finishes with a series of goals for improving your assessment and outcome measurement practice; these are divided into goals, or challenges, to be addressed by five different therapist groups: clinicians, managers, educators, researchers and students. Therapists are encouraged to review the goals in the sections that apply to them and to select some pertinent goals as the basis for identifying their own continuing professional development (CPD) plans. A CPD action plan worksheet is included for this purpose and an example of a completed CPD action plan is given. The chapter will also endeavour to answer the following questions: 'How do I set about identifying appropriate standardised tests for my service?' and 'How do I combine the best available evidence with my clinical experience and my knowledge of my client's preferences in order to implement the optimum assessment and measurement approach?'

IMPROVING ASSESSMENT AND MEASUREMENT PRACTICE: WHERE TO BEGIN?

As we have seen throughout this book, and especially in the chapters on validity (Chapter 6) and reliability (Chapter 7), knowledge of the psychometric properties of a measure is not just the concern of therapist researchers; it is also of immense relevance to any clinician who wishes to use a test to provide a baseline for treatment, a predictive or discriminative measure to guide decision-making or an outcome measure to evaluate the effects of intervention. However, the pressures of everyday practice, which for many therapists include demanding caseloads and waiting lists, can make it challenging for therapists to find the time to take a critical look at their assessment practice and to undertake the necessary work to make informed changes to provide a more efficient, valid and reliable assessment process for their clients. It is a matter of balancing the gold standard of measurement with the pragmatics of real, work-life situations. However, please remember that even if you feel that a few clients have lost out to some degree if you take time out for CPD to work on this area, very many clients should benefit from the resultant improvements in your practice in the future. To make improvements to your current assessment and measurement practice, I suggest you follow a straightforward eight-step process, outlined in Figure 11.1 (below). The rest of this chapter provides guidance related to the different steps in this process.

ANALYSING YOUR CURRENT ASSESSMENT PRACTICE

Therapists, as potential users of published tests, should undertake a similar process to a test developer when choosing the optimum approach for assessing their clients. For example, therapists should explicitly define their conceptualisation of the constructs they plan to measure so that they can compare their definition with the description of the constructs in any test manuals they are critiquing (Polgar, 1998). They also should start with a review of the relevant literature on the assessment/measurement of their client group and the constructs they wish to measure. When selecting an assessment approach for a client or group of clients, we need to consider:

- the level(s) of function to be assessed (see Chapter 9)
- the purpose(s) of the assessment (see Chapter 3)
- the data-collection method(s) (see Chapter 2)
- the use of standardised versus unstandardised tools (see Chapters 5, 6, 7 and 8)
- the level of measurement provided by assessment methods (see Chapter 4).

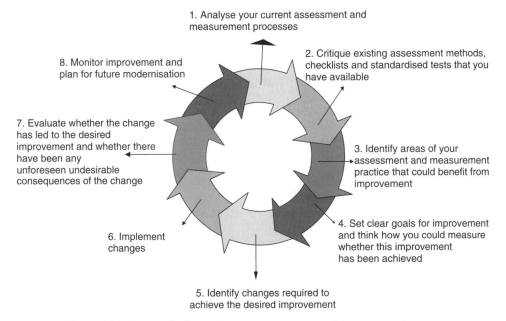

Figure 11.1 Process for improving your assessment and measurement process.

In step 1 (Figure 11.1), you need to analyse your current assessment and measurement process. Start by reflecting on the purpose of your service. If this is not clearly articulated, then a good starting point is to develop a written statement of purpose, called a 'service specification' (see Chapter 3, and especially Table 3.3). Once you are clear about the purpose of your service, review your existing assessment approaches and tests. Categorise what you currently have available (checklists, standardised tests etc.) and the assessment methods you currently use in terms of their purposes, data source, data-collection method, levels of function addressed and levels of measurement provided. Worksheets related to Chapters 2, 3, 4 and 9 will help you to do this. There are a number of simple techniques that you can use to help you structure an analysis of your current assessment process; two frequently used methods are SWOT and mapping, and these are described below.

SWOT

SWOT is an acronym for examining a service's Strengths, Weaknesses, Opportunities and Threats and using the results to identify priorities for action. It enables therapists to look at both internal factors (the strengths and weaknesses of your current assessment practice) and external factors (opportunities and threats that do, or may, affect your assessment process). If you have a mission statement/vision/service specification, use these as they can be helpful as a framework for examining SWOT. The advantages to using SWOT as a starting point for examining your own/your service's current assessment practice are that it:

- is one of the most widely used strategic planning tools in current use across a range of sectors and so is familiar to the majority of staff/stakeholders and not perceived as daunting
- provides a good starting point
- actively engages individuals or groups to share their views.

The disadvantages are that SWOT can often result 'in an over-long list of factors, general and often meaningless descriptions, a failure to prioritise issues and no attempt to verify conclusions . . .

[while] outputs once generated [are] rarely used' (Iles and Sutherland, 2001, p. 41). Therefore, in order to ensure SWOT analyses are useful, you need to pose a second level of questions. In relation to strengths and weaknesses, you should ask the following additional questions.

- What are the causes of this strength or weakness?
- What are the consequences of this?
- Do they help or hinder us in achieving an optimum assessment process for our clients?

In relation to opportunities and threats, you should pose the following additional questions (Iles and Sutherland, 2001).

- What impact is this likely to have on our assessment process?
- Will it help or hinder us in achieving an optimum assessment process for our clients?
- What must we do to respond to this opportunity or threat?

Please refer to Worksheet 11 (p. 413) to assist you with undertaking a SWOT analysis.

MAPPING YOUR CURRENT ASSESSMENT AND MEASUREMENT PROCESS

Mapping is an approach recommended by the NHS Modernisation Agency. A useful resource is their *Improvement Leader's Guide To Process Mapping, Analysis and Redesign* (NHS Modernisation Agency, 2002a). Process mapping is 'one of the most powerful ways for multi-disciplinary teams to understand the real problems in a service from the perspective of people using the service and their family or carers, and to identify opportunities for improvement. This is often described as *mapping the patient journey*' (Dementia Services Collaborative, 2004).

Definition of mapping

'Mapping is the process by which you represent the activities and steps experienced by the patient. This is a diagnostic and analytical process of discovering what actually happens. You can then use this information to find ways to improve how the patient experiences the care you deliver' (Fraser, 2002, p. 4).

There are a number of advantages for mapping your assessment process (Fraser, 2002), which makes it a worthwhile exercise if you wish to improve your assessment and measurement practice.

- It helps you to see the whole picture of the person's journey through your assessment process: what happens now and how do therapists, colleagues, clients and carers feel about the process? You might find that the client does not understand why a particular test is given or might find a test anxiety-provoking. The client might feel that he does not receive sufficient feedback about the results of a test. Therapists might value a test because it has good reliability and validity but not use it regularly because it takes too long to administer and tires the client.
- It identifies where the real problems are (bottlenecks, backlogs etc.). For example, you might discover that you have a long waiting list but find on initial assessment that a significant number of referrals are inappropriate. If so, you might consider a trial process to triage referrals as they are received by your service. You might have only one therapist trained to administer a particular standardised assessment and have bottlenecks occurring while clients wait to receive this assessment.
- It identifies any duplication of effort (e.g. wasted time and resources). For example, the occupational therapists, physiotherapists and speech therapists might be all collecting the same details about the person, their living situation and the history of the presenting

condition. Therapists might decide to seek informed consent from the client to share this information with the team or undertake a joint initial interview.
- It provides a baseline against which changes to your assessment process will be measured in order to evaluate whether any changes lead to a more effective and/or efficient assessment.

Therapists can use a range of methods for gathering information to help them map their clients' assessment/measurement process, for example by:

- looking through records to see what assessment and measurement data are collected, how they are collected and how they have been recorded
- physically following a person's journey (e.g. shadowing a client through an initial assessment process)
- interviewing the client and their carer about their experience of being assessed and measured
- seeing key personnel to get their view (e.g. doctors who receive a summary of the assessment results, such as the client's consultant or GP)
- getting all staff involved in the assessment process engaged in the mapping exercise and making it a team endeavour by having a stakeholder timeout to map the assessment process together, ideally involving clients and carers at this event.

There are several factors that can affect the success of your mapping exercise (Fraser, 2002) and are worth considering in advance.

- You need to engage all the people who are involved in the assessment pathway as participants in the mapping process (this includes client and carer representatives).
- It can be useful to include people who are not in your service/department but are still involved in the client process (e.g. GPs or consultants who refer clients to your service for assessment and to whom you send assessment reports).
- You need to seek agreement in advance from all stakeholders to provide required information. If you are just mapping your own assessment process, this will not be a problem but if you are part of a multidisciplinary team or provide assessment into a service, such as a memory assessment clinic for people with dementia, then looking at how your assessment fits into the whole process for the client will require liaison with other professionals.
- Define a clear start and end point for the process you are mapping and agree the level of detail from the outset (e.g. your starting point might be when the referral is received by the therapist and the end point might be when a final report detailing outcome measurement is sent to the referral source when the person is discharged from the therapy service).

Ideally, an analysis of therapy assessment should not be undertaken in isolation. Many therapists work as members of a team, and even where a therapist works in a discrete therapy service this service is likely to be one component of a client's clinical pathway. It is helpful to engage other team members or stakeholders in the analysis of assessment processes (also see Table 11.1 below re levels of engagement). Finally, mapping is a good method for fostering collaboration.

Welch (2002) provides a description of how process mapping was applied to occupational therapy activity within a medical admissions unit. She reports that process mapping proved to be a valuable approach and 'enabled the occupational therapy service to evaluate systematically the service being provided and to visualise the optimum pathway of care' (p. 158).

If you wish to map your assessment process, a useful resource to help you plan your mapping exercise is Fraser (2002). This book is a good introductory guide and covers how to get started, the process of mapping, analysing your results, taking action following a mapping exercise and how to facilitate a mapping exercise.

Having mapped the client's assessment journey, the therapist must then begin to analyse it, for example highlighting bottlenecks or areas of duplication. Within the Dementia Services Collaborative (DSC) model, once DSC teams have used mapping to identify areas for improvement within their journey they then use a PDSA cycle approach (see below) to test out change ideas on a small scale to see if they will bring about the required improvement.

IMPROVING YOUR ASSESSMENT PROCESS

Once you have identified the limitations in your current practice, you are ready to identify the changes required and to plan for making improvements to your assessment and measurement process. A number of service improvement models are in use across health and social care services and are helpful. The NHS Modernisation Agency recommends a model for service improvement (2002a) that draws upon the work of Langley *et al.* (1996). This model begins with three questions (NHS Modernisation Agency, 2002a, p. 10).

1. *What are we trying to accomplish?*
   Step 4 in Figure 11.1 requires the setting of improvement goals. You, your multidisciplinary team or your therapy service need to start with clear and focused goals for improving your assessment/measurement process. For example, a goal might be:

   All clients will be assessed twice using a standardised, valid, reliable and responsive outcome measure, first when they enter our service to provide a baseline and again on discharge to provide an evaluation of the effectiveness of our intervention.

2. *How will we know that a change is an improvement?*
   Step 7 in Figure 11.1 involves evaluating whether your changes have led to improved practice. This is a really important question because not all changes lead to enhanced service and some changes, which do provide the desired improvement, can have unexpected consequences. For example, your assessment process might be much more rigorous and meet your original improvement goal, but it also turns out to take much longer to administer leading to a slower throughput of clients through your service and increased waiting lists. As an example, you might measure your improvement goal through analysing whether:

   A standardised, valid, reliable and responsive measure is identified and applied across the service. Client records show evidence of baseline data on referral and outcome data at discharge. There is no increase in waiting list numbers or waiting times for our service.

3. *What changes can we make that result in improvement?*
   This question relates to step 5 in Figure 11.1, as it prompts the beginning of a planning cycle for change. You might already have a suitable standardised test(s) identified or a change in the current assessment process in mind. However, you might be starting from scratch and need to undertake a literature or Web-based search as a starting point.

THE PDSA CYCLE APPROACH

The PDSA cycle approach to service improvement has been recommended by the NHS Modernisation Agency (2002a) and widely used by clinical staff engaged in a range of clinical collaboratives, such as the DSC. The DSC (2004) states:

> Making improvements in services involves changing things, however, change can sometimes seem overwhelming or threatening for busy people doing demanding work. The PDSA method is a way of breaking down change into manageable chunks, testing each small part to make sure that things 'are' improving and no effort is wasted. The change ideas that a team wishes to try out may be based on research, feedback, theory, review, audit or simply practical ideas that have been proven to work elsewhere.

The PDSA process will help you with steps 5, 6, 7 and 8 of the Improvement Process (Figure 11.1). There are four simple steps to follow in a PDSA cycle process. These are:

1. P = plan: At this stage, therapists identify what change they think will result in an improvement to their assessment process and then they plan how they will test out that change. This stage involves thinking about the who, what, where and when of the improvement. Deciding how to measure the improvement is critical.
2. D = do: At this stage, therapists carry out their plan for improvement. This could be altering part of the assessment process or trying out a new standardised outcome measure. At this stage, therapists need to record any unexpected events, problems and make any useful observations. Towards the end of this stage, therapists should start analysing any data. This could involve auditing client records to see how many clients have been given the newly adopted measure or have been assessed following the new process, reviewing data on how many therapists have undertaken a particular training course, counting how many different clients each therapist has assessed using the new test or analysing the qualitative feedback (e.g. questionnaires) that the therapists have completed about clinical utility factors.
3. S = study: At this stage, therapists complete the analysis of all data they have collected to evaluate whether the change has been fully implemented and whether it has resulted in the desired improvement. Therapists reflect on whether there has been a significant improvement, whether their expectations matched the reality of what actually happened when implementing the planned change and whether, with hindsight, they would do anything differently.
4. A = act: At the final stage of the PDSA process, therapists agree what did and did not work. They consider what further changes or amendments are required to ensure the improvement is fully implemented and sustained. If appropriate, they plan the next PDSA cycle.

Modernising your whole assessment process, including both informal and standardised assessment data collection and assessment undertaken with all sources (client self-report, carer proxy, colleague proxy and observational data-collection methods), can be a big undertaking. To make it more achievable, I recommend breaking your assessment/measurement improvement project into small goals and undertaking a small PDSA cycle for each goal. This should mean that you divide your improvement project into bite-size chunks that feel more manageable and lead to faster results so you can celebrate the achievement of completed goals more quickly. For example, you might:

- begin with a PDSA cycle that focuses on the quality of referral information received by your service, review how this information is used (e.g. decisions made from referral data for prioritising referrals onto a waiting list), evaluate whether data collected are adequate for this purpose and implement the use of a referral form, which provides a uniform and adequate initial assessment at referral
- (with a second PDSA cycle) focus on client self-report assessment, and particularly on interview data gathered to provide a baseline
- (with further PDSA cycles) focus on outcome measurement.

RAID

RAID is another improvement model that has been used by the NHS Modernisation Agency (2002a), for example by their Clinical Governance Support Team. It stands for:

- R = review: therapists need to look at their current assessment process and measurement techniques and prepare their service for change (step 1 of Figure 11.1)

- A = agree: therapists need to ensure all stakeholders (e.g. clinicians, managers, other members of a multidisciplinary team, secretarial staff) are signed up to the proposed changes in the assessment process and/or measures used (an aspect of step 5 of Figure 11.1)
- I = implement: therapists then put in place the proposed changes, e.g. they purchase a standardised test, attend the related training course and implement it with clients (step 6 of Figure 11.1)
- D = demonstrate: at this stage, the therapists need to show that the changes made have led to improvements, e.g. they now have individual client and group data that show a standardised measure is being used and that enables the service to review whether interventions have had the desired/anticipated outcome, both on an individual client and service-population basis (step 7 of Figure 11.1).

The step of agreement is essential if any change is to be adopted wholeheartedly by stakeholders and is to lead to a sustainable change. There are different levels of agreement, and Senge (1990, cited by Iles and Sutherland, 2001) differentiates between commitment, enrolment and compliance. It is preferable to have considerable commitment for change from all stakeholders (also referred to as 'players' by Senge) but it is not always 'necessary for everyone to be as fully signed up as this' (Iles and Sutherland, 2001, p. 47). The different levels of agreement or resistance to change are defined in Table 11.1. It is useful to rate each of your stakeholders against these criteria if you can so that you are aware of the levels of support and resistance you might experience from colleagues when implementing your planned change.

Table 11.1 Commitment, enrolment and compliance. *Table 3: Commitment, enrolment and compliance (p. 47) in Iles V, Sutherland K (2001) Managing Change in the NHS. Organisational Change: A Review for Healthcare Managers, Professionals and Researchers. London, National Co-ordinating Centre for NHS Service Delivery and Organisation R & D (NCC SDO). Copied with kind permission from Valerie Iles and Kim Sutherland, with agreement from the SDO Programme. Based upon the work of P Senge (1990) The Fifth Discipline: The Art and Practice of the Learning Organization. London, Doubleday/Century Business*

Disposition	Stakeholders'/players' response to change
Commitment	Want change to happen and will work to make it happen. Willing to create whatever structures, systems and frameworks are necessary for it to work.
Enrolment	Want change to happen and will devote time and energy to making it happen within given frameworks. Act within the spirit of the frameworks.
Genuine compliance	See the virtue in what is proposed, do what is asked of them and think proactively about what is needed. Act within the letter of the frameworks.
Formal compliance	Can describe the benefits of what is proposed and are not hostile to them. They do what they are asked but no more. Stick to the letter of the framework.
Grudging compliance	Do not accept that there are benefits to what is proposed and do not go along with it. They do enough of what is asked of them not to jeopardise position. Interpret the letter of the framework.
Non-compliance	Do not accept that there are benefits and have nothing to lose by opposing the proposition. Will not do what is asked of them. Work outside framework.
Apathy	Neither in support of nor in opposition to the proposal, just serving time. Don't care about the framework.

SELECTING TESTS

The decision to use a particular assessment strategy or test should be conscious and the result of informed evidence-based reasoning. Nowadays, there is a wide choice of tests from which an individual therapist or occupational therapy/physiotherapy service can choose. It is critical that therapists select the most appropriate tests for their clients. Also, financial considerations often place limits upon the number of tests that can be purchased for a service. Therefore, careful consideration needs to be given before purchasing a test. Selecting a suitable measure from the vast and ever-growing body of literature 'requires objective criteria to make an informed choice' (Jeffrey, 1993, p. 394). Many clinicians find this a daunting task and do not know where to start when trying to find the right measure to evaluate the effectiveness of their services. The Chartered Society of Physiotherapy (CSP; 2001a) describes some of the problems that face clinicians looking for a measure. These can include:

- finding journal articles describing outcome measures and their application; this can be difficult because a proportion of articles of relevance do not mention the specific outcome measure in the title, summary or key words, which results in the article not being identified by a key word, database literature search
- (once you have identified journal articles on the right subject) the research reported being of varying quality: just because it is published does not mean the research was without flaws and so therapists need to develop critical appraisal skills and become informed consumers of research literature
- a scarcity of information on the psychometric properties of measures, studies involving small samples or different studies reporting quite conflicting results
- copyright restrictions on measures; these vary dramatically between tests: some measures are published in journal articles and are free and easily accessed, others can be obtained from the authors and used with their permission for free and yet a significant number of measures can only be obtained by purchasing the manual, forms and any standardised test equipment and might also require paying for training on the measure.

The national clinical guidelines for stroke, which were developed by the Intercollegiate Working Party for Stroke (Royal College of Physicians, 2002) provide some sensible advice on implementing changes to assessment. They state that:

> Local clinicians should:
>
> 1. agree which assessments are going to be used locally, in order to improve communication;
> 2. agree how frequently formal reassessment is going to occur;
> 3. not spend too much time and effort discussing and researching individual assessments (this can take years). It is important to allow some choice if there are strong views or equally good measures available. (section 4.1)

This section discusses ways of identifying potential tests and describes the process for undertaking a test critique with a detailed critique of the Parenting Stress Index (PSI; Abidin, 1995) given as an example. Test critique will assist therapists with steps 1 and 5 described in Figure 11.1. In step 1, you need to critique any published/standardised tests that you already have access to in your clinical setting. In step 5, you need to identify and critique potential new standardised tests to meet identified gaps and limitations in your current practice.

There are a number of avenues you can explore to identify potential measures for your service. These include:

- tapping the expertise of colleagues
- going to your local health care library and looking in the journals and books they have available

- searching the Internet as it has many useful sites on specific published measures and the assessments of different conditions and you can access online databases to search for information about measures, e.g. the CSP has a good outcome measures searchable database on its website (http://www.csp.org.uk); occupational therapy and physiotherapy organisations, the Department of Health and the World Health Organization websites are all good starting points
- undertaking a literature search (journal articles and reviews, textbooks, test manuals) on one or more of the health databases and requesting interlibrary loans for identified articles/books/book chapters) if they are not in journals available locally. Useful databases include:
  - CINAHL (Cumulative Index to Nursing and Allied Health Literature) is a database for nursing and allied health literature and can be found at http://www.cinahl.com; you may be able to access this through a hospital or university library or your service could explore getting a CD-ROM subscription or signing up for the CINAHL*direct*® online service.
  - PubMed is a database at the National Library of Medicine site found at http://www. ncbi.nlm.nih.gov/entrez/query.fcgi.
  - Medline Plus at http://medlineplus.gov/ is a useful health information site aimed at clients.
  - The contents of Wilma L. West Library are indexed in OTsearch, an online bibliographic database with over 27,000 records covering the literature of occupational therapy and its related subject areas. OTsearch is a fee-based subscription service. You may subscribe to OTsearch either as an individual or as an institution. Access it via the American Occupational Therapy Foundation website (http://www.aotf.org/) and follow the links to 'Institute for the Study of Occupation and Health', then to the 'Wilma West Library' and then to 'OTsearch'.
- attending conferences, study days, workshops and lectures related to assessment and measurement; if you cannot get the funding to attend, try to access the conference abstracts, or some conference/workshop providers sell the proceedings
- looking in catalogues produced by test publishers or visiting their stands if there is an exhibition at a conference or study day.

The cheapest and easiest way to begin your search is by talking to other therapists who are working with a similar client group or are already using the test you are interested in, or who are leading conference presentations and workshops on aspects of assessment. The CSP (2001a) recommends drawing upon the knowledge of colleagues and suggests that you:

- 'Ask around the practice or department.
- Speak to colleagues, especially including other professions.
- Ask a question on an internet discussion group' (p. 3).

Professional organisations often operate specialist sections, special interest groups (SIGs) and listservs, which are groups or networks of therapists meeting up or communicating via email to discuss like-minded subjects or clinical areas. For example, the College of Occupational Therapists (COT) recognises the following specialist sections.

- AOTMH: Association of Occupational Therapists in Mental Health
- COTSSIH: College of Occupational Therapists Specialist Section in Housing
- HOPE: Occupational Therapy in HIV/AIDS, Oncology, Palliative Care and Education
- NANOT: National Association of Neurological Occupational Therapists
- NAPOT: National Association of Paediatric Occupational Therapists
- NAROT: National Association of Rheumatology Occupational Therapists

- OTIP: Occupational Therapists in Independent Practice
- OTOP: Occupational Therapy for Older People
- OTPLD: Occupational Therapists working with People with Learning Disabilities
- OTTO: Occupational Therapy in Trauma and Orthopaedics
- OTWPP: Occupational Therapists in Work Practice and Productivity
- RISSOT: Rapid Intervention Specialist Section for Occupational Therapists

Links to each of these specialist sections can be followed from the COT website at: http://www. cot.co.uk/specialist/intro.php.

The CSP website also contains links to numerous groups and networks (go to http://www. csp.org.uk/), such as musculoskeletal groups, occupational groups, neurology groups, client groups, complementary therapy groups and specific interest groups. There is 'Interactive CSP', an online discussion forum for CSP members providing access to news, events, discussions and exchanges, documents and useful Web links. The American Physical Therapy Association (APTA) lists and provides links to a number of specialist sections (http://www.apta.org and follow links to 'Communities'), including:

- acute care
- aquatic physical therapy
- cardiovascular and pulmonary
- education
- geriatrics
- hand rehabilitation
- neurology
- oncology
- orthopaedic
- paediatrics
- private practice
- sports physical therapy.

EXPLORING THE LITERATURE FOR EXAMPLES OF TESTS AND TEST CRITIQUES

If you are new to conducting a literature search, seek advice from your librarian or from a colleague who is familiar with searching the literature, perhaps because they have undertaken a university module or degree or have been engaged in research. The CSP (2002b) provides a basic starting point for therapists, which can be downloaded from its website. The CSP (2001a) also has useful guidance on outcome measures, which can be downloaded from its website. The guidance covers subjects such as how to begin looking for a measure, details about the CSP outcome measures database and sections on how to choose a measure to use in your clinical practice, assessing the quality of a measure and how to know whether a measure is any good. The World Confederation for Physical Therapy (WCPT; 2002) has also published a useful article about how to tell whether an article is worth reading. This can be downloaded from its website at http://www.wcpt.org.

Some critiques already exist in the form of published reviews in books and journal articles. While writing this book, I have come across the following examples of useful test critiques and reviews.

EXAMPLE REVIEWS AND CRITIQUES IN BOOKS

- Asher (1996) provides an annotated index of many standardised and published occupational therapy assessments.

- Borg and Bruce (1991) in their chapter entitled 'Assessing psychological perform-ance factors' provide a useful table summarising assessment approaches and exam-ples that can be used for assessing psychological performance factors. They use the following table headings: category of test (e.g. self-report, observational scales, self-monitoring, projective tests and interview), typical format, perspective emphasised, characteristics and specific examples of published measures with full references.
- Cole *et al.*'s (1995) excellent book provides detailed test critiques for 60 measures, which are grouped under four domains: adult motor and functional activity measures, back and/or pain measures, cardiopulmonary measures and developmental measures.
- For therapists working with people suffering with back pain, the Chartered Society of Physiotherapy (2004) provides a useful resource that can be downloaded as a PDF file from the CSP website.
- For therapists working with people suffering from depression, the Chartered Society of Physiotherapy (2002a) provides a useful resource that can be downloaded as a PDF file from the CSP website. This document provides a list of outcome measures for physio-therapists to consider using to evaluate interventions aimed at improving levels of physi-cal activity, improving mood, reducing negative feelings of depression and anxiety, im-proving self-esteem and to measure health-related aspects of quality of life. Twenty-two measures are identified and a critique is provided for a recommended measure related to each of these aims of intervention. The critiques are divided into five areas: aims and content of the measure, user-centredness, properties, feasibility and utility.
- For therapists working with people with chronic fatigue syndrome (CFS) Cox (2000), in Chapter 10 of her book, critiques a number of measures used to assess people with CFS, including the SF-36, Health Fatigue Questionnaire, Profile of Fatigue Related Symptoms, Social Adjustment Questionnaire, Illness Management Questionnaire and Hospital Anxiety and Depression Scale.
- McDowell and Newell (1987) provide critiques of numerous assessments that they have grouped together based on content and explored in chapters on functional disability and handicap, psychological well-being, social health, quality of life and life satisfaction, pain measurements and general health measurements.
- Smith (1993, pp. 173–181, Table 7.1) provides brief summaries of tests for occupational therapists using the following headings: name, type, description, features and source and groups. Tests are reviewed depending on the client group or construct to be measured: manual dexterity and motor function tests, developmental tests, sensory integration tests, sensory integration and praxis tests, intelligence tests, psychological tests, stress tools and tests for young children and their families.
- Lewis and Bottomley (1994) provide two useful chapters in their text on geriatric physical therapy: Chapter 6 describes assessment instruments and Chapter 10 details patient evaluation.

EXAMPLE REVIEWS AND CRITIQUES IN JOURNAL ARTICLES

There are lots of good overview articles exploring research on different tests and test critiques in the therapy literature; a few good examples are:

- a review of outcome measures for a service provided by Jeffrey (1993), who was seeking to select appropriate measures for the West Lothian NHS Trust occupational therapy service, which included occupational therapy for adults and older adults who were physically ill, injured or disabled and/or had mental health problems.
- Carswell *et al.* (2004), who provide a very thorough review of research and clinical literature related to the Canadian Occupational Performance Measure (COPM); their

literature search identified 88 papers that were reviewed, 86 per cent of which examined the COPM in relation to its psychometric properties (19 papers), research outcomes (33 papers) or practice (33 papers). If you were thinking of using the COPM in your practice, this paper would be a very good place to start.

* Sturgess, Rodger and Ozanne (2002), who provide a detailed review of the use of self-report assessment with young children and present summaries of 12 self-report measures which have been used with child populations.

Another good place to search for possible measures is in test publishers' catalogues. The disadvantage of this is that there will almost certainly be some sort of charge for the measures listed. However, if you have some budget available to purchase standardised tests for your service, there are some worthwhile measures available. Test publishers often provide a global statement of the focus of their assessments. Jeffrey (1993) groups these into three main categories.

1. disorder-specific clinical or functional outcome measures
2. functional outcome measures suitable for people with a variety of disorders/diagnoses
3. comprehensive functional measures

Some catalogues specifically deal with tests suitable for occupational therapists and/or physiotherapists. Helpful catalogues also group tests according to age range (paediatric, adult, older adult etc.) and/or conditions (mental health, autistic spectrum disorders etc.) and/or domains (motor, cognitive, sensory, perceptual, behavioural, work placement etc.). You will usually find a brief overview of the test (100–200 words) and some summary information. For example, the Thames Valley Test Company (TVTC) 2004 catalogue provides summary information under the following headings: overview, authors, date published, age range, norms, administration, qualification, other languages, components, price and ISBN number. This helps you identify whether you and/or your staff will be qualified to administer the test, whether it may be designed for your client group, how long it should take to administer, whether it comes with standardised equipment and how much it will cost. The information about qualifications is particularly important as you do not want to waste time purchasing a test that you or your staff are not competent to use, and you will need to budget in advance for any additional training costs.

Most catalogues will contain a statement about the general and/or specific qualifications required for test administration, for example:

> Only those meeting the TVTC competency qualification guidelines detailed below should use [the] test. The test administrator must, as part of their academic or professional training, have successfully completed a course in test interpretation, psychometrics and measurement theory, educational statistics or a closely related field or hold certification from a suitable professional body providing training in ethical and competent use of psychological assessments. (Thames Valley Test Company, 2004, p. 35)

Many publishers list the professions qualified to use the test in their summaries; for example, the TVTC catalogue lists the qualifications of 'medical doctor, occupational therapist, physiotherapist' for practitioners wanting to use the Rivermead Assessment of Somatosensory Performance (RASP; Winward, Halligan and Wade, 2000). Some test publishers require purchasers to register with them before they can buy test materials and allocate a qualification code for different professional groups. For example, I had to register with the Psychological Corporation/Harcourt Education Ltd and was given a registration number and a qualification code. When looking for potential tests in their catalogue, I check for the qualification code first. If a test sounds relevant but has a different code, then I contact the publisher and clarify the qualification requirements and opportunities for specific training that would enable me/my staff to use the test. A few publishers/test developers insist therapists attend an approved training course before they can use their test; for example, Harrison Associates now organises training courses for the Assessment of Motor Process Skills and therapists have to purchase the five-day training course and the test manual and materials as a package.

Catalogue summaries can be a useful starting point, but as tests are often expensive it is usually worth looking at the test materials before you commit to purchasing them. You can either borrow a test from another service you know is using it or request a review copy from the publisher or ask if you can order the test on a sale-or-return basis. Some publishers will provide talks and demonstrations by representatives coming out to your service, as well as providing sample test materials on loan for a trial basis. Other publishers run training events on a specific test or groups of tests; for example, when the Structured Observational Test of Function (SOTOF; Laver and Powell, 1995) was published, I ran workshops for therapists to give them an overview of the content, development and administration of the SOTOF; some of these workshops were organised by the test publisher, NFER Nelson, some by the COT and others were commissioned directly by therapy services.

TEST CRITIQUE

Therapists are likely to experience some challenges in finding a perfect battery of standardised measures for their client group. The robustness of the psychometric properties of a test (such as its validity, reliability and responsiveness to change) need to be carefully weighed against the pragmatics of your clinical environment and reviewed in terms of face validity and clinical utility factors. This balancing of the scientific versus the practical factors is best undertaken through a formal process known as *test critique*. A number of structured checklists are provided by therapy authors for undertaking test critiques. For example, occupational therapists could refer to Law (2001). Law uses the headings: focus, clinical utility, scale construction, standardisation, reliability, validity, overall utility and materials used. Detailed descriptions are provided for rating each of these areas. Occupational therapists could also refer to the article by Jerosh-Herold (2005).

Physiotherapists could access the CSP website, which contains a searchable database of critiqued outcome measures of relevance to physiotherapists (Chartered Society of Physiotherapy, 2005). In these reviews, the following test critique headings have been used.

- summary of the test
- time to do (in minutes)
- training
- equipment
- cost
- distribution
- patient population
- locale
- reference
- development
- reliability
- responsiveness
- validity
- miscellaneous
- descriptors
- related website

As can be seen from this list, the first parts of the critique relate to areas of clinical usefulness.

- Will this test be of relevance to my patient population and the areas/locale in which I work?
- Can it be administered in the time I have available for this type of assessment?
- Will it be too expensive for my service to purchase and will I have to undergo additional training to use it?

The second part of the critique addresses the more scientific aspects of the critique and presents a summary and analysis of the test's psychometric properties.

When reviewing a potential test, I strongly advise you make a written summary of your review in the form of a test critique. This may seem time-consuming but can be useful for a number of reasons.

1. It helps you to review the test in a systematic manner and look for all the salient information that you need to make an informed decision as to whether this test will be useful in your practice/service.
2. It will help you to reflect on the evidence upon which the test is based and articulate your rationale for selecting or rejecting the test.
3. If you work in a multidisciplinary team, you may need to sell the usefulness of this measure to your colleagues, and providing a written summary of the test can strengthen your case for implementation.
4. A copy of the test critique can be placed in your CPD file as evidence of new learning: both learning about a new assessment and also, if this is your first test critique, as evidence for developing the skill of critiquing tests.
5. As tests are expensive, you may need to make a case to the budget holder for funding a purchase. If you need more than one copy of a test or there is expensive training involved, you may need to make a detailed business case.
6. If you leave the service, a copy of you critique can be kept in your service's records so that any future therapists can see the evidence for the measures they are inheriting.

A comprehensive test critique should involve the examination of many factors, including:

- the purpose of the test and ways in which it can be used
- data-collection method (such as observation, interview, questionnaire)
- perspective gained (self-report, proxy report or therapist viewpoint)
- test environments
- content, which includes the domains covered and levels of function addressed
- scoring method and levels of measurement used
- standardisation
- criteria used in a criterion-referenced measure or description of norms if a normative test
- psychometric properties (reliability and validity data)
- clinical utility and feasibility
- face validity
- qualifications needed for administration and training issues
- cost and accessibility.

If you cannot find a useful critique of the test you are interested in already undertaken by another therapist or published in the literature, then the following series of questions, provided in Box 11.1, will guide you in this process.

Box 11.1 Questions for undertaking a test critique (Chartered Society of Physiotherapy, 2002a; Greenhalgh *et al.*, 1998)

1. What is the stated purpose of the test?
2. Is there information about why and how the measure was developed?
3. For what population has the test been designed?
4. What levels of function does the test address?
5. In what environments can the test be administered?
6. Is the test standardised?
7. Is it a norm-referenced or a criterion-referenced test?
8. If norm-referenced, is the normative sample representative of the clients with whom you will use the test?
9. What scoring system is used and what level of measurement is provided by this scoring system? Are the scores easy to analyse and interpret?
10. Does the test have acceptable levels of reliability? What evidence is there about its reliability with your client population?
11. Has validity been established? What evidence is there about its validity with your client population?
12. Is there information about how responsive it is to meaningful clinical change?
13. Does the test have good face validity? How acceptable is it for you and your clients?
14. Does the test have good clinical utility and how feasible is it for use in clinical practice (e.g. time required for administration and scoring, cost of test manual, materials and forms, ease of administration and scoring)?
15. What qualifications are needed by the test administrator and is additional training required to administer the test?
16. How do you obtain a copy?

Once the critique has been undertaken, summarise your findings into a list of strengths and weaknesses in order to facilitate a comparison of possible options and to help you decide upon your final choice of what test to use for your service or specific client. Please refer to Worksheet 12 (pp. 414–7). I have undertaken a detailed critique as an example; this is shown in Table 11.2, and the process for undertaking this critique is described below. A good example of a test critique is provided by Brown, Rodger and Davis (2003) in their article providing an overview and critique of the Motor-Free Visual Perception Test – Revised.

AN EXAMPLE TEST CRITIQUE: THE PARENTING STRESS INDEX

My process for undertaking this test critique: I picked up a copy of the Psychological Corporation/Harcourt Assessment Company *Occupational Therapy and Physiotherapy 2004 Catalogue* from their exhibition stand at the COT's annual conference and asked their representative if they provided review copies of any of their tests. The company did have a system of roving tests that are loaned out for short periods for review purposes. I identified a number of potentially useful tests in the catalogue and emailed the company (their website is at http://www.tpc-international.com), who then requested I telephoned to discuss which tests I wanted to borrow and why. Within a few days the roving copies of test manuals, forms and equipment arrived. One of the tests Harcourt provided for me to review was the Parenting Stress Index (PSI; Abidin, 1995). I had ensured that within our service for older people with mental health problems we were assessing carer burden and stress and I had used care burden measures in several research projects. I was interested to review a stress index for another group of carers and to see how the PSI compared with the measures I already knew, such as the Strain Scale (Gilleard, 1984) and the Zarit Caregiver Burden Survey (Zarit, Reever and Bach-Peterson, 1980). The catalogue provided the following information on the PSI.

- Overview: Recognise stressful areas in parent–child interactions.
- Age range: adult.
- Qualification code: CL2.
- Administration: individual, 20–30 minutes; short form 10 minutes.

The publisher's brief description of the PSI was:

> Identify stressful areas in parent–child interactions with this updated screening and diagnostic instrument. The PSI was developed on the basis that the total stress a parent experiences is a function of certain salient child characteristics, parent characteristics and situations directly related to the role of being a parent. The PSI Short Form is a direct derivative of the 101-item full-length test and consists of a 36-item self-scoring questionnaire/profile. It yields a Total Stress score from three scales. (Psychological Corporation/Harcourt Assessment, 2004, p. 61)

I started by reading through the manual, item booklet and answer sheet and making notes on my test critique form (see Worksheet 12, pp. 414–7). I then like to try out tests myself if at all possible, by completing myself or role-playing test administration with a colleague, family member or friend. As I am a parent with two small children, this test was relevant to me; so I did it myself and answered the items in relation to my youngest child (then aged 14 months). In the manual, it had some normative data for fathers and the manual stated that 'the data from this sample would suggest that fathers earn lower stress scores on many PSI scales when compared to mothers' (Abidin, 1995, p. 25). In my clinical practice and research, I have found it useful to use assessments that can be scored by different people involved with my client: the older person and their spouse, the child and their parent, the parent and the child's teacher or in this case both parents. So I arm-twisted (gently!) my husband into completing the PSI too. This gave me two sets of data to try to score and interpret (mother's and father's scores for a child), some clinical utility and face validity information from doing it myself and a face validity perspective from a father. Based on the information in the manual and trying the test out informally at home, I decided it seemed a useful test. So I approached a mother with a two-year-old child with gross- and fine-motor skill developmental delay, hemi-hypertrophy and hearing problems. I explained that I was reviewing this test as an example for this book and asked her if she would be prepared to do the PSI and complete a face validity survey for me. This gave me a third set of data to score and some face validity feedback from a parent whose child was currently receiving occupational therapy and physiotherapy.

Few standardised measures available to therapists are completely ideal, and you are likely to identify limitations as well as strengths when conducting your own test critiques. Even if you do not find a perfect test, Stokes and O'Neill (1999) advise that 'it may be appropriate to employ an incompletely assessed tool as an alternative to a non-standardised assessment. This may lead to uniformity in the utilisation of scales within departments which in turn will aid in the full evaluation of scales through multi-centre research activities and stem the multitude of "in-house" scales' (p. 562). So if you find a standardised assessment that covers the assessment domains of interest and has some reasonable psychometric data, albeit with small sample sizes, then it is worth trying this measure. Even better would be to contribute to its ongoing development, perhaps by writing a letter to your professional journal outlining your experience using the test or approaching the test developer or publisher to give your ideas on what further studies would be helpful in your field.

Table 11.2 Test critique example: critique of the Parenting Stress Index

Critique area	Comments
Name of test, authors and date of publication	Parenting Stress Index (PSI). Reference: Abidin, RR (1995) Parenting Stress Index (3rd edn.) Professional Manual. Odessa, FL, Psychological Assessment Resources, Inc.
Publisher: Where to obtain test. Cost (if any)	UK distributor Harcourt Assessment, 2004 Catalogue (includes manual, 10 reusable item booklets, 25 hand-scored answer/ profile forms). (*Note*: I reviewed the full test version.) Short-form kit includes manual and 25 hand-scored answer/profile forms.
Population: For what population has the test been designed?	Adults: parents of children aged one month to 12 years. References are provided for research using the PSI with a wide range of child populations, including birth defects (e.g. spina bifida, congenital heart disease), communication disorders (e.g. hearing impairment, speech deficits), attention deficit hyperactivity disorder (ADHD), autism, developmental disability, learning disabled, premature infants, at risk/abused children and other health problems (e.g. asthma, diabetes, otitis media). Originally developed in the US with norms mainly based on a white American population, the PSI has since been used in a number of cross-cultural studies and has been translated into Spanish, Chinese, Portuguese, Finnish, Japanese, Italian, Hebrew, Dutch and French.
Purpose(s) of test: Stated purpose and uses	The manual states that the 'PSI was designed to be an instrument in which the primary value would be to identify parent-child systems that were under stress and at risk for the development of dysfunctional parenting behaviour or behaviour problems in the child involved' (Abidin, 1995, p. 6). Uses: the author describes the PSI as a screening and diagnostic tool, so the primary purpose is to provide descriptive information. Predictive validity studies (see below) allow for some predictive assessment uses. Several studies are summarised in the manual that have found the PSI to discriminate between different groups of children and of parents. Some of the test–retest reliability data show acceptable levels thus allowing for the full PSI to be used as an outcome measure for evaluative purposes, but coefficients varied considerably across four studies and careful attention should be paid to the length of the period between baseline testing and the follow-up evaluative test. However, the short-form (PSI/ SF) can be used as an evaluative measure with more confidence.
Data-collection method(s) used	Self-report tool. The parent is given a seven-page reusable item booklet containing a front sheet with scoring instructions and 120 questions. The parent circles his/her answer for each of the 101 PSI items and for the 19-item Life Stresses scale if required. The therapist then tears off the perforated edge and opens up the form. Inside, answers are transformed to numerical scores, which are summed and then plotted on the profile.
Level(s) of function addressed by test	Reflecting on the NCMRR model of levels of function/dysfunction, I think that most of the subscales address the societal limitation level because they address interactions between humans in their environment through exploration of the child–parent system, the parent–spouse system and the parent–social environment context. The test looks at domains such as role restriction and isolation, which clearly fall within the level of societal limitation. The PSI has two subscales that provide data at the impairment level: the Child Domain of Mood and the Parent Domain of Depression. The Parent subscale of Health covers the concept of health in a very broad way and might capture health problems at several levels, including the pathophysiological level.

(*continued*)

Table 11.2 *(Continued)*

Critique area	Comments
Testing environments where test can be used:	The PSI can be used as a clinical and/or research tool. References provided for research where the PSI has been applied in a range of settings, including well-child clinics/well-child-care paediatrics clinics, private paediatric group parenting clinic for consultation on child behaviour, early parenting groups for mothers abusing drugs and/or alcohol, preschool training project, parenting skills programme.
Scoring method and levels of measurement	For most items an ordinal scale is used. The majority of items are scored on a five-point Likert type scale: strongly agree, agree, not sure, disagree and strongly disagree. Some items use a four- or five-point scale with specific choices for that question (e.g. 'I feel that I am: 1. a very good parent; 2. a better than average parent; 3. an average parent; 4. a person who has some trouble being a parent; 5. not very good at being a parent'). The Life Stresses scale uses a dichotomous nominal two-point yes/no scale to rate whether any of the 19 listed events has occurred in the person's immediate family in the last 12 months (e.g. marriage, pregnancy, legal problems, began new job, death of immediate family member).
Qualifications needed to administer the test and additional training requirements/costs	Catalogue lists qualification code as 'CL2'. Manual states that non-graduates can administer the PSI but an examination and interpretation of PSI scores should be undertaken by people with 'graduate training in clinical counselling or educational psychology or in social work or related fields' (Abidin, 1995, p. 3).
Standardisation: Is it standardised? Test development details	Yes, the test has been standardised and comprises a standardised item booklet and answer sheet. I reviewed the third edition. Earlier editions were published in 1983 and 1990. Test development began in 1976. Content was based on a literature review of research in psychology and psychiatry into stressors linked to dysfunctional parenting. Out of the original 150 test items, 95 were related to at least one research study. Initial test development took place at the University of Virginia over three years during which the PSI was piloted on a group of 208 mothers of children under three years in a parenting clinic linked to a group of paediatricians in Virginia. Test went through several revisions. Factor analyses were conducted on PSI items and the final version of 101 items was finalised.
Is it a normative or criterion-referenced test? Details of criteria or norms	The PSI is a normative assessment. Original norms based on 2,633 mothers (age 16 to 61 years, mean age 30.9) of children aged one month to 12 years (mean 4.9 years; s.d. 3.1) and comprising 76% White, 11% African American, 10% Hispanic and 2% Asian women. The sample was drawn from several US states (Virginia, Massachusetts, New York City, North Carolina and Wisconsin) and from a range of settings: well-child-care paediatric clinics, public school day centres, health maintenance program one, private and public paediatric clinics and public schools. Opportunistic sample (not random or stratified). Norm data also presented for 200 fathers aged 18 to 65 years (mean age 32.1 years) comprising 95% White and 5% African American men. The manual reports: 'the data from this sample would suggest that fathers earn lower stress scores on many PSI scales when compared to mothers' (Abidin, 1995, p. 25). In the manual, norms are also presented for a sample of 223 Hispanic parents. References are given for cross-cultural studies for populations of Bermudan, Chinese, French Canadian, Hispanic, Irish, Israeli, Italian, Japanese and Portuguese parents. Percentile scores can be calculated for all PSI subscales, the Child Domain and the Parent Domain and the Total Stress Score.

(continued)

Table 11.2 (*Continued*)

Critique area	Comments
Reliability data	The PSI manual provides details of studies to evaluate the internal consistency and test–retest reliability of the PSI. Data are variable and details of studies brief making it difficult to draw firm conclusions about the reliability of the PSI and its use as an outcome measure. Test–retest reliability: the PSI manual provides brief summaries of four test–retest reliability studies. It is difficult to draw firm conclusions from the data and there was considerable variation across studies, both in terms of the period between the initial and post-test administrations and in the retest-reliability data obtained from each study. Accepted values for test–retest reliability are coefficients of 0.70 or above (Laver Fawcett, 2002; Opacich, 1991; Benson and Clark, 1982). Parent Domain scores are consistent across three of the four studies and fall just at an acceptable level: 0.69 (Zakreski, 1983, n = 54 parents, retest period over three months), 0.70 (Hamilton, 1980, n = 37 mothers, retest period one year), 0.71 (Burke, 1978, n = 15 mothers, retest period three weeks), with a much higher value of 0.91 reported by Abidin (1995, n = 30 mothers, retest periods one to three months). Across the four studies variability was found for the test–retest reliability of the Child Domain, which ranged from 0.55 Hamilton (1980) and 0.63 (Abidin, 1995), which would be perceived as unacceptably low levels of reliability, to 0.77 (Zakreski, 1983) and 0.82 (Burke, 1978), which are acceptable. Test–retest reliability data for the Total Stress Scoring was provided from three studies and ranged from 0.65 (Hamilton, 1980), which is slightly lower than acceptable levels, 0.88 (Zakreski,1983) to 0.96 (Abidin, 1995), which is a highly acceptable reliability level. Given the nature of the construct being studied, one would expect some changes to occur, especially over longer periods; so I would suggest a therapist consider the time intervals for re-assessment required to measure outcomes and look at the data for the study that used the most comparable retest period. Test–retest reliability data for the PSI short-form from two studies produced acceptable levels of reliability. Internal consistency: a table is given showing coefficient alpha calculations for the Child Domain, Parent Domain, Total Stress Score and all subscales calculated from the normative sample data (n = 2,633) and from a study by Hauenstein, Scarr and Abidin (1987) using a sample of 435. Accepted values for internal consistency are 0.80 or above (Laver Fawcett, 2002; Opacich, 1991; Benson and Clark, 1982). Coefficients from the normative sample ranged from 0.70 to 0.83 for the Child subscales and 0.90 for the Child domain (47 items) and 0.70 to 0.84 for the Parent subscales, 0.93 for the Parent domain (54 items) and 0.95 for the Total Stress Score (101 items). Abidin (1995) reports that Hauenstein and colleagues obtained similar values and their data range from 0.57 for the Health subscale to 0.95 for the Total Stress Score.

Table 11.2 (*Continued*)

Critique area	Comments
Validity data	Yes, various validity studies have been undertaken by the test developer and other researchers, and summaries and references are given in the manual.
	Content validity: content was initially based on a literature review. A panel of six professionals rated each item for relevance of content and adequacy of construction. A reference (Burke, 1978) is cited for more details of the initial content validation process. Factor analytic studies are reported and Abidin (1995) reports that data 'supports the notion that each subscale is measuring a moderately distinct source of stress' (p. 32).
	Concurrent validity: extensive research has been undertaken by different researchers; in Appendix C the manual lists references for research providing PSI correlations with 92 different measures including the Bayley Scales of Infant Development (three studies, e.g. Hanson and Hanline, 1990), the Beck Depression Inventory (nine studies, e.g. Donenberg and Baker, 1993), the Child Behaviour Checklist (18 studies, e.g. Kazdin, 1990) and the Peabody Picture Vocabulary Test – Revised (two studies, e.g. Wilfong, Saylor and Elksnin, 1991).
	Predictive validity: the manual provides details of a predictive validity study that 'examined the relationship of PSI scores to children's subsequent behavioural adjustment in a sample of 100 White, middle-class mothers with children between 6 and 12 months at the time of the initial testing with the families. They were followed up 4 1/2 years later' (Abidin, 1995, p. 37). The manual reports that the PSI 'Life stress, Child Domain, and the Parent Domain PSI scores were significant predictors of subsequent child functioning in relation to conduct disorders, social aggression, attention problems, and anxiety withdrawal' (Abidin, Jenkins and McGaughey, 1992, cited in Abidin, 1995, p. 38).
	Discriminative validity: references are given for studies using the PSI with a variety of clinical populations. For example, Moran et al. (1992) found that the PSI discriminated between children with developmental delay and normally developing children and Cameron and Orr (1989) found that the PSI discriminated between children with delayed mental development and the normative sample. Lafiosca (1981) reports that 'the PSI was able to identify correctly 100% of the parents of normal children and 60% of the parents of the children who were seen at a child development clinic, when the 90th percentile of the PSI Total Stress Score was used as a cut-off. Further, significant mean differences were found for the Total Stress Score, the Child and Parent Domain scores, and for the majority of subscales' (Abidin, 1995, p. 38).

(*continued*)

Table 11.2 (Continued)

Critique area	Comments
Clinical utility (ease of use and scoring, portability, cost, training issues, settings etc.)	The test can be used with a wide range of child–parent populations and can be administered during a clinic appointment or given to the parent to take home and complete independently. It could be used for in-patient, outpatient and community-based practice settings. The PSI manual is laid out in a logical way and it was easy to find the information I wanted when I needed it. The main text is well referenced and fairly easy to read. There are additional numbered references in the appendix and useful lists of 'PSI correlations with other measures' and for uses of 'PSI in research with special populations', which are cross-referenced to the numbered references. The manual reports the PSI takes approximately 20 minutes to complete. It took my husband and the mother, who tried the PSI for my critique, and myself less time, at about 15 minutes each. The three of us found it straightforward to complete and easy to understand. The test accounts for defensive responding and the therapist can easily calculate a defensive responding score for the Parent domain and interpret the data accordingly. The test allows for a small amount of missing data, and a formula is given for calculating subscale and domain scores if data are omitted. The therapist conversion of raw scores to subscale, domain, total stress and percentile scores was quite easy to do and it took me about 15 minutes to sum the scores in each subscale and domain, calculate the total score and plot scores on the profile to transform raw scores into percentiles. It took only another minute to look up the age-based norms in the appendix. The amount of time required for interpretation will depend on the complexity of the results and the therapist's familiarity with the PSI and manual. Chapter 3 'Interpretation and Interventions' provides helpful summaries related to each subscale and domain with guidance as to what percentile levels would indicate a need for further intervention/referral and with ideas for intervention approaches. As the scoring of responses is done on a separate form to the PSI item question booklet, the person completing it needs to keep careful track to correspond the item numbers on the answer form and item booklet; as most items are scored using the same scale (SA, A, NS, D, SD), it is quite easy to miss one out and continue going down the score sheet; it is only when the parent reaches a question with a different scoring format that he/she will realise that the item they are scoring on the answer sheet doesn't correspond with the item question in the booklet. The test is not cheap but neither is it very expensive. Therapists in a team/department could share one manual, and there are 10 reusable item booklets enabling 10 parents to be assessed simultaneously. No additional training is required and I would suggest a therapist allow at least one hour to familiarise herself with the manual and another hour to complete the PSI (or have a colleague, family member, friend complete an answer form) and score and interpret a practice set of data prior to using the test with clients.
Face validity (for therapists, clients, others receiving results)	I felt the PSI had good face validity, both as a therapist administering, scoring and interpreting the test and when completing it as a mother of two young children. I felt the questions were relevant to me as a mother. As a therapist, there was a clear theoretical base for the subscales and domains, and I felt I was assessing parents' perceptions of their children's behaviours and of their own situations and coping. I provided the mother, who tried the PSI for my critique, with a short face validity survey to complete on the PSI. She rated the PSI as 'Easy' (as opposed to difficult), 'Interesting' (as opposed to boring), 'Relevant' (as opposed to irrelevant) and 'Undemanding' (as opposed to stressful). She commented that the PSI was 'very interesting as it was about me for a change rather than just my child'. The mother did not find any questions unclear or ambiguous and answered all questions and indicated that there were no questions that she did not feel comfortable answering. When asked if she found it useful to reflect on the PSI questions, she answered: 'Yes, it made me think about a few of the answers I gave, perhaps highlighting a few areas.'

(continued)

Table 11.2 *(Continued)*

Critique area	Comments
Summary of strengths	Strong underlying research and theory base to the development of the PSI and uses in different cultures and with a wide range of conditions. Fairly easy to complete for most parents and not too time-consuming (about 15–20 minutes). Straightforward to score and plot profile (took about 15 minutes). Easy to covert raw score to percentiles on either profile or against age-based norms. Case examples and diagnostic group mean profiles allow for comparison. Manual contains useful information for interpreting scores and planning related intervention. Allows comparison of mother, versus father, perspectives of child and experience of stress related to parenting. A short form of the PSI, which the manual states takes about 10 minutes to complete, is available as a screening tool, if the 20-minute administration time is perceived as too long for a particular parent group (e.g. parents have difficulty with concentration) or service requirement (e.g. a service wanted to use the PSI as a screen with all parents). The short form has acceptable levels of test–retest reliability and could be used as an evaluative measure.
Summary of limitations	No British normative data but a wide range of cross-cultural studies indicate that the PSI norms are robust across different populations. Summaries of the psychometric studies are very brief with only a few sentences about the samples and the results and quite a few of the references cited for important psychometric studies are from unpublished work, making it very difficult for a therapist to access details of these studies. For example, Burke's (1978) unpublished doctoral dissertation is cited as providing 'a detailed description of the initial content validation of the PSI' and the reference for the internal consistency study by Hauenstein, Scarr and Abidin (1987) is referenced as an unpublished manuscript. I have concerns about the variability of the reliability data; results from four test–retest reliability studies ranged from 0.55, 0.63, 0.77 to 0.82 (see reliability section above) with half the data being at acceptable levels (over 0.70) and half the data raising causes for concern if the PSI is to be implemented for evaluative purposes (under 0.70). The reasons for the variability in these results are not discussed in the test manual and it is difficult to hypothesise about the causes of this variability as little detail is given about the methodology used in each study. To compound the problem, three of the four test–retest reliability studies referenced are from unpublished doctoral dissertations. The manual reports parents with at least fifth grade education were found to understand the instructions; parents with less formal education, learning disability or cognitive impairment might need support to ensure understanding.
Overall conclusion: Should test be adopted, piloted or rejected as an option for your service?	I would recommend this measure to therapists working in a wide range of paediatric settings. It is a good descriptive measure that provides a useful overview of the parent's perceptions of child behaviours and the parent's overall level and causes of parenting stress. I would suggest therapists obtain a review copy or borrow a copy of the PSI first to critique for their particular service and pilot with a few parents prior to purchase. The PSI has some predictive and discriminative use, but I recommend that therapists obtain and review the relevant research referenced in the manual before applying in this way. If the PSI is to be used as an evaluative measure, I would recommend therapists conduct their own test–retest reliability study for the time period that is likely to occur in their clinical practice between baseline assessment and outcome measurement to ensure that the PSI has adequate reliability for this purpose.

OBTAINING PERMISSION TO USE A TEST FOR YOUR CLINICAL PRACTICE OR FOR RESEARCH

Whether and from whom you need obtain permission depends on whether the test is in the public domain and whether there is a cost or training requirement for using the test. If a test has been purchased for use from the author or a publisher, then the permission to use it is implicit. However, you might inherit a test when you move to a new service or obtain a copy of a test at a workshop or from a colleague. In these cases, you need to track down who the author is, who has copyright and whether the test is published. If a test developer has sold the copyright to a publisher, then permission is sought from the publisher and usually you will be charged to use the test and all related materials. If the assessment has been printed in full in an article where the journal publishers require the author to sign over copyright of the article, then permission may need to be sought from the publisher of the journal. Sometimes the author may have maintained copyright of the instrument prior to publication of the article and permission then has to be obtained from both the author and the journal publisher. If the instrument has not been published in full (for example you access a copy being used for research during test development), then the author must be contacted.

MODIFYING A STANDARDISED TEST

If you cannot find a standardised instrument that meets your needs but do identify a standardised test that seems to address many of the factors that you require, then it may be worth considering whether part of this test could be used or whether you could tailor some aspects of the test to your client group's needs/service outcomes. However, changing standardised tests or only using part of a test battery should not be undertaken lightly. If the test were rigorously developed, then every aspect of that test (test items, format, data-collection method, instructions, scoring method) will have been carefully considered and its contribution to the overall content and reliability of the test will have been evaluated. You need to be aware that by omitting certain parts of the test or by changing a test item, instruction or scoring method the validity and reliability of the resultant test could be negatively affected. Therefore, you should treat the modified or shortened version of the test as a new test and should ideally conduct new psychometric evaluation to ensure that levels of validity and reliability are still clinically acceptable (Royeen, 1989).

If you plan to alter a test in any way, your proposed changes should be approved by the copyright holder/author prior to use. Be prepared for the author not granting permission to use the test if you plan to change the test in some way. Validity and reliability can be altered by changes to a test; so authors are right to be cautious about authorising changes without additional research to establish whether the change has affected the psychometric properties of the test. All permissions should be obtained in writing and kept safely in case required in future.

LINKING IMPROVING YOUR ASSESSMENT PRACTICE TO CONTINUING PROFESSIONAL DEVELOPMENT

Both occupational therapists and physiotherapists working in the UK have to be registered with the Health Professions Council (HPC). The HPC plans to introduce new standards for therapists around the undertaking and recording of CPD. In a recent summary of its consultation on CPD, the HPC states that 'the CPD process will be based on continuing learning and development with a focus on individual learning achievements and how these enhance service delivery'

(Health Professions Council, 2005, p. 3). The HPC will be looking for evidence of a range of CPD activities, which include:

   i. 'work-based learning, for example, reflective practice, clinical audit, significant event analysis, user feedback, membership of a committee, journal club;

  ii. professional activity, for example, member of specialist interest group, mentoring, teaching, expert witness, presentation at conferences;

 iii. formal/educational, for example, courses, undertaking research, distance learning, planning or running a course;

 iv. self-directed learning, for example, reading journals/articles, reviewing books/articles, updating knowledge via www/TV/press' (Health Professions Council, 2005, p. 9).

A number of these activities are helpful when undertaking a review of your current assessment practice and when critiquing the evidence to improve areas of your practice where you cannot demonstrate that the current methods you are using are the most effective and efficient available. The CSP provides guidance on CPD on its website (Chartered Society of Physiotherapy, 2004b). The COT also provides guidance on CPD activities on its website. The COT (2005b) recommends therapists maintain a CPD portfolio that includes the following five sections.

1. career history (CV) and current job description
2. personal development plan (PDP) and most current performance appraisal
3. reflection logs
4. sample achievements of learning (e.g. research paper, improved client outcomes in practice, design of new rehabilitation programme)
5. other (e.g. course certificates, letters from users, carers, colleagues etc.)

The COT (2005b) recommends that each therapists should have a PDP, which 'should reflect your learning goals for a specific time frame, your strategies to achieve these goals, timelines for pursuing these goals, and evidence of progress towards your goals'. The College has designed two templates that can be used to record your PDP and your reflections on learning (reflection logs), and these can be downloaded from its website at http://www.cot.co.uk.

    To begin setting yourself some PDPs for improving your assessment practice I have included a worksheet (see Worksheet 13, p. 418) and a series of goals for therapists related to assessment and measurement are presented below.

ASSESSMENT AND OUTCOME MEASUREMENT GOALS FOR EFFECTIVE PRACTICE

Therapists working in a wide variety of roles (clinician, researcher, manager, educator, therapy consultant or student) can all play a part in service modernisation by working to reduce barriers and facilitate the implementation of evidence-based, effective and efficient assessment processes with the administration of valid and reliable outcome measures at the heart of therapy practice. This will require changes in attitudes, knowledge, skills and behaviour. Cole *et al.* (1995) present a series of challenges for therapists in different roles, and I have used their work as the basis for developing CPD goals for occupational therapy and physiotherapy clinicians, managers, educators, researchers and students. I suggest you identify the role(s) you undertake and select from the goals as the basis for identifying your own CPD to improve your assessment practice, a worksheet (Worksheet 13, p. 418) is provided for this purpose and an example of a completed CPD action plan is provided in Table 11.3 below.

Table 11.3 Continuing professional development goals for improving assessment practice: an example

CPD Goal	Action plan	Comments/ideas	Date accomplished
Example: *As a clinician, I need to increase my application of standardised outcome measures*	1. Contact the Special Interest Group for therapists in my area and ask about appropriate standardised outcome measures for my client group.	1. I have copied a number of journal articles on potential assessments and placed in my CPD file: make time to read them!	1. Received emails from SIG members with recommendations for tests.
	2. Borrow/obtain at least two of the recommended measures and review the manuals and materials.	2. Perhaps we could set up a journal club for our department or within my MDT?	2. Following month, borrowed test from neighbouring hospital for a weekend and reviewed manual. Appears appropriate for our service.
	3. Pilot with at least five clients to evaluate clinical utility and face validity.		3. Two months later, organised to have sample test from publisher for two weeks and tried out with three clients.
	4. Use the Test Critique Worksheet to summarise my findings from actions 2 and 3		4. In the same month, completed test critique.
	5. If I find a suitable test that requires funding, make a business case for required resources.		5. Two months later, made business case to manager for funding to purchase two copies of the test for our department.
	Time scale one year. Review progress at my next annual appraisal		Test purchased nine months after initial emails received. Provided in-house training on test administration for colleagues the following month.

GOALS FOR CLINICIANS

- Clinicians need to increase their application of standardised outcome measures.
- Clinicians need to follow standards laid down for test users, e.g. the standards for test users produced by the American Physical Therapy Association (1991) or the *Hierarchy of competencies relating to the use of standardized instruments and evaluation techniques by occupational therapists* produced by the American Occupational Therapy Association (cited in Hopkins and Smith, 1993).
- Clinicians need to use the outcome data gathered to modernise and improve service provision for clients and carers.
- Clinicians need to work with other therapists (clinicians and researchers) to identify limitations in assessment practice and outcome measures and identify the need for improved measures.
- Clinicians need to share information on standardised tests and outcomes with other therapists and professionals working with similar client groups.
- Clinicians should become life-long learners who seek opportunities to attend courses or conferences where they can learn more about assessment and allocate CPD time for reading in order to stay up to date with the growing literature on standardised outcome measures for their client group.
- If you supervise students on placement, explain your rationale for your assessment process, share your clinical reasoning and encourage students to critique the standardised tests used within your service.

GOALS FOR THERAPY MANAGERS

For managers, Cole *et al.* (1995) identify five major challenges that I have expanded into the following goals for service improvement.

- Managers need to value outcome measurement as an integral part of providing an effective service. They must explicitly articulate this attitude to staff and encourage staff still using predominately non-standardised assessment to change their attitudes and behaviour and embrace evidence-based assessments.
- Managers need to ensure that therapists have received the appropriate training to administer the specific standardised assessments used in their service and ensure the staff, under their management, maintain the appropriate standards of test administration.
- Managers should encourage the sharing of data within departments and across services, including the development of computer systems. In the UK, this is an explicit goal of the development of a single assessment process (SAP; Department of Health, 2002a).
- Managers should formulate a well-articulated case to educate service leaders/managers and funding agencies that the information obtained from evidence-based outcome measures is essential for making informed decisions about competing resource allocation.
- Managers should take responsibility for collating service-wide data and providing information obtained from evidence-based outcome measures in a readily usable form.
- Managers should become life-long learners who seek opportunities to attend courses or conferences where they can learn more about assessment, measurement and service evaluation and allocate CPD time for reading in order to stay up to date with the growing literature on standardised outcome measures for their client population.

GOALS FOR EDUCATORS

- Educators need to ensure that a significant emphasis is placed on the curriculum for developing occupational therapy and physiotherapy students' attitudes, knowledge and skills related to assessment and outcome measurement and highlight that competence in assessment and evaluation is an essential part of providing a high-quality therapy service.

- Educators should teach occupational therapy and physiotherapy students how to undertake test critiques and provide role modelling by disseminating critical reviews of outcome measures.
- Educators need to encourage occupational therapy and physiotherapy students to engage in projects/assignments that examine the evidence base for published tests and for existing assessment processes, which they observe on clinical practice.
- Educators are needed to contribute to the identification of areas where practice can be improved and further development of measures is needed.

GOALS FOR OCCUPATIONAL THERAPY AND PHYSIOTHERAPY RESEARCHERS

- Researchers need to contribute to the identification of areas where practice can be improved and further development of measures is needed.
- Researchers need to undertake research to build upon the body of evidence for existing outcome measures, e.g. by conducting further validity and reliability studies or by obtaining normative data for different populations.
- Researchers need to take lead roles in the adaptation of existing measures and/or the development of new measures in areas where practice can be improved and further development of measures is needed to provide clinically useful, evidence-based outcome measures.

GOALS FOR OCCUPATIONAL THERAPY AND PHYSIOTHERAPY STUDENTS

- Students must understand and apply the principles of robust assessment and strive to base their assessment practice on the application of well-evidenced procedures and outcome measures.
- Students should strive to become life-long learners who stay up to date with the growing literature on standardised outcome measures for the client groups they interact with on placement and, once qualified, to continue a quest for knowledge and stay up to date on outcome measures for their client group.
- As therapists of the future, students should become proactive agents for change in the services where they undertake clinical placements and, when they qualify and start work, should share knowledge and skills, particularly in services where the application of outcome measures is not common practice, perhaps by running an in-service training event for colleagues or by implementing the use of standardised measures with their own caseload.

CONCLUSION: ACHIEVING AN EFFECTIVE AND EFFICIENT ASSESSMENT

The role of assessment is of paramount importance to occupational therapy and physiotherapy practice because assessment enables the therapist to describe the person's functional problems in the form of a therapy diagnosis, formulate a prognosis, use the diagnosis and prognosis as a baseline for treatment planning, monitor the person's responses during treatment and evaluate the effectiveness of the intervention (Law and Letts, 1989). The practice setting and the nature of the therapy service will place parameters around the type of assessment that is possible. Therapists need to be pragmatic in their choices, but also should lobby for improvements when restrictions place unacceptable limitations on the quality of the assessment that can be undertaken; a rushed, one-time assessment, for example, is rarely a sufficient baseline from which to plan effective treatment. No assessment of human functioning can be entirely objective, and therapists need to make careful observations, hypotheses and judgements – all of which could be open to some degree of error. Therefore, in order to ensure that their assessments are as valid and reliable as possible, therapists should endeavour to use standardised assessments where available. In the future, health professionals need to achieve a shift from the use of non-standardised, therapist-constructed assessments to well-researched, clinically useful, standardised measures. In a political environment that places increasing emphasis on quality, clinical governance and evidence-based practice, a greater use of standardised assessments should assist therapists to present more objective and precise findings and to evaluate their interventions in a reliable and sensitive manner. Therapists need to make time to critically examine all non-standardised assessments used within their service. Where these non-standardised assessments are found to be unsuitable for future practice, therapists need to review and trial potential standardised measures to replace them.

In summary, when selecting assessments for a service, care should be taken that a potential test has good face validity and clinical utility, in addition to thorough standardisation, established validity and acceptable levels of reliability. It should be remembered that a good test administration can be rendered useless if the results are not documented adequately and the results are not shared with the client and other relevant personnel; so, when planning an assessment, sufficient time should be allowed for scoring, interpretation, report writing and feedback.

Assessment should never be viewed in isolation, for it is not an end in itself. Assessment always should be at the heart of the initial interaction with a client and then should be interwoven as an important component of the whole intervention process, right through to a final evaluation when the client is discharged from the therapy service.

It is critical that we continue to review our assessment process and measurement tools on a regular basis. New research might be available that could strengthen or reduce the rationale for using a particular test. A recently published measure might be more reliable or responsive or have better face validity and clinical utility, making it a better choice for your client group. Your service might change, for example a different intervention approach could be implemented leading to the requirement for the measurement of different outcomes. It is very helpful to set a date for the next review of assessment and measurement and to identify a lead clinician who will prompt others when this review is due and facilitate the review process. For your service to thrive and to continually offer best practice, you need to develop a culture where it is acceptable and welcomed for everyone to question practice and to present and debate ideas. A question from a client, or a suggestion from a student or new member of staff, could lead you another step along the path of evidence-based practice.

STUDY QUESTIONS AND TASKS

11.1 Give an example of:
    a. a standardised self-report assessment
    b. a standardised proxy assessment
    c. a standardised observational assessment
       that would be appropriate for your client group and practice setting.
11.2 Choose a standardised test of interest and undertake a comprehensive test critique using Worksheet 12 (pp. 474–7) as a template.
11.3 Review the goals for improving assessment practice, select at least three goals of relevance to you and then complete Worksheet 13 (p. 418).
(*Note:* See note on p. 394.)

12

The Final Case Study
'Carol': Experience of a Chronic
Pain Service

This case study has been written to illustrate how a comprehensive and rigorous assessment process can be developed and implemented. The case describes both a physiotherapist's and an occupational therapist's approach to assessment and measurement. The case is provided to illustrate many of the points raised in previous chapters and show how these recommendations can be applied in practice. It is a detailed study so that students and novice therapists can see examples of how therapists frame and explain their assessment approaches. Some narrative is provided to show how an interview might be conducted. The case ends with some information about how the team have undertaken a service evaluation using both quantitative and qualitative data.

INTRODUCTION TO THE THERAPISTS AND THE CHRONIC PAIN SERVICE

THE PHYSIOTHERAPIST

Gail Brooke trained in Birmingham and qualified as a physiotherapist in 1973. While working in mental health services, she became interested in pain management and, in conjunction with a member of the psychology department, she surveyed GPs to evaluate the need for a Chronic Pain Service (CPS). She has led the development of the CPS in Harrogate since 1993. Gail works full-time, with half her post designated as manager of the CPS and as a physiotherapist in the CPS team and the other half as superintendent physiotherapist managing the physiotherapists within the Mental Health Directorate.

THE OCCUPATIONAL THERAPIST

Heather Shaw has been an occupational therapist for 25 years and qualified with a DipCOT in 1979. Heather has been a Senior I occupational therapist with the CPS team for about eight years and works part-time. She views client education as an essential part of the occupational therapy intervention offered by the CPS. She feels that it can be easy to become a generic therapist and works hard to maintain her core occupational therapy skills in her work with people with chronic pain.

THE CHRONIC PAIN SERVICE

The service was set up in 1993 and is staffed by a multidisciplinary team. All the staff work part-time within the team and the multidisciplinary team currently includes a consultant in anaesthetics, two occupational therapists, two physiotherapists, a clinical psychologist and two secretaries/team coordinators. The team is about to appoint another part-time physiotherapist and part-time psychologist and further developments of an intermediate care service are due to take place over the next 18 months. The aim of the Chronic Pain Service is to rehabilitate chronic pain sufferers, enabling them to take control of their lives rather than being controlled by the pain. The objectives for the service are to:

- offer a holistic approach to assessment and treatment
- improve fitness, mobility and posture and counteract the effects of disuse
- encourage sufferers in self-efficacy
- teach coping skills, such as pacing and relaxation
- improve stress management and sleep
- counteract unhelpful beliefs and improve mood and confidence
- avoid adverse drug effects and reduce intake of unhelpful drugs
- improve social relationships and reduce the effects of pain on the activities of daily living (ADL)
- educate the sufferer/carer/health professional on the factors influencing chronic pain
- encourage realistic expectations and a healthy acceptance of the client's condition.

The CPS team sees clients both individually and in groups and runs three pain management programmes known as Turnabout, Turnabout Active and Turnabout Easy. There are plans to expand the team in order to provide a service across the whole Primary Care Trust (PCT), and also to develop services for people with chronic fatigue syndrome (CFS)/myalgic encephalomyelitis (ME).

The team follows a biopsychosocial model of chronic pain (for example as described by Waddel, 1987, in relation to lower back disability). Cognitive behavioural therapy forms a major part of the intervention for the majority of clients seen by the CPS team. The team is also learning more about acceptance theory and the psychologist is due to attend a course to expand her knowledge of this model. Amongst others, the team draws upon an edited interdisciplinary text on pain management (Main and Spanswick, 2000) and Gifford (1998, 2000) Melzack (1987, 1975) and Wall (1996) and many others.

STANDARDISED MEASURES USED IN THE SERVICE

The team combines the use of standardised assessments, informal interview, observation and physical assessment, including the:

- Canadian Occupational Performance Measure (COPM; Law *et al.*, 1998). The COPM is a client-centred assessment that measures problems identified by the client himself. It engages the client right from the start of the therapeutic process and supports the idea that clients have some responsibility for their own health. It measures not only performance but also the client's satisfaction with performance. This means that as an assessment it fits in well with the CPS team's approach to the management of chronic pain. In terms of limitations, Heather reports the COPM is not regarded highly by the world of research as it does not use norms, it can be time-consuming to administer and the number rating system can be hard for some clients to grasp. (*Note:* see Chapter 2, p. 56 and p. 76 for a description of this measure.)
- Beck Depression Inventory (BDI; Steer and Beck, 1996; for the latest version BDI-II see Beck, Steer and Brown, 1996; Steer and Beck, 2004). The BDI can be self-administered or given as an interview. It comprises 21 items to assess the intensity of depression. Each item is a list of four statements arranged in increasing severity about a particular symptom of depression. The BDI is a short validated assessment tool that can be used to assess the level of depression. It takes about five minutes to complete. Its main strength for use in the CPS is that it alerts the team to suicide risk; however, a limitation is that it is affected by physical factors and so can give biased scores. The BDI relies on self-report, which can vary day by day.
- Beck Anxiety Inventory (BAI; Beck and Steer, 1990; Steer and Beck, 1997). The BAI allows a quick assessment of anxiety using a validated tool. Clients rate themselves on 21 items using a scale from 0 to 3. Each item is descriptive of subjective, somatic or panic-related symptoms of anxiety. It is developed for use with adults aged 17 to 80 years and takes between five and ten minutes to complete. Like the BDI, it is influenced by physical factors and may not give a true record of health anxiety. It also relies on self-report, which can vary day by day.
- McGill Pain Questionnaire (Melzack, 1975; also a modified short form is available, see Melzack, 1987). This is an internationally recognised questionnaire and is classed as a valid and acceptable instrument for moderate to severe or acute pain. It is translated into 15 languages. 'The McGill Pain Questionnaire consists primarily of 3 major classes of word descriptors, sensory, affective and evaluative, that are used by patients to specify subjective pain experience. It also contains an intensity scale and other items to determine the properties of pain experience' (Melzack, 1975, p. 277). The three measures included are: '(1) the pain rating index, based on two types of numerical values that can be assigned to each word descriptor, (2) the number of words chosen and (3) the present

pain intensity based on a 1–5 intensity scale' (p. 277). There are few limitations, but it does have restrictions for clients with communication problems.

- SF-36 Coping Questionnaire (Ware *et al.*, 1993). This questionnaire is a short-form health survey with 36 questions. It provides 'an 8-scale profile of functional health and well-being scores as well as psychometrically-based physical and mental health summary measures and a preference-based health utility index' (Ware, 2005, p. 1). It can be used across a wide range of age groups and diagnoses. The team uses it to identify the effect of pain on ADL and the impact of pain on social activities. It is also used to identify beliefs about pain, a picture of the individual's general health and the emotional impact of pain. (*Note:* there is also a 12-item short-form version, SF-12; see Ware, 2005.)
- Fear-avoidance Beliefs Questionnaire (FABQ; Waddell *et al.*, 1993). This is a self-report survey to explore the role of fear-avoidance beliefs in people with chronic lower-back pain and the link to disability.
- Functional Measurements/observations: These include joint range of movement (ROM), strength and an observation of how easily the client fulfils certain activities, e.g. dressing/undressing. Therapists also observe the quality of movement (e.g. whether it is jerky) and the person's ability to transfer and his gait.
- Pain Score: The interpretation of pain drawing and numeric rating scale used by the CPS was produced by Margolis, Tait and Krause (1986) and the reliability examined by Margolis, Chibnall and Tait (1988).

INTRODUCTION TO THE CASE: 'CAROL'

Gail and Heather have used their eight years' experience of working together in the CPS team to develop a typical case for this vignette. Carol is a 45-year-old married lady with a history of chronic back pain.

REFERRAL

The referral was made by a neurosurgeon within the district hospital. The letter was sent to the consultant with the CPS suggesting treatment with injections. The referral information told the team that Carol had a mild disc bulge at L4/5, but no nerve root entrapment. She had already had X-rays and an MRI (magnetic resonance imaging) scan and her nerve conduction tests were normal. The referral stated that Carol had tried physiotherapy in the past without success. She had been a nursing auxiliary but had not worked for several years owing to her pain. She had been unsuccessful in proving that her condition dated back to an accident lifting a client and had not received compensation from her previous employer. The neurosurgeon noted that she was 'quite low' and concluded the referral by saying, 'I see no need for surgery and I am unable to find any physical reason to account for the level of this lady's disability.'

INITIAL ASSESSMENT

There are two pathways to access the CPS. In a small number of cases, a referral may be made for a specific intervention (for example an epidural). People who have been referred to the team are sent a postal questionnaire, which is part of a triage process for allocating clients to assessment clinics and potential intervention programmes. Although Carol had been referred to the consultant for injections, the other information in the referral led the team to hypothesise that Carol might benefit from a full multidisciplinary team approach. She was, therefore, sent the Triage Questionnaire to complete. This was sent with a stamped addressed envelope along with a leaflet about the CPS and a leaflet about confidentiality, explaining that information is shared amongst team members.

The Triage Questionnaire contains some standardised tools, such as the BDI, BAI, McGill Pain Questionnaire and the SF-36. It also contains additional questions that have been developed by the team to obtain demographic information and a history of the condition, past treatments, medications used and outcomes.

The objectives for the initial triage assessment are to:

- obtain some baseline data to frame the main problems and decide which team members should conduct the first clinic-based assessment
- assess for risk of suicide
- check whether the client is too depressed to comply and fully benefit from the service
- assess the presence of mental health problems and highlight a potential need for psychological intervention
- obtain some preliminary information about the level of functional impairment and a profile of what the person used to do and activities that have been given up because of the pain
- obtain a history of the condition, previous treatments and responses to treatment
- provide insight, using the McGill Pain Questionnaire, into the client's perception of her pain both through the location and manner in which the person depicts her pain on the body drawings and by the choice of pain descriptors circled
- form useful hypotheses from the parts of the triage assessment that a person chooses to omit, as well as from the completed sections.

In the past, the team has received a few complaints about the questionnaire from clients. The team wanted to make the triage assessment more acceptable to clients, and so they involved the chairman of a group for clients, Action on Pain, in a review of the questionnaire in order to improve its face validity (see Chapter 6). He helped them to redesign the form and make the questions and format more user-friendly. He recommended removing a couple of questions, which had asked about employment and any history of sexual abuse, as these had been perceived as too intrusive by clients. The team felt the redesigned questionnaire was not as clinically useful as the previous version because some of the information was harder to interpret, and they now raise the removed questions in person during the first clinic assessment. However, they felt the revised triage assessment had better face validity, and the team has not received complaints from clients since it was changed.

Carol completed her self-assessment and posted it back to the team within a week. There are several different types of assessment clinic run by the team, including a full multidisciplinary team clinic in which the client is assessed by a doctor, physiotherapist, occupational therapist and psychologist. But clients can see any combination of staff in a clinic depending on their assessed needs, and there are some therapy/psychology-only clinics if it is felt the client does not need to see a doctor. The team meet once a week to evaluate triage assessment data and allocate new clients to the most appropriate assessment clinic. Team members share out the returned Triage Questionnaires to score the standardised tests during the meeting and then take it in turns to present the results of the questionnaire they have analysed.

Heather scored Carol's Triage Questionnaire. The BDI showed a moderate to high depression score of 20. Carol stated that she could not walk further than 50 yards and was no longer undertaking domestic activities of daily living (DADL). She had given up all social activities, apart from seeing her parents. She used to enjoy long walks and ballroom dancing with her husband two evenings a week. She had been forced to give up work for health reasons about nine years ago. Key results from her triage assessment were:

1. summary of SF-36, which indicated moderate functional impairment owing to her pain (e.g. difficulty with housework, shopping, walking more than 100 yards) and difficulty bathing and dressing and a decrease in her social activity.

2. BAI score of 20, which indicated a moderate to high level of anxiety.
3. the McGill Pain Questionnaire is a generic instrument aimed at specifying the qualities of pain, determine intensities implied by the use of words used to describe pain and acts as a measure looking at all dimensions of pain, which results in a pain-rating index. Words used are grouped into four subclasses:
   a. sensory
   b. affective
   c. evaluative
   d. miscellaneous

   In Carol's case, she circled 15/78 words used to describe pain and rated it as an intensity of 7 on a visual analogue scale (VAS). The drawing she completed indicated an emotional component to her pain with colouring outside of the area one would expect from her medical history.

After reviewing Carol's triage assessment, Heather provided a summary of the above to the team, which suggested that:

- there was evidence of emotional components to Carol's experience of her pain
- Carol seemed to be confused regarding her loss of role
- the BAI and BDI showed moderate levels of depression and anxiety
- from the history of her condition and treatment to date, previous physiotherapy appeared to have been unsuccessful.

The team concluded that a multidisciplinary team approach would be valuable for her, and Carol was invited to attend a Friday afternoon initial assessment clinic in order to be assessed by the team. The clinic is run by four members of the service: the consultant, the psychologist, one of the physiotherapists and one of the occupational therapists. The team usually sees three new clients in this clinic over a four- to five-hour period. During the initial assessment, each client spends about 40 minutes with each member of the team. The four professionals then meet to discuss their assessment findings and summarise a treatment plan. The client then returns to meet with the team and is either given a diagnosis or an explanation as to why a diagnosis cannot be made at this time. The team also explains a potential intervention plan and reaches a mutual agreement with the client regarding the proposed plan. The client is given a written copy of this plan.

Carol's husband, Jim, drove her to the clinic in his taxi and accompanied her up to the CPS reception. Carol asked whether Jim was required to sit in with her during her assessments. She was told that clients are usually seen individually but that her husband was welcome to wait with her and meet with the team at the end of the afternoon. This is because in the past the team has found that meeting individually with the client can lead to a more frank and open discussion. Carol and Jim decided that he should get back to work and she arranged to phone him when she was ready to be collected.

MULTIDISCIPLINARY TEAM HALF-DAY CLINIC ASSESSMENT PROCESS

The objectives for Carol's first clinic assessment were to:

- carry out a full, holistic assessment of needs and exclude any physical problems that may need further investigation
- provide a diagnosis or explanation of why pain is present and explain the difference between acute and chronic pain
- allow her the opportunity to ask questions and clarify any confusion regarding her situation that she may have

- formulate an agreed treatment plan
- clarify the client's understanding of the team's approach
- begin to develop a therapeutic relationship with the team by gaining client collaboration.

The team decided it was important for Carol to be seen by the consultant first. This was to find out if Carol was expecting to receive an injection at the clinic (as the neurosurgeon had made a referral specifically mentioning injections) and to explain that injections would not be prescribed without a full team assessment and might not be the best form of treatment.

MEDICAL ASSESSMENT

The consultant took a medical history and undertook a physical assessment. Carol had been experiencing pain for ten years following an accident when transferring a client during her work as a nursing auxiliary. She had given up work nine years ago and felt very bitter towards her past employer as she had lost her compensation case. Her X-ray had shown some signs of osteoarthritis, and the defence had argued that this might have been present before the accident and could be the cause of her symptoms. The team always ask about benefits because they have found that, for some clients, this can influence progress because of fears of losing any of their benefits. Carol reported that her husband was a taxi driver and the breadwinner and she did not claim any benefits. In terms of family history, her mother had chronic back pain and diabetes and had been bedridden on and off for years, while her father remained fit and well. She was the middle of three children; her younger brother had no medical problems, but her older sister had diabetes, like their mother, and Carol was very anxious that she also might develop diabetes in time. The doctor asked Carol about her previous medications and any side effects and about her current medications. He also assessed her knowledge of her condition to identify any misconceptions.

PHYSIOTHERAPY ASSESSMENT

After Carol had seen the consultant, she was passed over to the physiotherapist for assessment. Gail had noted from the referral information that Carol had received physiotherapy before but had not found it successful. She therefore hypothesised that Carol might not be interested in receiving further physiotherapy and might be resistant to the physiotherapeutic component of the planned CPS clinic assessment. It was, therefore, going to be really important to explain the physiotherapy role within the CPS team very clearly and describe the physiotherapeutic approach within the CPS. Gail would need to ask Carol about her previous physiotherapy treatment and might then need to explain how her proposed intervention within the CPS would differ from the service Carol might have received before within a more traditional outpatient physiotherapy clinic. In order to ensure realistic expectations, Gail would need to explain that the team was aiming to help her manage her pain and improve her quality of life, rather than offering her a complete cure and explain in simple terms the difference between acute pain and chronic pain and the way in which these are treated.

Gail's hypothesis proved correct. Carol questioned the use of further physiotherapy and told Gail that her previous physiotherapy had sometimes been very painful and had even made her condition feel worse. She also said that her previous physiotherapist had told her that she could not do anything more for her. Carol was disappointed that she would not be receiving the injection that she had expected and was concerned at what could be offered her as she felt she had tried most treatments available. Gail needed to be sensitive to these feelings and worked hard to start to develop some trust and rapport with Carol. She spent several minutes explaining her proposed assessment approach and the rationale for physiotherapy in Carol's case. Carol agreed to the assessment somewhat reluctantly, but still seemed unconvinced about future physiotherapy treatment.

Gail began with a physical assessment. This was based upon assessment methods she was taught while training and incorporated Maitland spinal manipulation assessment techniques (for example see Maitland *et al.*, 2000). This assessment process begins with a self-report assessment through taking a history of the problem and asking for a history of changes of movement and rest, and about any variation of symptoms. She explored movements carried out with difficulty and asked for Carol to identify the level at which pain is felt. Through the history taking, she tried to identify whether Carol experienced stress about movement. Gail asked questions to ascertain what improved pain and also what made the pain worse. The second part of the assessment process involves observational techniques through undertaking a physical examination to differentiate sources of symptoms. Gail tested for normal movements and observed bony land marks, position of feet and weight transference, posture (for example note if there is lordosis, swing back, flatback, kyphosis, pole head), level of ischial crests, gluteal and waist folds, level of ischial tuberosities. She tested straight-leg raising, neural tests, sacro-iliac joint rocking and femoral stretch. Gail undertook palpation, noting tension in muscles, heat, tightness and a lack of movement of vertebra at specific levels. She also assessed changes in sensation. Throughout the assessment, Gail was looking for yellow flags and ensuring there were no red flags as per the Clinical Standards Advisory Group (CSAG; 1994) guidelines on back pain (also see Watson and Kendall, 2000; Roberts, 2000).

Gail examined Carol's joint function and observed her mobility, posture and gait. Carol was very fearful of movement and needed constant reassurance during the assessment and encouragement to comply with Gail's instructions. She walked stiffly carrying weight on her right leg, her knees were held slightly flexed and she had over pronation of her feet. Her lumbar movement was restricted and Gail found reduced mobility of the L4/5 vertebra. Carol reported a generalised ache in her lumbar spine. She had shortened hamstrings. Gail found increased muscle tone on palpation and tender spots around L4/5 and L3/4. Carol had poor posture with a flattened lumbar spine, slight kyphosis and poke head. There was no sign of neural tension, but muscles were tight and slightly swollen. On examination, Carol had a reduced range of lumbar flexion, extension and side flexion. During the assessment, Gail observed the way Carol transferred on and off the chair and the plinth. She also observed informally how Carol managed to get undressed and redressed and noted the speed and quality of her movements. (Gail finds that a person's appearance can be very informative, for example a person may present to clinic looking neat and tidy, but when she undresses for the assessment may be wearing dirty underwear or have a strong body odour, and this can be indicative of self-neglect and mental health problems.) During these informal observations, Gail was looking out for pain behaviours (as described by Waddel, 1987). Carol displayed grimacing, rubbing and groaning during the assessment. Carol reported that her pain was relieved to some degree by heat, massage and not staying in one position too long. She said that her pain got worse when she tried to exercise and when she was lifting, shopping or walking.

Gail often assesses reflexes and skin sensation, but did not need to do this on this occasion as the consultant had said he would include this in his medical assessment. She also omitted detailed questioning about the performance of ADL, as this was to be covered by the occupational therapist, and did not explore emotional issues or the potential for somatisation of mental health disorders as Carol was to see the psychologist.

Gail asked Carol to rate her pain on a scale of one to 10, in which one would be no pain at all and 10 would be the worse pain that she could imagine. Carol said that she had a constant pain level of 4/10, which she always felt in her neck and shoulders and she described this as an aching pain. This ache increased to 6/10 when she tried to do anything, such as working on her computer. Carol said her pain rating went up further to 9/10 when she experienced a spasm of pain, which she got several times a day. She was incapacitated by these spasms and had to lie down with her wheat pack (which she heats up in the microwave) until the spasm had passed and she had recovered. Gail then asked Carol to rate her level of disability on a 10-point scale, with one equal to being able to do everything she wanted and 10 meaning that she was unable to do anything. Carol rated her usual disability level at 7/10 but said this went up to 10/10 or more when she had spasms.

During the assessment, Gail was looking for clues to Carol's stressors and also to what might motivate her. (Gail sees therapists as detectives who are trying to find out what makes a person tick and to seek a way in to help change their behaviour in order to influence their health; this way in can be unique to the individual and is a key component to building a successful therapeutic relationship.) She asked Carol a bit more about the strategies she had tried to deal with her pain. From her response, Gail judged that Carol had a very passive approach to managing her pain and had waited for doctors and therapists to offer medication and physically focused treatments. She also appeared to have lost a lot of confidence.

Gail concluded her assessment by asking Carol: 'What are you hoping to get out of seeing us today?'

When Carol replied 'a cure', Gail responded: 'Do you think that's realistic?'

Carol shrugged and rather resignedly said: 'I guess not.'

Gail continued: 'So what would be the next best thing for you then?'

After a minute's reflection, Carol said: 'I just want to find some way of dealing with this awful pain and would love to get a good night's sleep.'

Gail's general impression of Carol was that she was very tense and anxious, a general worrier and a bit of a perfectionist. (During the assessment process, Gail is matching the person's described symptoms with the physical findings from the assessment and looking for any discrepancies.)

At the end of the assessment, Gail provided Carol with a brief summary of her findings. It was important to focus on building trust and rapport with Carol because of her negative feelings towards physiotherapy and to validate her pain. Only an explanation that she felt would be acceptable was made at this point in time as further discussion with the team would decide the final explanation and treatment plan to be suggested to Carol. Gail said that she felt Carol was generally unfit because she was fearful of movement as this had increased her pain in the past. This had affected her posture; her muscles were sore and out of condition, and this added to her pain problem. She asked Carol if she agreed with this summary and asked her if it had affected her in any other way. Carol replied she was less confident than she used to be.

Gail often starts her client education intervention during the first assessment, and in this instance she gave a description of a prolapsed disc and described what happens when a disc is injured. The focus of this initial client education was to begin to dispel some misconceptions Carol had about her discs and spine. This had to be handled with tact; because Carol had been a nursing auxiliary, she thought she had a good knowledge of the physical body, but Gail had picked up on several inaccuracies and needed to start re-educating Carol about how her body worked.

Gail concluded by saying that the whole team would meet with her after she had seen the occupational therapist and psychologist and would talk to her about potential treatment approaches then. She then escorted Carol to the waiting area and let Heather know that Carol was available for her occupational therapy assessment.

OCCUPATIONAL THERAPY ASSESSMENT

Heather asked Carol if she had seen an occupational therapist in the past. Carol replied: 'I've never had an occupational therapist before; what are you going to do for me?' Heather explained what occupational therapists do and her role within the CPS. She explained to Carol that: 'Occupational therapists are interested in what you do and the problems the pain causes you in the activities you need, want or expect to do in the course of a day. Occupational therapists usually focus on the day-to-day activities that people need, want or expect to do in order to help them do as much as they can despite any difficulties they may have. Within the CPS, this means learning to pace, which involves managing an activity so that you can do things without causing a flare up of pain. The other focus of my work is often around people's life balance, encouraging a return to valued roles and helping people deal with stress management issues. This could involve filling in a pacing diary to identify activities that trigger pain. Once I have a baseline for a client's tolerance levels for their daily activities, I will support them to gradually increase their activity. We set goals for activity levels and tolerance times, and these are increased when each level has been achieved comfortably.'

Heather focuses her assessment process around what a person can and cannot do in daily life. Therefore, she uses a standardised, client-centred, self-report measure as the focus of her first assessment; this is the COPM (Law *et al.*, 1991) and she uses it as both a descriptive measure to identify problems and priorities for treatment and as an outcome measure to evaluate clinically relevant changes following intervention.

Heather began her assessment process with an informal interview to build rapport and learn about Carol and her life. She started by asking Carol about her family and tried to identify Carol's key roles and responsibilities. Carol had been married to Jim for 25 years. She had a son, Paul, who was 24 years old and lived about 10 miles away with his girlfriend. She also had a daughter, Sarah, who was 20 and still living at home. Heather used the COPM to explore Carol's ability to perform self-care, productivity and leisure activities and to identify how satisfied Carol felt with her performance in these three occupational areas. (Heather expands on the assessment of the client's ability to perform activities by exploring how long a person can tolerate performing an activity before the pain gets worse.) Heather helped Carol to identify areas that were problematic and to rate which of these were the most important for her to improve. (In addition to the traditional self-care areas on the COPM, Heather also asks her clients about their sleep and about areas of tension in their lives.)

Carol said that her husband and daughter now did all the shopping, cooking and ironing and most of the housework. Carol reported that her pain had got much worse over the last 18 months and that she had gradually stopped doing things that made her pain worse, like driving more than a couple of miles, anything that she needed to stand to do, like cooking, anything that was heavy work, like vacuuming or mopping, and anything that involved walking for more than a few yards, like shopping. She said that she still tried to do some light housework, such as dusting, but could only manage to do this for very short periods. Heather asked her how long she could continue with dusting before she had to stop. Carol responded by saying: 'I keep going as long as I can. I don't like to give in; so I do it for as long as I can.'

Heather probed further to clarify her tolerance: 'So how many minutes on average can you manage when you're dusting?'

Carol said: 'Well, it all depends on whether I get a spasm or not; when I get spasms, they are excruciating and I have to stop immediately and usually end up going to bed with a hot-water bottle for a couple of hours before I can do anything again.'

Heather questioned further: 'But if you don't have a spasm, then how long will you manage to dust for?'

Carol replied: 'Well, it does depend on whether I'm having a bad day or not. I try to keep going as long as I can.'

To which Heather asked: 'So on a good day what would be the longest you could manage?'

Carol said: 'On a really good day, I might manage to dust the living room, and that takes me about 15 minutes if I push myself really hard.'

In terms of leisure interests, Carol painted a picture of herself 10 years before as a very fit woman who went on long hikes with her husband and children in the Yorkshire Dales most weekends and who had loved to go ballroom dancing with Jim at least twice a week. She had not managed either of these leisure pursuits since her accident 10 years before and now perceived herself as being very unfit. They had purchased a computer six months ago and Carol was trying to occupy her time by learning some basic computer skills, such as using the Internet to email her son, and she had been wondering about Internet shopping but had been nervous about giving her credit-card details online and was anxious as to whether goods would really be delivered. She said she liked the computer but it made her neck and shoulder pain much worse within about 10 minutes.

Carol's husband was a taxi driver and she said this meant he worked shifts and was not always around to help her when she was having spasms. However, Carol described him as 'very supportive and helpful when he is at home' and said that he worked his shifts so that he could pop home to cook Carol some tea if her daughter was going to be out. Heather ascertained that Carol was feeling quite guilty that her family was doing so much around the house and felt that she had lost one of her primary roles as a homemaker. She thought she was a burden on her family and worried that Sarah might have chosen to leave home by now had she not needed her help so much. Carol appeared to be close to her husband and grateful for his support.

She said: 'I don't know what I'd do without Jim; he's been so fantastic.' She became upset and angry when referring to her lost compensation claim: 'Jim is working too hard; now I can't work he has to work much longer hours just to bring in enough money. I didn't earn much when I was nursing, but it helped. That's why I needed my compensation – so Jim wouldn't have to work so hard.'

Heather then helped Carol to identify some realistic outcomes.

'How would people know you were getting better?' she asked her.

Carol replied: 'Well, I'd be back at work.'

Heather continued: 'Well, that would be much better and I'm not talking about a magic-wand treatment, rather how would people know you were a bit better?'

'Well, Jim would think I was a bit better if I had a good night's sleep and that would be great for him too because my tossing and turning disturbs his sleep as well.' Heather identified improving sleep as the first goal and continued: 'And what other things would show you were a bit better?'

Carol replied: 'People would see me out walking again. I hate being stuck in doors, as I used to love getting out into the countryside for walks most weekends.'

'So increasing your walking tolerance will be a second goal, and what else do you want to improve?' continued Heather.

'It would be good to be cooking a meal sometimes and to be able to go shopping with my daughter. I can't manage the heavy grocery shopping but I'd like to get out to buy clothes or presents for my family.'

Carol also identified that she was getting tense and irritable with the pain and that Jim would like it if she was less snappy.

Like Gail, Heather began her summary by validating Carol's pain and her frustration with her level of disability. She then explained further about the possible occupational therapy interventions, which would aim to help Carol manage her pain and gradually increase her activities. Heather explained that she could not take Carol's pain away but would work with her to teach her how to manage her pain better in order to do the things that she wanted to be able to do. The intervention would not be a hands-on treatment. Carol would be expected to take a lead role in her treatment programme and would be taught techniques and strategies to try out by herself at home. Heather explained that they would be trying to re-educate Carol's nervous system and would build up her ability by introducing pacing and a relaxation technique. This would involve seeing Carol for about three therapy sessions. During this intervention Heather planned to:

- explain what pacing is and how it affects pain
- provide Carol with an activity diary to complete daily (this would enable patterns of activity and triggers for pain to be identified)
- teach Carol a relaxation technique that would enable her muscles to recover between activity and would probably help her sleep.

At this point, Carol said to Heather: 'You haven't asked me where the pain is or what my pain is like. Do you want me to explain my symptoms to you?'

Heather responded: 'Have you explained the location and type of pain already to the doctor and the physiotherapist?'

'Oh yes; they both asked me all about it,' she replied.

'Well, we don't want clients to waste time and energy repeating the same story over and over again; so each team member focuses on a different part of your assessment. As an occupational therapist, my focus is on what you can and can't do, and also what you have given up doing because of the pain and what you would like to be doing again. In the information that we sent out to you was a leaflet about confidentiality and sharing information; have you had a chance to read it?'

Carol confirmed: 'Yes, I got it and I have read it through.'

'So you understand, then, that we work closely as a team and will share the results of our individual assessments so we can form a comprehensive picture of your condition. When we have our meeting, the doctor and physiotherapist will tell the rest of the team about your pain symptoms,' explained Heather.

At the end of the assessment, Carol and Heather mutually agreed that her goals would be to:

- increase the length of time she was able to sleep
- increase her tolerance on the computer, aiming for sessions of 30 minutes
- increase the distance she could walk, aiming to walk from home to the postbox two streets away to post her own bills and letters
- improve her pain management so she could prepare a one-course meal for her family
- manage her pain to go on a one-hour shopping trip with her daughter
- learn to reduce tension through relaxation techniques.

Heather used the COPM to record baseline scores out of 10 for the first five goals. Carol rated her ability to sleep as 3/10 and said her level of satisfaction with the quality and amount of her sleep was very low; so she rated this as only 1/10 for satisfaction. In terms of her ability to use the computer, she gave herself 2/10 and also rated her satisfaction as 2/10. She felt a tiny bit better about her ability to walk and gave this 3/10 for performance but as she used to go on long hikes with her family at weekends she felt very dissatisfied with her current walking tolerance and so only rated this 1/10 for satisfaction. Carol hardly ever prepared meals anymore; so this goal was set baseline scores of 1/10 for both performance and satisfaction. Finally, she rated her ability to go shopping as 3/10 and her satisfaction with this activity as 2/10 (see Table 12.3, p. 386, for a summary of Carol's COPM baseline scores).

Heather's impression was that Carol was quite physically focused and her expectations of treatment were unrealistic. She also wondered if her family were overly supportive and whether they had taken over too much responsibility for household chores, shopping and cooking, leading Carol to experience a sense of loss of role within the family. It was going to be important to encourage Carol to share her goals with her family and for them to support her to do more at home.

IDENTIFICATION OF PROBLEMS TO BE THE FOCUS OF THERAPY

Table 12.1 lists the therapy problems for Carol to work on that the two therapists identified.

Table 12.1 Identified problems for therapy intervention

Physiotherapy problem list	Occupational therapy problem list
1. Poor general fitness	1. Poor pacing skills
2. Poor posture	2. High tension levels
3. Myofascial pain	3. Loss of role
4. Chronic pain syndrome/anxiety re future	4. High dependence on others
	5. Decreased social activities

MULTIDISCIPLINARY TEAM MEETING WITH CAROL

The team got back together when they had all finished their individual assessments with Carol. Gail's and Heather's findings and diagnoses were discussed with the other team members and the therapists suggested some individual treatment followed by a Turnabout pain management programme. The team diagnosed Carol as having myofascial pain and chronic pain syndrome. Each team member summarised their findings.

SUMMARY OF THE RESULTS OF OTHER TEAM MEMBERS' ASSESSMENTS

Psychologist

The psychologist identified the following problems.

- low mood, but not clinically depressed
- low self-esteem
- guilt regarding not being able to carry out role
- external locus of control

Doctor

The doctor said that he agreed with Gail's findings and felt there was no further pathology to be concerned about. He felt Carol was on a suitable medication regime.

Gail and Heather then proposed individual treatment plans for Carol.

Box 12.1 Carol's individual treatment plans

Occupational therapy (Heather)
1. Instruction in pacing and relaxation.
2. Education aimed at improving Carol's motivation to engage in a pain management approach.

Physiotherapy (Gail)
1. Teaching an individual programme of exercise aimed at improving Carol's posture and fitness and decreasing her fear of movement and further injury.
2. Basic education regarding chronic pain and the need for exercise and encouraging her to participate in a pain management programme.
3. Suggestion that in future a referral to the gym or a Pilates group may be of benefit.

The team agreed to Gail and Heather's plans and Carol and her husband were invited in to discuss the findings and plan. They explained to Carol how tension, worry and guilt can play a significant part in the vicious cycle of pain. At this point, Carol became quite defensive and questioned: 'Are you saying it's all in my head?'

The team again validated Carol's pain and problems and explained their Biopsychosocial model (Waddell, 1992) in simple terms, saying that they take an approach which looks at the way a person's body and mind work in tandem and how the body and mind can influence each other, both positively and negatively. They explore how the pain affects the whole person (for example their social life, physical relationships and activity) and how pain can make a person feel down in the dumps and more irritable. The team explained to Carol that as in the past she had received symptomatic relief which obviously had not worked (and they confirmed this was Carol's perception too) the team would offer her an approach which would not be a cure but would help her to change some aspects of her life and her behaviour in order to learn to cope with the pain and gain some control over her life.

Carol was given the opportunity to ask questions at the end of her meeting with the team. Her main question was: 'So you're saying there's no cure for me?' The team explained that at the moment there was no cure and that evidence suggested that the best way of managing chronic pain was the plan they were suggesting. The team then described the Turnabout programme to Carol and her husband, and provided her with a leaflet about the programme. They explained that she would receive individual physiotherapy and occupational therapy to start with and that the therapists would be aiming towards her joining a Turnabout group within six months. She was asked if she preferred appointments to be arranged for both occupational therapy and physiotherapy sessions at the same time, and Carol said she would prefer this. Carol was seen by Gail and Heather on the same day for her first appointment but found it very tiring to have two individual therapy sessions back to back and so future sessions were booked on different days.

INDIVIDUAL TREATMENT SESSIONS WITH THE PHYSIOTHERAPIST

Gail started Carol's intervention by providing her with a TENS (transcutaneous electrical nerve stimulation) machine to use at home. This was to give Carol a pain management intervention that she could control herself to encourage her to take a more active approach to controlling her pain. Gail demonstrated to Carol how to use the machine. Carol then tried to put it on herself and adjusted the controls to experience different levels of input. Gail assessed that Carol would be competent to use the TENS independently and suggested that Carol borrow a machine to trial at home, particularly when she was experiencing the acute pain associated with her spasms.

Next, Gail talked to Carol about her fear of movement and reassured her that some gentle exercise would be beneficial. Gail continued her educational role and was keen to correct any continuing misconceptions. Carol had a fear that her spine 'was crumbling' and thought that her disc had 'slipped out'. Gail used a model of the spine and discs to show Carol how the discs and spine worked. Gail wanted to work with Carol on the movements and activities that were the most difficult for her and which she was either modifying or avoiding altogether.

Physiotherapists teach people how to exercise despite chronic pain. The aim was for Carol to build up all-round fitness levels so she could resume normal everyday activities with greater ease. She taught Carol a series of exercises aimed at improving her posture, increasing flexibility and stretching her hamstrings. Carol practised these exercises in front of Gail, who monitored and corrected her technique until she felt that Carol would be able to perform the exercises effectively on her own at home. Carol was given a handout with diagrams and instructions to remind her of the exercise regime, and they mutually agreed the number of repetitions that Carol should try to undertake each day.

They ended the session with a discussion about the potential benefits of acupuncture. The aim of using acupuncture is to reduce the level of pain in order to enable a client to carry out the pacing, relaxation and exercises taught by the therapist. Gail and Carol mutually agreed that Carol would receive a trial of four acupuncture sessions.

At Carol's second appointment, Gail wanted to evaluate any benefits or problems related to the use of the TENS machine. Self-report was the best form of assessment. Carol reported that she had managed to put on the TENS machine herself and had used it frequently and found it helped her to bear the acute spasms of pain. Carol reported that she felt her pain reduced when she was using the TENS machine and said she was able to relax more in the evening when she was using it. Gail therefore advised Carol to purchase her own TENS machine. Carol felt this would be worthwhile and said she was happy to do this. She asked for advice on specifications and where she might be able to purchase one.

Gail then asked Carol how she had managed with her exercise regime. Carol reported that she had been motivated and with encouragement from her husband and daughter had done at least a few of the exercises every day. She admitted that she had not always achieved the agreed number of repetitions for every exercise as she felt some were harder than others. Gail asked Carol to demonstrate how she was doing her exercises so that she could monitor Carol's technique and assess whether she was still restricted by fear of movement. She corrected Carol's technique on a couple of exercises and reiterated the educational messages about Carol's spine that they had discussed in the first session. Gail then suggested increasing the number of repetitions on the exercises she was managing well and encouraged aiming for the original number of repetitions set for the other exercises. Gail reiterated the need for the regular exercise programme and explained that although Carol might feel progress was slow the benefits of improving her posture, flexibility and strength would be significant if she persevered. At the end of the second appointment, Gail discussed the group Turnabout programme and explained its purpose and content in more depth. Carol said that she was interested in attending Turnabout although a bit nervous about being in a group.

INDIVIDUAL TREATMENT SESSIONS WITH THE OCCUPATIONAL THERAPIST

Heather had decided that the main focus of her sessions would be on teaching Carol pacing and relaxation techniques. She also planned to work with Carol on building self-esteem, assertiveness, communication skills and confidence. An aspect of this would involve correcting errors in Carol's thinking. She intended to support Carol to look at replacing previous leisure activities, like her ballroom dancing, and to encourage her to resume walking.

At the first session, Heather provided neutral information using a motivational interviewing technique to help reduce resistance. Information was given about pacing. Heather described how this had helped others and also explained how to overcome the difficulties that can be found when trying to pace. Pacing involves the occupational therapist teaching people how to set personal goals and then break them down into mini goals with a systematic plan of how to achieve them. The aim was for Carol to resume whatever activities she wished to undertake. She was told that this may include everyday activities, hobbies, leisure pursuits and work (including voluntary work and other responsibilities), and Heather reminded Carol of the treatment goals they had set together at the end of her first assessment. Pacing involved Carol gradually building up her chosen activity in a steady and systematic way so that eventually she could achieve her personal goals despite the pain. Heather set a first homework task of a pacing diary. Carol was asked to keep an Activity Diary, in which she would record what she did, how long she engaged in the activity and her pain levels during the activity. This would enable Heather and Carol to establish baseline tolerances for different activities and then to work to increase Carol's tolerance. In particular, Heather asked Carol to note how she managed activities that they had identified as her treatment goals during the assessment. Carol was asked to bring this Activity Diary with her to her next occupational therapy appointment.

Heather provided the rationale for learning a relaxation technique. (Muscle tension is a common response to pain and stress. Heather teaches a variety of relaxation techniques for clients to practise frequently and be able to use in different circumstances. These skills help people with chronic pain to manage challenging situations, movements or activities, including sleeping difficulties, more easily. Relaxation techniques can be used effectively alongside pacing to enable clients to build up the amount of exercise or activity they can undertake with greater ease.) Carol agreed to try this approach, and abdominal breathing techniques were taught. All the information Heather had shared with Carol on pacing and relaxation techniques were backed up by handouts, which Carol was to refer to at home. As a second homework task, Carol was instructed to practise the relaxation technique daily.

At the second occupational therapy individual treatment session, Heather started by asking Carol to share her Activity Diary. They went through Carol's diary entries and Heather encouraged Carol to discuss what she had learnt through filling in her diary. Together, they then identified specific activities to pace, particularly activities that were linked to Carol's treatment goals. Using the times and pain levels recorded in the diary, Heather established baseline tolerances for the focus activities. She instructed Carol that these were to be increased by a maximum of 10 per cent at a time so that tolerance times are achieved comfortably. For example, if Carol had managed an activity, such as walking, for 10 minutes, she would aim to increase this by 10 per cent, which would be an additional one minute, giving a goal time of 11 minutes for the activity. Homework was set on pacing specific activities identified after discussion. Heather described how this could be achieved by using the example of meal preparation. Carol was shown how to break down the task of preparing a meal for her family. She was to attempt this task in different stages and to think carefully about the menu chosen, how easy this would be to prepare, whether she would need to go shopping for ingredients, how long it should take to prepare and timing the preparation. Heather encouraged Carol to think how she could pace the cooking by spreading out the meal preparation; for example, could any tasks, such as preparing vegetables, be done in advance?

Heather then explored how Carol had managed with the relaxation technique. Carol said that she found the breathing technique hard to start with but was excited to find she was getting the hang of it and reported that she was more able to relax. Heather encouraged Carol to keep this up.

Heather encouraged her to progress to the stage of preparing to change. Many people with chronic pain have already developed some strategies to manage their pain. Heather's aim was to further develop the helpful strategies Carol was already using, support her to reduce the unhelpful ones and teach her new strategies and support her to practise these until they became habitual behaviours. Changing the way a person does things can take a long time and for people with chronic pain may need to be a life-long process. Carol's work with staff at the CPS was an important starting point for these changes. Heather took on an educational role by explaining to Carol about the Stages of Change model and encouraging her to identify where she was in the process (Prochaska and DiClemente, 1982, 1986, 1992; Prochaska, DiClemente and Norcross, 1998). Carol was still at the early stage of contemplating a change. Heather emphasised that much of the work would need to be done by Carol at home, where she could start to put into practice the strategies in her normal, daily life.

Gail and Heather liaised outside the individual therapy sessions regarding their treatment approaches and Carol's response to particular interventions. They then reinforced the messages and techniques that the other therapist was using during their next sessions in order to ensure that Carol received consistent messages from each member of the CPS team. Gail and Heather discussed Carol's progress and agreed that she was ready to be allocated to the next Turnabout programme.

THE GROUP INTERVENTION PROGRAMME: TURNABOUT

The Turnabout programme is aimed at breaking the common vicious cycle experienced by many pain sufferers and improving the individual's quality of life. Carol was asked to attend three days per week for four weeks. The four-week programme is shown in Figures 12.1 and 12.2. Therapists find that this programme gives clients a reason to get up and go to the Turnabout session, which in turn can help prepare them for returning to the routine of going out to work.

The Turnabout programme is led by the team's psychologist, but all CPS team members participate and outside speakers are also invited to participate in the programme. Throughout the programme, team members teach a number of different skills. Effective pain management

TIMES	Monday	Wednesday	Friday	Monday	Wednesday	Friday
8.30–11.00	Getting to know you	Exercise theory and practice	Exercise	Stress and its influence on pain	Exercise on prescription	Joints exercise
11.00						
11.15–12.00	What is pain ↓	Pacing ↓	Triggers/ behaviours/ consequences	Pain theory	Disability employment adviser	Life balance roles
12.00–12.30				Relaxation	Relaxation	Relaxation
12.30–1.30						
1.30–2.30	Fitness assessments	Introduction to relaxation stages of change		Goal setting and rewards	Communication	
2.30						
2.45–4.30	Using art to communicate about your pain	Back care and posture		Hydrotherapy	Depression	

NB – all sessions are negotiable

Figure 12.1 Turnabout programme: weeks 1 and 2.

involves integrating all of the skills taught on the programme to address the challenge of living with chronic pain. None of the skills taught are designed to cure the pain but, applied together and over the long term, aim to improve a person's quality of life. During Turnabout, Carol took part in a programme of educational and fitness sessions and received group-based instruction in pain coping strategies. In the Turnabout programme, Heather led group sessions on pacing, communication, stress management, life balance and goal setting. This supported Carol to build on the work she had undertaken in her individual occupational therapy sessions. In addition to input from CPS staff, outside speakers talked about several topics, including returning to work, disability benefits and complementary therapies. As the team feel it important that family and friends understand the concepts of the programme, Carol's husband and daughter were invited to attend one session with her.

TIMES	Monday	Wednesday	Friday	Monday	Wednesday	Friday
8.30–11.00	Neurology	Injury and healing exercise	Exercise	Exercise	Exercise	Fitness reassessment
11.00						
11.15–12.00	Tests and examinations ↓	Medication ↓	Thinking	Citizens Advice Bureau ↓	Worry-busting and problem-solving ↓	Life balance roles
12.00–12.30						
12.30–1.30						
1.30–2.30	Volunteers organiser	Friends/relatives group ↓		Massage	Sleep	
2.30						
2.45–4.30	Hydrotherapy			Relationships	Setbacks and flare ups	

NB – all sessions are negotiable

Figure 12.2 Turnabout programme: weeks 3 and 4.

During the Turnabout programme, the clients undertake an exercise circuit that involves arm lifts with weights, back raises, press-ups against a wall, sit-ups lying on the floor, time on the treadmill and on the bike and step-ups. Results from each part of the circuit are plotted onto graphs so that clients have a visual record of their progress. This enables clients to reflect on peaks and troughs and to see the benefits of pacing. Each group member is supported to develop a personal plan to steadily and systematically build up each exercise. The aim is to show participants what they can achieve and have them complete the Turnabout programme with the ability and confidence to continue to improve their own fitness into the future. Practice in a group with other chronic pain sufferers enabled Carol to improve her fitness, balance and flexibility in a supportive environment.

Gail uses some fitness measures to evaluate clients' progress during the Turnabout programme. The measures she uses are based on research by Vicky Harding at St Thomas' Hospital and have been agreed by the Physiotherapy Pain Association (http://www.ppaonline. co.uk). For example, see Harding, *et al.*'s (1994) paper on the development of a battery of measures for assessing physical functioning of chronic pain clients and their website for the INPUT pain management unit at Guy's and St Thomas' Hospital in London (http://www. inputpainunit.net). The fitness measures used were:

- a three-minute measured walk (measured in laps)
- one-minute measured step-ups (stepping on and off a block)
- one-minute measured sit-ups (chair to standing).

During these assessments, Gail also observes for and records pain behaviours. Gail measures outcome using the three fitness tests at the end of the Turnabout programme and at reviews.

Towards the end of the Turnabout programme, clients are asked to write a completion story, to share with staff and group members on the last day of the programme. For their completion story, they are asked to describe what they were like before the programme and what they are like now, to identify what they liked most and least about the programme, to assess where they are in the change model and to make plans for the future, including setting some specific goals to be achieved by their six-week review. Carol's completion story is provided in Box 12.2.

Box 12.2 Carol's completion story

What were you like before the programme?
- I was quite depressed and isolated. I felt no one understood the problems I had. I felt very guilty that my family had to do so much for me.

What has changed?
- Knowing I am not alone and that others understand has lifted my mood. I feel I now have a toolbox to use to help me get back some of the things I have lost.

What did you enjoy most about the programme?
- Meeting with others with similar problems. Being believed and understood. Also the fun and laughter.

What did you enjoy least about the programme?
- I found it hard to concentrate for such long periods of time.

Carol's goal planning built upon the earlier goals she had set with Heather at her first assessment and so the original COPM baseline scores were still relevant for measuring outcomes. Carol's goals are shown in Table 12.2 (below).

Table 12.2 Carol's goal planning

Goal planning: Occupational area	Carol's goals
A. Work (paid/unpaid, e.g. voluntary work)	1. Increase time spent at computer 2. Cook more meals for family (3 times per week)
B. Pleasurable/leisure activities	3. More shopping trips with daughter 4. Go for a massage
C. Daily exercise	5. Take a short walk daily 6. Continue with exercises regime every other day
D. Social activities	7. Get back in touch with at least one friend 8. Go out with husband once a fortnight
E. Other	9. Use relaxation technique daily, especially to improve sleep

OUTCOME MEASUREMENT AND DISCHARGE

At the end of the Turnabout programme, Heather reassessed Carol's progress using both a standardised measure (the COPM) and an informal measure (Carol's completion story). Gail re-assessed using the three fitness tests and found that Carol's ability to perform these tests had increased.

- Carol's measured walk had increased from four laps to six laps during a timed three-minute period.
- Carol's sitting to standing measure improved from eight to 11 during a timed one-minute test.
- Carol's step-ups improved from 10 to 14 during a timed one-minute test.

In addition, a graph of her performance on the exercise circuit demonstrated a change in her approach to exercise indicative of better pacing.

FIRST FOLLOW-UP EVALUATION

Six weeks after completing the Turnabout programme, the group were invited to return for a half day. In the first six weeks, group members were expected to have tried integrating pain management strategies into their own everyday lives. At the follow-up session, Carol and her fellow group members discussed how they were managing since finishing the programme. Staff used a problem-solving approach to encourage the group to share their achievements and discuss difficulties and possible solutions. It was a chance for Carol to review her personal goals and think about the next steps that she needed to take in order to work towards her long-term goals. In addition to the group follow-up session, Carol was re-assessed individually by her therapists.

Carol reported that she had experienced a flare up about three weeks after she had been discharged from the programme, but she said she had been doing well up until then. Carol explained that this flare up had put 'me in a panic that I was going back to square one', and she admitted that she had forgotten to look at her setback plan. However, she explained that over the six-week period she had used some of the skills taught on the programme, especially pacing and relaxation techniques. Carol was pleased that, since the flare up had subsided, she had been successful with her meal-preparation goal and reported that she was now cooking a few meals each week for the family. She was also increasing the amount of time spent on her computer.

Heather provided positive encouragement for the gains Carol had made and the goals she had achieved. Heather and Carol went through her flare-up plan and discussed what Carol should do next time she had a flare up and planned how Carol would pace and return to her previous level of activity after a setback. Staff talked to Carol about how to access exercise on prescription (Department of Health, 2001c).

Carol was asked to consider whether she wanted to set any new goals to achieve in the long term. She said she would like to return to work eventually. Heather asked her to think about a stepping stone to this long-term goal, and Carol agreed that she would explore a non-strenuous volunteer job part-time. She also set the goal of starting some sort of evening class to learn a new skill. Carol was given the phone number of her local voluntary services organiser. This contact could be useful for two reasons: to link Carol to potential support networks and community groups and also to encourage her to explore volunteering as a way of resuming some productive activities and perhaps even prepare for returning to some sort of paid employment on a part-time basis.

SIX-MONTH FOLLOW-UP EVALUATION

Carol returned to the CPS for a review six months after her discharge from the Turnabout programme. This gave her another opportunity to reflect on her progress and review the integration of pain management strategies into her daily life and consider the benefits and any challenges she was experiencing. Carol was asked to think about her longer-term goals and was encouraged to set some new goals for the future.

At her review, Carol told Heather: 'I'm now feeling like I've got the hang of the pacing. I'm much more laid back about the housework and leave it, rather than expecting my husband and daughter to do it, when it is not done. Then often in a day or two I can mange to do a bit of housework again and catch up on chores.'

Carol also reported that she had enrolled on an evening class to learn digital camera photography. Carol reported that she was continuing to exercise on a regular basis, was doing more than when she first came to the clinic and was using relaxation to help her sleep.

She said: 'I feel like I'm getting my life back. I still get down at times, especially if I start to think about how I used to be, but I'm getting much better at stopping negative thoughts. I don't brood as much and I'm being more positive. Seeing what the others achieved in our Turnabout group made me feel I wanted to try harder.'

At the six-month review appointment, Heather re-administered the COPM to obtain Carol's follow-up scores for both performance and satisfaction on her five goal areas; her baseline (initial assessment) and follow-up (six-month post-discharge) scores are shown in Table 12.3).

From these individual scores, Heather took the average of scores across the five goal areas to produce total COPM scores for performance and satisfaction (these results are shown in Table 12.4).

In order to examine clinical outcome, Heather then calculated Carol's change scores. This is done by subtracting the total score at time 1 (baseline) from the total score at time 2 (in this case at six months).

Table 12.3 Carol's COPM results at six months

Goal area	Performance baseline	Satisfaction baseline	Performance at 6 months	Satisfaction at 6 months
Sleep	3	1	6	7
Using computer	2	2	5	5
Walking	3	1	5	6
Preparing meals	1	1	7	7
Shopping	3	2	5	6

Table 12.4 Carol's combined COPM scores for five goal areas

	Time 1 COPM score for 5 goals		Time 2 COPM score for 5 goals
Performance baseline	2.4	Performance outcome	5.6
Satisfaction baseline	1.4	Satisfaction outcome	6.2

CAROL'S COPM CHANGE SCORES

For overall performance, Carol had a follow-up score of 5.6, which minus the baseline of 2.4 gave a change score of 3.2, which indicated clinically significant improved performance across her five goal areas. Carol had a total satisfaction score of 6.2, which minus her baseline satisfaction score of 1.4 gave a change score of 4.8. These change scores indicated clinically significant improvement in both areas, with Carol's level of satisfaction increasing more than her perceived change in performance; this finding is usual. Validity studies conducted on the COPM have indicated that a change score of two or more represents an outcome that is considered clinically important by the client, family and therapist (Carswell *et al.*, 2004; Law *et al.*, 1998). Carol's change scores were above two for both performance and satisfaction, indicating clinically important change following intervention.

At the time that Carol attended, reviews were conducted at six weeks, six months and two years, but as only 50 per cent of clients return for their two-year follow-up, the team is changing to a six-month and then a one-year review. Further follow-up reviews for Carol were planned at six months and two years. Carol did not attend the two-year review as she telephoned to say that she was unable to attend as she had a part-time job. During her phone call, she said she had made friends with one of the other members of her Turnabout group and they continued to see each other regularly and support each other. Overall, Carol said she was 'finding life much improved'. The last contact with Carol was when the team received a postcard from her, which she had sent them while on holiday in Spain, to say she was having a lovely time and was enjoying life again.

SERVICE REVIEW

Every two years, the team undertakes an analysis of COPM baseline and follow-up scores for all their individual clients and for all groups that have undertaken one of the three Turnabout programmes (Turnabout, Turnabout Active and Turnabout Easy). The team uses this data to produce graphs to illustrate CPS service outcomes.

COPM data showed significant improvement for clients being seen individually and in Turnabout pain management programmes (see Table 12.5). Data also showed there had been no drop-outs from programmes.

Table 12.5 Group COPM data for the CPS Turnabout pain management programmes

	Clinically significant improvement		Not clinically significant improvement		Negative scores	
	Performance	Satisfaction	Performance	Satisfaction	Performance	Satisfaction
Individual	76%	73%	24%	27%	0	0
Turnabout	79%	84.2%	21%	15.8%	0	0
Turnabout Easy	74%	87%	21%	13%	4.3	0
Turnabout Active	69.2%	77%	30.9%	23%	0	0

At the end of each Turnabout session, clients are asked to complete a feedback sheet on the content, presentation and handouts for that day. At the end of each programme, the therapists meet for a debriefing session to review client feedback and to reflect on what the therapists thought went well and what they feel could be improved. As a result of service review, the format of the Turnabout programme has now been changed from three times per week for four weeks to twice a week for six weeks. Programme feedback has led the team to introduce more active 'moving about' activities and techniques after group members complained of sitting too long. The CPS has also established a pre-programme Turnabout information session so that people have a better understanding of what is on offer and can make a more informed choice as to which of the programmes will best suit them. Staff received feedback about the quality of some of the handout material and the team has organised a re-printing of illegible handouts. Handouts are now being scrutinised by a client group.

Brief Answers to Study Questions

Study questions have been provided at the end of Chapters 2 through to 11. This section provides some brief answers to these questions.

CHAPTER 2

2.1 Direct measures involve observations, standardised assessment and client self-report. Indirect methods can include referral information, client records and reports from the person's carer or family members or from other professionals or service providers who are working with the client.

2.2 Three sources for gathering assessment data are:
- self-report from client
- proxy/informant report
- direct observation undertaken by the therapist

2.3 Self-report data can be collected by interview, asking the client to keep a journal or the use of standardised or unstandardised checklists and questionnaires.

2.4 Types of informants/proxies include:
- the person's primary carer
- other members of the therapist's multidisciplinary team
- other health professionals involved with the client's care
- other professionals working with the client

2.5 Methods for collecting proxy/informant report data include interviewing the proxy face to face or over the telephone, through case conferences, ward rounds and team meetings or via written data (e.g. letters, standardised or unstandardised checklists and questionnaires, referrals, medical notes and assessment reports).

2.6 The three phases of an interview are initiation, development and closing.

2.7 The factors that might influence the outcome of an interview are perceptual factors, such as how sensory stimuli affect the way the other person is perceived, conceptual factors (which include the therapist's knowledge base), role issues (which include the way each person perceives the role he or she is to play in the interview) and self-esteem issues (which involve the way each person feels about himself or herself) (Fidler, 1976, cited by Smith, 1993), environmental factors, the influence of the therapist, the influence of the client and the nature of the dynamic interactions between therapist and client (Borg and Bruce, 1991).

2.8 An advantage of collecting self-report data is that you gain insight into the client's perspectives, values, beliefs and priorities, which helps you to develop meaningful, client-centred treatment goals and plans. A disadvantage of collecting self-report data is that this method is not ideal for people with communication difficulties or people who lack insight.

CHAPTER 3

3.1 If I were choosing a suitable discriminative assessment for my clinical practice, the factors I would consider are the quality of the normative data and the relevance of the normative sample to my client group so that I could generalise with confidence from the normative data in the test manual to my clients. I would also review the test manual and associated research literature for evidence of discriminative validity.

3.2 Predictive assessment is undertaken by therapists to predict the future ability or state of a client or to predict a specific outcome in the future (Adams, 2002).

3.3 Therapists need to detect change in functioning over time, and evaluative assessment is undertaken to monitor a person's progress during rehabilitation and to determine the effectiveness of the intervention. It is critical to use objective and sensitive measures of outcome because 'any subjective estimate, especially if made by the clinician who has invested time, effort and perhaps more in treating the client, is likely to be unreliable' (de Clive-Lowe, 1996, p. 359). Standardised outcome measures are more likely to be valid, reliable and sensitive to change than so-called home-grown assessments.

3.4 Therapists need to undertake evaluations of their services because this can help to 'show that the intervention offered by the service is appropriate and effective; indicate areas where service development might be required or additional resources deployed; enable changes that lead to an improvement in consumer satisfaction; show that a contracted service has been provided; and indicate effective use of health resources' (Austin and Clark, 1993, p. 21).

CHAPTER 4

4.1 Both nominal and ordinal scales assign numbers to categorical data; however, with ordinal scales the categories can be assigned to some sort of rank order. This means a nominal scale is sufficient to measure the proportion of a population who has a particular characteristic or who achieves a particular outcome, while an ordinal scale can describe how one test score compares with another.

4.2 A ratio scale has a fixed origin or absolute zero point. This means that a ratio scale can be used to tell us how proportionally different one test score is from another test score.

4.3 In an interval scale, scores are classified by both order and by a known and equal interval between points (Lichtman *et al.*, 1989). This means an interval scale has rank order and the distances between the numbers have meaning with respect to the property being measured. An interval scale enables us to define how one test score differs from another.

4.4 Rasch analysis allows us 'to convert observed counts of ordinal data (raw scores) into an approximately equal-interval number line' (Fisher, 1993, p. 320). This enables us to compare how much more or less the person exhibits of the construct or behaviour being measured (Hayley *et al.*, 1998).

CHAPTER 5

5.1 A standardised test is a measurement tool that is published and has been developed for a specific purpose and for use with a particular client group. A standardised test should have detailed instructions explaining how and when it should be administered and scored. It should give guidance on how to interpret scores. The exact test materials should be listed or included. The test manual should provide results of investigations to evaluate the test's psychometric properties. If it is a norm-referenced test, the normative sample should be described and normative data should be provided to enable comparison with clients' scores.

5.2 A criterion-referenced test is used to evaluate a client against pre-defined criteria. With criterion-referenced tests, performance/attributes are not compared to those of other people (as with norm-referenced tests); they are evaluated only against the defined criterion. Criterion-referenced tests produce raw scores that have a direct, interpretable meaning. The person's score is interpreted by comparing it with a pre-specified standard of performance or against specific content and/or skills. Therapists use criterion-referenced tests to judge whether their clients have mastered the required standards (e.g. to judge whether the person has sufficient independence to be safe to be discharged to live alone at home).

5.3 Norm-referenced tests are used to determine clients' placement on a normal distribution curve. This enables therapists to evaluate the score obtained by an individual against the scores of a peer group whose performance has been described using a normative sample and to establish whether this score is significantly above or below what would be expected for a person of the same age, gender and sociocultural background. The test author should provide guidance for using the normative data to judge whether a person's attribute or performance represents a problem that will require some sort of intervention or further referral for support.

5.4 The standard deviation (σ) is a measure of the spread or extent of variability of a set of scores around their mean. It is the average amount a score varies from the average score in a series of scores. The standard deviation reflects the degree of homogeneity of the group with respect to the test item in question. In therapy measurement, standard deviations are used to indicate the degree to which a person's performance on the test is above or below average. Some tests use standard deviations to provide a cut-off point at which a person's performance is said to be dysfunctional or at which a specific deficit is considered to be present.

CHAPTER 6

6.1 The use of an expert panel is one method to examine the content validity of a test. The expert panel are given a copy of the draft test and asked to rate the relevance and acceptability of each test item. When matching test items to the performance domain to be measured by the test, experts can either make a dichotomous decision (i.e. the item either is or is not an aspect of the performance to be assessed) or experts rate the degree of match between the test item and the performance domain (e.g. using a five-point scale where 5 = an excellent match and 1 = no match). Another method used to help establish content validity is a content analysis of relevant research literature on the domain that is to be tested. This requires a clear definition of all the variables to be measured by the test, parameters to be set for the scope of the literature search and agreement about what is to be recorded in the content analysis of the literature. For a helpful example of a content validity study that provides clear details of the methodology followed, refer to the study by Clemson, Fitzgerald and Heard (1999).

6.2 Construct validity involves the extent to which an assessment can be said to measure a theoretical construct or constructs.

6.3 One type of criterion-related validity is concurrent validity and this is evaluated by comparing test data for the same sample of clients on two or more measures that have been designed to measure the same or similar content or constructs. Another type of criterion-related validity is predictive validity, which develops a hypothesis between the test scores and some future state or ability and then tests this hypothesis by studying whether the results obtained by the test directly predict the amount/frequency/timing of the domain or construct of interest.

6.4 Predictive validity relates to the accuracy with which a test predicts some future event. Predictive validity is important to therapists because they often need to make predictions, such as the person's function in a wide range of activities from observation of just a few activities, or the person's functioning in the future, such as upon discharge, or their function in a different environment.

6.5 Face validity relates to whether a test appears to measure what it is intended to measure as judged by clients taking the test, their family members, managers and other professionals who will see the test results. Therapists should consider face validity because if therapists are to be client-centred in their practice then the client's perception of any assessment process or standardised test as being relevant and meaningful is critical.

6.6 If I wanted to evaluate a test's clinical utility, I would examine the cost of the test, whether there are additional training requirements, the length of administration time, how long and how difficult it is to score and whether it is portable and I would then make a judgement of the overall usefulness of the test in my clinical setting.

CHAPTER 7

7.1 Reliability refers to the stability of test scores over time and across different examiners (de Clive-Lowe, 1996).

7.2 In*ter*-rater reliability is the level of agreement between or among *different* therapists (raters) administering the test, while in*tra*-rater reliability is the consistency of the judgements made by the *same* therapist (rater) over time.

7.3 Test–retest reliability is the correlation of scores obtained by the same person on two administrations of the same test and is the consistency of the assessment or test score over time (Anastasi, 1988).

7.4 An acceptable correlation coefficient for test–retest reliability is considered to be 0.70 or above, anything above 0.80 would be considered good and above 0.86 would be considered very high.

7.5 Responsiveness is the measure of efficiency with which a test detects clinical change (Wright, Cross and Lamb, 1998). Responsiveness is important when measuring outcomes because a test may have good test–retest reliability but not be sensitive to the small amount of change that a therapist and client would consider to be clinically significant. When using outcome measures, the therapist should ensure that the test used is responsive to picking up both the type and amount of change in behaviour or function that is anticipated, or desired, as the result of intervention.

CHAPTER 8

8.1 The factors I should discuss with my clients prior to assessment to ensure I have gained their informed consent are:
- the purpose of the proposed assessment/standardised test/measurement
- how the assessment results will be used and what decisions or treatment plans will be guided by the results
- who will be given access to the results of the assessment/test/measurement and what form the results will take
- what will be involved (interview, observations, standardised tests, everyday tasks)
- whether the person will need to get undressed and their right to a chaperone
- who will be involved in the assessment (carer, relatives, other health/social care providers, teacher etc.)
- where the assessment/test/measurement will be undertaken
- how long the assessment/test/measurement should take
- the purpose and use of photographs and videos.

8.2 To ensure I achieve an effective and efficient assessment, I need to consider the timing of the assessment, the optimum environment for conducting the assessment and must check I have all of the necessary test materials and equipment. I need to clarify my and the client's expectations of the proposed assessment and obtain the person's informed consent. I also need to think about how I will engage the person and his carer and build rapport to facilitate the development of an effective therapeutic relationship.

8.3 In order to build rapport with my client, I could use physical and verbal mirroring, a similar pace of communication and tone of voice to the client and maintain good eye contact to show I am actively listening. During an initial interview, I could use clean language questions to help unpackage any descriptions or metaphors used by the person to explain his feelings, problems, experiences or symptoms. I could also make time for informal interactions with the person, such as fetching him from the ward to the therapy department, and use this time for informal conversation to put him at ease and get to know him a little.

CHAPTER 9

9.1 Applying a model of function can assist your assessment process in a number of ways. It is useful to categorise the person in terms of levels of function/dysfunction and to use the boundaries of a defined level to help focus further data collection. Hierarchies describing levels of function/dysfunction can be useful for identifying and comparing the levels, domains and scope of different or apparently similar tests. When working as a member of a multidisciplinary team, models can be useful to help you to identify your primary level or domain of concern and for the team to identify areas where there is overlap in the assessment data collected and any gaps or omissions where a level of functioning has not been adequately assessed by team members. Humans are very complex, and therapy assessment needs to encompass a vast field of phenomena from neurons and cells and to organs, such as the brain and eyes, to the person as a whole and to the interaction between people and their physical and social environments. Some models provide a framework for viewing all these disparate phenomena (e.g. as an inter-related continuum or an ordered hierarchy).

9.2 The 10 levels in the hierarchy of living systems (Christiansen, 1991, p. 16) are:
   1. atom
   2. molecules
   3. cells
   4. organs
   5. person
   6. family group
   7. organisations
   8. societies
   9. *Homo sapiens*
   10. biosphere.

9.3 In the ICF model, body functions are defined as physiological functions of body systems, including psychological functions, and body structures are defined as anatomical parts of the body such as organs, limbs and their components, while impairments are defined as problems in body function or structure such as a significant deviation or loss (World Health Organization, 2002).

9.4 In the ICF model, activity is defined as the execution of a task or action by an individual, and activity limitations are seen as the difficulties an individual may have in executing activities. Participation is viewed as involvement in a life situation, and participation restrictions are problems a person may experience in involvement in life situations.

9.5 The five levels proposed by the NCMRR (1992) model of function and dysfunction are:

- societal limitation level: dysfunction is caused by restriction, attributable to social policy or barriers (structural or attitudinal), which limits fulfilment of roles or denies access to services and opportunities that are associated with full participation in society
- disability level: dysfunction is defined in terms of an inability or limitation in performing socially defined tasks and activities, within a physical and social environmental context, resulting from internal or external factors and their interplay
- functional limitation level: dysfunction is exhibited by a restriction or lack of ability, resulting from impairment, to perform an action or skill in the manner or range considered normal for stage of development and cultural background
- impairment level: dysfunction is exhibited as loss and/or abnormality of cognitive, emotional or anatomical structure or function; including all losses or abnormalities, not just those attributable to the initial pathophysiology
- pathophysiology level: dysfunction is exhibited by interruption of/or interference with normal physiological and developmental processes or structures.

CHAPTER 10

10.1 Clinical reasoning involves 'the mental strategies and high level cognitive patterns and processes that underlie the process of naming, framing and solving problems and that enable the therapist to reach decisions about the best course of action. Clinical reasoning translates the knowledge, skills and values of the therapist into action' (College of Occupational Therapists, 2003a, p. 51) and ensures that physiotherapists practise physiotherapy and occupational therapists practise occupational therapy and not some other form of intervention.

10.2 The type of questions that therapists attempt to answer through pragmatic reasoning include questions about the referral source and reason for referral, who will be paying for the treatment, expectations of the outcome of therapy, the level of support the client has from family/carers, the amount of time the therapist will have available to work with this client, the clinically and client-based environments that will be available for therapy and what standardised tests, equipment and adaptations the therapist can access to support the therapeutic process, the expectations of her manager, supervisor and multidisciplinary colleagues and her own clinical competencies and whether these will be sufficient to provide the client with the therapy he needs (Schell, 1998).

10.3 The four components of diagnostic reasoning are cue acquisition, hypothesis generation, cue interpretation and hypothesis evaluation (Rogers and Holm, 1991).

10.4 Reflections on my practice can be documented as diary entries, reflective journals, significant incident analyses, case analyses, clinical stories and notes from supervision, mentorship or peer reflection sessions. These should be kept in my portfolio of continuing professional development.

CHAPTER 11

11.1–11.3 Answers to these questions will be unique to your clinical practice or placement. Depending on the area of practice, you may find relevant examples in this text or you may need to undertake a literature search or talk to your clinical supervisor/colleagues to identify suitable examples.

Worksheets

The following pages contain templates for worksheets that I developed to assist students and therapists to reflect on the content of the chapters and apply various principles of assessment and outcome measurement to their own practice. These are photocopiable masters.

Worksheet 1: Evidence-based practice

Question	Comments
Do you currently base your assessment practice on evidence?	Yes, all assessments are evidence-based.
	Partly, some assessments are evidence-based.
	No, none of the assessments used is evidence-based.
What else, apart from evidence, do you use to guide your assessment decisions/practice?	
Think of an instance where you changed your assessment practice based on evidence (e.g. acquired from journal article, conference presentation or course)	What was your previous practice?
	What was the evidence that convinced you to change?
	What changes did you make?
	What have been the outcomes of the change?
What other areas of your current assessment practice could benefit from being changed?	Do you need to seek more evidence related to these areas of assessment?

Principles of Assessment and Outcome Measurement for Occupational Therapists and Physiotherapists: Theory, Skills and Application by Alison Laver Fawcett © 2007
John Wiley & Sons Ltd.

Worksheet 2: Reflecting on data-collection methods

Data-collection method	What data do you currently collect using this method?	What decisions do you need to make from these data?	What assessments (standardised or unstandardised) do you currently use to collect data using this method?	Is this assessment method adequate? YES or NO	List potential assessments that you could use to collect data using this method
Observation					
Self-report from client					
Proxy report (other professional, next of kin, other carer)					

Principles of Assessment and Outcome Measurement for Occupational Therapists and Physiotherapists: Theory, Skills and Application by Alison Laver Fawcett © 2007
John Wiley & Sons Ltd.

Worksheet 3: Reflecting on the purposes of assessment

Purpose of assessment	What data do you currently collect related to each purpose?	What decisions do you need to make from these data?	What assessments (standardised or unstandardised) do you currently use to collect data for this assessment purpose?	Is this assessment method adequate? YES or NO	List potential assessments that you could use to collect data for this assessment purpose
Descriptive assessment					
Evaluative assessment (outcome measure)					
Predictive assessment					
Discriminative assessment					
Service evaluation					

Principles of Assessment and Outcome Measurement for Occupational Therapists and Physiotherapists: Theory, Skills and Application by Alison Laver Fawcett © 2007 John Wiley & Sons Ltd.

Worksheet 4: Reflecting on levels of measurement

Level of measurement	What level of measurement is provided by each of the assessments (standardised and unstandardised) that you are using in your clinical practice? List the tests/assessment methods for each level	Are you using data in an appropriate way for the level of measurement? Identify any issues or limitations in current assessment practice	List potential assessments that you could use to collect data at this level of measurement. This is particularly important if the majority of your assessment data are collected at the lower nominal and ordinal levels
Nominal			
Ordinal			
Interval			
Ratio			

Principles of Assessment and Outcome Measurement for Occupational Therapists and Physiotherapists: Theory, Skills and Application by Alison Laver Fawcett © 2007 John Wiley & Sons Ltd.

Worksheet 5: Basic checklist for reflecting on the adequacy of standardisation

Name of test:
Full reference:

Is there a test manual?   YES   NO

Does the test manual describe the test development process?   YES   NO

Does the test manual describe the purpose of the test and the client group for whom the test has been developed?   YES   NO

Does the test manual provide details of psychometric studies undertaken to establish reliability and validity?   YES   NO

Does the test manual describe the materials needed for test administration or are these included as part of the test package?   YES   NO

Does the test manual describe the environment that should be used for testing?   YES   NO

Is there a protocol for test administration that provides all the instructions required to administer the test?   YES   NO

Is there guidance on how to score each test item?   YES   NO

Is there a scoring form for recording scores?   YES   NO

Is there guidance for interpreting scores?   YES   NO

If it is a norm-referenced test, is the normative sample well described?   YES   NO   NOT APPLICABLE

Are there norm-tables from which you can compare a client's score with the distribution of scores obtained by the normative group?   YES   NO

Worksheet 6: Reflecting on validity (page 1)

Name of test:
Full reference:

Is there evidence of **content validity**?   YES   NO
Describe study, brief summary of method (e.g. content analysis of literature, expert panel review), any sample details and findings:

Do you feel confident that this test measures what it says it does?   YES   NO

Have the domains to be measured been weighted to reflect their relative importance to the overall content area?   YES   NO

Is this test attempting to measure a theoretical construct?   YES   NO

If yes, is there evidence of **construct validity**?   YES   NO

Describe study and findings: method (e.g. exploring the relationship between hypothesised variables, factor analysis), sample used, statistics calculated, results:

Is the level of construct validity acceptable for your clinical practice?   YES   NO

Worksheet 6: Reflecting on validity (continued, page 2)

Name of test:

Does this test attempt to distinguish between individuals/groups, diagnostic categories etc.?

If yes, is there evidence of **discriminative validity**?   YES   NO

Describe study and findings: method, sample size, clinical sample used, statistics calculated, results:

Is the level of discriminative validity adequate for your clinical practice?   YES   NO

Was this test originally developed as a research tool or for use in a different clinical setting?   YES   NO

If yes, is there evidence of **external validity**?

Describe study and findings: method, sample size, clinical sample used, statistics calculated, results:

Are you confident that this test will be valid for your clinical setting?   YES   NO

Name of test:

Is there evidence of **criterion-related validity**?   YES   NO

Is the test used to make predictions about future ability, functioning in a different environment etc.?

If yes, is there evidence of **predictive validity**?   YES   NO

Describe study and findings: method, sample size, clinical sample used, statistics calculated, results:

What would be the likely consequences and problems associated with your predictions not being valid?

Is the predictive validity adequate for your clinical setting?   YES   NO

Does this test measure the same or similar traits/behaviours as other existing and recognised test(s)?   YES   NO

If yes, is there evidence of **concurrent validity**?   YES   NO

Describe study and findings: method, concurrent measure(s), sample size, clinical sample used, statistics calculated, results:

Is the level of concurrent validity adequate for your clinical setting?   YES   NO

Worksheet 6: Reflecting on validity (continued, page 4)

Name of test:

Is there evidence of **face validity**?   YES   NO

Describe study and findings: method, sample size, clinical sample used, statistics calculated, results:

Do you think this test will be acceptable to your clients, their families and colleagues who will view the results?   YES   NO

If yes, is there evidence of **clinical utility**?   YES   NO

Describe study and findings: method, sample size, clinical sample used, statistics calculated, results:

Are you confident that this test will be useful in your clinical setting?   YES   NO

Worksheet 7: Reflecting on reliability (page 1)

Name of test:
Full reference:

Is there evidence of **test–retest reliability**?   YES   NO
Describe study and findings: method, sample size, clinical sample used, statistics calculated, results:

Is the level test–retest of reliability adequate (0.70 or above) or good (0.80 or above)?

Do you feel confident that you can apply this test reliably over time?   YES   NO

Is there evidence of **inter-rater reliability**?   YES   NO
Describe study and findings: method, rater/therapist, sample size and description, clinical sample used, statistics calculated, results:

Is the level of inter-rater reliability adequate (0.80 or above) or good (0.90 or above)?

Do you feel confident that you can apply this test reliably across different therapist raters?   YES   NO

Principles of Assessment and Outcome Measurement for Occupational Therapists and Physiotherapists: Theory, Skills and Application by Alison Laver Fawcett © 2007 John Wiley & Sons Ltd.

Worksheet 7: Reflecting on reliability (continued, page 2)

Name of test:

Is there evidence of **internal consistency**?   YES   NO
Describe study and findings: method, sample size, clinical sample used, statistics calculated, results:

Is the level of internal consistency adequate (0.85 or above)?

Do you feel confident that the test items have homogeneity?

If the test has a parallel (equivalent) form, is there evidence of **parallel form reliability**?   YES   NO
Describe study and findings: method, sample size, clinical sample used, statistics calculated, results:

Is the level of parallel form reliability adequate (0.70 or above) or good (0.80 or above)?

Do you feel confident that the parallel form can be used reliably?   YES   NO

Worksheet 7: Reflecting on reliability (continued, page 3)

Name of test:

Test specificity:
Is there evidence of test specificity?   YES   NO
Describe study and findings: method, sample size, clinical sample used, statistics calculated, results:

What is the false positive rate?

What would be the likely consequences and problems associated with a person being wrongly identified as having a problem on this measure?

Is the test specificity adequate for your clinical setting?   YES   NO

Test sensitivity:
Is there evidence of **test sensitivity**?   YES   NO
Describe study and findings: method, sample size, clinical sample used, statistics calculated, results:

What is the true positive and/or false negative rate?

What would be the likely consequences and problems associated with a person not being identified as having a problem on this measure?

Is the test sensitivity adequate for your clinical setting?   YES   NO

Principles of Assessment and Outcome Measurement for Occupational Therapists and Physiotherapists: Theory, Skills and Application by Alison Laver Fawcett © 2007
John Wiley & Sons Ltd

Worksheet 7: Reflecting on reliability (continued, page 4)

Name of test:

Responsiveness to change:
Is there evidence of responsiveness to change?   YES   NO

Describe study and findings: method, sample size, clinical sample used, statistics calculated, results:

Do you feel confident that this test can detect the type and amount of anticipated and/or desired change in your client group?   YES   NO

Floor and ceiling effects:
Is there evidence that the test has floor and/or ceiling effects?   NO EFFECTS   FLOOR EFFECTS   CEILING EFFECTS   BOTH

Describe study and findings: method, sample size, clinical sample used, statistics calculated, results:

Do you think that these effects will result in any of your clients failing or passing all test items?   YES   NO

Standard error of measurement (SEM):
Does the test manual/related literature report on SEM?   YES   NO

Does it provide details on how you would use the SEM to calculate a confidence interval for a client's score?   YES   NO

Do you feel confident about calculating confidence intervals using this test?   YES   NO

Principles of Assessment and Outcome Measurement for Occupational Therapists and Physiotherapists: Theory, Skills and Application by Alison Laver Fawcett © 2007

Worksheet 8: Checklist for preparing for an assessment

TO DO LIST	Tick when completed or mark as not applicable (N/A)	Notes
• Discussed purpose of assessment/measurement with client		
• Discussed purpose of assessment/measurement with carer		
• Obtained informed consent		
• Identified optimum timing for the assessment		
• Contacted and liaised with other people who need to be involved (colleagues for joint assessments, carer, parent, teacher etc.)		
• Organised time, date and venue and informed client and any others involved		
• Checked the environment (hazards, lighting, temperature, furniture) and set the environment up ready for the assessment		
• Got the test instructions and test materials		
• Got pens/pencils for recording and if needed for assessment		
• Got a stopwatch and checked it is working		
• Got a calculator and checked it is working		
• Battery of tests: checked all the component parts are present and in their correct bags/places		
• Got any consumables required (paper, food, drink, ingredients for a cooking assessment etc.)		
• Have the right aids/equipment needed for assessment		
• Checked if the person uses a hearing aid and checked it is on and working		
• Checked if the person uses visual aids and checked these are being used		
• (left blank for any other things you need to add)		

Principles of Assessment and Outcome Measurement for Occupational Therapists and Physiotherapists: Theory, Skills and Application by Alison Laver Fawcett © 2007 John Wiley & Sons Ltd.

Worksheet 9.1: Reflecting on the levels of function therapists need to consider: applying the NCMRR model

Level of function/ dysfunction National Center for Medical Rehabilitation Research (NCMRR; 1992)	What data do you currently collect related to this level of function?	What decisions do you need to make from these data?	What assessments (standardised or unstandardised) do you currently use to collect data related to this level of function?	Is this assessment method adequate? YES or NO	List potential assessments that you could use to collect data related to each level of function
Societal limitation					
Disability					
Functional limitation					
Impairment					
Pathophysiology					

Worksheet 9.2: Reflecting on the levels of function therapists need to consider: applying the ICF model

ICF dimension *International Classification of Functioning, Disability and Health (WHO, 2002)*	What data do you currently collect related to this dimension?	What decisions do you need to make from these data?	What assessments (standardised or unstandardised) do you currently use to collect data related to this dimension?	Is this assessment method adequate? YES or NO	List potential assessments that you could use to collect data related to each dimension
Body function and structure and impairments					
Activity and activity limitations					
Participation and participation restrictions					
Environmental factors					

Principles of Assessment and Outcome Measurement for Occupational Therapists and Physiotherapists: Theory, Skills and Application by Alison Laver Fawcett © 2007 John Wiley & Sons Ltd.

Worksheet 10: Clinical reasoning: writing a therapy diagnostic statement

Client's name	
Descriptive component:	
Explanatory component:	
Cue component: As evidenced by the following **symptoms** described by client and/or proxy	
Cue component: As evidenced by the following **signs** identified through observational assessment	
Pathologic component:	

Worksheet 11: Analysing your current assessment process SWOT analysis

Strengths of your current assessment process:

Weaknesses of your current assessment process:

Opportunities to support improving your assessment process:

Threats to achieving an optimum assessment process for your clients:

Principles of Assessment and Outcome Measurement for Occupational Therapists and Physiotherapists: Theory, Skills and Application by Alison Laver Fawcett © 2007 John Wiley & Sons Ltd.

Worksheet 12: Test critique form (page 1)

Critique area	Comments
Name of test, authors and date of publication:	
Publisher: where to obtain test: **Cost** (if any):	
For what population has the test been designed?	
Purpose(s) of test: Stated purpose and uses:	
Data-collection method(s) used:	
Level(s) of function addressed by test:	

Worksheet 12: Test critique form (continued, page 2)

Critique area	Comments
Testing environments where test can be used:	
Scoring method and levels of measurement:	
Qualifications needed to administer the test and additional training requirements/costs:	
Standardisation: Is it standardised? Development details	
Is it a **norm-** or **criterion-referenced test?** Details of criteria or norms:	

Principles of Assessment and Outcome Measurement for Occupational Therapists and Physiotherapists: Theory, Skills and Application by Alison Laver Fawcett © 2007
John Wiley & Sons Ltd.

Worksheet 12: Test critique form (continued, page 3)

Critique area	Comments
Reliability data:	
Validity data:	
Clinical utility: (ease of use and scoring, portability, cost, training issues, settings etc.)	

Worksheet 12: Test critique form (continued, page 4)

Critique area	Comments
Face validity: (for therapists, clients, others receiving results)	
Summary of strengths:	
Summary of limitations:	
Overall conclusion: Should test be adopted, piloted or rejected as an option for your service?	

Principles of Assessment and Outcome Measurement for Occupational Therapists and Physiotherapists: Theory, Skills and Application by Alison Laver Fawcett © 2007 John Wiley & Sons Ltd.

Worksheet 13: Continuing professional development goals for improving assessment practice

CPD goal	Action plan	Comments/ideas	Date accomplished

Glossary

Assessment: is the overall process of selecting and using multiple data-collection tools and various sources of information to inform decisions required to guide therapeutic intervention during the whole therapy process. Assessment involves interpreting information collected to make clinical decisions related to the needs of the person and the appropriateness and nature of therapy. Assessment involves the evaluation of the outcomes of therapeutic interventions.

Baseline assessment: comprises the initial data gathered at the start of therapeutic intervention. Baseline data can be used to guide the nature of the required intervention. A baseline forms the basis for comparison when measuring outcomes to evaluate the effects of intervention.

Case method: 'is a problem-solving process that fosters the application of knowledge for defining and resolving problems. Data are collected, classified, analysed and interpreted in accordance with a clinical frame of reference and transformed into a definition of the problem and subsequently an action plan' (Line, 1969, cited by Rogers, 2004, p. 17).

Ceiling effect: occurs when the person scores the maximum possible score on a test and the test does not reflect the full extent of his ability.

Clinical effectiveness: 'the degree to which a therapeutic outcome is achieved in real-world patient populations under actual or average conditions of treatment provision' (Maniadakis and Gray, 2004, p. 27).

Clinical judgement: 'the ability of professionals to make decisions within their own field of expertise using the working knowledge that they have acquired over time. It is based on both clinical experience and the theoretical principles embedded in their professional knowledge base but it may remain highly subjective' (Stewart, 1999, p. 417).

Clinical reasoning: involves 'the mental strategies and high level cognitive patterns and processes that underlie the process of naming, framing and solving problems and that enable the therapist to reach decisions about the best course of action. Clinical reasoning translates the knowledge, skills and values of the therapist into action and ensures that ... therapists practise ... therapy and not some other form of intervention' (College of Occupational Therapists, 2003a, p. 51).

Clinical utility: 'the overall usefulness of an assessment in a clinical situation' (Law, 1997, p. 431).

Coefficient of equivalence: is obtained from two sets of scores drawn from parallel (equivalent/alternate) test forms (Crocker and Algina, 1986).

Comparative scaling: with comparative scaling items being rated are directly compared with each other in some way; items might be rated in terms of which is the best, the most difficult, the most frequently occurring or the preferred option (e.g. 'Do you prefer the colour blue or red?').

Concurrent validity: is 'the extent to which the test results agree with other measures of the same or similar traits and behaviours' (Asher, 1996, p. xxx); sometimes referred to as *congruent validity*.

Conditional reasoning: relates to the therapist thinking about 'the whole condition, including the person, the illness, the meanings the illness has for the person, the family, and the social and physical contexts in which the person lives' (Mattingly and Fleming, 1994a, p. 18).

Conscious use of self: is a key therapeutic tool used by therapists and 'involves a planned interaction with another person in order to alleviate fear or anxiety; provide reassurance; obtain necessary information; give advice; and assist the other individual to gain more appreciation, expression, and functional use of his or her latent inner resources' (Mosey, 1981, p. 95).

Construct: 'a product of scientific imagination, an idea developed to permit categorization and description of some directly observable behaviour' (Crocker and Algina, 1986, p. 230).

Construct validity: the extent to which an assessment can be said to measure a theoretical construct(s) and 'the ability of an assessment to perform as hypothesized' (Law, 1997, p. 431).

Contact assessment: this is a stage of assessment defined by the Department of Health as part of a single assessment process (SAP) and 'refers to a contact between an older person and health and social services where significant needs are first described or suspected ... At contact assessment basic personal information is collected and the nature of the presenting problem is established and the potential presence of wider health and social care needs is explored' (Department of Health, 2002c, p. 3).

Content validity: the degree to which an assessment measures what it is supposed to measure judged on the appropriateness of its content as judged by 'the comprehensiveness of an assessment and its inclusion of items that fully represent the attribute being measured' (Law, 1997, p. 431).

Content validity index (CVI): the overall CVI for a test is calculated by dividing the proportion of items judged by an expert panel to have content validity by the total number of items in a test, and the CVI for each item on a test is the proportion of experts who rated that item as valid (see Clemson, Fitzgerald and Heard, 1999).

Correlation: is a 'measure of association that indicates the degree to which two or more sets of observations fit a linear relationship' (McDowell and Newell, 1987, p. 327).

Criterion-referenced test: is a test that examines performance against pre-defined criteria and produces raw scores that are intended to have a direct, interpretable meaning (Crocker and Algina, 1986).

Criterion-related validity: is the effectiveness of a test in predicting an individual's performance in specific activities; this is measured by comparing performance on the test with a criterion, which is a direct and independent measure of what the assessment is designed to predict.

Deductive reasoning: involves reasoning from the general to the particular (or from cause to effect). The deductive reasoning process begins with statements that are accepted as true and then applies these held 'truths' to a new situation to reach a conclusion and is therefore seen as reasoning based on facts.

Descriptive assessment: is an assessment that provides information which describes the person's current functional status, problems, needs and/or circumstances.

Diagnostic reasoning: involves the therapist creating a clinical image of the person through cue acquisition, hypothesis generation, cue interpretation and hypothesis evaluation (Rogers and Holm, 1991).

Diagnostic statement: a statement made by therapists at the end of an assessment process that consists of four components: 'descriptive (functional problem) + explanatory (aetiology of the problem) + cue (signs and symptoms) + pathological (medical or psychiatric)' (Rogers, 2004, p. 19).

Differential diagnosis: is the systematic method used by health care professionals to identify the causes of a person's problems and symptoms (sometimes abbreviated DDx or ΔΔ in therapy and medical notes).

Discriminative test: is a measure that has been developed to 'distinguish between individuals or groups on an underlying dimension when no external criterion or gold standard is available for validating these measures' (Law, 2001, p. 287).

Discriminative validity: relates to whether a test provides a valid measure to distinguish between individuals or groups.

Domain: is a collection of issues that are related; in terms of assessment it is usually the set of functions/activities/behaviours from which test items are selected.

Ecological validity: addresses the relevance of the test content, structure and environment to the population with whom the test is used (Laver, 1994).

Efficacy: 'the degree to which a therapeutic outcome is achieved in a patient population under rigorously controlled and monitored circumstances, such as controlled clinical trials' (Maniadakis and Gray, 2004, p. 27).

Equivalent form reliability: the correlation between scores obtained for the same person on two (or more) forms of a test (also known as parallel form/alternate form reliability).

Evaluation: is a component of a broader assessment process that involves the collection of data to enable the therapist to make a judgement about the amount of a specific construct of interest (such as degree of range of movement, or level of independence in an activity of daily living) or to make a judgement about the value of an intervention for delivering the desired outcome for a person or the value of a service for delivering outcomes of relevance to the client population. Evaluation often involves data being collected at two time points in order to measure effect and also can involve the translation of observations to numerical scores.

Evaluative assessment: is a process used to detect change in function over time and is undertaken to monitor a client's progress during rehabilitation and to determine the effectiveness of the intervention.

Evaluative test: is an instrument 'used to measure the magnitude of longitudinal change in an individual or group on the dimension of interest' (Law, 2001, p. 287).

Evidence-based medicine (EBM): 'is the conscientious, explicit, and judicious use of current best evidence in making decisions about the care of individual patients. The practice of evidence-based medicine means integrating individual clinical expertise with the best available external clinical evidence from systematic research' (Sackett *et al.*, 1996, p. 71).

Evidence-based practice (EBP): 'encourages the integration of high quality quantitative and qualitative research with the clinician's clinical expertise and the client's background, preferences and values. It involves the client in making informed decisions and should build on, not replace, clinical judgement and experience' (OTseeker, 2005).

External validity: is 'the extent to which findings can be generalised to other settings in the real world' (Lewis and Bottomley, 1994, p. 602).

Face validity: whether a test *seems* to measure what it is intended to measure (Asher, 1996); in particular face validity concerns the acceptability of a test to the test taker (Anastasi, 1988).

Factorial validity: factorial validity relates to the factorial composition of a test. It is the correlation between a test and the identified major factors that determine test scores (Anastasi, 1988).

False negative result: a false negative occurs when a person who has a deficit is not identified as having that deficit through his performance on the test.

False positive result: occurs when someone who does not have a deficit is identified on a test as having the deficit.

Floor effect: occurs when a person obtains the minimum score on a test and the test does not reflect the full extent of the person's deficits.

Frequency distribution: is a table of scores (either presented from high to low, or low to high) providing the number of people who obtain each score or whose scores fall in each score interval.

Generalisability: is the ability to make inferences from a sample to the population, given the scale you have selected; in assessment, it is the ability to make inferences from the results obtained for a sample of the population used to produce normative data to the results of an individual client tested in your practice environment.

Heuristics: is a mental short-cut used in judgement and decision-making. It is a problem-solving technique in which the most appropriate solution is selected using rules, and usually these are simplified and used for processing information on a rule-of-thumb, trial-and-error basis.

Hypothesis: is a tentative explanation of the cause(s) of observed dysfunction (Rogers and Holm, 1991).

Inductive generalisation: is a form of reasoning that proceeds from a premise about a sample of people to a conclusion about the whole population. So if a proportion of the sample has a particular attribute, then it is generalised that the same proportion of the total population has that same attribute.

Inductive reasoning: is a system of reasoning based on observation and measurements and involves observing patterns and using those observations to make generalisations.

Informed consent: before undertaking an assessment or treatment intervention therapists have a duty to obtain the client's consent; informed consent is when the client has been given sufficient information to enable him to make an informed decision, and he has been able to understand and weigh up the information provided and been given the space to act under his own free will.

Initial assessment: 'is the first step in the ... therapy process following referral; the art of gathering relevant information in order to define the problem to be tackled, or identify the goal to be attained, and to establish a baseline for treatment planning' (College of Occupational Therapists, 2003a, p. 54).

Instrument: 'is a device for recording or measuring' (American Occupational Therapy Association, cited by Hopkins and Smith, 1993a, p. 914).

Internal consistency: is the degree to which test items all measure the same behaviour or construct.

Inter-rater reliability: is the level of agreement between or among different therapists (raters) administering the test.

Interval scale: has a constant, common unit of measurement and the gap, or 'interval', between each position on the scale is kept the same. However, the units of measurement and the zero point on an interval scale are arbitrary (Hunter, 1997).

Intra-rater reliability: is the consistency of the judgements made by the same therapist (rater) over time.

Item: 'The term "item" is used to refer to individual questions or response phrases in any health measurement. It replaces the more obvious term "question" simply because not all response categories are actually phrased as questions: some use rating scales, others use agree/disagree statements' (McDowell and Newell, 1987, p. 328).

Kappa: is a statistical method used to produce a 'coefficient of agreement between two raters; kappa expresses the level of agreement that is observed beyond the level that would be expected by chance alone' (McDowell and Newell, 1987, p. 328).

Likelihood ratio: 'is an approach to summarizing the results of sensitivity and specificity analyses for various cutting points on diagnostic and screening tests. Each cutting produces a value for the true positive rate (i.e. sensitivity) and the false positive rate (i.e. specificity). The ratio of true to false positives is the likelihood ratio for each cutting point' (McDowell and Newell, 1987, p. 328).

Mapping: 'is the process by which you represent the activities and steps experienced by the patient. This is a diagnostic and analytical process of discovering what actually happens. You can then use this information to find ways to improve how the patient experiences the care you deliver' (Fraser, 2002, p. 4).

Mean: is, in measurement, the average score obtained by a group of people on a test and is calculated by adding the scores obtained by all people taking the test and then dividing this total by the number of obtained scores.

Measurement: is the data obtained by measuring. Measuring is undertaken by therapists to ascertain the dimensions (size), quantity (amount) or capacity of a trait, attribute or characteristic of the person that is required by the therapist to develop an accurate picture of the person's needs and problems to form a baseline for therapeutic intervention and/or to provide a measure of outcome. A measurement is obtained by applying a standard scale to variables, thus translating direct observations or client/proxy reports to a numerical scoring system.

Moral reasoning: relates to 'a more philosophical enquiry about norms and values, about ideas of right and wrong, and about how therapists make moral decisions in professional work. Moral issues have to be resolved through reflective thinking and problem solving because guidelines to ethics cannot cope with specific instances' (Barnitt, 1993, p. 402).

Narrative reasoning: is a reasoning process that 'uses story making and story telling to assist the therapist in understanding the meaning of disability or disease to the client' (Unsworth, 1999, p. 48).

Nominal scale: is a scale that simply uses numbers to classify a characteristic and is used to identify differences without quantifying or ordering those differences (Polgar, 1998); therefore, the numbers used in a nominal scale do not have any meaning except in the context in which they are being used (Hunter, 1997).

Non-comparative scaling: with this, each item in the scale is rated/scored independently of all the other items. This might be in terms of how well the item can be performed, how frequently the item occurs or how the person feels about that item. For example, how well can you get dressed? How often do you go out with friends? How do you feel about the colour red?

Norm-referenced test: is a test used to evaluate performance against the scores of a peer group whose performance has been described using a normative sample.

Norms: are sets of scores from clearly defined samples of a population (Kline, 1990). A wider definition refers to them as 'a standard, a model, or pattern for a specific group; an expected type of performance or behaviour for a particular reference group of persons' (American Occupational Therapy Association, cited by Hopkins and Smith, 1993b, p. 914).

Objective data: are 'facts or findings which are clearly observable to and verifiable by others, as reflecting reality' (American Occupational Therapy Association, cited by Hopkins and Smith, 1993a, p. 914).

Obtained score: is the score achieved by a person taking a test.

Occupational diagnosis: 'refers to both the cognitive processes used by the occupational therapy practitioner to formulate a statement summarizing the client's occupational status, and the outcome of that process, the diagnostic statement' (Rogers, 2004, p. 17).

Ongoing assessment: 'is an integral part of the process of intervention in which information is collected and used to examine the client's progress or lack of progress, to monitor the effects of intervention and to assist the therapist's clinical reasoning process' (College of Occupational Therapists, 2003a, p. 56).

Ordinal scale: is used to rank the order of the scores, and adjacent scores indicate that the parameter being measured is either better/greater or worse/less than the other (Hunter, 1997).

Outcome: is the observed or measured consequence of an action or occurrence; in a therapeutic process, it is the end result of the therapeutic intervention.

Outcome measure: is a standardised instrument used by therapists to establish whether their desired therapeutic outcomes have been achieved.

Outcome measurement: is a process undertaken to establish the effects of an intervention on an individual or the effectiveness of a service on a defined aspect of the health or well-being of a specified population; it is achieved by administering an outcome measure on at least two occasions to document change over time in one or more trait, attribute or characteristic to establish whether that trait/attribute/characteristic has been influenced by the intervention to the anticipated degree to achieve the desired outcome.

Parallel form reliability: is the correlation between scores obtained for the same person on two (or more) forms of a test (also known as equivalent form or alternate form reliability).

Patterns: refer to 'patterns of behaviour, patterns of conversations, patterns of clinical outcomes or the patterns of anything that can be counted such as waiting lists, prescribing or demand' (NHS Modernisation Agency, 2004, p. 12).

PDSA cycle: is a service improvement method recommended by the NHS Modernisation Agency (2002a): P = plan, D = do, S = study, A = act (see Chapter 11, pp. 342–3).

Pragmatic reasoning: is a reasoning process used by therapists to facilitate an understanding about how the personal context and the practice setting affect the assessment and treatment processes they implement. It takes into account organisational, political and economic constraints and opportunities that place boundaries around the assessment and treatment that a therapist may undertake in a particular practice environment (Schell and Cervero, 1993; Unsworth, 1999).

Predictive assessment: is undertaken by therapists to predict the future ability or state of a client or to predict a specific outcome in the future (Adams, 2002).

Predictive test: is a measure that has been designed to 'classify individuals into a set of pre-defined measurement categories, either concurrently or prospectively, to determine whether individuals have been classified correctly' (Law, 2001, p. 287).

Predictive validity: is 'the accuracy with which a measurement predicts some future event, such as mortality' (McDowell and Newell, 1987, p. 329).

Procedural reasoning: is an 'umbrella term that describes a therapist's thinking when working out what a client's problems are and what procedures may be used to reduce the effect of those problems' (Unsworth, 1999, p. 54).

Process: is the therapeutic practice that transforms inputs (such as materials, staff, equipment) into outputs (therapy outcomes).

Process goal: is 'what the therapist hopes to achieve during the process of intervention. This may be action by the therapist or a change in the therapist's knowledge, skills or attitudes' (College of Occupational Therapists, 2003a, p. 57).

Proxy: is formally defined as 'a person or agency or substitute recognized by law to act for, and in the best interest of, the patient' (Centre for Advanced Palliative Care, 2005), but in the context of therapy assessment the term is used more widely to refer to an informant (e.g. carer, professional) who has knowledge about the circumstances or condition of the client who is able to share that knowledge with the person's permission or without breaking laws of confidentiality.

Proxy report: is information given to the therapist by someone who knows the client and is also sometimes referred to as an informant interview (Borg and Bruce, 1991).

RAID cycle: is a service improvement method recommended by the NHS Modernisation Agency (2002a): R = review, A = agree, I = implement, D = demonstrate (see Chapter 11, pp. 342–3).

Rapport: should be understood, within the context of a therapy assessment process, to be the ability of the therapist to place the person at his ease by building a relationship based on mutual understanding and empathy and can also be understood as a means of facilitating a person's cooperation with the assessment process by encouraging a conscious feeling of trust in the therapist.

Ratio scale: has a constant unit of measurement, a uniform interval between points on the scale and has a true zero at its origin (Hunter, 1997).

Raw score: is the actual numerical score (e.g. the number of correctly answered items that a person obtains on a test). In some tests, it is transformed to provide additional data (e.g. it could be transformed into a standard score or percentile rank).

Reflective practice: is a process by which the therapist, as a practitioner, stops and thinks about her practice, consciously analyses her decision-making processes and draws on theory and relates it to what she does in practice. This process of critical analysis and evaluation refocuses the therapist's thinking on her existing knowledge to generate new knowledge and ideas. This may lead to a change in her actions, behaviour, assessment approach, treatments and/or learning needs (Chartered Society of Physiotherapy, 2006b).

Reliability: refers to the stability of test scores over time and across different examiners (de Clive-Lowe, 1996).

Reliability coefficient: is a statistic used to indicate the extent to which a test is a stable instrument that is capable of producing consistent results; it is usually expressed as a correlation coefficient between 0 and 1 and can be cited with a positive or negative sign (ranging from +1.0 to −1.0).

Responsiveness to change: refers to the measure of efficiency with which a test detects clinical change (Wright, Cross and Lamb, 1998).

Scale: provides a means of recording something that can be rated in terms of levels, amounts or degrees. Therapists use scales to rate the presence or severity of a problem, such as a symptom, or to rate the person's level of independence in a needed or chosen occupation, activity or task. Scales can be categorised into one of four levels of measurement: nominal, ordinal, interval or ratio. Numbers are frequently assigned as scores in scales. How these numerical scores can be used and interpreted depends upon the level of measurement used in the scale.

Sensitivity: is 'the ability of a measurement or screening test to identify those who have a condition, calculated as a percentage of all cases with the condition who were judged by the test to have the condition: the "true positive' rate"' (McDowell and Newell, 1987, p. 330).

Service outcomes: are measures of the overall occupational therapy or physiotherapy service's efficiency and effectiveness.

Service structures: refer to the 'layout of equipment, facilities and departments as well as organisational structures such as maps showing roles, committees, working groups etc.' (NHS Modernisation Agency, 2004, p. 12).

Social perception: is the process by which someone infers other people's motives and intentions from observing their behaviour and deciding whether the causes of the behaviour are internal or situational. Social perception helps people make sense of the world, organise their thoughts quickly and maintain a sense of control over the environment. It helps people feel competent, masterful and balanced because it helps them predict similar events in the future (Lefton, Boyles and Ogden, 2000, p. 457).

Specialist assessment: is a stage of assessment defined by the Department of Health as part of a single assessment process and is defined as 'an assessment undertaken by a clinician or other professional who specialises in a branch of medicine or care e.g. stroke, cardiac care, bereavement counselling' (Department of Health, 2001a, p. 160).

Specificity: is 'the ability of a measurement to correctly identify those who do not have the condition in question' (McDowell and Newell, 1987, p. 330).

Stakeholders: are 'those individuals, groups, and parties that either affect or who are affected by the organization. Stakeholders as a general rule, include all internal and external customers and are involved or consulted as a part of the strategic planning process so that their views, needs and concerns are given consideration during development of organizational goals, objectives and strategies, and also to provide input related to programmatic outcome measures' (Centre for Advanced Palliative Care, 2005).

Standard error of measurement (SEM): is the estimate of the 'error' associated with a person's obtained score on a test when compared with his hypothetical 'true' score.

Standardised: means to be 'made standard or uniform; to be used without variation; suggests an invariable way in which a test is to be used, as well as denoting the extent to which the results of the test may be considered to be both valid and reliable' (American Occupational Therapy Association, cited by Hopkins and Smith, 1993a, p. 914).

Standardised test/measure/assessment/instrument: is a 'published measurement tool, designed for a specific purpose in a given population, with detailed instructions provided as to when and how it is to be administered and scored, interpretation of the scores, and results of investigations of reliability and validity' (Cole *et al.*, 1995, p. 22).

Subjective data: are observations 'not rigidly reflecting measurable reality; may imply observer bias; may not be verifiable by others in the same situation' (American Occupational Therapy Association, cited by Hopkins and Smith, 1993a, p. 914).

Test critique: is a critical review and discussion about a test and usually describes the purpose, format, content, psychometric properties and strengths and limitations of the test.

Test elements: 'are all the aspects of the measurement process that can affect the obtained data. For example, the elements of questionnaires include individual items, response formats, and instructions. The elements of behavioral observation include observation codes, time sampling parameters, and the situations in which observation occurs' (Haynes, Richard and Kubany, 1995, p. 2).

Test manual: is a booklet containing information about the development of a test, details of the method and results of any studies undertaken to establish the test's psychometric properties, and tables for any normative data. Some test manuals also contain background theoretical information, example case histories and suggestions for treatment planning linked to possible results that might be obtained from the test.

Test protocol: is a document that describes the specific procedures which must be followed when undertaking that test.

Test–retest reliability: is the correlation of scores obtained by the same person on two administrations of the same test and is the consistency of the assessment or test score over time (Anastasi, 1988).

Theoretical reasoning: is reasoning based upon knowledge acquired from sources such as textbooks and lectures and relates to generalisations and what the therapist can predict (Unsworth, 1999).

Validity: is the 'extent to which a measurement method measures what it is intended to' (McDowell and Newell, 1987, p. 330).

List of Abbreviations

ACS	Activity Card Sort
ADL	activities of daily living
AIMS	Alberta Infant Motor Scale
AIMS	Arthritis Impact Measurement Scale
AMPS	Assessment of Motor Process Skills
ANOVA	analysis of variance
A-ONE	Arnadottir OT-ADL Neurobehavioural Evaluation
AOTA	American Occupational Therapy Association
APTA	American Physical Therapy Association
AusTOMs-OT	Australian Therapy Outcome Measures for Occupational Therapy
BAI	Beck Anxiety Inventory
BAOT	British Association of Occupational Therapists
BBS	Beck Scale for Suicide Ideation
BDI	Beck Depression Inventory
BHS	Beck Hopelessness Scale
BI	Barthel Index
CANTAB	Cambridge Neuropsychological Test Automated Battery
CAOT	Canadian Association of Occupational Therapists
CAPE	Clifton Assessment Procedures for the Elderly
CAS	complex adapting system
CDR	Clinical Dementia Rating
CGAT	Clinical Governance Assessment Toolkit
CHART	Craig handicap assessment and reporting techniques
CINAHL	Cumulative Index to Nursing and Allied Health Literature
CMHT	community mental health team
CNS	central nervous system
COPM	Canadian Occupational Performance Measure
COT	College of Occupational Therapists
COTA	Community Occupational Therapists and Associates
COTNAB	Chessington Occupational Therapy Neurological Assessment Battery
CPD	continuing professional development
CPS	Chronic Pain Service
CRQ	Chronic Respiratory Disease Questionnaire
CSP	Chartered Society of Physiotherapy
CVI	content validity index
DADL	domestic activities of daily living
DCD	developmental coordination disorder

DCDQ	Developmental Coordination Disorder Questionnaire
DoH	Department of Health
DSC	Dementia Services Collaborative
EBM	evidence-based medicine
EBP	evidence-based practice
EDPS	Electronic Descriptive Pain Scale
FABQ	Fear-avoidance Beliefs Questionnaire
FACE	Functional Assessment of Care Environment
FAMS	Functional Assessment of Multiple Sclerosis Quality of Life Instrument
FCA	Functional Capacity Assessment
FIM	Functional Independence Measure
GCT-R	General Clerical Test – Revised
GDS	Geriatric Depression Scale
GMFM	Gross Motor Function Measure
HPC	Health Professions Council
IADL	instrumental activities of daily living
ICF	International Classification of Functioning, Disability and Health
ICIDH-1	International Classification of Impairments, Disabilities and Handicaps
IMCA	independent mental capacity advocate
KTA	Kitchen Task Assessment
LEC	Life Experiences Checklist
LSI-P	Life Satisfaction Index – Parents
MBPC	Memory and Behaviour Problems Checklist
MEAMS	Middlesex Elderly Assessment of Mental State
MMSE	Mini Mental State Examination
MMT	manual muscle testing
MOHO	Model of Human Occupation
MPQ PPI	McGill Pain Questionnaire's Present Pain Intensity
NAROT	National Association of Rheumatology Occupational Therapists
NCMRR	National Council for Medical Rehabilitation Research
NICE	National Institute of Clinical Excellence
NSF	National Service Framework
NYAS	National Youth Advocacy Service
OPHI	Occupational Performance History Interview
OPMH	older people's mental health
PALS	Patient Advocacy and Liaison Service
PEDI	Pediatric Evaluation of Disability Inventory
PSI	Parenting Stress Index
PSMS	Physical Self-maintenance Scale
RASP	Rivermead Assessment of Somatosensory Performance
RCP	Royal College of Physicians
RMI	Rivermead Mobility Index
ROM	range of movement
RPAB	Rivermead Perceptual Assessment Battery
SAFER Tool	Safety Assessment of Function and the Environment for Rehabilitation
SAP	single assessment process
s.d.	standard deviation
SDAT	senile dementia of the Alzheimer's type
SEM	standard error of measurement
SFA	School Function Assessment
SIB	Severe Impairment Battery
SIGN	Scottish Intercollegiate Guidelines Network

SIP	Sickness Impact Profile
SMMSE	Standardised Mini-mental State Examination
SOPP	Standards of Physiotherapy Practice
SOTOF	Structured Observational Test of Function
SRU	stroke rehabilitation unit
SSI	Scale for Suicide Ideation
TIM	total integration model
TOM	Therapy Outcomes Measure
VAS	visual analogue scale
VAPS	visual analogue pain scale
WAD	whiplash-associated disorder
WCPT	World Confederation for Physical Therapy
WeHSA	Westmead Home Safety Assessment
WFOT	World Federation of Occupational Therapy
WHO	World Health Organization

References

Abidin RR (1995) *Parenting Stress Index: Professional Manual* (3rd edn.). Odessa, FL, Psychological Assessment Resources.

Adams J (2002) The purpose of outcome measurement in rheumatology. *British Journal of Occupational Therapy* **65**(4), 172–174.

Ager A (1990) *The Life Experiences Checklist (LEC)*. Windsor, NFER-Nelson.

AGILE (2004) Chartered physiotherapists working with older people, http://www.agile-uk.org, accessed 31.03.06.

Allport DA (1968) Phenomenal simultaneity and the perceptual moment hypothesis. *British Journal of Psychology* **59**(4), 395–406.

Allport F (1955) *Theories of Perception and the Concept of Structure*. London, John Wiley & Sons.`

American Occupational Therapy Association (1989) *Uniform Terminology for Occupational Therapy* (2nd edn.). Rockville, MD, AOTA.

American Occupational Therapy Association (1984) Hierarchy of competencies relating to the use of standardized instruments and evaluation techniques by occupational therapists. *American Journal of Occupational Therapy* **38**(12), 803–804.

American Occupational Therapy Association (1979) *Uniform Terminology for Reporting Occupational Therapy Services*. Rockville, MD, AOTA.

American Physical Therapy Association (1991) Standards for test users. *Physical Therapy* **71**(8), 613/69–619/75.

Anastasi A (1988) *Psychological Testing* (6th edn.). New York, Macmillan.

Anderson T (1992) Reflections on reflecting with families. In S McNamee, KJ Gergen (eds), *Therapy as Social Construction*. London, Sage Publications.

answers.com (2006a) Scale construction decisions, http://www.answers.com/main/ntquery?me thod=4&dsid=2222&dekey=Scale+%28social+sciences%29&gwp=8&curtab=2222_1&l inktext=Scale%20(social%20sciences, accessed 14.10.06.

answers.com (2006b) Standard deviation, http://www.algebra.com/~pavlovd/wiki Standard_deviation, accessed 14.10.06.

Arnadottir G (1990) *The Brain and Behavior: Assessing Cortical Dysfunction Through Activities of Daily Living*. St Louis, CV Mosby.

Asher IE (1996) *Occupational Therapy Assessment Tools: An Annotated Index* (2nd edn.). Bethesda, MD, AOTA.

Atkins RM (2004) The foot. In P Pynsent, J Fairbank, A Carr (eds), *Outcome Measures in Orthopaedics and Orthopaedic Trauma* (2nd edn.). London, Arnold.

Austin C, Clark CR (1993) Measures of outcome: for whom? *British Journal of Occupational Therapy* **56**(1), 21–24.

Baldwin W (2000) Information no one else knows: the value of self-report. In AA Stone, JS Turkkan, CA Bachrach, JB Jobe *et al.* (eds), *The Science of Self-report: Implications for Research and Practice*. Mahwah, NJ, Lawrence Erlbaum Associates.

Barlow DH, Hayes SC, Nelson RO (1984) *The Scientist Practitioner: Research and Accountability in Clinical and Educational Settings*. London, Allyn & Bacon.

Barnitt R (1993) Deeply troubling questions: the teaching of ethics in undergraduate courses. *British Journal of Occupational Therapy* **56**(11), 401–406.

Bartram D (1990a) Reliability and validity. In Beech JR, Harding L (eds), *Testing People: A Practical Guide to Psychometrics*. Windsor, NFER-Nelson.

Bartram D (1990b) Introduction. In Beech JR, Harding L (eds), *Testing People: A Practical Guide to Psychometrics*. Windsor, NFER-Nelson.

Baum CM (1995) The contribution of occupation to function in persons with Alzheimer's disease. *Journal of Occupational Science (Australia)* 2(2), 59–67.

Baum CM (1993) The effects of occupation on behaviours of persons with senile dementia of the Alzheimer's type and the carers. Unpublished doctoral thesis, George Warren Brown School of Social Work, Washington University, St Louis.

Baum CM, Edwards DF (1993) Cognitive performance in senile dementia of the Alzheimer type: the Kitchen Task Assessment. *American Journal of Occupational Therapy* 47(5), 431–436.

Baum CM, Perlmutter M, Edwards DF (2000) Measuring function in Alzheimer's disease. *Alzheimer's Care Quarterly* 1(3), 44–66.

Bayley N (1993) *Bayley Scales of Infant Development*. San Antonio, TX, The Psychological Corporation.

Beck AT, Kovacs M, Weissman A (1979) Assessment of suicidal intention: the Scale for Suicide Ideation. *Journal of Consulting and Clinical Psychology* 47, 343–352.

Beck AT, Steer RA (1991) *Manual for the Beck Scale for Suicide Ideation (BBS)*. London, The Psychological Corporation.

Beck AT, Steer RA (1990) *Beck Anxiety Inventory Manual*. London, The Psychological Corporation.

Beck AT, Steer RA (1988) *Manual for Beck Hopelessness Scale*. San Antonio, TX, The Psychological Corporation.

Beck AT, Steer RA, Brown GK (1996) *Beck Depression Inventory* (2nd edn.). San Antonio, TX, The Psychological Corporation.

Beck AT, Steer RA, Kovacs M, Garrison B (1985) Hopelessness and eventual suicide: a 10-year prospective study of patients hospitalised with suicidal ideation. *American Journal of Psychiatry* 142(5), 559–563.

Beery K (1997) *Developmental Test of Visual Motor Integration* (4th edn.). Parsippany, NJ, Modern Curriculum Press.

Belsey J, Snell T (2003) What is evidence-based medicine? What is...? Hayward Medical Communications, 1(2), http://www.evidence-based-medicine.co.uk/ebmfiles/Whatisebm.pdf, accessed, 25.10.06.

Bender MP (1990) Test review – Clifton assessment procedures for the elderly. In JR Beech, L Harding (eds), *Assessment of the Elderly*. Windsor, NFER-Nelson.

Benner P (1984) *From Novice to Expert: Excellence and Power in Clinical Nursing*. London, Addison-Wesley.

Bennett AE, Ritchie K (1975) *Questionnaires in Medicine: A Guide to Their Design and Use*. London, Oxford University Press.

Benson J, Clark F (1982) A guide for instrument development and validation. *American Journal of Occupational Therapy* 36(12), 789–800.

Berg KO, Maki BE, Williams JI, Holliday PJ, Wood-Dauphinee SL (1992) Clinical and laboratory measures of postural balance in an elderly population. *Archives of Physical Medicine and Rehabilitation* 73, 1073–1080.

Berg KO, Wood-Dauphinee S, Williams JI, Gayton D (1989) Measuring balance: preliminary development of an instrument. *Physiotherapy Canada* 41(6), 304–310.

Berg L (1988) Clinical Dementia Rating (CDR). *Psychopharmacology Bulletin* 24(4), 637–639.

Bergner M, Bobbitt RA, Carter WB, Gibson BS (1981) The Sickness Impact Profile: development and final revision of a health status measure. *Medical Care* 19, 787–805.

Blank A (2001) Patient violence in community metal health: a review of the literature. *British Journal of Occupational Therapy* 64(12), 584–589.

Borg B, Bruce MA (1991) Assessing psychological performance factors. In C Christiansen, C Baum (eds), *Occupational Therapy: Overcoming Human Performance Deficits*. Thorofare, NJ, Slack.

Boud D, Keogh R, Walker D (1985) *Reflection: Turning Experience into Learning*. New York, Kogan Page.

Boulding KE (1968) General systems theory: the skeleton of science. In W Buckley (ed.), *Modern Systems Research for the Behavioral Scientist*. Chicago, Aldine.

Brooke P (2000) The 6-CIT Kingshill version 2000 and 4-item GDS, http://www.kingshill-re-search.org/kresearch/6cit.ASP, accessed 16.10.06.

Brooke P, Bullock R (1999) Validation of the 6-item Cognitive Impairment Test. *International Journal of Geriatric Psychiatry* **14**(11), 936–940.

Brown GT, Rodger S, Davis A (2003) Motor-Free Visual Perception Test – Revised: an overview and critique. *British Journal of Occupational Therapy* **66**(4), 159–167.

Browne JE, O'Hare NJ (2001) Review of different methods for assessing standing balance. *Physiotherapy* **87**(9), 489–495.

Bruce DG, Divine A, Prince RL (2002) Recreational physical activity levels in healthy older women: the importance of fear of falling. *Journal of the American Geriatric Society* **50**(1), 84–89.

Bruce E (2000) Looking after well-being: a tool for evaluation. *Journal of Dementia Care* **Nov/Dec**, 25–27.

Burke WT (1978) The development of a technique for assessing the stresses experienced by parents of young children. Unpublished doctoral dissertation, University of Virginia, Charlottesville. Cited in Abidin RR (1995) *Parenting Stress Index: Professional Manual* (3rd edn.). Odessa, FL, Psychological Assessment Resources.

Burnham M (1999) Effective group memory therapy for people with dementia. *Signpost* **3**(4), 2–4.

Burtner P, Wilhite C, Bordegaray J, Moedl D *et al.* (1997) Critical review of visual perceptual tests frequently administered by pediatric therapists. *Physical and Occupational Therapy in Pediatrics* **17**(3), 39–61.

Bury T, Mead J (1998) Evidence-based healthcare: a practical guide for therapists. Boston, Butterworth-Heinemann.

Cambridge Cognition (2006) Thinking ahead, http://www.cantab.com/cantab/site/home.acds?context=1306318&instanceid=1306319, accessed 08.10.06.

Cameron SJ, Orr RR (1989) Stress in families of school-aged children with delayed mental development. *Canadian Journal of Rehabilitation* **2**, 137–44.

Campbell AJ, Robertson MC, Gardner MM, Norton RN *et al.* (1997) Randomised control-led trial of a general practice programme of home based exercise to prevent falls in elderly women. *British Medical Journal* **315**(7373), 1065–1069.

Canadian Association of Occupational Therapists (2006) Canada's Occupational Therapy Resources site, http://www.otworks.ca/default.asp?pageid=781, accessed 10.08.06.

Canadian Association of Occupational Therapists (1991) *Occupational Therapy Guidelines for Client-centred Practice*. Toronto, CAOT.

Capra F (1982) *The Turning Point: Science, Society and the Rising Culture*. New York, Simon & Schuster.

Carnevali DL, Thomas MD (1993) *Diagnostic Reasoning and Treatment Decision Making in Nursing*. Philadelphia, JB Lippincott.

Carr J (2001) Reform of the Mental Health Act 1983: implications of safety, capacity and com-pulsion. *British Journal of Occupational Therapy* **64**(12), 590–594.

Carr P (1999) *Thesis Collection: The National Collection of Unpublished Occupational Therapy Research*. London, COT.

Carswell A, McColl MA, Baptiste S, Law M *et al.* (2004) The Canadian Occupational Performance Measure: a research and clinical literature review. *Canadian Journal of Occupational Therapy* **71**(4), 210–222.

Case-Smith H (2001) Development of childhood occupations. In H Case-Smith (ed.), *Occupational Therapy for Children*. St Louis, CV Mosby.

Cella DF, Dineen K, Arnason B, Reder A *et al.* (1996) Validation of the Functional Assessment of Multiple Sclerosis Quality of Life Instrument. *Neurology* **47**(1), 29–39.

Centre for Advanced Palliative Care (2005) Lexicon on the CAPC manual, http://64.85.16.230/educate/content/elements/lexicon/, accessed 26.10.05.

Chamberlain E, Evans N, Neighbour K, Hughes J (2001) Equipment: is it the answer? An audit of equipment provision. *British Journal of Occupational Therapy* **64**(12), 595–600.

Chandler JM, Duncan PW, Kochersberger G, Studenski S (1998) Is lower extremity strength gain associated with improvement in physical performance and disability in frail, community dwelling elders? *Archives of Physical Medicine and Rehabilitation* **79**(1), 24–30.

Chang JT, Morton SC, Rubenstein LZ, Mojica WA *et al.* (2004) Interventions for the prevention of falls in older adults: systematic review and meta-analysis of randomized clinical trials. *British Medical Journal* **328**(7441), 680.

Chapparo C (1979) Sensory integration for adults workshop. Cited in Hilko Culler K (1993) Home and family management. In HL Hopkins, HD Smith (eds), *Willard and Spackman's Occupational Therapy* (8th edn.). Philadelphia, JB Lippincott.

Chard G (2004) International Classification of Functioning, Disability and Health. *British Journal of Occupational Therapy* **67**(1), 1.

Chartered Society of Physiotherapy (2006a) Garner report, http://www.csp.org.uk/director/effectivepractice/healthinformatics.cfm, accessed 18.04.06.

Chartered Society of Physiotherapy (2006b) Reflective practice, http://www.csp.org.uk/director/careersandlearning/continuingprofessionaldevelopment/reflectivepractice.cfm, accessed 20.10.06.

Chartered Society of Physiotherapy (2005) Outcomes measures searchable database, http://www.csp.org.uk/director/effectivepractice/outcomemeasures/database.cfm, accessed 22.10.05.

Chartered Society of Physiotherapy (2005b) *Standards of Physiotherapy Practice (SOPP)*. London, CSP, http://www.csp.org.uk/director/effectivepractice/standards.cfm, accessed 07.12.06.

Chartered Society of Physiotherapy (2004a) Physiotherapy Pain Association (PPA) recommendations for low back pain-related functional limitation outcome measures, http://admin.csp.org.uk/admin2/uploads/-38c9a362-ed71ce5fa5–7f10/csp_outcomemeasures_clef04.pdf, accessed 21.03.05.

Chartered Society of Physiotherapy (2004b) Outcomes model: demonstrating competence through evidence of CPD, http://www.csp.org.uk/uploads/documents/csp_cpd_outcomes-model.pdf, accessed 22.10.05.

Chartered Society of Physiotherapy (2002a) Outcome measures for people with depression, http://admin.csp.org.uk/admin2/uploads/-38c9a362-ed71ce5fa5–7dcb/csp_outcomemeasures_clef05.pdf, accessed 21.03.05.

Chartered Society of Physiotherapy (2002b) Literature searching: a user's guide, http://www.csp.org.uk/libraryandinformation/publications/html/library_info_papers/csp_literature_search.cfm, accessed 21.03.05.

Chartered Society of Physiotherapy (2002c) Rules of professional conduct, http://admin.csp.org.uk/admin2/uploads/37536023-ec2dfbfabd–7bd2/csp_rules_conduct.pdf, accessed 03.08.05.

Chartered Society of Physiotherapy (2002d) *Physiotherapy Assistants Code of Conduct*. London, CSP.

Chartered Society of Physiotherapy (2001a) Outcome measures, http://admin.csp.org.uk/admin2/uploads/-38c9a362-ed71ce5fa5–7f12/csp_outcomemeasures_clef03.pdf, accessed 21.03.05.

Chartered Society of Physiotherapy (2001b) Specialisms and specialists: guidance for developing the clinical specialist role, http://www.csp.org.uk/uploads/documents/csp_physioprac_pa23.pdf, accessed 07.08.06.

Chartered Society of Physiotherapy (2000) *General Principles of Record Keeping and Access to Health Records.* London, CSP.

Chia SH (1996) The use of non-standardised assessments in occupational therapy with children who have disabilities: a perspective. *British Journal of Occupational Therapy* **59**(8), 363–364.

Chow WH (2001) An investigation of carers' burden: before and after a total hip replacement. *British Journal of Occupational Therapy* **64**(10), 503–508.

Christiansen C (1991) Occupational therapy – intervention for life performance. In C Christiansen, C Baum (eds), *Occupational Therapy: Overcoming Human Performance Deficits.* Thorofare, NJ, Slack.

Christiansen C, Baum C (eds) (1991) *Occupational Therapy: Overcoming Human Performance Deficits.* Thorofare, NJ, Slack.

Clabby J, O'Connor R (2004) Teaching learners to use mirroring: rapport lessons from neuro-linguistic programming. *Family Medicine* **36**(8), 541–543.

Clark CA, Corcoran M, Gitlin LN (1995) An exploratory study of how occupational therapists develop therapeutic partnerships with family caregivers. *American Journal of Occupational Therapy* **49**(7), 587–594.

Clarke C, Sealey-Lapes C, Kotsch L (2001) *Outcome Measures: Information Pack for Occupational Therapy.* London, COT.

Clemson L (1997) *Home Fall Hazards and the Westmead Home Safety Assessment.* West Brunswick, Australia, Coordinates Publications.

Clemson L, Fitzgerald MH, Heard R (1999) Content validity of an assessment tool to identify home fall hazards: the Westmead Home Safety Assessment. *British Journal of Occupational Therapy* **62**(4), 170–179.

Clifford P (2003) An infometric approach to mental health outcome measurement. Unpublished doctoral thesis, Psychology Department, University College London.

Clifford P (2002) The FACE Assessment and Outcome System. Nottingham, FACE Recording and Measurement Systems, http://www.facecode.com/tools.html, accessed 16.10.06.

Clinical Standards Advisory Group (1994) *Report on Back Pain.* London, HMSO.

Clouston T (2003) Narrative methods: talk, listening and representation. *British Journal of Occupational Therapy* **66**(4), 136–142.

Cohn ES, Czycholl C (1991) Facilitating a foundation for clinical reasoning: in self-paced instruction for clinical education and supervision (SPICES). Rockville, MD, AOTA.

Colborn AP, Robertson SC (1997) Outcomes in occupational therapy: perspectives and suggestions for research. *Occupational Therapy Practice* **2**(6), 36–39.

Cole B, Finch E, Gowland C, Mayo N (1995) *Physical Rehabilitation Outcome Measures.* London, Williams and Wilkins.

College of Occupational Therapists (2006) *COT/BAOT Briefings: Record Keeping: Issues of Responsibility.* London, COT.

College of Occupational Therapists (2005a) *Occupational Therapy Standard Terminology Project Report.* London, COT.

College of Occupational Therapists (2005b) CPD tools, http://www.cot.co.uk/members/education/lifelong_learning/cpd_tools.php, accessed 22.10.05.

College of Occupational Therapists (2005c) *COT/BAOT Quality Briefing 42: Assessments and Outcome Measures.* London, COT.

College of Occupational Therapists (2005d) *COT/BAOT Quality Briefing 39: Effective Practice.* London, COT.

College of Occupational Therapists (2005e) *COT/BAOT Quality Briefing 41: Governance in Health and Social Care.* London, COT.

College of Occupational Therapists (2005f) *Code of Ethics and Professional Conduct for Occupational Therapists.* London, COT.

College of Occupational Therapists (2004) *Guidance on the Use of the International Classification of Functioning, Disability and Health (ICF) and the Ottawa Charter for Health Promotion in Occupational Therapy Services.* London, COT.

College of Occupational Therapists (2003a) *Occupational Therapy Defined as a Complex Intervention*. London, COT.

College of Occupational Therapists (2003b) *Professional Standards for Occupational Therapy Practice*. London, COT.

College of Occupational Therapists (2000) *Producing Clinical Guidelines for Occupational Therapy Practice*. London, COT.

College of Occupational Therapists (1993) *Statement on Consent to Treatment (SPP 195)*. London, COT.

Collen FM, Wade DT, Robb GF, Bradshaw CM (1991) The Rivermead Mobility Index: a further development of the Rivermead Motor Assessment. *International Disability Studies* **13**(2), 50–54.

Community Occupational Therapists and Associates (1991) *Safety Assessment of Function and the Environment for Rehabilitation (SAFER Tool)*. Toronto, COTA.

Cooper B, Rigby P, Letts L (1995) Evaluation of access to home, community and workplace. In Trombly CA (ed.), *Occupational Therapy for Physical Dysfunction* (4th edn.). Baltimore, Williams and Wilkins.

Corr S (2003) Evaluate, evaluate, evaluate. *British Journal of Occupational Therapy* **66**(6), 235.

Coster W (1998) Occupation-centred assessment of children. *American Journal of Occupational Therapy* **52**(5), 337–345.

Coster W, Deeney T, Haltiwanger J, Haley S (1998) *School Function Assessment*. San Antonio, TX, The Psychological Corporation.

Coster WJ, Hayley SM (1992) Conceptualization and measurement of disablement in infants and young children. *Infants and Young Children* **4**(4), 11–22.

Cox DL (2000) *Occupational Therapy and Chronic Fatigue Syndrome*. London, Whurr.

Craik FIM (1977) Age differences in human memory. In JE Birren, KW Schaie (eds), *Handbook of the Psychology of Aging*. New York, Van Nostrand Reinhold.

Crammond HJ, Clark MS, Smith DS (1989) The effect of using the dominant or non-dominant hand on performance of the Rivermead Perceptual Assessment Battery. *Clinical Rehabilitation* **3**, 215–221.

Creek J (1996a) Making a cup of tea as an honours degree subject. *British Journal of Occupational Therapy* **59**(3), 128–130.

Creek J (ed) (1996b) *Occupational Therapy and Mental Health: Principles Skills and Practice*. Edinburgh, Churchill Livingstone.

Crocker L, Algina J (1986) *Introduction to Classical and Modern Test Theory*. Fort Worth, TX, Holt, Rinehart and Winston.

Cromack TR (1989) Measurement considerations in clinical research. In CB Royeen (ed.), *Clinical Research Handbook: An Analysis for the Service Professions*. Thorofare, NJ, Slack.

Cronbach L (1960) Validity. In CW Harris (ed.), *Encyclopedia of Educational Research*. New York, Macmillan.

Cup EH, Scholte OP, Reimer WJ, Thijssen MC, van Kuyk-Minis MA (2003) Reliability and validity of the Canadian Occupational Performance Measure in stroke patients. *Clinical Rehabilitation* **17**(4), 402–409.

Dalton P (1994) *Counselling People with Communication Problems*. London, Sage Publications.

Day L, Fildes B, Gordon I, Fitzharris M *et al.* (2002) Randomised factorial trial of falls prevention among older people living in their own homes. *British Medical Journal* **325**(7356), 128–141.

de Bruin AF, Diederiks JPM, de Witte LP, Stevens FC, Philipsen H (1994) The development of a short generic version of the Sickness Impact Profile. *Journal of Clinical Epidemiology* **47**(4), 407–418.

de Clive-Lowe S (1996) Outcome measurement, cost-effectiveness and clinical-audit: the importance of standardised assessment to occupational therapists in meeting these new demands. *British Journal of Occupational Therapy* **59**(8), 357–362.

DeGangi GA (1995) *Test of Attention in Infants*. Dayton, OH, Southpaw Enterprises.

DeGangi GA, Greenspan SI (1989) *Test of Sensory Functions in Infants*. Los Angeles, Western Psychological Services.

DeGangi GA, Poisson S, Sickel RZ, Santman Wiener A (1995) *Infant and Toddler Symptom Checklist*. Tucson, AZ, Therapy Skill Builders/The Psychological Corporation.

Dementia Services Collaborative (2004) What is a PDSA cycle?, http://www.neyh.csip.org.uk/dementia-services-collaborative/improvement-tools/pdsa-cycles.html, accessed 23.10.06.

Denshire S, Mullavey-O'Byrne C (2003) Named in the lexicon: meanings ascribed to occupational therapy in personal and professional life spaces. *British Journal of Occupational Therapy* **66**(11), 519–527.

Department of Health (2006a) Mental Capacity Act 2005 – summary, http://www.dh.gov.uk/PublicationsAndStatistics/Bulletins/ChiefExecutiveBulletin/ChiefExecutiveBulletinArticle/fs/en?CONTENT_ID=4108436&chk=z0Ds8/, accessed 04.10.06.

Department of Health (2006b) Introduction to the single assessment process, http://www.dh.gov.uk/PolicyAndGuidance/HealthAndSocialCareTopics/SocialCare/SingleAssessmentProcess/SingleAssessmentProcessArticle/fs/en?CONTENT_ID=4015630&chk=MBIL%2B1, accessed 16.10.06.

Department of Health (2004) Standards for better health: health care standards for services under the NHS, http://www.dh.gov.uk/assetRoot/04/13/29/91/04132991.pdf, accessed 16.10.06.

Department of Health (2003) *Implementing the NSF for Older People Falls Standard: Support for Commissioning Good Services*. London, TSO, http://www.dh.gov.uk/PublicationsAndStatistics/Publications/PublicationsPolicyAndGuidance/PublicationsPolicyAndGuidanceArticle/fs/en?CONTENT_ID=4071478&chk=8RlsvY, accessed 16.10.06.

Department of Health (2002a) *The Single Assessment Process: Guidance on Local Implementation*. London, DoH, http://www.dh.gov.uk/assetRoot/04/07/93/12/04079312.PDF, accessed 16.10.06.

Department of Health (2002b) Single Assessment Process (SAP) Annex B: key implications for older people and professionals: key implications for therapists, http://www.dh.gov.uk/PolicyAndGuidance/HealthAndSocialCareTopics/SocialCare/SingleAssessmentProcess/SingleAssessmentProcessArticle/fs/en?CONTENT_ID=4076541&chk=riuwvo, accessed 16.10.06.

Department of Health (2002c) Annex E: stages of assessment, http://www.dh.gov.uk/PolicyAndGuidance/HealthAndSocialCareTopics/SocialCare/SingleAssessmentProcess/SingleAssessmentProcessArticle/fs/en?CONTENT_ID=4073350&chk=SQMmkJ, accessed 16.10.06.

Department of Health (2002d) Annex F: domains and sub-domains of the Single Assessment Process, http://www.dh.gov.uk/assetRoot/04/07/33/78/04073378.pdf, accessed 16.10.06.

Department of Health (2001a) *National Service Framework for Older People*. London, DoH. http://www.dh.gov.uk/assetRoot/04/07/12/83/04071283.pdf, accessed 16.10.06.

Department of Health (2001b) Consent: what you have a right to expect: a guide for adults, http://www.dh.gov.uk/PublicationsAndStatistics/Publications/PublicationsPolicyAndGuidance/PublicationsPolicyAndGuidanceArticle/fs/en?CONTENT_ID=4005204&chk=q9IGT, accessed 01.04.06.

Department of Health (2001c) Exercise on prescription for NHS patients, http://www.dh.gov.uk/PublicationsAndStatistics/PressReleases/PressReleasesNotices/fs/en?CONTENT_ID=4010718&chk=LWsNgu, accessed 24.10.06.

Department of Health (2000) *Reforming the Mental Health Act*. White Paper Cm. 5016–I. London, TSO.

Department of Health (1999a) *Review of the Mental Health Act 1983: Report of the Expert Committee (chair: G Richardson)*. London, DoH.

Department of Health (1999b) *For the Record: Managing Records in NHS Trusts and Health Authorities*. London, DoH, http://www.dh.gov.uk/assetRoot/04/08/23/3904082339.pdf, accessed 10.10.06.

Department of Health (1998a) *Modernising Social Services*. London, TSO.

Department of Health (1998b) *The New NHS: Modern, Dependable*. London, TSO.

Department of Health (1998c) *Health Services Circular (HSC) 1998/153 Using Electronic Patient Records in Hospitals: Legal Requirement and Good Practice*. London, DoH, http://www.dh.gov.uk/PublicationsAndStatistics/LettersAndCirculars/HealthServiceCirculars/HealthServiceCircularsArticle/fs/en?CONTENT_ID=4004847&chk=ZdIiPM, accessed 21.04.06.

Donabedian A (1980) *The Definition of Quality and Approaches to Its Assessment*. Ann Arbour, MI, Health Administration Press.

Donaghy M, Morss K (2000) Guided reflection: a framework to facilitate and assess reflective practice within the discipline of physiotherapy. *Physiotherapy Theory and Practice* **16**(1), 3–14.

Donenberg G, Baker BL (1993) The impact of young children with externalising behaviors on their families. *Journal of Abnormal Child Psychology* **21**(2), 179–198.

Donnelly S (2002) The Rivermead Perceptual Assessment Battery: can it predict functional performance? *Australian Occupational Therapy Journal* **49**(2), 71–81.

Drever J (1973) *A Dictionary of Psychology* (revised by H Wallerstein). Middlesex, Penguin.

Dreyfus HL, Dreyfus SE (1986) *Mind Over Machine: The Power of Human Intuition and Expertise in the Era of the Computer*. New York, Free Press.

Duncan P, Studenski S, Chandler J, Prescott B (1992) Functional reach: predictive validity in a sample of elderly male veterans. *Journal of Gerontology* **47**(3), 93–98.

Duncan P, Weiner D, Chandler J, Studenski S (1990) Functional reach: a new clinical measure of balance. *Journal of Gerontology* **45**(6), M192–197.

Dunn W (2002) *Infant/Toddler Sensory Profile: User's Manual*. San Antonio, TX, Therapy Skill Builders.

Dunn W (2000) *Best Practice Occupational Therapy: In Community Service with Children and Families*. Thorofare, NJ, Slack.

Eakin P (1989a) Assessments of activities of daily living: a critical review. *British Journal of Occupational Therapy* **52**(1), 11–15.

Eakin P (1989b) Problems with assessments of activities of daily living. *British Journal of Occupational Therapy* **52**(2), 50–54.

EASY-Care (2006a) History and development, http://www.shef.ac.uk/sisa/easycare/html/what_is_easycare/easy_history.html, accessed 24.03.06.

EASY-Care (2006b) What is EASY-Care?, http://www.shef.ac.uk/sisa/easycare/easy-text.html, accessed 18.03.06.

Edgeworth JA, Robertson IH, McMillan TM (1998) *The Balloons Test*. Bury St Edmunds, Thames Valley Test Company.

Enderby P (1998) *Therapy Outcome Measures*. San Diego, Singular.

Enderby P, John A (1997) *Therapy Outcome Measures: Speech-language Pathology Technical Manual*. London, Singular.

Enderby P, John A, Petherham B (1998) *Therapy Outcome Measures Manual: Physiotherapy, Occupational Therapy*. San Diego, Singular.

Eva G, Paley J (2004) Numbers in evidence. *British Journal of Occupational Therapy* **67**(1), 47–49.

Fairgrieve E (1992) Ways of using the Movement ABC. In SE Henderson, DA Sugden (eds), *Movement Assessment Battery for Children*. London, The Psychological Corporation.

Field MJ, Lohr KN (1992) *Guidelines for Clinical Practice: From Development to Use*. Washington, National Academy Press.

Fisher AG (2003a) *Assessment of Motor and Process Skills. Volume 1: Development, Standardization and Administration Manual* (5th edn.). Fort Collins, CO, Three Star Press.

Fisher AG (2003b) *Assessment of Motor and Process Skills. Volume 2: User Manual* (5th edn.). Fort Collins, CO, Three Star Press.

Fisher AG (1993) The assessment of IADL motor skills: an application of many-faceted Rasch Analysis. *American Journal of Occupational Therapy* **47**(4), 319–329.

Fisher AG, Bryze K, Hume V (2002) *School AMPS*. Fort Collins, CO, Three Star Press.

Fisher AG, Short-DeGraff M (1993) Improving functional assessment in occupational therapy: recommendations and philosophy for change. *American Journal of Occupational Therapy* **47**(3), 199–201.

Fitzpatrick R (2004) Measures of health status, health-related quality of life and patient satisfaction. In P Pynsent, J Fairbank, A Carr (eds), *Outcome Measures in Orthopaedics and Orthopaedic Trauma* (2nd edn.). London, Arnold.

Fleming MH (1994a) The therapist with a three-track mind. In C Mattingly and MH Fleming (eds), *Clinical Reasoning: Forms of Inquiry in a Therapeutic Practice*. Philadelphia, FA Davis.

Fleming MH (1994b) Procedural reasoning: addressing functional limitations. In C Mattingly and MH Fleming (eds), *Clinical Reasoning: Forms of Inquiry in a Therapeutic Practice*. Philadelphia, FA Davis.

Fleming MH (1991) Clinical reasoning in medicine compared with clinical reasoning in occupational therapy. *American Journal of Occupational Therapy* **45**(11), 988–996.

Folio R, Fewell RR (1983) *Peabody Developmental Motor Scales and Activity Cards*. Hingham, MA, DLM Teaching Resources.

Folstein MF, Folstein SE, McHugh PR (1975) Mini Mental State: a practical method for grading the cognitive state of patients for the clinician. *Journal of Psychiatry Research* **12**(3), 189.

Foster (2002) Skills for practice. In A Turner, M Foster, SE Johnson (eds), *Occupational Therapy and Physical Dysfunction: Principles, Skills and Practice* (5th edn.). London, Churchill Livingstone.

Fraser SW (2002) *The Patient's Journey: Mapping, Analysing and Improving Healthcare Processes*. Chichester, Kingham Press.

Freeman JA (2002) Treatment and management of a patient with multiple sclerosis. In C Partridge (ed.), *Bases of Evidence for Practice: Neurological Physiotherapy*. London, Whurr.

Friedman PJ, Richmond DE, Baskett JJ (1988) A prospective trial of serial gait speed as a measure of rehabilitation in the elderly. *Age and Ageing* **22**(4), 27–30.

Fugl-Meyer AR, Jaasko L, Leyman I, Olsson S, Steglind S (1975) The post-stroke hemiplegic patient: a method for the evaluation of physical performance. *Scandinavian Journal of Rehabilitation Medicine* **7**(1), 13–31.

Gardner M (1996) *Test of Visual Perceptual Skills (Non-motor) – Revised*. Hydesville, CA, Psychological and Educational Publications.

Gardner MM, Buchner DM, Robertson MC, Campbell AJ (2001) Practical implementation of an exercise-based falls prevention programme. *Age and Ageing* **30**(1), 77–83.

Garner R, Rugg S (2005) Electronic care records: an update on the Garner Project. *British Journal of Occupational Therapy* **68**(3), 131–134.

Gibbs G (1988) *Learning by Doing: a Guide to Teaching and Learning Methods*. Oxford, Further Education Unit, Oxford Polytechnic.

Gifford L (ed.) (2000) *Topical Issues in Pain 2: Biopsychosocial Assessment and Management, Relationships and Pain*. Falmouth, CNS Press.

Gifford L (ed.) (1998) *Topical Issues in Pain 1: Whiplash: Science and Management; Fear Avoidance Beliefs and Behaviour*. Falmouth, CNS Press.

Gift AG (1989) Validation of a vertical visual analogue scale as a measure of clinical dyspnoea. *Rehabilitation Nursing* **14**(6), 323–325.

Gilleard CJ (1984) *Living with Dementia: Community Care of the Elderly Mentally Infirm*. Beckenham, Croom Helm.

Gillespie LD, Gillespie WJ, Robertson MC, Lamb SE *et al.* (2003) *Interventions for Preventing Falls in Elderly People* (Cochrane Review). In The Cochrane Library, Issue 4. Chichester, John Wiley & Sons.

Golding E (1989) *The Middlesex Elderly Assessment of Mental State (MEAMS)*. Bury St Edmunds, Thames Valley Test Company.

Gowland C, Stratford P, Ward M, Moreland J *et al.* (1993) Measuring physical impairment and disability with the Chedoke–McMaster Stroke Assessment. *Stroke* **24**(1), 58–63.

Granger CV, Hamilton BB, Linacre JM, Heinemann AW, Wright BD (1993) Performance profiles of the functional independence measure. *American Journal of Physical Medicine and Rehabilitation* **72**(2), 84–89.

Green D, Bishop T, Wilson N, Crawford S *et al.* (2005) Is questionnaire-based screening part of the solution to waiting lists for children with development coordination disorder? *British Journal of Occupational Therapy* **68**(1), 2–10.

Greenhalgh J, Long AF, Brettle AJ, Grant MJ (1998) Reviewing and selecting outcome measures for use in routine practice. *Journal of Evaluation in Clinical Practice* **4**(4), 339–350.

Griffin EM (1997) *A First Look at Communication Theory.* New York, McGraw-Hill.

Griffiths S, Schell D (2002) Professional context. In A Turner, M Foster, S Johnson (eds), *Occupational Therapy and Physical Dysfunction: Principles, Skills and Practice* (5th edn.). London, Churchill Livingstone.

Guyatt G, Berman LB, Townsend M, Pugsley SO, Chambers LW (1987) A measure of quality of life for clinical trials in chronic lung disease. *Thorax* **42**(10), 773–778.

Hagedorn R (1997) *Foundations for Practice in Occupational Therapy.* New York, Churchill Livingstone.

Hall AD, Fagen RE (1956) Definition of a system. *General Systems Yearbook* **1**, 18–28.

Hamilton EB (1980) The relationship of maternal patterns of stress, coping, and support to quality of early infant–mother attachment. Unpublished doctoral dissertation, University of Virginia, Charlottesville. Cited in Abidin RR (1995) *Parenting Stress Index: Professional Manual* (3rd edn.). Odessa, FL, Psychological Assessment Resources.

Hammell KW (2004) Deviating from the norm: a sceptical interrogation of the classificatory practices of the ICF. *British Journal of Occupational Therapy* **67**(9), 408–411.

Hammell KW (2003) Changing institutional environments to enable occupation among people with severe physical impairments. In L Letts, P Rigby, D Stewart (eds), *Using Environments to Enable Occupational Performance.* Thorofare, NJ, Slack.

Hanson MJ, Hanline MF (1990) Parenting a child with a disability: a longitudinal study of parental stress and adaptation. *Journal of Early Intervention* **14**(3), 234–248.

Harding VH, Williams AC, Richardson PH, Nicholas MK *et al.* (1994) The development of a battery of measures for assessing physical functioning of chronic pain patients. *Pain* **58**(3), 367–375.

Hauenstein E, Scarr S, Abidin RR (1987) Detecting children at risk for developmental delay: efficacy of the Parenting Stress Index in a non-American culture. Unpublished manuscript, University of Virginia, Charlottesville. Cited in Abidin RR (1995) *Parenting Stress Index: Professional Manual* (3rd edn.). Odessa, FL, Psychological Assessment Resources.

Hayley SM, Coster WJ, Ludlow LH (1991) Pediatric functional outcome measures. *Physical Medicine and Rehabilitation Clinics of North America* **2**, 689–723.

Hayley SM, Coster WJ, Ludlow LH, Haltiwanger JT, Andrellos PJ (1998) *Pediatric Evaluation of Disability Inventory (PEDI): Development, Standardization and Administration Manual: Version 1.0.* Boston, Boston University.

Hayley SM, Coster WJ, Ludlow LH, Haltiwanger JT, Andrellos PJ (1992) *Pediatric Evaluation of Disability Inventory: Development, Standardization and Administration Manual.* Boston, New England Medical Center.

Haynes SN, Richard DCS, Kubany ES (1995) Content validity in psychological assessment: a functional approach to concepts and methods. *Psychological Assessment* **7**(3), 238–347.

Health Professions Council (2006) *Your Guide to Our Standards for Continuing Professional Development.* London, HPC.

Health Professions Council (2005) Continuing professional development – key decisions, http://www.hpc-uk.org/publications/consultations/index.asp?id=76, accessed 22.10.05.

Heaton J, Bamford C (2001) Assessing the outcomes of equipment and adaptations: issues and approaches. *British Journal of Occupational Therapy* **64**(7), 346–356.

Henderson A (1991) Measurement and knowledge development. In Symposium on Measurement and Research 16th–18th October 1991. University of Illinois at Chicago, unpublished paper.

Henderson S, Sugden D (1992) *Movement Assessment Battery for Children.* London, The Psychological Corporation.

Higgs J (1990) Developing knowledge: a process of construction, mapping and review. *New Zealand Journal of Physiotherapy* **20**, 23–30.

Higgs J, Bithell C (2001) Professional expertise. In J Higgs, A Titchen (eds), *Practice Knowledge and Expertise in the Health Professions*. Oxford, Butterworth-Heinemann.

Higgs J, Jones M (2000) Clinical reasoning in the health professions. In J Higgs, M Jones (eds), *Clinical Reasoning in the Health Professions* (2nd edn.). Oxford, Butterworth-Heinemann.

Hilko Culler K (1993) Home and family management. In HL Hopkins and HD Smith (eds), *Willard and Spackman's Occupational Therapy* (8th edn.). Philadelphia, JB Lippincott.

Hill J (1993) Activities of daily living. In HL Hopkins and HD Smith (eds), *Willard and Spackman's Occupational Therapy* (8th edn.). Philadelphia, JB Lippincott.

Hogan K, Orme S (2000) Measuring disability: a critical analysis of the Barthel Index. *British Journal of Therapy and Rehabilitation* **7**(4), 163–167.

Hopkins H, Smith H (eds) (1993a) *Willard and Spackman's Occupational Therapy* (8th edn.). Philadelphia, JB Lippincott.

Hopkins HL, Smith HD (1993b) Appendix G: hierarchy of competencies relating to the use of standardized instruments and evaluation techniques by occupational therapists produced by the American Occupational Therapy Association. In HL Hopkins and HD Smith (eds), *Willard and Spackman's Occupational Therapy* (8th edn.). Philadelphia, JB Lippincott.

Hughes S (1983) *Orthopaedics and Traumatology* (3rd edn.). London, Hodder & Stoughton.

Hunt SM, McEwen J, McKenna SP (1985) Measuring health status: a new tool for clinicians and epidemiologists. *Journal of the Royal College of General Practitioners* **35**(273), 185–188.

Hunter J (1997) Outcome, indices and measurements. In CJ Goodwill, MA Chamberlain, C Evans (eds), *Rehabilitation of the Physically Disabled Adult*. Cheltenham, Stanley Thornes.

Hurley BF, Roth SM (2000) Strength training in the elderly. *Sports Medicine* **30**(4), 249–268.

Iles V, Sutherland K (2001) Managing change in the NHS. Organisational change: a review for healthcare managers, professionals and researchers. London, National Co-ordinating Centre for NHS Service Delivery and Organisation R & D (NCC SDO), http://www.sdo.lshtm.ac.uk, accessed 01.05.04.

Jacobs K (1993) Occupational therapy performance areas: section 2B1 work assessments and programming. In HL Hopkins and HD Smith (eds), *Willard and Spackman's Occupational Therapy* (8th edn.). Philadelphia, JB Lippincott.

Jeffrey LIH (1993) Aspects of selecting outcome measures to demonstrate effectiveness of comprehensive rehabilitation. *British Journal of Occupational Therapy* **56**(11), 394–400.

Jensen GM, Gwyer J, Hack LM, Shepard F (2000) Research report: expert practice in physical therapy. *Physical Therapy* **80**(1), 28–43, http://www.ptjournal.org/pt_journal/PTJournal/January2000/v80n1p28.cfm, accessed 07.08.06.

Jerosh-Herold C (2005) An evidence-based approach to choosing outcome measures: a checklist for the critical appraisal of validity, reliability and responsiveness studies. *British Journal of Occupational Therapy* **68**(8), 347–353.

Jette AM (1995) Outcomes research: shifting the dominant research paradigm in physical therapy. *Physical Therapy* **75**(11), 965–970.

Jette AM (1994) Physical disablement concepts for physical therapy research and practice. *Physical Therapy* **74**(5), 380–386.

Johns C (2004) Foreword. In S Tate, M Sills (eds), *The Development of Critical Reflection in the Health Professions*. London, School of Integrated Health, LTSN/HSAP, http://www.health.ltsn.ac.uk/publications/occasionalpaper/occasionalpaper04.pdf, accessed 10.10.06.

Jones L (1991) Symposium on methodology: the standardized test. *Clinical Rehabilitation* **5**, 177–180.

Katz N (1988) Interest Checklist: a factor analytical study. *Occupational Therapy in Mental Health* **8**(1), 45–55.

Kazdin AE (1990) Premature termination from treatment among children referred for anti-social behavior. *Journal of Child Psychology and Psychiatry and Allied Disciplines* **31**(3), 415–425.

Khanna R (2004) Reflective practice within the occupational therapy curriculum. In S Tate, M Sills (eds), *The Development of Critical Reflection in the Health Professions*. London, LTSN/HSAP, http://www.health.ltsn.ac.uk/publications/occasionalpaper/occassionalpaper04.pdf, accessed 30.07.06.

Kielhofner G (2002) *Model of Human Occupation* (3rd edn.). Baltimore, Lippincott, Williams and Wilkins.

Kielhofner G (1992) *Conceptual Foundations of Occupational Therapy*. Philadelphia, FA Davis.

Kielhofner G (1985) *A Model of Human Occupation: Theory and Application*. Baltimore, Williams and Wilkins.

Kielhofner G (1978) General systems theory: implications for theory and action in occupational therapy. *American Journal of Occupational Therapy* **32**(10), 637–645.

Kielhofner G, Burke J (1980) A Model of Human Occupation, part one: conceptual framework and content. *American Journal of Occupational Therapy* **34**(9), 572–581.

Kielhofner G, Forsyth K (1997) The Model of Human Occupation: an overview of current concepts. *British Journal of Occupational Therapy* **60**(3), 103–110.

Kielhofner G, Henry AD (1988) Development and investigation of the Occupational Performance History Interview. *American Journal of Occupational Therapy* **42**(8), 489–498.

King CA, Bithell C (1998) Expertise in diagnostic reasoning: a comparative study. *British Journal of Therapy and Rehabilitation* **5**(2), 78–87.

Klein RM, Bell BJ (1982) *Klein–Bell Activities of Daily Living Scale*. Seattle, WA, Health Sciences Centre for Educational Resources, University of Washington.

Kline P (1990) How tests are constructed and selecting the best test. In JR Beech and L Harding (eds), *Testing People*. Windsor, NFER-Nelson.

Kline P (1986) *A Handbook of Test Construction*. London, Methuen.

Knox V, Evans AL (2002) Evaluation of the functional effects of a course of Bobath therapy in children with cerebral palsy: a preliminary study. *Developmental Medicine & Child Neurology* **44**(7), 447–60.

Lafiosca T (1981) The relationship of parent stress to anxiety, approval, motivation and children's behaviour problems. Unpublished doctoral dissertation, University of Virginia, Charlottesville. Cited in Abidin RR (1995) *Parenting Stress Index: Professional Manual* (3rd edn.). Odessa, FL, Psychological Assessment Resources.

Laliberte Rudman DL, Tooke J, Glencross T, Eimantes T *et al.* (1998) Preliminary investigation of the content validity and clinical utility of the predischarge assessment tool. *Canadian Journal of Occupational Therapy* **65**(1), 3–11.

Lane D (2006) Normal distribution: hyperstat online statistics textbook, http://davidmlane.com/hyperstat/normal_distribution.html, accessed 16.10.06.

Langley G, Nolan K, Nolan T, Norman C, Provost L (1996) *The Improvement Guide: A Practical Approach to Enhancing Organisational Performance*. San Francisco, Jossey-Bass.

Larin H, Wessel J, Al-Shamlan A (2005) Reflections of physiotherapy students in the United Arab Emirates during their clinical placements: a qualitative study. *BMC Medical Education* **5**(3), http://www.biomedcentral.com/1472-6920/5/3, accessed 30.07.06.

Laver AJ (1996) The occupational therapy intervention process. In KO Larson, RG Stevens-Ratchford, LW Pedretti, JL Crabtree (eds), *ROTE: The Role of Occupational Therapy with the Elderly: A Self-Paced Clinical Course*. Bethesda, MD, AOTA.

Laver AJ (1994) The development of the Structured Observational Test of Function (SOTOF). Unpublished doctoral thesis, University of Surrey, Guildford (held at the College of Occupational Therapists library, London).

Laver AJ (1990) Test review: the Rivermead Perceptual Assessment Battery. In JR Beech, L Harding (eds), *Assessment of the Elderly*. Windsor, NFER-Nelson.

Laver AJ, Baum CM (1992) Areas of occupational therapy assessment related to the NCMRR model of dysfunction. In AJ Laver (1994) The Development of the Structured Observational Test of Function (SOTOF). Unpublished doctoral thesis, University of Surrey, Guildford.

Laver AJ, Huchinson S (1994) The performance and experience of normal elderly people on the Chessington Occupational Therapy Neurological Assessment Battery (COTNAB). *British Journal of Occupational Therapy* **57**(4), 137–142.

Laver AJ, Powell GE (1995) *The Structured Observational Test of Function (SOTOF)*. Windsor, NFER-Nelson.

Laver AJ, Unsworth C (1999) Evaluation and intervention with simple perceptual impairment (agnosias). In C Unsworth (ed.), *Cognitive and Perceptual Dysfunction: A Clinical Reasoning Approach to Evaluation and Intervention*. Philadelphia, FA Davis.

Laver Fawcett AJ (2002) Assessment. In A Turner, M Foster, S Johnson (eds), *Occupational Therapy and Physical Dysfunction: Principles, Skills and Practice*. London, Churchill Livingstone.

Law M (2001) Appendix 2: outcome measures rating form guidelines. In M Law, C Baum, W Dunn (eds), *Measuring Occupational Performance: Supporting Best Practice in Occupational Therapy*. Thorofare, NJ, Slack.

Law M (1997) Self care. In J Van Deusen, D Brunt (eds), *Assessment in Occupational Therapy and Physical Therapy*. London, WB Saunders.

Law M (1993) Evaluating activities of daily living: directions for the future. *American Journal of Occupational Therapy* **47**(3), 233–237.

Law M, Baptiste S, Carswell-Opzoomer A, McColl MA *et al.* (1991) *Canadian Occupational Performance Measure*. Toronto, CAOT.

Law M, Baptiste S, Carswell A, McColl MA *et al.* (1994b) *Canadian Occupational Performance Measure* (2nd end.). Ottawa, CAOT.

Law M, Baum C (2001) Measurement in occupational therapy. In M Law, C Baum, W Dunn (eds), *Measuring Occupational Performance: Supporting Best Practice in Occupational Therapy*. Thorofare, NJ, Slack.

Law M, Baptiste S, Carswell A, McColl M *et al.* (1998) *The Canadian Occupational Performance Measure* (3rd edn.). Ottawa, CAOT.

Law M, Letts L (1989) A critical review of scales of activities of daily living. *American Journal of Occupational Therapy* **43**(8), 522–528.

Law M, Baum C, Dunn W (eds) (2001) *Measuring Occupational Performance: Supporting Best Practice in Occupational Therapy*. Thorofare, NJ, Slack.

Law M, Cooper B, Strong S, Stewart D *et al.* (1996) The person-environment-occupation model: a transactive approach to occupational performance. *Canadian Journal of Occupational Therapy* **63**(1), 9–23.

Law M, Polatajko H, Pollock N, McColl MA *et al.* (1994) Pilot testing of the Canadian Occupational Performance Measure: clinical and measurement issues. *Canadian Journal of Occupational Therapy* **61**(4), 191–197.

Law M, Russell D, Pollock N, Rosenbaum P *et al.* (1995) A comparison of intensive neurodevelopmental therapy plus casting and a regular occupational therapy program for children with cerebral palsy. Unpublished thesis. Hamilton, ON, Neurodevelopmental Clinical Research Unit, McMaster University.

Lawley J, Thompkins P (2000) *Metaphors in Mind: Transformation Through Symbolic Modelling*. Lisburn, UK, The Developing Company Press.

Lawley J, Thompkins P (1997) Less is more: the art of clean language, http://www.anlp.org/index.asp?CatName=Magazine&CatID=9, accessed 16.10.06.

Lawton MP, Brody EM (1969) Assessment of older people: self-maintaining and instrumental activities of daily living. *Gerontologist* **9**(3), 179–186.

Lefton LA, Boyles MC, Ogden NA (2000) *Psychology*. Toronto, Prentice Hall.

Letts L, Bosch J (2001) Measuring occupational performance in basic activities of daily living. In M Law, C Baum, W Dunn (eds), *Measuring Occupational Performance: Supporting Best Practice in Occupational Therapy*. Thorofare, NJ, Slack.

Letts L, Law M, Pollock N, Stewart D *et al.* (1999) *A Programme Evaluation Workbook for Occupational Therapists: An Evidenced-based Practice Tool*. Ottawa, CAOT.

Letts L, Scott S, Burtney J, Marshall L, McKean M (1998) The reliability and validity of the Safety Assessment of Function and the Environment for Rehabilitation (SAFER Tool). *British Journal of Occupational Therapy* **61**(3), 127–132.

Levine RE, Brayley CR (1991) Occupation as a therapeutic medium: a contextual approach to performance intervention. In C Christiansen, C Baum (eds), *Occupational Therapy: Overcoming Human Performance Deficits*. Thorofare, NJ, Slack.

Lewis CB, Bottomley JM (1994) *Geriatric Physical Therapy: A Clinical Approach*. Norwalk, CT, Appleton & Lange.

Lewis SC (1989) *Elder Care in Occupational Therapy*. Thorofare, NJ, Slack.

Liang MH (1995) Evaluating measurement responsiveness. *Journal of Rheumatology* **22**(6), 1191–1192.

Lichtman M, Barokas J, Kaplan SH, Royeen CB (1989) Distribution of variables in clinical research. In CB Royeen (ed.), *Clinical Research Handbook: An Analysis for the Service Professions*. Thorofare, NJ, Slack.

Lincoln NB, Edmans J (1989) A shortened version of the Rivermead Perceptual Assessment Battery. *Clinical Rehabilitation* **3**(3), 199–204.

Lunz ME, Stahl JA (1993) The effect of rater severity on person ability measure: a Rasch model analysis. *American Journal of Occupational Therapy* **47**(4), 311–317.

Mackay DM (1968) The informational analysis of questions and commands. In W Buckley (ed.), *Modern Systems Research for the Behavioural Scientist: A Sourcebook*. Chicago, Aldine.

Mackenzie L, Byles J, Higginbotham N (2000) Designing the Home Falls and Accidents Screening Tool (Home FAST): selecting the items. *British Journal of Occupational Therapy* **63**(6), 260–269.

MacRae A (2005) Mental health of the older adult. In E Cara and A MacRae (eds), *Psychosocial Occupational Therapy: A Clinical Practice* (2nd edn.). Albany, OR, Thomson Delmar Learning.

Mahoney F, Barthel D (1965) Functional evaluation: the Barthel Index. *Maryland State Medical Journal* **14**(Feb), 61–65.

Main CJ, Spanswick CC (eds) (2000) *Pain Management: An Interdisciplinary Approach*. London, Churchill Livingstone.

Maitland GD, Hengeveld E, Banks K, English K (eds) (2000) *Maitland's Vertebral Manipulation* (6th edn.). Sydney, Butterworth-Heinemann.

Maniadakis N, Gray A (2004) Economic evaluation. In P Pynsent, J Fairbank, A Carr (eds), *Outcome Measures in Orthopaedics and Orthopaedic Trauma* (2nd edn.). London, Arnold.

Margolis RB, Chibnall JT, Tait RC (1988) Test–retest reliability of the pain drawing instrument. *Pain* **33**(1), 49–51.

Margolis RB, Tait RC, Krause SJ (1986) A rating system for use with pain drawings. *Pain* **24**(1), 57–65.

Marino RJ, Shea JA, Stineman MG (1998) The Capabilities of Upper Extremity Instrument: reliability and validity of a measure of functional limitation in tetraplegia. *Archives of Physical Medicine and Rehabilitation* **79**(12), 1512–1521.

Maslow A (1943) Theory of human motivation. *Psychological Review* **50**, 370–396. For the full paper see: http://psychclassics.yorku.ca/Maslow/motivation.htm, or for a summary: http://en.wikipedia.org/wiki/Maslow's_hierarchy_of_needs, accessed 01.01.06.

Mathias S, Nayak USL, Isaacs B (1986) Balance in elderly patients: the 'get up and go' test. *Archives of Physical Medicine and Rehabilitation* **67**(6), 387–389.

Matsutsuyu J (1969) The Interest Checklist. *American Journal of Occupational Therapy* **23**(4), 323–328.

Matthey S, Donnelly S, Hextell D (1993) The clinical usefulness of the Rivermead Perceptual Assessment battery: statistical considerations. *British Journal of Occupational Therapy* **56**(10), 365–370.

Mattingly C (1994a) Occupational therapy as a two-body practice: the lived body. In C Mattingly, MH Fleming (eds), *Clinical Reasoning: Forms of Inquiry in a Therapeutic Practice*. Philadelphia, FA Davis.

Mattingly C (1994b) The narrative nature of clinical reasoning. In C Mattingly, MH Fleming (eds), *Clinical Reasoning: Forms of Inquiry in a Therapeutic Practice*. Philadelphia, FA Davis.

Mattingly C (1991) What is clinical reasoning? *American Journal of Occupational Therapy* **45**(11), 979–986.

Mattingly C, Fleming MH (1994a) *Clinical Reasoning: Forms of Inquiry in a Therapeutic Practice*. Philadelphia, FA Davis.

Mattingly C, Fleming MH (1994b) Interactive Reasoning: collaborating with the person. In C Mattingly, MH Fleming (eds), *Clinical Reasoning: Forms of Inquiry in a Therapeutic Practice*. Philadelphia, FA Davis.

Mayers C (2003) The development and evaluation of the Mayers' Lifestyle Questionnaire 2. *British Journal of Occupational Therapy* **66**(9), 388–395.

Mayers C (2002) *The Mayers' Quality of Life Scale*. York, York St John College.

Mayers C (2000) Quality of life: priorities for people with enduring mental health problems. *British Journal of Occupational Therapy* **63**(12), 591–566.

Mayers C (1998) An evaluation of the use of the Mayers' Lifestyle Questionnaire. *British Journal of Occupational Therapy* **61**(9), 393–398.

Mayers C (1995) Defining and assessing quality of life. *British Journal of Occupational Therapy* **58**(4), 146–150.

Mayo N, Cole B, Dowler J, Gowland C, Finch E (1994) Use of outcome measures in physiotherapy: a survey of current practice. *Canadian Journal of Rehabilitation* **7**, 81–82.

McAvoy E (1991) The use of ADL indices by occupational therapists. *British Journal of Occupational Therapy* **54**(10), 383–385.

McCormack GL, Llorens LA, Glogoski C (1991) Culturally diverse elders. In Kiernat JM (ed.), *Occupational Therapy and the Older Adult*. Aspen, CO, Gaithersburg.

McDonald R, Surtees R, Wirz S (2004) The International Classification of Functioning, Disability and Health provides a model for adaptive seating interventions for children with cerebral palsy. *British Journal of Occupational Therapy* **67**(7), 293–302.

McDowell I, Newell C (1987) *Measuring Health: A Guide to Rating Scales and Questionnaires*. Oxford, Oxford University Press.

McFayden AK, Pratt J (1997) Understanding the statistical concepts of measures of work performance. *British Journal of Occupational Therapy* **60**(6), 279–284.

McGruder J (2004) Disease models of mental illness and aftercare patient education: critical observations from meta-analyses, cross-cultural practice and anthropological study. *British Journal of Occupational Therapy* **67**(7), 310–318.

McKee KJ, Philp I, Lamura G, Prouskas C et al. (2003) The COPE Index: a first stage assessment of negative impact, positive value and quality of support of caregiving in informal carers of older people. *Ageing and Mental Health* **7**(1), 39–52.

McQuay HJ (2004) The measures of pain. In P Pynsent, J Fairbank, A Carr (eds), *Outcome Measures in Orthopaedics and Orthopaedic Trauma* (2nd edn.). London, Arnold.

Meenan RF, Gertman PM, Mason JH (1980) Measuring health status in arthritis: Arthritis Impact Measurement Scales. *Arthritis Rheumatism* **23**(2), 146–152.

Meenan RF, Gertman PM, Mason JH, Dunaif R (1982) The Arthritis Impact Measurement Scales: further investigations of a health status measure. *Arthritis Rheumatism* **25**(9), 1048–1053.

Melzack R (1987) The short-form McGill Pain Questionnaire. *Pain* **30**(2), 191–197.

Melzack R (1975) The McGill Pain Questionnaire: major properties and scoring methods. *Pain* **1**(3), 277–299.

Missiuna C, Pollock N, Law M (2004) *Perceived Efficacy and Goal Setting System (PEGS)*. San Antonio, TX, The Psychological Corporation.

Model of Human Occupation (2006) Introduction to MOHO, http://www.moho.uic.edu/intro.html, accessed 10.08.06.

Mollineux M (ed) (2004) *Occupation for Occupational Therapists*. Oxford, Blackwell.

Molloy DW, Alemayehu E, Roberts R (1991) Reliability of a standardised mini-mental state examination compared with traditional mini-mental state examination. *American Journal of Psychiatry* **148**(1), 102–105.

Moran G, Pederson DR, Pettit P, Krupka A (1992) Maternal sensitivity and infant–mother attachment in a developmentally delayed sample. *Infant Behavior & Development* **15**(44), 427–442.

Mosey AC (1991) Common vocabulary. *Occupational Therapy Journal of Research* **11**, 67–68.

Mosey AC (1981) *Occupational Therapy: Configuration of a Profession*. New York, Raven Press.

Mountain G, Lepley D (1998) *Finding and Using the Evidence Base*. London, COT.

Muir Gray JA (2001) *Evidence-based Health Care*. Edinburgh, Churchill Livingstone.

Murdock C (1992) A critical evaluation of the Barthel Index: part 1. *British Journal of Occupational Therapy* **55**(3), 109–111.

Nagi SZ (1991) Disability concepts revisited: implications for prevention. In AM Pope, AR Tarlov (eds), *Disability in America: Toward a National Agenda for Prevention*. Washington, National Academy Press.

National Association of Rheumatology Occupational Therapists (2005) Occupational therapy in the management of inflammatory rheumatic diseases, http://www.cot.co.uk/members/publications/guidelines/pdf/inflammatory1.pdf, accessed 10.10.06.

National Co-ordinating Centre for NHS Service Delivery and Organisation R & D (2001) Managing change in the NHS: organisational change, http://www.sdo.lshtm.ac.uk/managingchange.html, accessed 16.10.06.

National Center for Medical Rehabilitation Research (1992) *Report and Plan for Medical Rehabilitation Research to Congress*. Bethesda, MD, NCMRR/US Department of Health and Human Services, National Institutes of Health.

Neale M (2004) Why I have difficulty with standardised assessments and outcome measures. *NANOT News: Journal of the National Association of Neurological Occupational Therapists* **24**(winter), 25–26.

NHS Executive (1996) *Clinical Guidelines*. Leeds, NHSE.

NHS Information Authority (2003) Clinical Governance Assessment Toolkit (CGAT), http://www.icservices.nhs.uk/clinicalgovernance/pages/default.asp, accessed 16.10.06.

NHS Modernisation Agency (2006) *NHS Modernisation Agency Collaboration Tools*. London, DoH.

NHS Modernisation Agency (2004) *Improvement Leader's Guide to Working in Systems*. London, DoH.

NHS Modernisation Agency (2002a) *Improvement Leader's Guide to Process Mapping, Analysis and Redesign*. London, DoH.

NHS Modernisation Agency (2002b) *Improvement Leader's Guide to Measurement for Improvement*. London, DoH.

NHS Modernisation Agency (2002c) *Improvement Leader's Guide for Involving Patients and Carers*. London, DoH.

Norkin CC, White DJ (1975) Measurement of joint motion: a guide to goniometry. Philadelphia, FA Davies. For details of third edition published in 2003 go to: http://www.matthewsbooks.com/productdetail.aspx?pid=8036NOR0972&close=false, accesed 07.01.06.

Norusīs MJ (1992) *SPSS/PC+: Base System User's Guide, Version 5.0*. Chicago, SPSS Inc.

Norusīs MJ (1991) *The SPSS Guide to Data Analysis for SPSS/PC+* (2nd edn.). Chicago, SPSS Inc.

Oakley F, Kielhofner G, Barris R, Reichler RK (1986) The Role Checklist: development and empirical assessment of reliability. *Occupational Therapy Journal of Research* **6**(3), 157–170.

O'Brien MT (1993) Multiple sclerosis: stressors and coping strategies in spousal caregivers. *Journal of Community Health Nursing* **10**(3), 123–35.

Opacich KJ (1991) Assessment and informed decision making. In C Christiansen, C Baum (eds), *Occupational Therapy: Overcoming Human Performance Deficits*. Thorofare, NJ, Slack.

Ostensjo S, Carlberg EB, Vollestad NK (2004) Motor impairments in young children with cerebral palsy: relationship to gross motor function and everyday activities. *Developmental Medicine & Child Neurology* **46**(9), 580–589.

OTseeker (2005) What is evidence-based practice?, http://www.otseeker.com/tutorial.htm, accessed 26.10.06.

Ottenbacher KJ, Tomchek SD (1993) Reliability analysis in therapeutic research: practice and procedures. *American Journal of Occupational Therapy* **47**(1), 10–16.

Partridge C, Johnston M (1989) Perceived control of recovery from physical disability: measurement and prediction. *British Journal of Clinical Psychology* **28**(1), 53–59.

Pattie A (1988) Measuring levels of disability: the Clifton Assessment Procedures for the Elderly. In JP Wattis, I Hindmarch (eds), *Psychological Assessment of the Elderly*. London, Hodder & Stoughton.

Pattie AH, Gilleard CJ (1979) *Manual of the Clifton Assessment Procedures for the Elderly (CAPE)*. London, Hodder & Stoughton.

Payne S (2002) Standardised tests: an appropriate way to measure the outcome of paediatric occupational therapy? *British Journal of Occupational Therapy* **65**(3), 117–122.

Payton OD (1985) Clinical reasoning process in physical therapy. *Physical Therapy* **65**(9), 924–928.

Penn RD, Savoy SM, Corcos D, Latash M *et al.* (1989) Intrathecal baclofen for severe spinal spasticity. *New England Journal of Medicine* **320**(23), 1517–1521.

Perry A, Morris M, Unsworth C, Duckett S *et al.* (2004) Therapy outcome measures for allied health practitioners in Australia: the AusTOMs. *International Journal for Quality in Health Care* **16**(4), 285–291.

Phillips C, Thompson G (2003) What is cost-effectiveness? What is...? Hayward Medical Communications, **1**(3), http://www.evidence-based-medicine.co.uk/ebmfiles/Whatiscosteffect.pdf, accessed 25.10.06.

Philp I (2000) EASY-Care: A systematic approach to the assessment of older people. *Geriatric Medicine* **30**(5), 15–19.

Piper MC, Pinnell LE, Darrah J, Maguire T, Byrne PJ (1992) Construction and validation of the Alberta Infant Motor Scale (AIMS). *Canadian Journal of Public Health* **83**(suppl 2), S46–S50.

Platt W, Bell B, Kozak J (1998) Functional Mobility Profile: a tool for measuring functional outcome in chronic care clients. *Physiotherapy Canada* **50**(1), 47–74.

Podsiadlo D, Richardson S (1991) The timed 'up and go': a test of basic functional mobility for frail elderly persons. *Journal of the American Geriatrics Society* **39**(2), 142–148.

Polgar JM (1998) Critiquing assessments. In ME Neistadt, EB Crepeau (eds), *Willard & Spackman's Occupational Therapy* (9th edn.). Philadelphia, Lippincott, Williams and Wilkins.

Pollock N, McColl MA (1998) Assessment in client-centred occupational therapy. In Law M (ed.), *Client-centered Occupational Therapy*. Thorofare, NJ, Slack.

Pollock N, Stewart D (1998) Occupational performance needs of school-aged children with physical disabilities in the community. *Physical and Occupational Therapy in Pediatrics* **18**(1), 55–68.

Pollock N, Stewart D (1996) *Occupational Performance Needs of School-aged Children with Physical Disabilities in the Community*. Hamilton, ON, Neurodevelopmental Clinical Research Unit, McMaster University.

Pope AM, Tarlow AR (1991) *Disability in America: Toward a National Agenda for Prevention.* Washington, National Academy Press.

Portney LG, Watkins MP (1993) *Foundations of Clinical Research: Applications to Practice.* Norwalk, CT, Appleton & Lange.

Prochaska JO, DiClemente CC (1992) Stages of change in the modification of problem behaviors. In M Hersen, RM Eisler, PM Miller (eds), *Progress on Behavior Modification.* Sycamore, IL, Sycamore Press.

Prochaska JO, DiClemente CC (1986) Toward a comprehensive model of change. In W Miller and N Heather (eds), *Addictive Behaviors: Processes of Change.* New York, Plenum Press.

Prochaska JO, DiClemente CC (1982) Transtheoretical therapy: toward a more integrative model of change. *Psychotherapy: Theory, Research and Practice* **19**(3), 276–288.

Prochaska JO, DiClemente CC, Norcross JC (1998) Stages of change: prescriptive guidelines for behavioral medicine and psychotherapy. In GP Koocher, JC Norcross, SS Hill III (eds), *Psychologists' Desk Reference.* Oxford, Oxford University Press.

Psychological Corporation/Harcourt Assessment (2004) *Occupational Therapy and Physiotherapy Catalogue.* London, TPC/Harcourt Assessment.

Pynsent P (2004) Choosing an outcome measure. In P Pysent, J Fairbank, A Carr (eds), *Outcome Measures in Orthopaedics and Orthopaedic Trauma* (2nd edn.). London, Arnold.

Pynsent PB (ed.) (1993) *Outcome Measures in Orthopaedics.* London, Butterworth-Heinemann.

Reinauer H (1998) AWMF and Clinical Guideline Program in Germany. Paper delivered at the International Conference on Clinical Practice Guidelines (4 September 1998, Frankfurt/Main), http://www.uni-duesseldorf.de/WWW/AWMF/konfer/iccpg-hr.htm, accessed 10.12.05.

Renwick RM, Reid DT (1992a) *Life Satisfaction Index – Parents (LSI-P).* Toronto, Department of Occupational Therapy, University of Toronto.

Renwick RM, Reid DT (1992b) Life satisfaction of parents of adolescents with Duchenne muscular dystrophy: validation of a new instrument. *Occupational Therapy Journal of Research* **12**, 296–312.

Research and Development Group (1997) Buzz words: some definitions to highlight similarities and differences. *Occupational Therapy News* **5**(10), 7.

Richards S (2002) Foreword. In A Turner, M Foster, SE Johnson (eds), *Occupational Therapy and Physical Dysfunction: Principles, Skills and Practice* (5th edn.). London, Churchill Livingstone.

Richardson J (2001) The EASY-Care assessment system and its appropriateness for older people. *Nursing Older People* **13**(7), 17–19.

Rivett DA, Higgs J (1997) Hypothesis generation in the clinical reasoning behavior of manual therapists. *Journal of Physical Therapy Education* **11**(1), 40–45.

Roberts AE (1996) Approaches to reasoning in occupational therapy: a critical exploration. *British Journal of Occupational Therapy* **59**(5), 233–236.

Roberts GW (2004) New horizons in occupational therapy. In R Watson and L Swartz (eds), *Transformation Through Occupation.* London, Whurr.

Roberts L (2000) Flagging the danger signs of low back pain. L Gifford (ed.), *Topical Issues in Pain 2: Biopsychosocial Assessment and Management Relationships and Pain: Physiotherapy Pain Association Yearbook.* Falmouth, CNS Press.

Robertson MC, Campbell AJ, Gardner MM, Devlin N (2002) Preventing injuries in older people by preventing falls: a meta-analysis of individual-level data. *Journal of the American Geriatric Society* **50**(5), 905–911.

Robinson BC (1983) Validation of a Caregiver Strain Index. *Journal of Gerontology* **38**(3), 344–48.

Rodger S, Ziviani J, Watter P, Ozanne A *et al.* (2003) Motor and functional skills of children with developmental coordination disorder: a pilot investigation of measurement issues. *Human Movement Science* **22**(4–5), 461–78.

Rogers JC (2004) Occupational diagnosis. In M Mollineux (ed.), *Occupation for Occupational Therapists.* Oxford, Blackwell.

Rogers JC (1983) Eleanor Clarke Slagel Lectureship – 1983: clinical reasoning: the ethics, science, and art. *American Journal of Occupational Therapy* **37**(9), 601–616.

Rogers JC, Holm MB (1991) Occupational therapy diagnostic reasoning: a component of clinical reasoning. *American Journal of Occupational Therapy* **45**(11), 1045–1053.

Rogers JC, Holm MB (1989) The therapist's thinking behind functional assessment I. In CB Royeen (ed.), *AOTA Self Study Series Assessing Function.* Rockville, MD, AOTA.

Rogers JC, Masagatani G (1982) Clinical reasoning of occupational therapists during the initial assessment of physically disabled patients. *Occupational Therapy Journal of Research* **2**(5), 195–219.

Roskell C (1998) Clinical reasoning in physiotherapy development. *British Journal of Therapy and Rehabilitation* **5**(2), 60–61.

Royal College of Physicians (2002) National clinical guidelines for stroke, http://www.rcplondon.ac.uk/pubs/books/stroke/index.htm, accessed 25.02.05.

Royeen CB (1989) *Clinical Research Handbook: An Analysis for the Service Professions.* Thorofare, NJ, Slack.

Rubenstein LZ, Josephson KP, Trueblood PR, Loy S *et al.* (2000) Effects of a group exercise program on strength, mobility, and falls among fall prone elderly men. *Journal of Gerontology* **55a**(6), M317–M321.

Rundshagen I, Schnabel K, Standl S, Schulte am Esch J (1999) Patients' vs. nurses' assessments of postoperative pain and anxiety during patient or nurse controlled analgesia. *British Journal of Anaesthesia* **82**(3), 374–378.

Russell DJ (1987) Validation of a gross motor measure for children with cerebral palsy. Unpublished Master of Science thesis. Hamilton, ON, McMaster University.

Russell DJ, Rosenbaum P, Gowland C, Hardy S, Cadman D (1990) Validation of a gross motor measure for children with cerebral palsy. *Physiotherapy Canada* **42**(suppl 3), 2.

Russell DJ, Rosenbaum P, Gowland C, Hardy S *et al.* (1993) *Gross Motor Function Measure Manual* (2nd edn.). Hamilton, ON, McMaster University.

Russell DJ, Rosenbaum PL, Cadman DT, Gowland C *et al.* (1989) The Gross Motor Function Measure: a means to evaluate the effects of physical therapy. *Developmental Medicine and Child Neurology* **31**(3), 341–352.

Ryan SE, McKay EA (eds) (1999) *Thinking and Reasoning in Therapy: Narratives from Practice.* Cheltenham, Stanley Thornes.

Sackett DL, Rosenberg WMC, Muir Gray JA, Haynes RB, Richardson WS (1996) Editorial: evidence-based medicine: what it is and what it isn't. *British Medical Journal* **312**(7023), 71–72.

Sarle WS (1997) Measurement theory: frequently asked questions. Version 3, ftp://ftp.sas.com/pub/neural/measurement.html, accessed 04.06.06.

Sarno J, Sarno M, Levita E (1973) The functional life scale. *Archives of Physical Medicine and Rehabilitation* **54**(5), 214–220.

Saslow CA (1982) *Basic Research Methods.* New York, Random House.

Saxton J, McGonigle KL, Swinhart AA, Boller F (1993) *Severe Impairment Battery (SIB).* Bury St Edmunds, Thames Valley Test Company.

Schell BB (1998) Clinical reasoning: the basis of practice. In ME Neistadt and EB Crepeau (eds), *Willard & Spackman's Occupational Therapy* (9th edn.). Philadelphia, Lippincott, Williams and Wilkins.

Schell BA, Cervero RM (1993) Clinical reasoning in occupational therapy: an integrative review. *American Journal of Occupational Therapy* **47**(7), 605–610.

Schoemaker MM, van der Wees M, Flapper B, Verheij-Jansen N *et al.* (2001) Perceptual skills of children with developmental coordination disorder. *Human Movement Science* **20**(1–2), 111–33.

Schön DA (1983) *The Reflective Practitioner: How Professionals Think in Action.* Aldershot, Averbury.

Scudds RA, Fishbain DA, Scudds RJ (2003) Concurrent validity of an electronic descriptive pain scale. *Clinical Rehabilitation* **17**(2), 206–208.

Sealey C (1998) *Clinical Audit Information Pack.* London, COT.

Sewell L, Singh SJ (2001) The Canadian Occupational Performance Measure: is it a reliable measure in clients with chronic obstructive pulmonary disease? *British Journal of Occupational Therapy* **64**(6), 305–310.

Shanahan M (1992) Objective and holistic: occupational therapy assessment in Ireland. *Irish Journal of Occupational Therapy* **22**(2), 8–10.

Sherr Klein B (1997) *Slow Dance: A Story of Stroke, Love and Disability.* Toronto, Knopf.

Siegel S (1956) *Nonparametric Statistics for the Behavioural Sciences.* London, McGraw-Hill Kogakusha.

Siegel S, Castellan J (1988) *Nonparametric Statistics for the Behavioural Sciences.* London, McGraw-Hill Book Company.

Skruppy M (1993) Activities of daily living evaluations: is there a difference in what the patient reports and what is observed? *British Medical Journal* **11**(3), 13–25.

Slater DY, Cohn ES (1991) Staff development through analysis of practice. *American Journal of Occupational Therapy* **45**(11), 1038–1044.

Smith G (2006) The Casson Memorial Lecture 2006: telling tales: how stories and narratives co-create change. *British Journal of Occupational Therapy* **69**(7), 304–311.

Smith HD (1993) Assessment and evaluation: an overview. In HL Hopkins and HD Smith (eds), *Willard & Spackman's Occupational Therapy* (8th edn.). Philadelphia, Lippincott.

Smyth MM, Mason UC (1998) Use of proprioception in normal and clumsy children. *Developmental Medicine & Child Neurology* **40**(10), 672–681.

Spiegel TM, Spiegel JS, Paulus HE (1987) The joint alignment and motion scale: a simple measurement of joint deformity in patients with rheumatoid arthritis. *Journal of Rheumatology* **14**(5), 887–892.

Stanley M, Buttfield J, Bowden S, Williams C (1995) Chessington Occupational Therapy Neurological Assessment Battery: comparison of performance of people aged 50–65 years with people aged 66 and over. *Australian Occupational Therapy Journal* **42**, 55–65.

Starey N (2003) What is clinical governance? What is it…? Hayward Medical Communications, **1**(12), http://www.evidence-based-medicine.co.uk/ebmfiles/WhatisClinGov.pdf, accessed 15.12.05.

Steer RA, Beck AT (2004) Beck Depression Inventory II. In WE Craighead, CB Nemeroff (eds), *The Concise Corsini Encyclopedia of Psychology and Behavioral Science* (3rd edn.). New York, John Wiley & Sons.

Steer RA, Beck AT (1997) Beck Anxiety Inventory. In CP Salaquett, RJ Wood (eds), *Evaluating Stress: A Book of Resources.* Lanhan, MD, The Scarecrow Press.

Steer RA, Beck AT (1996) Beck Depression Inventory (BDI). In LI Sederer, B Dickey (eds), *Outcomes Assessment in Clinical Practice.* Baltimore, Williams & Wilkins.

Stephenson R (2002) The complexity of human behaviour: a new paradigm for physiotherapy? *Physical Therapy Reviews* **7**(4), 243–258.

Stevens SS (1946) On the theory of scales of measurement. *Science* **103**(2684), 677–680.

Stewart S (1999) The use of standardised and non-standardised assessments in a social service setting: implications for practice. *British Journal of Occupational Therapy* **62**(9), 417–423.

Stokes EK, O'Neill D (1999) The use of standardised assessments by physiotherapists. *British Journal of Therapy and Rehabilitation* **6**(11), 560–565.

Strong J, Ashton R, Crammond T, Chant D (1990) Pain intensity, attitude and function in back pain patients. *Australian Occupational Therapy Journal* **37**(4), 1786–1791.

Sturgess J, Rodger S, Ozanne A (2002) A review of the use of self-report assessment with young children. *British Journal of Occupational Therapy* **65**(3), 108–116.

Sumsion T (2000) A revised occupational therapy definition of client centred practice. *British Journal of Occupational Therapy* **63**(7), 304–309.

Swain J (2004) Interpersonal communication. In S French, J Sim (eds), *Physiotherapy: A Psychosocial Approach* (3rd edn.). London, Elsevier Butterworth-Heinemann.

Sykes JB (ed.) (1983) *The Concise Oxford Dictionary of Current English* (7th edn.). Oxford, Oxford University Press.

Tate S, Sills M (2004) *The Development of Critical Reflection in the Health Professions*. London, LTSN/HSAP, http://www.health.ltsn.ac.uk/publications/occasionalpaper/occasionalpaper04.pdf, accessed 30.07.06.

Teri L, Truax P, Logsdon R, Uomoto J *et al.* (1992) Assessment of behavioral problems in dementia: the revised Memory and Behavior Problems Checklist. *Psychology and Aging* 7(4), 622–631.

Thames Valley Test Company (2004) *Thames Valley Test Company 2004 Catalogue*. Bury St Edmunds, TVTC.

Thom KM, Blair SEE (1998) Risk in dementia: assessment and management: a literature review. *British Journal of Occupational Therapy* 61(10), 441–447.

Thomas KW, Kilmann RH (1974) *The Thomas–Kilmann Conflict Mode Instrument*. New York, Xicom.

Thorpe K (2004) Reflective learning journals: from concept to practice. *Reflective Practice* 5(3), 327–343.

Tinetti ME (1986) Performance-oriented assessment of mobility problems in elderly patients. *Journal of the American Geriatrics Society* 34(2), 119–126.

Tinetti ME, Inouye SK, Gill TM, Doucette JT (1995) Shared risk factors for falls, incontinence and functional independence: unifying the approach to geriatric syndromes. *Journal of the American Medical Association* 272(17), 1348–1353.

Tinetti ME, Williams TF, Mayewski R (1986) Fall risk for elderly patients based on the number of chronic disabilities. *American Journal of Medicine* 80(3), 429–434.

Toft B (2001) *External Inquiry into the Adverse Incident that Occurred at Queens Medical Centre Nottingham 4th January 2001*. London, DoH.

Toft B, Reynolds S (in press) *Learning from Disasters: A Management Approach* (3rd edn.). London, Palgrave Macmillan.

Townsend E, Ryan B, Law M (1990) Using the World Health Organization's international classification of impairments, disabilities and handicaps in occupational therapy. *Canadian Journal of Occupational Therapy* 57(1), 16–25.

Trombly C (1993) Anticipating the future: assessment of occupational function. *American Journal of Occupational Therapy* 47(3), 253–257.

Tullis A, Nicol M (1999) A systematic review of the evidence for the value of functional assessment of older people with dementia. *British Journal of Occupational Therapy* 62(12), 554–563.

Turner A (2002) Patient? Client? Service user? What's in a name? *British Journal of Occupational Therapy* 65(8), 355.

Tursky B, Jamner LD, Friedman R (1982) The Pain Perception Profile: a psychophysical approach to the assessment of pain report. *Behavior Therapy* 13, 376–394.

Tyerman R, Tyerman A, Howard P, Hadfield C (1986) *The Chessington Occupational Therapy Neurological Assessment Battery Introductory Manual*. Nottingham, Nottingham Rehab Limited.

University of Bradford (2002) *Well Being Profile*. University of Bradford: Bradford Dementia group, http://www.brad.ac.uk/acad/health/dementia/intro.php, accessed 24.06.06.

Unsworth CA (2005) Measuring outcomes using the Australian Therapy Outcome Measures for Occupational Therapy (AusTOMs-OT): data description and tool sensitivity. *British Journal of Occupational Therapy* 68(8), 354–366.

Unsworth C (2000) Measuring the outcome of occupational therapy: tools and resources. *Australian Occupational Therapy Journal* 47(4), 147–158.

Unsworth C (1999) *Cognitive and Perceptual Dysfunction: A Clinical Reasoning Approach to Evaluation and Intervention*. Philadelphia, FA Davis.

Unsworth C, Duncombe D (2004) *AusTOMs for Occupational Therapy Manual*. Melbourne, La Trobe University.

Vitale BA, Nugent PM (1996) *Test Success: Test Taking Techniques for the Healthcare Student.* Philadelphia, FA Davis.

Von Bertalanffy L (1968) *General Systems Theory: Foundations Development Applications.* London, Penguin Press.

Wade DT (1992) *Measurement in Neurological Rehabilitation.* Oxford, Oxford University Press.

Wade DT (1988) *Stroke: Practical Guides for General Practice 4.* Oxford, Oxford University Press.

Waddell G (1992) Biopsychosocial analysis of low back pain. *Clinical Rheumatology* **6**(3), 523–557.

Waddell G (1987) A new clinical model for the treatment of low back pain. *Spine* **12**(7), 632–644.

Waddell G, Newton M, Henderson I, Somerville D, Main CJ (1993) A Fear-avoidance Beliefs Questionnaire (FABQ) and the role of fear-avoidance beliefs in chronic low back pain and disability. *Pain* **52**(2), 157–168.

Wall PD (1996) Editorial comment: back pain and the workplace I. *Pain* **65**(5), 5.

Ware JE (2005) SF-36 Health Survey update, http://www.sf-36.org/tools/sf36.shtml, accessed 02.10.05.

Ware JE, Snow KK, Kosinski M, Gandek B (1993) *SF-36 Health Survey: Manual and Interpretation Guide.* Boston, The Health Institute, New England Medical Center.

Warren A (2002) An evaluation of the Canadian Model of Occupational Performance and the Canadian Occupational Performance Measure in mental health practice. *British Journal of Occupational Therapy* **65**(11), 515–521.

Waterlow JA (2005) Pressure ulcer risk assessment and prevention, http://www.judy-waterlow. co.uk/index.htm, accessed 16.10.06.

Watson P, Kendall N (2000) Assessing psychosocial yellow flags. In L Gifford (ed.), *Topical Issues in Pain 2: Biopsychosocial Assessment and Management Relationships and Pain: Physiotherapy Pain Association Yearbook.* Falmouth, CNS Press.

Watson R (2004) New horizons in occupational therapy. In R Watson and L Swartz (eds), *Transformation Through Occupation.* London, Whurr.

Watson R, Fourie M (2004) Occupation and occupational therapy. In R Watson and L Swartz (eds), *Transformation Through Occupation.* London, Whurr.

Welch A (2002) Process mapping occupational therapy activity within a medical admissions unit. *British Journal of Occupational Therapy* **65**(4), 158–164.

Welford AT (1993) The Gerontological Balance Sheet. In J Cerella, J Rybash, W Hoyer, ML Commons (eds), *Adult Information Processing: Limits on Loss.* London, Academic Press.

Wheatley CJ (1996) Evaluation and treatment of cognitive dysfunction. In LW Pedretti (ed.), *Occupational Therapy: Practice Skills for Physical Dysfunction.* St Louis, CV Mosby.

Whelan E, Speake B (1979) Scale for Assessing Coping Skills. In E Whelan, B Speake (eds), *Learning to Cope.* London, Souvenir Press.

White P (2004) Using reflective practice in physiotherapy curriculum. In S Tate, M Sills (eds), *The Development of Critical Reflection in the Health Professions.* London, School of Integrated Health, LTSN/HSAP, http://www.health.ltsn.ac.uk/publications/occasionalpaper/ occasionalpaper04.pdf, accessed 30.07.06.

Whiteneck GG, Charlifue SW, Gerhart KA, Overholser JD, Richardson GN (1992) Quantifying handicap: a new measure of long-term rehabilitation outcomes. *Archives of Physical Medicine and Rehabilitation* **73**(6), 519–26.

Whiting S, Lincoln N (1980) An ADL assessment for stroke patients. *British Journal of Occupational Therapy* **43**(Feb), 44–46.

Whiting S, Lincoln N, Bhavnani G, Cockburn J (1985) *The Rivermead Perceptual Assessment Battery (RPAB).* Windsor, NFER-Nelson.

Whitney SL, Poole JL, Cass SP (1998) A review of balance instruments for older adults. *American Journal of Occupational Therapy* **52**(8), 666–671.

Wilcox A (1994) A study of verbal guidance for children with developmental co-ordination disorder. Unpublished Master's thesis, London, ON, University of Western Ontario.

Wilcoxon F (1945) Individual comparisons by ranking methods. *Biometrics* **1**(6), 80–83.

Wilfong EW, Saylor C, Elksnin N (1991) Influences on responsiveness: interactions between mothers and their premature infants. *Infant Mental Health Journal* **12**(1), 31–40.

Wilson BN, Kaplan BJ, Crawford SG, Campbell A, Dewey D (2000) Reliability and validity of a parent questionnaire on childhood motor skills. *American Journal of Occupational Therapy* **54**(5), 484–493.

Wilson PH, McKenzie BE (1998) Information processing deficits associated with developmental coordination disorder: a meta-analysis of research findings. *Journal of Child Psychology and Psychiatry* **39**(6), 829–840.

Winward CE, Halligan PW, Wade DT (2000) *Rivermead Assessment of Somatosensory Performance (RASP)*. Bury St Edmunds, Thames Valley Test Company.

Wolf H (1997) Assessments of activities of daily living and instrumental activities of daily living: their use by community-based health service occupational therapists working in physical disability. *British Journal of Occupational Therapy* **60**(8), 359–364.

World Confederation for Physical Therapy (2006a) A message from the WCPT president, http://www.wcpt.org/about/index/php, accessed 10.10.06.

World Confederation for Physical Therapy (2006b) Description of physical therapy, http://www.wcpt.org/common/docs/WCPTPolicies.pdf, accessed 08.10.06.

World Confederation for Physical Therapy (2006c) Description of physical therapy: what characterises physical therapy?, http://www.wcpt.org/policies/description/character, accessed 24.06.06.

World Confederation for Physical Therapy (2003) Evidence-based practice: an overview. London, WCPT, http://www.wcpt.org/common/docs/102kn_ebp.pdf, accessed 20.03.05.

World Confederation for Physical Therapy (2002) Reading tips for the clinician: how to tell whether an article is worth reading. London, WCPT, http://www.wcpt.org/common/docs/102kn_reading1.pdf, accessed 20.03.05.

World Federation of Occupational Therapy (2005) Definitions of occupational therapy, draft 7. August 2005, http://www.wfot.org/Document_Centre/default.cfm, accessed 26.10.05.

World Health Organization (2004) International Statistical Classification of Diseases and Related Health Problems (ICD-10). Geneva, WHO. Can be downloaded from the WHO Website at: http://www.who.int/occupational_health/publications/en/oehicd10.pdf, accessed 14.10.06

World Health Organization (2002) *Towards a Common Language for Function, Disability and Health: International Classification of Functioning, Disability and Health (ICF)*. Geneva, WHO, http://www3.who.int/icf/beginners/bg.pdf, accessed 21.02.06.

World Health Organization (1997) *ICIDH-2 International Classification of Impairments, Activities and Participations: A Manual of Dimensions of Disablement and Functioning. Beta-1 Draft for Field Trials*. Geneva, WHO.

World Health Organization (1992) *ICD-10 Classification of Mental and Behavioural Disorders*. Geneva, WHO.

World Health Organization (1980) *International Classification of Impairments, Disabilities and Handicaps: A Manual of Classification Relating to the Consequences of Disease*. Geneva, WHO.

Worsfold C, Simpson JM (2001) Standardisation of a three-metre walking test for elderly people. *Physiotherapy* **87**(3), 125–132.

Wright BD, Linacre JM (1989) Observations are always ordinal; measurement, however, must be interval. *Archives of Physical Medicine and Rehabilitation* **70**(12), 857–860.

Wright BD, Masters GN (1982) *Rating Scale Analysis*. Chicago, MESA Press.

Wright J, Cross J, Lamb S (1998) Physiotherapy outcome measures for rehabilitation of elderly people: responsiveness to change of the Rivermead Mobility Index and Barthel Index. *Physiotherapy* **84**(5), 216–221.

Yerxa E, Burnett-Beaulieu S, Stocking S, Azen S (1988) Development of the satisfaction with performance scales questionnaire. *American Journal of Occupational Therapy* **42**(4), 215–221.

Zakreski JR (1983) Prematurity and the single parent: effects of cumulative stress on child development. Unpublished doctoral dissertation, University of Virginia, Charlottesville. Cited in Abidin RR (1995) *Parenting Stress Index: Professional Manual* (3rd edn.). Odessa, FL, Psychological Assessment Resources.

Zarit SH, Todd PA, Zarit JM (1986) Subjective burden of husbands and wives as caregivers: a longitudinal study. *Gerontologist* **26**(3), 260–266.

Zarit SH, Reever KE, Bach-Peterson J (1980) Relatives of the impaired elderly: correlates of feelings of burden. *Gerontologist* **20**(6), 649–655.

Index